Orthopaedic
Hand Trauma

Orthopaedic Hand Trauma

Adam E. M. Eltorai, MD, PhD

Department of Orthopedic Surgery
Medstar Union Memorial Hospital
The Warren Alpert Medical School of Brown University
Providence, Rhode Island

Edward Akelman, MD

Vincent Zecchino Professor and Chairman
Department of Orthopaedics
The Warren Alpert Medical School of Brown University
Surgeon-in-Charge
Department of Orthopaedics
Rhode Island Hospital & Miriam Hospital
Providence, Rhode Island

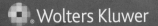. Wolters Kluwer

Philadelphia • Baltimore • New York • London
Buenos Aires • Hong Kong • Sydney • Tokyo

Acquisitions Editor: Brian Brown
Product Development Editor: Stacey Sebring
Editorial Coordinator: Lauren Pecarich/Jeremiah Kiely
Marketing Manager: Dan Dressler
Production Project Manager: Barton Dudlick
Design Coordinator: Stephen Druding
Manufacturing Coordinator: Beth Welsh
Prepress Vendor: S4Carlisle Publishing Services

9 8 7 6 5 4 3 2 1

Printed in China

Library of Congress Cataloging-in-Publication Data

Names: Eltorai, Adam E. M., editor. | Akelman, Edward, editor.
Title: Orthopaedic hand trauma / edited by Adam Eltorai, MD, Edward Akelman, MD.
Description: Philadelphia : Wolters Kluwer Health, [2020]
Identifiers: LCCN 2018049411 | ISBN 9781496372741 (paperback)
Subjects: LCSH: Hand—Surgery. | Hand—Wounds and injuries. | Orthopedic
    emergencies. | BISAC: MEDICAL / Orthopedics.
Classification: LCC RD778 .O78 2020 | DDC 617.5/75044—dc23
LC record available at https://lccn.loc.gov/2018049411

shop.lww.com

CCS0119

"For Ashley. Always."—Adam E. M. Eltorai

*"I dedicate this book to the many medical students; ortho-
paedic, plastic surgery, and general surgery residents; as
well as my hand surgery colleagues and friends who have
taught me so much about hand surgery over my career.
None of the educational work that I do and have done
could have been accomplished without the unwavering
love and support from my wife, Vickie, and my two sons,
Christopher and Matthew."—Edward Akelman*

Section Editors

Joseph A. Gil, MD
Hand Surgery Fellow
Department of Orthopedic Surgery
Mayo Clinic
Rochester, Minnesota

Christopher Got, MD
Assistant Professor of Orthopedic Surgery
Warren Alpert Medical School of Brown University
Providence, Rhode Island

Andrea Halim, MD
Assistant Professor
Yale Department of Orthopedics
Yale University/New Haven Hospital
New Haven, Connecticut

Robin Kamal, MD
Assistant Professor
Department of Orthopedic Surgery
Stanford University
Palo Alto, California

Craig Rodner, MD
Associate Professor
Department of Orthopedic Surgery
University of Connecticut
Farmington, Connecticut

Contributors

Ngozi Mogekwu Akabudike, MD
Assistant Professor
Department of Orthopaedics
University of Maryland Medical
  School
Attending Physician
Department of Orthopaedics
University of Maryland Medical
  Center
Baltimore, Maryland

Edward Akelman, MD
Vincent Zecchino Professor and
  Chairman
Department of Orthopaedics
The Warren Alpert Medical School of
  Brown University
Surgeon-in-Charge
Department of Orthopaedics
Rhode Island Hospital & Miriam
  Hospital
Providence, Rhode Island

Erez Avisar, MD
Chief
Hand & Upper Extremity Surgery Unit
Assaf Harofeh Medical Center
Tzrifin, Beer Yaakov, Israel

Hisham M. Awan, MD
Associate Professor
Department of Orthopaedics
The Ohio State University
Chief of the Division of Hand Surgery
Department of Orthopaedics
The Ohio State University Wexner
  Medical Center
The Ohio State University Wexner
  Medical Center
Columbus, Ohio

Omri Ayalon, MD
Assistant Clinical Professor
Division of Hand and Upper
  Extremity Surgery
Department of Orthopedic Surgery
NYU Langone Medical Center
New York, New York

Paul C. Baldwin III, MD
Attending Surgeon
Orthopaedic Surgery
Hughston Clinic
Fleming Island, Florida
Orthopaedic Trauma and Upper
  Extremity Surgeon
Orthopaedic Surgery
Orange Park Medical Center
Orange Park, Florida

**James D. Bedford, MSc, FRCS
(Plast), Br Dip Hand Surg**
Consultant Hand Surgeon
Department of Plastic Surgery
Wythenshawe Hospital
Manchester, United Kingdom

Kathryn Ashley Bentley, MD
Hand and Upper Extremity Fellow
Orthopaedic Surgery
The University of Alabama
  Birmingham
Birmingham, Alabama

Alan R. Blackburn II, MD, MS
Hand Fellow
Department of Orthopaedic Surgery
University of Pittsburgh Medical
  Center
Pittsburgh, Pennsylvania

Jonathan D. Boyle, MD
Chief Resident
Department of Orthopaedic Surgery
John Peter Smith Hospital
   Orthopaedic Surgery Residency
Fort Worth, Texas

Andrew Campbell, MD
Chief Resident
Orthopaedic Surgery
The Ohio State University
Wexner Medical Center
Columbus, Ohio

Matthew B. Cantlon, MD
Orthopaedic Surgeon
Department of Orthopaedic Surgery
ONS Foundation for Clinical
   Research and Education
Greenwich, Connecticut

Niki L. Carayannopoulos, DO
Department of Orthopaedics
Houston Methodist Hospital
The University of Texas Medical
   Branch at Galveston
Galveston, Texas

Nileshkumar M. Chaudhari, MD
Assistant Professor
The University of Alabama at Birmingham
Birmingham, Alabama

David J. Ciufo, MD
Resident
Department of Orthopaedic Surgery
   and Rehabilitation
University of Rochester Medical Center
Rochester, New York

Andrew Coskey, MD
Resident
The University of Texas Medical
   Branch at Galveston
Galveston, Texas

Nisha J. Crouser, MD
Surgical Intern
Department of Surgery

The Ohio State University
Wexner Medical Center
Columbus, Ohio

Timothy P. Crowley, MBChB, MSc, MRCS (Glasg)
Specialist Registrar
Department of Plastic Surgery
Royal Victoria Infirmary
Newcastle upon Tyne, United Kingdom

D. Nicole Deal, MD
Associate Professor
Head Hand Division
Department of Orthopaedic Surgery
Department of Plastic Surgery
Co-Director, UVA Hand Center
Director, Plastic Surgery Hand
   Fellowships
University of Virginia Health System
Charlottesville, Virginia

Ethan W. Dean, MD
Orthopaedic Surgery Resident
Department of Orthopaedics and
   Rehabilitation
University of Florida
Orthopaedic Surgery Resident
Department of Orthopaedics and
   Rehabilitation
UF Health Shands Hospital
Gainesville, Florida

Katherine M. Dederer, MD
Resident Physician
Department of Orthopaedic Surgery
University of North Carolina Hospitals
University of North Carolina at
   Chapel Hill
Chapel Hill, North Carolina

Hannah A. Dineen, MD
Resident
Orthopaedic Surgery Department
University of North Carolina Hospitals
University of North Carolina at
   Chapel Hill
Chapel Hill, North Carolina

Seth D. Dodds, MD
Associate Professor, Hand and Upper
    Extremity Surgery
Department of Orthopaedics
University of Miami, Miller School of
    Medicine
Miami, Florida

Patricia A. Drace, MD
Associate Clinical Professor
Department of Orthopaedic Surgery
University of Arizona College of
    Medicine – Phoenix
Orthopaedic Hand Upper Extremity
    Surgeon
Department of Orthopaedic Surgery
Phoenix Children's Hospital
Phoenix, Arizona

Reid W. Draeger, MD
Assistant Professor
Department of Orthopaedics
University of North Carolina School
    of Medicine
Assistant Professor
Department of Orthopaedics
University of North Carolina
    Healthcare
Chapel Hill, North Carolina

John C. Elfar, MD
Michael and Myrtle E. Baker
    Endowed Professor
Vice Chair Department of
    Orthopaedics and Rehabilitation
Director, Center for Orthopaedic
    Research and Translational Science
    (CORTS)
The Pennsylvania State University
    College of Medicine and Milton S.
    Hershey Medical Center
Hershey, Pennsylvania

Brooks Ficke, MD
Resurgens Orthopaedics
Atlanta, Georgia

John R. Fowler, MD
Assistant Professor
Department of Orthopaedic Surgery
University of Pittsburgh School of
    Medicine
Pittsburgh, Pennsylvania

Ryan M. Garcia, MD
Orthopedic Surgeon
OrthoCarolina Hand Center
Charlotte, North Carolina

Michael S. Gart, MD
Plastic and Reconstructive
    Surgeon, Hand and Upper
    Extremity Surgeon
OrthoCarolina Hand Center
Charlotte, North Carolina

Christopher Got, MD
Assistant Professor of Orthopedic
    Surgery
The Warren Alpert Medical School of
    Brown University
Providence, Rhode Island

Beatrice L. Grasu, MD
Resident
Department of Orthopaedic Surgery
MedStar Union Memorial Hospital
Baltimore, Maryland

Michael Guju, BS, MS
Medical Student
Tampa General Hospital
University of South Florida Morsani
    College of Medicine
Tampa, Florida

Steven C. Haase, MD
Associate Professor
Department of Surgery
Michigan Medicine
Ann Arbor, Michigan

Mark Henry, MD
Hand & Wrist Center of Houston
Houston, Texas

Rachel C. Hooper, MD
House Officer
Division of Plastic Surgery
Department of Surgery
Michigan University Medical Center
Ann Arbor, Michigan

Evan H. Horowitz, BSc
Medical Student, MS4
Department of Orthopaedics and
    Sports Medicine
University of South Florida Morsani
    College of Medicine
Medical Student, MS4
Department of Orthopaedics
Tampa General Hospital
Tampa, Florida

James Paul Hovis, MD
Resident Physician
Department of Orthopaedics
University of Maryland School of
    Medicine
Baltimore, Maryland

Margaret Jain, MD
Attending Surgeon
Orthopedic Surgery
The Doctor's Clinic
Silverdale, Washington

Edward W. Jernigan, MD
Resident Physician
Department of Orthopaedic Surgery
University of North Carolina at
    Chapel Hill
Chapel Hill, North Carolina

Emily E. Jewell, MD
Resident
Department of Orthopaedic Surgery
University of North Carolina Hospitals
University of North Carolina at
    Chapel Hill
Chapel Hill, North Carolina

Tamara John, MD
Surgical Fellow
Department of Orthopaedic Surgery

University of Pennsylvania
Surgical Fellow, Hand Surgery
Department of Orthopaedic Surgery
Hospital of the University of
    Pennsylvania
Philadelphia, Pennsylvania

Julie Johnson, MD
Orthopaedic Resident
Department of Orthopaedics
University of Pittsburgh Medical
    Center
Pittsburgh, Pennsylvania

Christopher M. Jones, MD
Hand and Upper Extremity Fellow
The Curtis National Hand Center
MedStar Union Memorial Hospital
Baltimore, Maryland
Hand and Upper Extremity Surgeon
Department of Orthopedic Surgery
Anne Arundel Medical Center
Annapolis, Maryland

Joseph J.King, MD
Assistant Professor
Department of Orthopaedic Surgery
University of Florida
Gainesville, Florida

Alan R. Koester, MD
Chief of Orthopedic Surgery
Cabell Huntington Hospital
Assistant Professor
Vice Chair of Orthopedic Surgery
Joan C. Edwards School of
    Medicine
Marshall University
Huntington, West Virginia

Lisa M. Kruse, MD
Assistant Professor
Department of Orthopedics and
    Rehabilitation
University of Wisconsin School of
    Medicine and Public Health
Physician

Department of Orthopedics and Rehabilitation
University of Wisconsin Hospital and Clinics
Madison, Wisconsin

Kenrick C. Lam, MD
Resident
The University of Texas Medical Branch at Galveston
Galveston, Texas

Steven T. Lanier, MD
Plastic Surgery Chief Resident
Division of Plastic Surgery
Northwestern University Feinberg School of Medicine
Chicago, Illinois

Alex C. Lesiak, MD, MS
Upper Extremity Fellow
Department of Orthopedic Surgery
University of Pittsburgh Medical Center
Pittsburgh, Pennsylvania

Daniel R. Lewis, MD
Clinical Instructor OrthoCarolina Hand Fellowship
OrthoCarolina
Charlotte, North Carolina
Assistant Professor
Department of Orthopedic Surgery
Carolinas Medical Center/Atrium Health
Charlotte, North Carolina

David M. Lichtman, MD
Professor of Hand Surgery
Department of Orthopaedic Surgery
John Peter Smith Hospital Orthopaedic Surgery Residency
Fort Worth, Texas

Jason S. Lipof, MD
Department of Orthopaedic Surgery and Rehabilitation
University of Rochester Medical Center

Department of Orthopaedic Surgery and Rehabilitation
Strong Memorial Hospital
Rochester, New York

Bryan Loeffler, MD
Assistant Professor
OrthoCarolina Hand Center
Assistant Professor
Department of Orthopedic Surgery
Atrium–Carolinas Medical Center
Charlotte, North Carolina

Anthony LoGiudice, MD
Fellow, Hand and Upper Extremity
Department of Orthopaedics
Ohio State University
Columbus, Ohio

Sohaib K. Malik, MD
Orthopaedic Surgical Resident
Marshall Orthopaedics
Joan C. Edwards School of Medicine at Marshall University
Orthopaedic Surgical Resident
Marshall Orthopaedics
Cabell Huntington Hospital
Huntington, West Virginia

Adam S. Martin, MD
Resident
Orthopaedic Surgery
The Ohio State University
Columbus, Ohio

Robert C. Matthias, Jr., MD
Assistant Clinical Professor
Department of Orthopedic Surgery
University of Florida
Gainesville, Florida

Roshan Melvani, MD
Resident Physician
Department of Orthopaedics and Sports Medicine
MedStar Union Memorial Hospital
Baltimore, Maryland

Christian A. Merrill, MD, MBA
Orthopedic Surgery Resident
Department of Orthopedic Surgery
University of Connecticut
Farmington, Connecticut

Rachel Michael, MD
Resident
Othopaedic Surgery
University of Toledo Medical Center
Toledo, Ohio

Michael Moustoukas, MD
Orthopedic Surgeon
Kennedy White Orthopedic Center
Sarasota, Florida

James R. Mullen, MD
Hand Surgery Fellow
Department of Orthopaedic Surgery
NYU Langone Medical Center
New York, New York

Thao Nguyen, MD
Resident
Department of Orthopaedics
University of Maryland School of
    Medicine
University of Maryland Medical
    Center
Baltimore, Maryland

Timothy R. Niacaris, MD, PhD
Assistant Professor of Hand
    Surgery
Department of Orthopaedic Surgery
John Peter Smith Hospital
    Orthopaedic Surgery Residency
Fort Worth, Texas

Steven R. Niedermeier, MD
Clinical Instructor Housestaff
Orthopaedic Surgery
The Ohio State University
Wexner Medical Center
Columbus, Ohio

Tiffany J. Pan, MD
Fellow
Department of Orthopaedic Surgery
University of Pittsburgh Medical
    Center
Pittsburgh, Pennsylvania

Maharsh K. Patel, MD
Chief Resident
Department of Orthopaedic Surgery
University of Florida
Gainesville, Florida

William F. Pientka II, MD
Assistant Professor of Hand Surgery
Department of Orthopaedic Surgery
John Peter Smith Hospital
    Orthopaedic Surgery Residency
Fort Worth, Texas

Craig M. Rodner, MD
Associate Professor
Department of Orthopaedic Surgery
University of Connecticut
Farmington, Connecticut

Joseph A. Rosenbaum, MD
Hand Surgery Fellow
Mary S. Stern Fellowship
Cincinnati, Ohio

Robert Ryu, MD
Clinical Instructor Housestaff
Orthopaedics
The Ohio State University Wexner
    Medical Center
Columbus, Ohio

Ardalan Sayan, MD
Resident
Department of Orthopaedics
Joan C. Edwards School of
Medicine
Marshall University
Cabell Huntington Hospital
Huntington, West Virginia

Roy E. Schneider, MS
Manager of Biomedical Illustration
  and VIR Development
Orthopedic Surgery
The Doctor's Clinic
Silverdale, Washington

**Francisco A. Schwartz-
  Fernandes, MS, MD, MBA**
Associate Professor of Orthopaedics
  and Sports Medicine
Department of Orthopaedics and
  Sports Medicine
University of South Florida
Tampa, Florida

Vishavpreet Singh, MD
Resident
Department of Orthopaedics
Joan C. Edwards School of
  Medicine
Marshall University
Cabell Huntington Hospital
Huntington, West Virginia

Andrew D. Sobel, MD
Hand and Microsurgery Fellow
Department of Orthopedic Surgery
Washington University in St. Louis
Hand and Microsurgery Fellow
Department of Orthopedic Surgery
Barnes-Jewish Hospital
St. Louis, Missouri

Mark K. Solarz, MD
Assistant Professor of Orthopaedics
  and Sports Medicine
Department of Orthopaedics and
  Sports Medicine
Lewis Katz School of Medicine at
  Temple University
Philadelphia, Pennsylvania

Mikael Starecki, MD
Attending Surgeon
Orthopaedic Surgery
Resurgens Orthopaedics
Austell, Georgia

**Susan Stevenson, MBChB, PhD,
  FRCS (PLAST)**
Consultant Hand Surgeon
Department of Plastic Surgery
Royal Victoria Infirmary
Newcastle upon Tyne, United
  Kingdom

**Matthew S. Torkington,
  MBChB, FRCS (Orth)**
Consultant Trauma and Orthopaedic
  Surgeon
Department of Orthopaedics
Glasgow Royal Infirmary
Glasgow, Scotland

Sarah Turner, MCSP
Clinical Specialist Hand Therapist
GradDip Physiotherapy
Wythenshawe Hospital
Manchester, United Kingdom

**David J. Warwick, MD, BM,
  DIMC, Eur Dip Hand Surg,
  FRCS, FRCS (Orth)**
Honorary Professor
Faculty of Medicine
University of Southampton
Consultant Hand Surgeon
Department of Orthopaedics
University Hospital Southampton
Southampton, United Kingdom

Tiffany Y. Wu, MD
Hand Surgeon
Orthopedic Surgery Department
Orlin & Cohen Orthopedic Group
Garden City, New York

Preface

Patients with suspected hand injuries require urgent and sometimes emergent evaluation to determine if serious complicating conditions exist. Such conditions, including any neurovascular injury, often require immediate surgical consultation. *Orthopaedic Hand Trauma* is a concise and user-friendly book, covering the most common hand injuries. This quick-reference guide includes bulleted text and easy-to-follow algorithms, protocols, and images (illustrations, radiographs, and photographs), acting as a "pocket consultant" to provide the most up-to-date information when you need it most. Organized by anatomic structure, each chapter includes mechanism of injury, evaluation, acute treatment, definitive treatment, and potential problems.

Adam E. M. Eltorai

Contents

Section 1: Assessment of Acute Hand Injury

Section Editors: Joseph A. Gil and Robin Kamal

Chapter 1: History and Physical Examination 1
Craig M. Rodner and Christian A. Merrill

Chapter 2: Imaging 16
Daniel R. Lewis

Chapter 3: Anesthesia 24
Rachel C. Hooper and Steven C. Haase

Chapter 4: General Concepts: Indications for Surgery 35
Ethan W. Dean and Robert C. Matthias, Jr.

Section 2: Bone and Joint Injuries

Section Editor: Christopher Got

Chapter 5: Phalanx Fractures.................................49
Joseph A. Rosenbaum and Hisham M. Awan

Chapter 6: Phalanx Dislocations.............................57
Joseph A. Rosenbaum and Hisham M. Awan

Chapter 7: Mallet Fractures..................................64
Andrew D. Sobel

Chapter 8: Digital Collateral Ligament Injury.................. 77
Steven T. Lanier and Michael S. Gart

Chapter 9: Base of the Thumb Fractures 89
Thao Nguyen and Ngozi Mogekwu Akabudike

Chapter 10: Thumb Collateral Ligament Injury 102
James Paul Hovis and Ngozi Mogekwu Akabudike

Chapter 11: Metacarpal Fractures 115
Joseph A. Rosenbaum and Hisham M. Awan

Chapter 12: Metacarpophalangeal Dislocations.............122
Joseph A. Rosenbaum and Hisham M. Awan

Chapter 13: Malunion and Nonunion of Fingers and Hand... 127
Tiffany Y. Wu and John R. Fowler

Chapter 14: Scaphoid Fractures 134
Adam S. Martin and Hisham M. Awan

Chapter 15: Perilunate Dislocations 146
Michael Moustoukas and Nileshkumar M. Chaudhari

Chapter 16: Hook of Hamate Fractures. 151
Katherine M. Dederer and Reid W. Draeger

Chapter 17: Hamate Body Fracture. 161
Kenrick C. Lam, Andrew Coskey, and Niki L. Carayannopoulos

Chapter 18: Pisiform Fractures. 173
Mikael Starecki and James R. Mullen

Chapter 19: Carpal Bone Malunions and Nonunions 176
Paul C. Baldwin and John R. Fowler

Chapter 20: Scapholunate Ligament Injury and Dorsal
Intercalated Segment Stability 183
Mark Henry

Chapter 21: Lunotriquetral Ligament Injuries,
Midcarpal Instability, and Volar Intercalated
Segment Instability 192
William F. Pientka II, Jonathan D. Boyle, Timothy R. Niacaris, and
David M. Lichtman

Chapter 22: Avascular Necrosis of the Hand and Wrist 205
Michael Guju, Evan H. Horowitz, and Francisco A. Schwartz-Fernandes

Chapter 23: Wrist Dislocation 216
Brooks Ficke and Nilesh Kumar M. Chaudhari

Chapter 24: Acute Triangular Fibrocartilage
Complex Tears 227
Tamara John and Seth D. Dodds

Chapter 25: Salvage Procedures of the Wrist. 242
Edward W. Jernigan and Reid W. Draeger

Chapter 26: Distal Radius Fractures 254
Kathryn Ashley Bentley and Nilesh Kumar M. Chaudhari

Chapter 27: Distal Radius Malunion. 268
Anthony LoGiudice and Hisham M. Awan

Chapter 28: Distal Ulna Fractures. 281
Adam S. Martin and Hisham M. Awan

Chapter 29: Distal Radioulnar Joint Injuries 291
Adam S. Martin and Hisham M. Awan

Chapter 30: Galeazzi Fractures. 305
Maharsh K. Patel and Joseph J. King

Section 3: Tendon Injuries

Section Editor: Craig Rodner

Chapter 31: Extensor Tendon Injuries 313
Mark Henry

Chapter 32: Mallet Finger.................................... 321
Steven R. Niedermeier and Hisham M. Awan

Chapter 33: Sagittal Band Rupture (Traumatic Extensor
Tendon Dislocation)... 329
Matthew S. Torkington and David J. Warwick

Chapter 34: Flexor Tendon Injuries........................... 337
Andrew Campbell and Hisham M. Awan

Chapter 35: Jersey Finger 344
Nisha J. Crouser, Steven R. Niedermeier, and Hisham M. Awan

Section 4: Nerve Injuries

Section Editors: Joseph A. Gil and Robin Kamal

Chapter 36: Peripheral Nerve Injury and Repair Principles .. 351
D. Nicole Deal and Patricia A. Drace

Chapter 37: Digital Nerve Injury............................. 368
Rachel Michael, Roy E. Schneider, and Margaret Jain

Chapter 38: Median Nerve Injuries 378
Sohaib K. Malik and Alan R. Koester

Chapter 39: Ulnar Nerve Injuries............................ 385
Vishavpreet Singh, Ardalan Sayan, and Alan R. Koester

Chapter 40: Radial Nerve Injuries........................... 397
Lisa M. Kruse and Bryan Loeffler

Section 5: Hand and Wrist Infections

Section Editor: Craig Rodner

Chapter 41: Gustilo Classification........................... 407
Tiffany J. Pan and John R. Fowler

Chapter 42: Pulp Space Infections 413
Omri Ayalon and Matthew B. Cantlon

Chapter 43: Paronychial Infections.......................... 419
Timothy P. Crowley and Susan Stevenson

Chapter 44: Pyogenic Flexor Tenosynovitis................. 425
Emily E. Jewell and Reid W. Draeger

Chapter 45: Septic Arthritis. 438
Alan R. Blackburn II and John R. Fowler

Chapter 46: Web Space Infections 443
Tiffany J. Pan and John R. Fowler

Chapter 47: Palmar Space Infections 448
Hannah A. Dineen and Reid W. Draeger

Chapter 48: Cellulitis 464
Julie Johnson and John R. Fowler

Chapter 49: Bite Wounds. 467
Mark Henry

Chapter 50: Osteomyelitis. 474
Julie Johnson and John R. Fowler

Section 6: Other Traumatic Injuries

Section Editor: Andrea Halim

Chapter 51: Compartment Syndrome 479
Roshan Melvani and Christopher M. Jones

Chapter 52: Nail Bed Injury 491
Andrew D. Sobel

Chapter 53: Fingertip Amputations 504
Robert Ryu and Hisham M. Awan

Chapter 54: Replantation. 515
Michael S. Gart

Chapter 55: The Mangled Hand 529
Jason S. Lipof and John C. Elfar

Chapter 56: High-Pressure Injection Injuries 538
Erez Avisar

Chapter 57: Ring Avulsion Injuries 543
Evan H. Horowitz, Michael Guju, and Francisco A. Schwartz-Fernandes

Chapter 58: Upper Extremity Gunshot Wounds 552
Alex C. Lesiak and John R. Fowler

Chapter 59: Burns. 557
Ryan M. Garcia and Michael S. Gart

Chapter 60: Frostbite 562
Michael S. Gart

Section 7: Appendix

Section Editor: Andrea Halim

Chapter 61: Hand and Wrist Anatomy........................573
Mark K. Solarz and Robert C. Matthias, Jr.

Chapter 62: Rehabilitation and Splinting.................... 605
James D. Bedford and Sarah Turner

Chapter 63: How to Remove a Tight Ring 623
John C. Elfar and David J. Ciufo

Chapter 64: Vascular Evaluation of the Hand.............. 629
Christopher M. Jones and Beatrice L. Grasu

Index 653

CHAPTER

1

History and Physical Examination

Craig M. Rodner and Christian A. Merrill

INTRODUCTION

The aim of this chapter is to provide a systematic guide and template on which to perform a history and physical (H&P) examination in the setting of hand and wrist trauma. For all hand and wrist injuries, obtaining a thorough H&P is essential to establishing the correct diagnosis and making the appropriate treatment decision.

HISTORY

The mechanism of injury can provide insightful knowledge about the type of injury sustained in a hand or wrist trauma patient. It is important to assess whether the injury is blunt or penetrating in nature and whether or not this is high-energy versus a low-energy type of injury. This can provide context to the type and extent of injury sustained and various other structures that may be damaged in the acute trauma patient. The chief complaint, whether it be acute or more chronic in nature or potentially a sequela from a previously sustained trauma, should be investigated. The pain must be carefully examined for location, onset, duration, intensity, character, frequency, aggravating and relieving factors, night or rest pain, and radiating symptoms. Additionally, any associated symptoms such as catching, clicking, locking, weakness, numbness, or temperature sensitivities should be addressed. For both acute and chronic pathologies, the history of prior and current treatments should be examined. Any motor or sensory deficits should be inquired about.

Additionally, the patient's handedness, occupation, and current work status should be ascertained. This information can add valuable insight into how this injury can affect the patient's life and livelihood. With regard to past medical history and past surgical history, any history related to the afflicted extremity should be obtained; furthermore, any conditions that may increase the risk for infection, wound healing capacity, or vascular conditions should be documented. Social history should include any smoking, alcohol, or illicit drug use. Allergies and vaccination status, in particular tetanus updates, should be inquired about as well.

PHYSICAL EXAMINATION

- When performing the physical examination (PE), it is always important to remove all jewelry, clothing, bandages, splints, or other impedances such that the entire extremity could be examined. It is important to take a systematic approach to examining the fingers, hand, and wrist. The contralateral limb can always provide a reference for examination and can be examined first. It is often best to have the patient demonstrate the site of maximum pain by pointing with one finger and then approach this site last during examination.
- Inspection
  - Traumatic wound
    - Type—laceration, crush, inoculation, penetrating, avulsion, necrotic, caustic, burn
    - Size—estimate/measure (cm)
    - Shape—linear, stellate, complex, poke-hole, injection
    - Location—volar, dorsum, zone of injury (Figure 1.1)
    - What is exposed? Subcutaneous tissue, fat, muscle, tendon, bone, nerves, vessels
  - Swelling—diffuse versus localized
  - Deformity
    - Natural resting position of hand—gentle flexion at the metacarpophalangeal (MCP), proximal interphalangeal (PIP), and distal interphalangeal (DIP) joints
    - Natural resting position of wrist—slight extension and ulnar deviation
    - Coronal, sagittal, rotational deformities notable to contralateral
  - Skin—color changes, hair loss, scar, wounds/sinus tracts

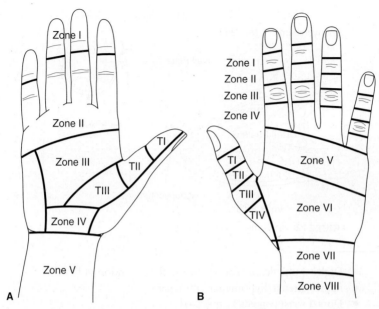

FIGURE 1.1 Flexor (A) and extensor (B) tendon zones of injury.

- Atrophy
  - Hand—thenar, hypothenar, interosseous musculature
  - Forearm—flexor and extensor compartments
- Palpation—assess tenderness, defects, step-offs, fluctuance, wounds
  - Hand—metacarpals, phalanges, MCPs, PIPs, and DIPs (Figures 1.2 and 1.4)
  - Nail—eponychium, paronychium, nail plate, and nail bed (Figure 1.3)

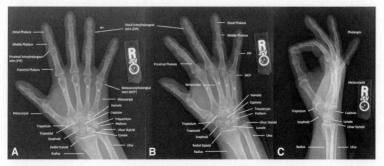

FIGURE 1.2 Radiograph of right hand including posteroanterior (PA) (A), oblique (B), and lateral (C) views and labeled osseous anatomy.

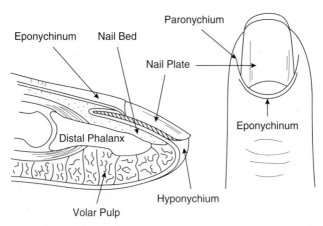

FIGURE 1.3 Anatomy of the nail bed.

- Digit—pulp, flexor tendon sheath, flexor tendon pulleys
- Palm—thenar/hypothenar eminence
- Dorsal wrist (Figures 1.2 and 1.4)
  - Distal radius—radial styloid, Lister tubercle
    - Distal radioulnar joint (DRUJ)
  - Distal ulna—ulna head, ulnar styloid
    - Triangular fibrocartilage complex
  - Carpal bones—scaphoid (proximal pole and waist), lunate, trapezium, trapezoid, capitate, hamate
  - Carpometacarpal joints—thumb, index, middle, ring, small finger
  - Extensor compartments: (1) abductor pollicis longus (APL) and extensor pollicis brevis (EPB); (2) extensor carpi radialis brevis (ECRB) and longus (ECRL); (3) extensor pollicis longus (EPL); (4) extensor digitorum communis (EDC) and extensor indicis proprius (EIP); (5) extensor digiti minimi (EDM); (6) extensor carpi ulnaris (ECU)
    - Anatomic snuff box—between first and second extensor compartment
- Volar wrist (Figures 1.2 and 1.4)
  - Carpal bones—scaphoid (tuberosity), trapezial ridge, pisiform, hook of hamate
  - Tendons—flexor carpi radialis (FCR), palmaris longus, flexor carpi ulnaris (FCU)
  - Neurovascular—radial and ulnar artery; median and ulnar nerve

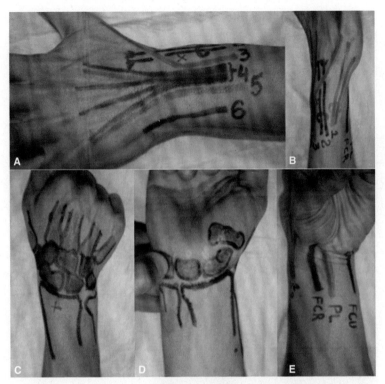

FIGURE 1.4 Palpable anatomic landmarks of the volar and dorsal wrist and hand—dorsal extensor compartment and tendons (A), radial wrist (B), dorsal wrist with osseous anatomy outlined (C), volar wrist with osseous anatomy outlined (D), volar wrist with flexor carpi radialis (FCR), palmaris longus (PL), and flexor carpi ulnaris (FCU) demonstrated (E).

- Mass—tenderness, consistency, mobility, compressibility, transillumination, pulsatileness, sinus tract
- Probing—explore wound with cotton tip applicator
■ Range of motion —assess both passive and active; assess smoothness of motion, abnormal movement, lack of movement, rotational deformity, scissoring (Table 1.1)
  - Passive tenodesis—fingers will flex with wrist passively extended and extend with passive flexion of the wrist (assess for tendon laceration) (Figure 1.5)
    ◆ Lack of tenodesis—disruption of tendon or musculotendinous junction

TABLE 1.1 **Normal Range of Motion**

Hand and Wrist Motion	Range of Motion (°)
Thumb MCP: palmar add/abduction	Contact-45
Thumb MCP radial add/abduction	Contact-60
Thumb MCP: extension–flexion	10-55
Thumb IP: extension–flexion	15 hyperextention -80
Finger DIP: extension–flexion	0-80
Finger PIP: extension–flexion	0-100
Finger MCP: extension–flexion	45 hyperextention -90
Wrist flexion	0-60
Wrist extension	0-75
Radial deviation	0-15
Ulnar deviation	0-40
Pronation	0-70
Supination	0-85

Abbreviations: DIP, distal interphalangeal; IP, interphalangeal; MCP, metacarpophalangeal; PIP, proximal interphalangeal.

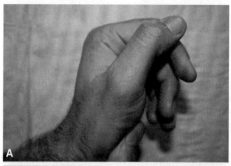

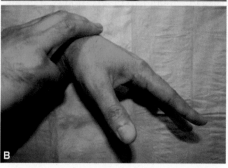

FIGURE 1.5 Clinical depiction of the passive tenodesis effect moving wrist from extension (A) to flexion (B).

- Hand—make full fist, open completely
  - ◆ All fingertips should touch palm, fingertips point toward scaphoid tubercle (assess rotational deformities)
- Wrist—move in all planes of motion
- ■ Muscular examination (Table 1.2)
  - Flexors
    - ◆ FCR—make a fist and flex wrist, ulnar deviation of the wrist is indicative of weak or incompetent FCR. Strength against resistance in wrist flexion and radial deviation.
    - ◆ FCU—make a fist and flex wrist, radial deviation of the wrist is indicative of weak or incompetent FCU. Strength against resistance in wrist flexion and ulnar deviation.
    - ◆ Flexor digitorum superficialis (FDS)—flex PIP joint of each individual digit while all other digits' MCP joint is stabilized in extension (Figure 1.6)
      - ∗ Prevents flexor digitorum profundus (FDP) from flexing because of quadriga effect because FDP tendons are connected to a single unit compared to FDS
    - ◆ FDP—flex DIP joint of each individual digit while PIP joint is stabilized in extension (Figure 1.7)
    - ◆ Flexor pollicis longus—flex interphalangeal (IP) joint of thumb while stabilizing thumb at proximal phalanx
  - Extensors
    - ◆ APL—hand supinated on table, radially abduct thumb in plane of hand
    - ◆ EPB—extend proximal phalanx of thumb while IP joint of thumb flexed
    - ◆ EPL—extend IP joint of thumb with proximal phalanx stabilized; hand pronated on table, lift thumb off table
    - ◆ EDC—extend fingers at MCP joint with wrist stabilized in extension
      - ∗ Sagittal band incompetence—able to maintain MCP extension but cannot obtain actively
    - ◆ EIP—extend index finger with other fingers flexed and wrist in extension
    - ◆ EDM—extend small finger with all other fingers flexed and wrist in extension
    - ◆ ECRL and ECRB—make a fist and extend wrist, ulnar deviation of the wrist is indicative of weak or incompetent ECRL and/or ECRB. Strength against resistance in wrist extension and radial deviation.

TABLE 1.2 **Motor Physical Examination Summary**

Muscle	Test	Nerve
FCR	Resisted wrist flex, radial deviation	Median
FCU	Resisted wrist flex, ulnar deviation	Ulnar
FDS	Flex PIP, all others extended	Median
FDP	Flex DIP, PIP stabilized	AIN: index and middle Ulnar: ring and small
FPL	Flex thumb IP	AIN
APL	Radially abduct in plane of hand	PIN
EPB	Extend proximal phalanx of thumb, IP flexed	PIN
EPL	Extend IP thumb; lift thumb from pronated hand off table	PIN
EDC	Extend MCP, wrist extended	PIN
EIP	Extend index finger, all others flexed	PIN
EDM	Extend small finger, all others flexed	PIN
ECRL and ECRB	Resisted wrist extension, radial deviation	ECRL: radial ECRB: deep radial
ECU	Resisted wrist extension, ulnar deviation	PIN
AP	Hand supinated, thumb straight up in air, patient brings down	Ulnar
OP	Touch tips of fingers w/thumb	Recurrent median
APB	Hand supinated, thumb straight up in air, patient keeps up	Recurrent median
FPB	Flex MCP thumb, IP extended	Superficial: recurrent median Deep: ulnar
ADM	Abduct small finger	Deep ulnar
ODM	Opposes small finger	Deep ulnar
Interossei	Dorsal: abduct fingers Palmar: adduct fingers	Dorsal: deep ulnar Palmar: deep ulnar
Lumbricals	Flex MCP, PIP, and DIP extended	Index and middle: deep median Ring and small: ulnar

Abbreviations: ADM, abductor digiti minimi; AIN, anterior interosseous nerve, branch of median nerve; AP, adductor pollicis; APB, abductor pollicis brevis; APL, abductor pollicis longus; DIP, distal interphalangeal; ECRB, extensor carpi radialis brevis; ECRL, extensor carpi radialis longus; ECU, extensor carpi ulnaris; EDC, extensor digitorum communis; EDM, extensor digiti minimi; EIP, extensor indicis proprius; EPB, extensor pollicis brevis; EPL, extensor pollicis longus; FCR, flexor carpi radialis; FCU, flexor carpi ulnaris; FDP, flexor digitorum profundus; FDS, flexor digitorum superficialis; FPL, flexor pollicis longus; IP, interphalangeal; MCP, metacarpophalangeal; ODM, opponens digiti minimi; OP, opponens pollicis; PIN, posterior interosseous nerve, branch of deep radial nerve from radial nerve; PIP, proximal interphalangeal.

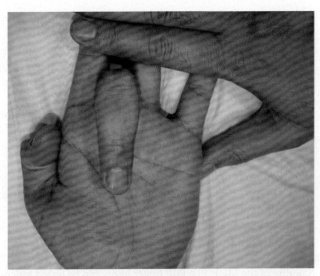

FIGURE 1.6 Physical examination of flexor digitorum superficialis.

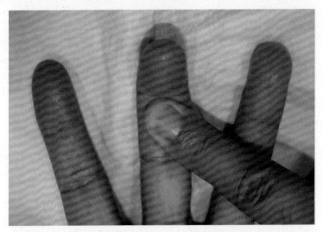

FIGURE 1.7 Physical examination of flexor digitorum profundus.

- ECU—make a fist and extend wrist, radial deviation of the wrist is indicative of weak or incompetent ECU. Strength against resistance in wrist extension and ulnar deviation.
- Intrinsics
  - Adductor pollicis—hand supinated on table, thumb palmarly abducted (straight in air), resistance applied to ulnar aspect

of thumb (patient brings it down); "OK" sign with index and middle finger
- Opponens pollicis—touch tips of all fingers with thumb tip
- Abductor pollicis brevis—hand supinated on table, thumb palmarly abducted (straight in air), resistance applied to radial aspect of thumb (patient keeps it up)
- Flexor pollicis brevis—flex MCP joint of thumb with IP joint in extension
- Abductor digiti minimi—abduct small finger
- Opponens digiti minimi—oppose small finger to thumb
- Interosseous muscles:
  * Dorsal—abduct fingers away from midline, spread fingers
  * Palmar—adduct fingers toward midline, close fingers
- Lumbricals—flex MCP joints while keeping PIP and DIP joints extended (intrinsic-plus position)

- Stability
  - Stability of the MCP, PIP, DIP finger joints can be tested for competency of the radial and ulnar collateral ligaments by stabilizing the joint and then applying a radial or ulnar directed force to test the respective ligaments.
    - Thumb—test ulnar collateral ligament both at full extension (accessory ligament) and at ~30° of flexion (proper ligament).
  - DRUJ stability—Ballottement test—stabilize distal radius with one hand, then translate the distal ulna dorsally and volarly with the other hand; compare with contralateral side (Figure 1.8)
- Sensory (Figure 1.9)
  - Light touch—finger, paper clip, and/or cotton swab
    - Semmes–Weinstein monofilament—objective sensitivity testing
  - Two-point discrimination—can assess both static and dynamic; can use special testing device or paper clip (Table 1.3)
  - Median—palmar aspect of radial 3½ digits, dorsal aspect of radial 3½ digits distal to DIP
  - Ulnar—palmar aspect of ulnar 1½ digits, dorsal aspect of ulnar 1½ digits
  - Radial—dorsal aspect of radial 2½ digits up to the DIP
  - Volar wrist—medial antebrachial cutaneous nerve (MABC), lateral antebrachial cutaneous nerve (LABC), and palmar cutaneous branches of median and ulnar nerves
  - Dorsal wrist—dorsal sensory branch of ulnar nerve, superficial radial nerve, MABC, LABC, and posterior antebrachial cutaneous nerve

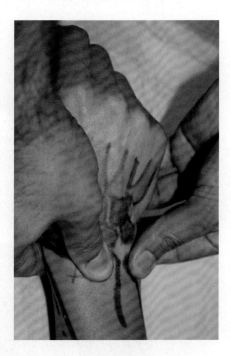

FIGURE 1.8 Physical examination of distal radial ulnar joint performing ballottement test.

- Vascular
  - Palpate radial and ulnar artery
  - Allen test—tests radial and ulnar artery perfusion to hand. Make fist, occlude both radial and ulnar artery, until hand is pale, release one artery and assess reperfusion (~5 seconds). Repeat with other artery to assess patency.
  - Perfusion—capillary refill, rough assessment of digital perfusion, less than 3 seconds considered normal
  - Doppler—can assess if concerned for vascular injury
- Specialty tests—(Table 1.4)

SUMMARY

The H&P of hand and wrist trauma requires a systematic approach to achieve an appropriate diagnosis and treatment plan. A detailed history of the chief complaint combined with thorough PE, understanding of anatomic landmarks, and possible pathology all aid in the recognition and care of these traumatic injuries.

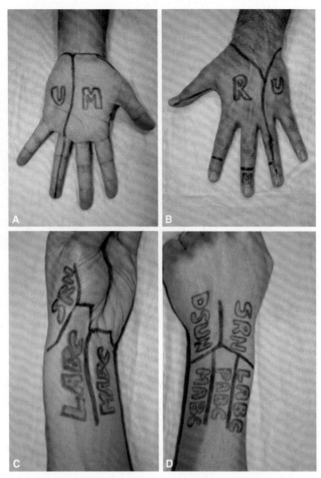

FIGURE 1.9 Clinical depiction of sensory nerve distribution of hand and wrist—volar hand (A), dorsal hand (B), volar wrist (C), and dorsal wrist (D); ulnar nerve (U), median nerve (M), radial nerve (R), superficial radial nerve (SRN), lateral antebrachial cutaneous nerve (LABC), medial antebrachial cutaneous nerve (MABC), dorsal sensory ulnar nerve (DSUN), posterior antebrachial cutaneous nerve (PABC).

TABLE 1.3 Two-Point Discrimination

Scale for Two-Point Discrimination	Discrimination Distance
Normal	Less than 6 mm
Fair	6-10 mm
Poor	11-15 mm
Anesthetic/absent	Absent sensation

TABLE 1.4 Specialty Hand and Wrist Examination Maneuvers

Name	Maneuver	Testing Outcome
Card test	Ask patient to grasp card between fingers by adducting toward midline and prevent examiner from removing	Tests the ulnar nerve and palmar interossei; positive if easily removed
Finger abduction	Ask patient to abduct fingers away from midline against resistance	Tests ulnar nerve and dorsal interossei; positive if unable to abduct or weakness
Froment sign	Ask patient to pinch card between thumb and radial border of index finger and prevent examiner from removing	Tests ulnar nerve and AP; positive if easily removed or if patient substitutes FPL by flexing thumb IP joint to resist removal of card
"OK" sign	Ask patient to make "OK" sign or an "O" by opposing thumb and index finger and prevent examiner from breaking "O" ring	Tests AIN, FPL, and FDP to index finger; positive if able to break "O" with little to no resistance
Thumb CMC grind test	Axially load the thumb MC against the trapezium	Detects CMC joint pathology such as arthritis; positive if significant pain
Bunnell–Littler test	Measure patient's passive PIP joint flexion with MCP fully extended and compare to MCP in 90° of flexion	Tests intrinsic tightness; if PIP joint flexion is greater when MCP joint is flexed it demonstrates intrinsic tightness (opposite for extrinsic tightness)
Elson test	Place patient's finger with palm down over edge of table with PIP flexed to 90°, then have patient extend finger against resistance	Test competency of the central slip of EDC tendon; DIP joint is rigidly extended with incompetency of central slip of EDC, supple DIP if intact
Anteroposterior drawer test	Examiner stabilizes distal forearm of patient with one hand and the MCs with other hand while applying anterior and posterior translating forces	Tests relative stability of the radiocarpal joint; positive if increased translation compared to the contralateral side
DRUJ compression test	Examiner compresses ulnar head against sigmoid notch while forearm is passively supinated and pronated	Tests DRUJ pathology; pain and tenderness with maneuver can suggest DRUJ pathology

(continued)

TABLE 1.4 Specialty Hand and Wrist Examination Maneuvers (*continued*)

Name	Maneuver	Testing Outcome
Finkelstein test	Patient makes fist over flexed thumb, examiner ulnarly deviates wrist	Pain and tenderness suggestive of first dorsal compartment inflammation (De Quervain tenosynovitis)
Pisotriquetral grind test	Patient slightly flexes and ulnarly deviates wrist while examiner grasps pisiform with thumb and index finger and grinds it over the triquetrum	Tests pisotriquetral pathology; positive if pain and tenderness present
Phalen test	Have patient maximally flex wrists or press dorsum of hands together to maintain wrist flexion for 1 min	Tests compression of median nerve for carpal tunnel syndrome; positive if paresthesias, numbness, tingling present in median nerve distribution
Scaphoid (Watson) shift	Patient's wrist and forearm in relaxed position while examiner applies dorsally directed force on scaphoid with thumb while the other hand moves the patient's wrist from an extended and ulnar deviation to flexion and radial deviation	Tests scapholunate instability; positive if presence of significant pain, catching, clicking, hypermobility, grinding compared to the contralateral side
LT Ballottement test (Reagan test)	Examiner attempts to translate the lunate and triquetrum in opposite directions in dorsal and volar plan	Tests LT stability; positive if hypermobility and tenderness compared to contralateral side
Kleinman shear test	Examiner stabilizes lunate with one hand, other hand applies a dorsally directed force to pisotriquetral joint	Tests LT stability; positive if pain, clicking, abnormal motion compared to contralateral side
Pivot shift test	Examiner stabilizes patient's wrist in full supination and then moves from radial deviation to ulnar deviation while attempting to sublux the distal carpus ulnarly	Tests midcarpal joint stability; positive if subluxation of capitate is noted
Midcarpal shift test	Examiner stabilizes patient's forearm with one hand and then moves wrist from radial to ulnar deviation while applying an axial load through the metacarpals	Tests midcarpal joint stability; positive if pain, clicking, subluxation, reproduction of symptoms compared to contralateral side

Abbreviations: AIN, anterior interosseous nerve; AP, adductor pollicis; CMC, carpometacarpal; DIP, distal interphalangeal; DRUJ, distal radioulnar joint; EDC, extensor digitorum communis; FDP, flexor digitorum profundus; FPL, flexor pollicis longus; IP, interphalangeal; LT, lunotriquetral; MC, metacarpal; MCP, metacarpophalangeal; PIP, proximal interphalangeal.

SUGGESTED READINGS

Browner B, Levine A, Jupiter J, Trafton P, Krettek C. Fractures and dislocations of the hand. In: Jupiter JB, Axelrod TS, Belsky MR, eds. *Skeletal Trauma: Basic Science, Management, and Reconstruction*. Philadelphia, PA: WB Saunders; 2018:chap 38.

Browner B, Levine A, Jupiter J, Trafton P, Krettek C. Fractures and dislocations of the carpus. In: Ruby LK, Cassidy C, eds. *Skeletal Trauma: Basic Science, Management, and Reconstruction*. Philadelphia, PA: WB Saunders; 2018:chap 39.

Browner B, Levine A, Jupiter J, Trafton P, Krettek C. Fractures of the distal radius. In: Cohen MS, Jupiter JB, McMurtry RY, eds. *Skeletal Trauma: Basic Science, Management, and Reconstruction*. Philadelphia, PA: WB Saunders; 2018:chap 40.

Court-Brown CM, Heckman JD, McQueen MM, Ricci WM, Tornetta P, McKee MD. Hand fractures and dislocations. In: Henry MH, ed. *Rockwood & Green's Fractures in Adults*. 8th ed. Philadelphia, PA: Wolters Kluwer; 2015:chap 30.

Court-Brown CM, Heckman JD, McQueen MM, Ricci WM, Tornetta P, McKee MD. Carpus fractures and dislocations. In: Duckworth AD, Ring D, eds. *Rockwood & Green's Fractures in Adults*. 8th ed. Philadelphia, PA: Wolters Kluwer; 2015:chap 31.

Court-Brown CM, Heckman JD, McQueen MM, Ricci WM, Tornetta P, McKee MD. Fractures of the distal radius and ulna. In: McQueen MM, ed. *Rockwood & Green's Fractures in Adults*. 8th ed. Philadelphia, PA: Wolters Kluwer; 2015:chap 32.

Kenney RJ, Hammert WC. Physical examination of the hand. *J Hand Surg*. 2014;39(11):2324-2334.

Kleinman WB. Physical examination of the wrist: useful provocative maneuvers. *J Hand Surg*. 2015;40(7):1486-1500.

Lee DH, Mignemi ME, Crosby SN. Fingertip injuries: an update on management. *J Am Acad Orthop Surg*. 2013;21(12):756-766.

Peterson SL, Peterson EL, Wheatley MJ. Management of fingertip amputations. *J Hand Surg*. 2014;39(10):2093-2101.

2   Imaging

Daniel R. Lewis

Radiographic imaging is essential in diagnosing most traumatic injuries of the musculoskeletal system. Unfortunately, poorly taken radiographs or medically unnecessary advanced imaging can lead to a delayed diagnosis or misdiagnosis. A fundamental knowledge of how to obtain and interpret proper skeletal imaging is paramount to the treating clinician. Even more important is the clinical examination of the patient, which identifies the anatomic location of concern and establishes a differential diagnosis to guide further evaluation.

RADIOGRAPHS[1,2]

Standard Views

- Finger examinations should include at a minimum a posteroanterior (PA) and a lateral view. The joint spaces on PA views should be visible and symmetric. Lateral views should be taken with minimal to no rotation.
- The basic radiographic examination of the hand and wrist includes, at a minimum, orthogonal views in the PA and lateral planes.
- For optimal results, the shoulder should be abducted to 90° and the hand placed on the imaging cassette for PA views. This allows for neutral rotation views, which are optimal for anatomic measurements. The PA view is extremely useful for initial survey of the wrist and hand. Fractures of the radius and ulna, carpus, metacarpals, and phalanges can be identified. The type of fracture, presence of comminution, displacement, angulation, and ulnar variance may be measured. This view also aids in the evaluation of carpal alignment in the coronal plane, including scapholunate diastasis and the alignment of the carpal rows (Gilula arcs). Radial height, inclination, and ulnar variance can also be measured (Figure 2.1).
- The anteroposterior (AP) plane may be used if range of motion of the extremity is limited.
- An optimal lateral radiograph of the wrist will show the pisiform superimposed over the scaphoid tuberosity. The alignment of the distal

radius articular surface, including location and position of fracture fragments and articular tilt, can be demonstrated. The lateral view is also extremely valuable for identifying dislocations of the carpus (eg, perilunate injuries) and carpometacarpal (CMC) joints. Important intercarpal measurements, including scapholunate and radiolunate angles, can also be performed.

- An oblique radiograph performed in 45° of pronation can be performed to evaluate fractures of the scaphoid, the scaphotrapezial-trapezoidal joint, dorsal triquetral avulsion fractures, and dorsoulnar corner fractures of the radius.
- Supinated 45° oblique films may be taken to evaluate the pisotriquetral joint and fourth and fifth CMC joints.

Specialized Views

The following are common specialized views that aid in the diagnosis of specific anatomic locations often performed by orthopedic clinicians.

- The scaphoid view is PA wrist view taken with the wrist in maximal ulnar deviation, which extends the scaphoid and brings it into full profile. The radiograph beam may be angled between 0° and 30° to obtain a series.

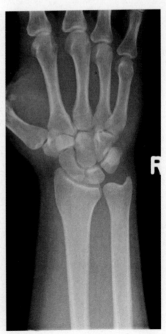

FIGURE 2.1 Standard zero rotation posteroanterior radiograph of the wrist. Note medial position of the ulnar styloid and ulnar positive variance.

- Bilateral clenched or pencil grip PA wrist films are the most sensitive radiographs to evaluate scapholunate diastasis secondary to dynamic scapholunate instability.
- The first CMC joint views are true AP (or hyperpronated PA) and lateral of the thumb and CMC joint and are often used to determine joint congruity and the presence of arthritis.
- The second and third CMC joints will be seen best on a lateral wrist film with the wrist in flexion and slightly supinated.
- The hook of hamate view is performed with the wrist in the lateral position with maximal radial deviation and slight supination. The thumb should be abducted palmarly as much as possible to allow adequate viewing of the entire hamate hook (Figure 2.2).

MRI OF THE WRIST AND HAND[3-6]

The use and advancement of magnetic resonance imaging (MRI), particularly 3-T magnets, dedicated wrist coils, and gadolinium arthrography, have provided a powerful tool in clinicians' armamentarium. Although

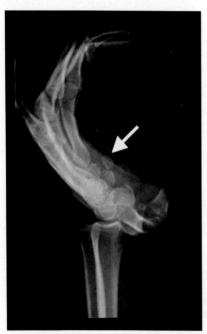

FIGURE 2.2 Hook of hamate view. Nonunion of hamate hook identified.

MRI is useful as a diagnostic tool, it should not supplant the importance of obtaining the patient's history and clinical examination.

- **MRI of the fingers**
  - Flexor tendons—Best seen on axial and sagittal images. Low signal on T1 and T2 sequences. Complete tears demonstrate discontinuity of signal and retraction. Avulsions will also show retraction consistent with anatomic description by Leddy and Packer. Strains and linear tears will show varying degrees of signal changes.
  - Flexor retinaculum (pulleys)—Best seen on axial and sagittal images. Injuries are demonstrated by increased signal or disruption and most often occur in A1–A4 pulleys. However, the entire retinaculum may be affected.
  - Extensor tendons—MRI is often useful to diagnose sagittal band tears. Sagittal bands are best seen on axial images. These extend from the extensor tendons dorsally at the metacarpophalangeal joints and extend palmarly to the volar plates. Injuries will be seen as signal changes or subluxation/dislocation of the extensor tendon.
  - Ligaments—Collateral ligaments are best seen on coronal images, and volar plates are best visualized on the sagittal images. Intrasubstance and more commonly insertional tears are demonstrated by increased signal or displacement.
- **MRI of the wrist**
  - Osseous structures—Fractures and bone contusions of the wrist and hand typically appear as low signal (dark) on T1 sequences and high signal on T2 images. MRI is particularly useful and has the highest sensitivity for identifying occult fractures.
  - Ligaments—The anatomy of the intrinsic and extrinsic wrist ligaments is visible on standard MRI; however, sensitivity to pathology is improved with the addition of intra-articular gadolinium. A high linear signal often shows the dye passing through the tear and into the adjacent joint in complete ligamentous tears. Displacement from ligamentous insertions and increased signal within the ligament are seen with avulsions and partial tears, respectively (Figure 2.3).
  - Triangular fibrocartilage complex (TFCC)—The TFCC appears as a low signal structure on all MRI sequences. Degeneration increases with age and may be seen as intermediate signal within the TFCC substance without a definite tear. Arthrography increases the sensitivity for TFCC tears, which are demonstrated by a high linear signal traversing the ulnocarpal joint to the distal radioulnar joint. Tears of the deep distal radioulnar joint ligaments (ligamentum subcruentum)

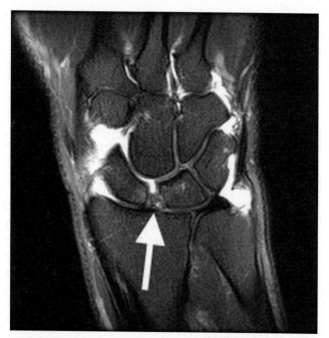

FIGURE 2.3 Magnetic resonance arthrogram demonstrates passage of gadolinium from the radiocarpal joint to the midcarpal joint, scapholunate diastasis, and scapholunate ligament disruption.

will show increased signal or disruption most commonly at the ulnar fovea (Figure 2.4).

- Tendons—Wrist and finger flexors and extensors are well demonstrated on all sequences. With complete tears, the tendon will often appear coiled and retracted with increased signal on T2 sequences. Intrasubstance tears may have linear or globular medium to high signal changes within the tendon. Tendonitis, if moderate to severe, will have a high signal fluid ring surrounding the affected tendon on T2 sequences.
- Avascular necrosis (AVN)—MRI can be used to determine and assess the presence of AVN prior to radiograph changes. The administration of intravenous gadolinium improves the sensitivity for AVN. AVN often appears as low signal on T1- and high signal on T2-weighted images when edema is present; however, the T2 sequences may also demonstrate low signal if the normal bone marrow is replaced with fibrosis. The signal abnormality typically affects the entire bone and there may be a mixture of signal (low to intermediate) depending upon the stage of AVN.

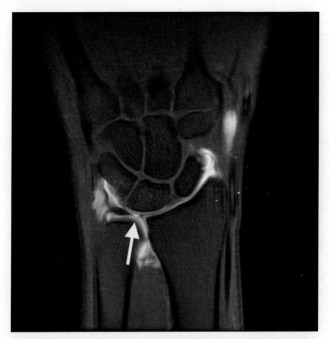

FIGURE 2.4 Magnetic resonance arthrogram demonstrates dye passing through a triangular fibrocartilage complex tear from the ulnocarpal joint to the distal radioulnar joint.

- **Computerized tomography (CT) scans**
  - The addition of 2D and 3D reconstructed images has provided a valuable tool in the evaluation and treatment of complex skeletal trauma.
  - CT scans of the hand and wrist in the traumatic setting is often utilized to:
    - Understand fracture patterns and displacement for clinical planning.
    - Detect the presence or absence of osseous healing.
      - CT reconstructed images of the scaphoid are superior to wrist images to assess scaphoid anatomy and healing (Figure 2.5).
    - Assess bone structure and stock for delayed surgical reconstructions.
    - Determine the presence of occult fractures (although MRI has demonstrated higher sensitivity and specificity).
    - Evaluate degenerative changes.
- **Ultrasound (US)**[7]
  - US is emerging as a valuable diagnostic modality given its portability, relatively low cost, ability to visualize most osseous and soft tissues

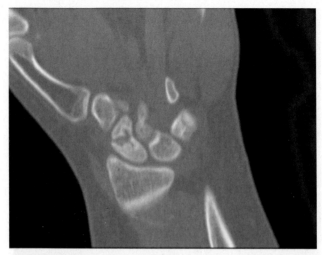

FIGURE 2.5 Coronal reconstructed wrist computerized tomography image demonstrates scaphoid nonunion and local bone resorption.

of the hand and wrist, and ability for real-time and dynamic evaluation of anatomic structures.

- Tissue that is dense, such as cortical bone and tendons, is hyperechoic and appears light. Hypoechoic tissue, such as muscle, appears dark.
- US is often used to evaluate:
  - Flexor and extensor tendon injuries and instability (ie, extensor carpi ulnaris)
  - Flexor pulley injuries
  - Ligaments of the hand and wrist injuries
  - Blood vessel and nerve injuries
  - Occult fractures
  - Hematomas
  - Foreign bodies
  - Location of injections

REFERENCES

1. Frank ED. *Merrill's Atlas of Radiographic Positioning and Procedures*. 12th ed. St Louis, MO: Mosby; 2011.
2. Long BW, Rafert JA. *Orthopaedic Radiography*. Philadelphia, PA: WB Saunders; 1995.

3. Dewan AK, Chhabra B, Khanna AJ, Anderson MW, Brunton LM. Magnetic resonance imaging of the hand and wrist: techniques and spectrum of disease. *J Bone Joint Surg Am.* 2013;95:e68(1-12).
4. Steinbach SS, Smith DK. MRI of the wrist. *J Clin Imaging.* 2000;24:298-322.
5. Ringler MD. MRI of wrist ligaments. *J Hand Surg Am.* 2013;38A:2034-2046.
6. Gupta P, Lenchik L, Wuertzer SD, Pachilke DA. High resolution 3-T MRI of the fingers: review of anatomy and common tendon and ligament injuries. *Am J Roentgenol.* 2015;2014:W314-W323.
7. Starr HM, Sedgley MD, Means KR, Murphy MS. Ultrasonography for hand and wrist conditions. *J Am Acad Orthop Surg.* 2016;24:544-554.

3 Anesthesia

Rachel C. Hooper and Steven C. Haase

TYPES OF ANESTHESIA

- Local anesthesia ("WALANT")
- Local anesthesia plus intravenous sedation (also known as monitored anesthesia care [MAC])
- Intravenous regional anesthesia (Bier block)
- Regional nerve block (wrist, elbow, brachial plexus)
- General anesthesia

GENERAL CONSIDERATIONS

- Comorbidities and general health
  - Deeper anesthetics result in a greater physiologic stress.
- Age, temperament, and maturity level
  - Able to keep still, follow directions?
  - Sedation may be difficult to titrate in children.
- Anxiety, attitude, and emotional status
  - Anxious patients may require sedation even for small procedures.
- Anatomic site and duration of procedure (need for tourniquet?)
  - Awake patients generally tolerate brachial tourniquet for 20 minutes or less.
  - Forearm tourniquet may be more comfortable for longer periods.
  - Finger tourniquets cause negligible discomfort if digit is blocked.

KEYS TO SUCCESS

- Patient education—discuss anesthesia options in detail before surgery
- Teamwork—work with anesthesia colleagues to obtain most comfortable situation for your patient

LOCAL ANESTHETICS[1]

- Mechanism of action—reversibly block nerve impulses by reducing cells' permeability to sodium
  - Formulated as water-soluble hydrochlorides
  - Must transition to lipid-soluble form to enter cells and take effect
  - Acidic environment (infection/inflammation) favors water-soluble form and decreases efficacy
- Two basic types—amides and esters
  - *Tip—Amides contain an "i" in the name before the "-caine." Esters do not!*
  - Amides (eg, lidocaine, bupivacaine)—most common class
  - Esters (eg, procaine, tetracaine)—used less often
- Duration of action/maximum safe dose—vary based on lipid solubility as well as addition of epinephrine
  - Epinephrine reduces drug diffusion/absorption, prolonging duration of action and increasing maximum safe dose.
  - Calculating maximum safe dose depends on patient weight, drug volume, and drug concentration.
  - *Tip—Move the decimal one place to the right to convert % to mg/mL (1.0% = 10 mg/mL)*
  - For rapid onset *plus* long duration, consider using a 1:1 mixture of lidocaine + bupivacaine!

Generic name	Brand name	Type	Speed of onset	Duration	Max safe dose without epinephrine	Max safe dose with Epinephrine
Lidocaine	Xylocaine	Amide	Rapid	1-2 h	5 mg/kg	7 mg/kg
Bupivacaine	Marcaine	Amide	Slow	8-12 h	2.5 mg/kg	3 mg/kg
Procaine	Novocain	Ester	Rapid	0.25-0.5 h	8 mg/kg	10 mg/kg
Tetracaine	Tetravisc	Ester	Slow	2-3 h	1.5 mg/kg	2.5 mg/kg

- *Allergies*—true allergies to local anesthetics are rare
  - More often, "reactions" are related to syncope or epinephrine-related palpitations.
  - True allergic reactions may occur in response to:
    - Para-aminobenzoic acid (PABA)—metabolite of methylparaben, a preservative included in multidose vials to prevent microbial growth
    - Sulfites—inorganic compounds included in epinephrine-containing products to prevent oxidation of the vasopressor

- ◆ **The Drug Itself**—amides and esters can both provoke allergies
  - ✳ Esters may be more common, because procaine metabolizes to PABA
- In case of a true allergy:
  - ◆ If drug is known—OK to use a *different* drug (amide or ester); cross-reactivity is rare
  - ◆ If drug is unknown—patient may require allergy testing
- *Resistance[2]*
  - True "resistance" to local anesthetics is also rare, and usually anecdotal:
    - ◆ Patients with Ehlers–Danlos syndrome—several reports of failed regional blocks
    - ◆ Patients with exposure to scorpion venom (affects sodium channels)—anecdotal reports
    - ◆ Patients/families with genetic mutation in *SCN5A* gene (responsible for opening and closing sodium channels)
- *Toxicity*—all local anesthetics are central nervous system depressants and may potentiate other depressants
  - Early symptoms (serum > 5 µg/mL)—perioral numbness, facial tingling, restlessness, vertigo, tinnitus, slurred speech
  - Life-threatening symptoms (serum > 10 µg/mL)—tonic–clonic seizures, coma, respiratory arrest, cardiovascular collapse
  - Treatment
    - ◆ ABCs—airway, breathing, circulation
    - ◆ Seizures—treat with thiopental or diazepam
    - ◆ Cardiac toxicity
      - ✳ Bupivacaine has greater potential for direct cardiac toxicity than other agents.
      - ✳ Antidote = lipid emulsion (20%)—bolus 1.5 mL/kg over 1 minute, then infuse at 0.25 mL/kg/min
    - ◆ Anaphylaxis—diphenhydramine, subcutaneous epinephrine, intravenous steroids

LOCAL ANESTHESIA ("WALANT")[3]

- *Wide Awake Local Anesthesia No Tourniquet (WALANT)* is a term increasingly used
  - No intravenous (IV) sedation
    - ◆ No anesthesiologist, no anesthesia charges
    - ◆ No need to be NPO for surgery

- Select patients may drive themselves home
- Able to talk with patient during procedure:
  - Improved patient education/understanding
  - Able to elicit active motion to test intraoperative function
- Need a cooperative patient
- Need to inject local anesthesia without sedation
  - To reduce pain of injection:
    - ▲ Inject *slowly* (eg, 10 mL over 5-10 minutes)
    - ▲ Use a small needle (25- to 30-gauge)
    - ▲ Add *sodium bicarbonate (8.4%)* to local anesthetic
      - ❖ Typical formulation is 10:1 ratio of anesthetic-to-bicarbonate
      - ❖ Decreases acidity, reducing pain and speeding onset of anesthetic
- No tourniquet
  - Less pain and discomfort
  - Less time constraints
  - Bleeding is minimized by addition of *epinephrine* to the local anesthetic
    - Epinephrine does not stop *all* bleeding—will still be mildly oozing
    - Maximum hemostatic effect is about 20 to 30 minutes after injection.
- Epinephrine—typically formulated as 1:100 000 (10 µg/mL) or 1:400 000 (2.5 µg/mL)
  - Safety has been proved in multiple studies.
  - Use with caution in patients with cardiopulmonary comorbidities, Raynaud phenomenon, and/or peripheral vascular occlusive disease.
  - Antidote = *phentolamine* (α-blocker)
    - Dosing for digit ischemia ("white finger" syndrome)—inject 1.5 mg subcutaneously around digit base
    - Onset of action is generally about 1.5 hours.
    - May need to be repeated if ischemia relapses.

DIGITAL BLOCK TECHNIQUES

- Anatomy—each finger is innervated by two volar and two dorsal digital nerves; whichever technique is utilized must address all nerve branches to be successful.
- Dorsal versus volar?

- Historically, many felt dorsal injections would be less painful.
- Newer evidence shows no difference in reported pain or preference for dorsal versus volar.
- *Classic Techniques*[4]
  - *Transthecal*—injection delivered via the flexor tendon sheath, usually accessed at the palmar-digital crease; only about 2 mL of injection is required (Figure 3.1).
    - Avoid using epinephrine with this technique, as "white finger" may result.
    - Although very fast and effective, patients often complain of long-lasting finger discomfort after this technique is used.
  - *Transmetacarpal*—injection delivered at the level of the distal palmar crease, placing about 2 mL at each of the common digital nerves at the level of the metacarpal necks (Figure 3.1)
    - May require dorsal supplementation to block the dorsal digital nerves
  - *Subcutaneous*—inject in the subcutaneous tissue around base of digit (Figure 3.2)
    - Theoretical risk of circulatory compromise has been disproven by multiple studies.
- *"SIMPLE" Technique (**S**ingle subcutaneous **I**njection in the **M**iddle of the **P**roximal phalanx with **L**idocaine and **E**pinephrine)*—a variant of subcutaneous technique popularized for WALANT surgery[5]

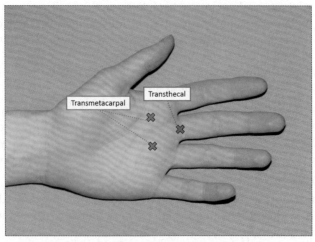

FIGURE 3.1 Transthecal and tansmetacarpal techniques.

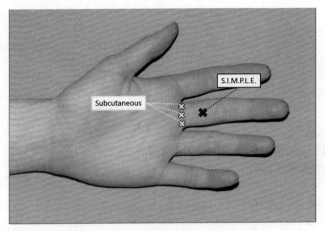

FIGURE 3.2 Subcutaneous and SIMPLE techniques.

- An injection of 2 mL in this location can provide sensory block (Figure 3.2).
- Additional injections along the digit are required for hemostasis when using epinephrine instead of tourniquet.

LOCAL PLUS INTRAVENOUS SEDATION (MAC)

- MAC is typically selected for patients with increased anxiety—or other factors—who may have difficulty coping with "wide awake" surgery
  - *Tip—Patients with tremors and/or movement disorders often exhibit reduction in these actions with light sedation, which can be helpful if the motion is counterproductive during surgery.*
- Agents commonly used:
  - Midazolam (Versed)—sedative, often causes some amnesia
  - Fentanyl (Duragesic, Sublimaze)—narcotic used for relief of severe pain, quick-acting
  - Propofol (Diprivan)—sedative with quick onset and rapid recovery, also reduces memory for events
- With this level of sedation, anesthesia monitoring is required
  - Airway—patients must be NPO because of risk of aspiration
  - Breathing—oxygenation must be monitored, especially in those patients at risk for sleep apnea (eg, high body mass index)
  - Circulation—heart rate and blood pressure must be monitored

- Communication between surgeon and anesthesiologist/nurse anesthetist is critical:
  - Continuous administration of sedatives is usually not required.
  - A sedation "bolus" at time of local anesthetic injection may be all that is required.
  - If the patient needs to be fully awake to follow commands intraoperatively, be sure to avoid long-acting agents.

INTRAVENOUS REGIONAL ANESTHESIA (BIER BLOCK)

- Typically selected for cases lasting between 30 and 120 minutes where dense, extensive anesthesia of the extremity is required
- Requires anesthesia monitoring; typically accompanied by at least light sedation
- Basics of technique:
  - Place a double-cuff tourniquet on upper arm and peripheral IV distally in the hand.
    - Test both cuffs prior to proceeding, to be sure tourniquet is in good working order.
  - Elevate and exsanguinate arm from fingertips to tourniquet, using Esmarch bandage or similar device.
  - Inflate distal cuff, then proximal cuff to 250 mm Hg each. Once proximal cuff is inflated, deflate distal cuff only, then remove Esmarch wrap. Confirm proximal cuff is up and working properly before injecting medication.
  - Slowly inject local anesthetic via peripheral IV in the hand
    - 0.5% lidocaine (max dose 3 mg/kg) and 0.5% prilocaine (max dose 6 mg/kg) are the most commonly used agents (low cardiac toxicity).
      - *Tip—Typical dose = 30 to 50 mL of 0.5% lidocaine for an adult patient*
      - *Tip—Do **not** use epinephrine; do **not** use other local anesthetics.*
  - Discontinue IV catheter once medication is completely instilled.
    - *Tip—Allow 10 minutes after instillation for IV anesthetic to have full effect.*
  - Prep and drape; proceed with surgery
  - If patient shows signs of tourniquet pain, inflate distal cuff (confirm inflation!) and then deflate proximal cuff. This effectively shifts the

tourniquet pressure to an area of the upper arm that should be anesthetized, eliminating much of the tourniquet pain for the patient.

- Plan ahead! Once both the cuffs are deflated, the anesthetic effect will disappear quickly. Additional local anesthesia will need to be injected to assist with wound closure and postoperative pain. Make sure total dose of lidocaine is within safe parameters.
- Safe deflation—typically, tourniquet can be safely deflated after 40 minutes, based on metabolism of lidocaine. Safe timing may vary for other drugs/dosages.
  - *Tip—If surgery concludes before 40 minutes of tourniquet time, may be able to "flash" the tourniquet (quickly cycle between deflation and inflation) intermittently, allowing lidocaine to enter the systemic circulation gradually. Need to consult with anesthesia colleagues before doing this.*

REGIONAL NERVE BLOCK

- *Wrist block*
  - Typically used for cases where individual digital blocks are inefficient or impractical.
  - Can anesthetize the entire hand by addressing three nerves: median, ulnar, and superficial radial.
    - Median nerve—typically accessed at volar wrist, proximal to wrist crease, between palmaris and flexor carpi radialis (Figure 3.3).
      - *Tip—Alternatively, injecting just ulnar to palmaris will typically place the needle ulnar to the median nerve, but still within the carpal tunnel.*
    - Ulnar nerve—typically accessed at the level of the ulnar head/neck; inject just deep to flexor carpi ulnaris tendon; aspirate before injecting, given proximity to ulnar artery (Figure 3.3).
    - Radial nerve—typically accessed at dorsal/radial wrist, near extensor carpi radialis longus, may be several branches across this area, so a broad area is typically injected (Figure 3.4).
  - *Caution*—Should only perform these blocks in an awake and alert patient. If patient reports neuropathic pain (shooting, burning, tingling, electric shock type symptoms), then your needle must be repositioned. NEVER risk injecting directly into a nerve, as nerve damage will ensue. Goal is to place medication AROUND the nerves, not INTO the nerves.

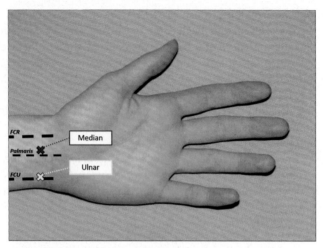

FIGURE 3.3 Wrist block, median and ulnar nerves. FCR, flexor carpi radialis; FCU, flexor carpi ulnaris.

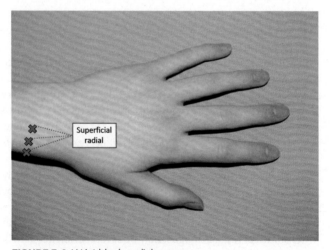

FIGURE 3.4 Wrist block, radial nerve.

- *More proximal blocks (brachial plexus/elbow)*
  - Typically performed by anesthesiologists using ultrasound guidance; these techniques are beyond the scope of this chapter.
  - Can provide pain control for as long as 12 to 18 hours, depending on the medication injected.

> ◆ *Tip—For even longer-lasting pain control, discuss placement of an indwelling catheter to slowly infuse local anesthetic over time; these can remain in place for several days in select patients.*

- Contraindicated in patients with coagulopathy and in patients taking anticoagulant medications.

GENERAL ANESTHESIA

- Typically selected for procedures requiring complete patient relaxation, muscle paralysis, and/or surgery at multiple sites or multiple extremities, where use of regional and/or local anesthesia techniques alone is not practical.
- Requires control of airway with endotracheal tube (ETT) or laryngeal mask airway (LMA).
  - LMA apparatus fits over glottic structures but does not provide as much airway protection as a cuffed ETT.
  - ETT is required for patients needing muscle paralysis for surgery and in those with significant history of gastroesophageal reflux disease.
- Components typically used for general anesthesia:
  - Inhalation agents (nitrous oxide, isoflurane, sevoflurane)
  - Intravenous sedatives (midazolam, propofol)
  - Muscle relaxants (succinylcholine, cisatracurium, rocuronium)
- General anesthesia poses more risk than alternative forms of anesthesia:
  - Postoperative nausea and vomiting (affects one-third of patients)
  - Airway compromise (eg, laryngospasm, aspiration)
  - Cardiopulmonary side effects
  - Malignant hyperthermia (rare reaction to succinylcholine and/or inhalational agents)
    - ◆ *Tip—This is an emergency situation. Need to stop all potential causative agents and administer dantrolene (Dantrium) to treat this condition.*

ACKNOWLEDGMENTS

The authors would like to thank Ava Haase for her help in creating the figures in this chapter.

REFERENCES

1. Becker DE, Reed KL. Local anesthetics: review of pharmacological considerations. *Anesth Prog.* 2012;59(2):90-102.

2. Clendenen N, Cannon AD, Porter S, Robards CB, Parker AS, Clendenen SR. Whole-exome sequencing of a family with local anesthetic resistance. *Minerva Anestesiol.* 2016;82(10):1089-1097.

3. Lalonde D, Eaton C, Amadio PC, Jupiter JB. Wide-awake hand and wrist surgery: a new horizon in outpatient surgery. *Instr Course Lect.* 2015;64:249.

4. Wolfe S, Pederson W, Kozin SH. *Green's Operative Hand Surgery.* 6th ed. Philadelphia, PA: Churchill Livingstone; 2011.

5. Wheelock ME, LeBlanc M, Chung B, et al. Is it True that injecting palmar finger skin hurts more than dorsal skin? New level 1 evidence. *Hand.* 2011;6(1):47-49.

General Concepts: Indications for Surgery

Ethan W. Dean and Robert C. Matthias, Jr.

INTRODUCTION

- Hand and wrist injuries are very common presenting complaints in the acute care setting.
- Categories of injury
  - Fracture or dislocation
  - Tendon injury
  - Nerve injury
  - Infection
  - Soft tissue damage or amputation
  - Vascular injury
  - Any combination of the above
- Selection of appropriate treatment strategy requires a thorough history, physical examination, and relevant imaging studies.
- Optimum treatment requires individualized approach to the patient:
  - Age
  - Occupation
  - Functional status
  - Presence of comorbidities
  - Ability to cooperate in treatment strategy
- Common questions posed to the treating provider:
  - Which conditions can be definitively managed in the acute care setting?
  - Which conditions warrant referral to a hand specialist?
  - Which conditions require emergent operative management?
- Principles of surgical management:
  - Restore maximal function of the injured hand or wrist
  - Prevent further loss of function
  - Expectation that ultimate outcome will be equivalent or better than the nonoperative alternative
  - Restore normal anatomy when possible

- Must consider risks of surgery including:
  - Soft tissue damage
  - Infection
  - Necessity for secondary procedures (eg, implant removal)
  - Iatrogenic injury or technical failure
  - Further decompensation in acutely ill patients
- Although many acute hand and wrist injuries may ultimately require surgical intervention, relatively few are considered emergent.
  - Important to appropriately triage
  - Determine which injuries may be appropriate for management in the subacute setting
  - If in doubt, discuss with hand specialist to aid in decision-making

EMERGENT INDICATIONS FOR SURGERY

- Surgical emergency
  - Medical emergency for which a delay in surgical management could result in permanent impairment or death
  - Few hand and wrist injuries are life-threatening; however, many can result in significant functional impairment if not treated in a timely fashion
- In general, hand or wrist conditions that may require emergent operative intervention include, but are not limited to:
  - Compartment syndrome
  - Open fractures or dislocations
  - Acute compressive neuropathy
  - Traumatic amputation
  - Infection
  - High-pressure injection injury
  - Vascular injury
- **Compartment syndrome** (see Chapter 51)
  - Increase in pressure within a limited space (usually a fascial compartment), which limits the perfusion and function of the tissues in that space
  - Mechanisms include, but are not limited to:
    - ◆ Fracture (most common)
      - ✳ Distal radius fractures in adults
      - ✳ Supracondylar humerus fractures in children

- ◆ Crush injury or soft tissue contusion
- ◆ Arterial injury
- ◆ Limb compression (eg, tight cast or splint)
- ◆ Burns
- If missed, can result in rapid tissue necrosis, subsequent fibrosis, contracture (ie, Volkmann ischemic contracture), and loss of function
- Diagnosis is primarily clinical:
  - ◆ Pain out of proportion to clinical situation
  - ◆ Pain with passive stretch of fingers
    - ✳ Most sensitive finding
  - ◆ Paresthesias
  - ◆ Paralysis
  - ◆ Swelling/tense compartments
  - ◆ Absence of peripheral pulses
    - ✳ Almost always a late finding
  - ◆ Hand may rest in the intrinsic minus position
    - ✳ Metacarpophalangeal (MCP) joints extended and proximal interphalangeal joints flexed
- Direct measurement of compartment pressure may be indicated if examination equivocal or if patient unresponsive or unreliable
  - ◆ Performed with specialized instrument (eg, Stryker Intra-Compartmental Pressure Monitor or equivalent)
  - ◆ Surgical intervention generally indicated for:
    - ✳ Value within 30 mm Hg of diastolic blood pressure
      - ▲ Accounts for effects of systemic hypertension or hypotension
    - ✳ Absolute value of 30 to 45 mm Hg
      - ▲ Falling out of favor
        - ❖ May lead to unnecessary fasciotomies
        - ❖ May lead to failure to perform needed fasciotomies
  - ◆ Often technique dependent
    - ✳ Should be performed by experienced provider
- Unequivocal diagnosis of compartment syndrome should prompt emergent decompressive fasciotomy
  - ◆ Increase in time to surgery has been shown to result in worse outcomes.
- **Open fracture or dislocation**
  - Communication of a fracture or joint space with the external environment
    - ◆ Typically graded by Gustilo classification (see Chapter 41)

- All open injuries should receive adequate infection prophylaxis as soon as possible:
  - Coverage for typical skin bacteria (Gram-positive cocci)
    - Usually a first-generation cephalosporin (eg, cefazolin)
  - Add Gram-negative coverage for higher grade injury
    - Often an aminoglycoside (eg, gentamicin)
  - Add high-dose penicillin for soil or barnyard contamination
  - Add fluoroquinolone for fresh water or salt water wounds
  - Antitetanus prophylaxis
- Need for emergent operative intervention often depends on degree of contamination.
  - Risk of infection directly related to adequacy of debridement
  - Injuries with extensive gross contamination often cannot be adequately debrided at the bedside
    - Remove any large, easily visible foreign bodies
    - Irrigate copiously with sterile saline or water
    - Cover with moist sterile dressing until reassessment in the operating room (OR)
- Select open hand fractures may be appropriate for irrigation and debridement in the acute care setting with definitive management as an outpatient
  - Absence of contamination
  - Small wounds
    - <1 cm in size or "poke hole" wound
  - Ability to obtain close outpatient follow-up
- Any open hand fracture generally warrants discussion with hand specialist.
- **Acute compressive neuropathy**
  - Direct or indirect pressure on a nerve as a result of acute trauma
    - Causes local nerve ischemia with resulting paresthesias, pain, and weakness
    - Risk of long-term or permanent deficits if neglected
  - Acute carpal tunnel syndrome
    - Acute compression of the median nerve as it traverses the carpal tunnel at the wrist
    - Presentation
      - Numbness and tingling in thumb, index, long, and radial half of ring fingers
      - Rapidly progressive pain and paresthesias in the median nerve distribution
        - Symptom onset occurs over a period of hours/days versus weeks/months with chronic carpal tunnel syndrome

- ◆ Causes:
  - ✳ Hand/wrist fractures or dislocations
    - ▲ Lunate or perilunate dislocations (see Chapter 15)
      - ◈ Lunate may dislocate into carpal tunnel and compress median nerve
    - ▲ Distal radius fractures (see Chapter 26)
  - ✳ Postoperative
    - ▲ Most commonly after fixation of distal radius fractures
  - ✳ Hemorrhage into the carpal tunnel secondary to:
    - ▲ Trauma
    - ▲ Coagulopathy
- ● First-line treatment
  - ◆ If secondary to fracture/dislocation:
    - ✳ Reduce as soon as possible
    - ✳ Should be performed by an experienced provider
      - ▲ Reduction of lunate/perilunate dislocations often challenging
  - ◆ Neurologic symptoms generally improve with successful reduction.
- ● Emergent carpal tunnel release or open fracture reduction may be indicated with:
  - ◆ Failure of closed reduction
  - ◆ Worsening of median nerve symptoms despite reduction
  - ◆ Progressive symptoms in the absence of fracture or dislocation
- ■ **Traumatic amputation** (see Chapter 53)
  - ● Mechanisms
    - ◆ Sharp transection
      - ✳ Most favorable replant profile
    - ◆ Blunt transection
    - ◆ Avulsion (eg, ring avulsion)
    - ◆ Crush
      - ✳ Least favorable replant profile
  - ● Preserve any potentially salvageable amputated tissue
    - ◆ Two primary methods:
      - ✳ Wrap in gauze moistened with sterile saline or Ringer lactate and place on ice
      - ✳ Immerse in sterile saline or Ringer lactate in a plastic bag and submerge bag in ice
  - ● Key question guiding treatment—Is replant indicated?
    - ◆ Complex and multifactorial decision
    - ◆ Replants performed by specialized team at limited number of facilities

- Time-sensitive
- Early assessment by hand surgeon recommended to help guide treatment
- Relative indications for replant:
  - Thumb amputation at any level
  - Multiple amputated digits
  - Partial hand amputation (through palm)
  - Amputation at wrist or forearm level
  - Amputation of individual digit distal to flexor digitorum superficialis insertion
  - Almost any amputated part in a child
- Unfavorable factors
  - Crush or mangling injury
  - Amputation at multiple levels (segmental amputation)
  - Presence of serious medical comorbidities
  - Vascular disease
  - Amputation of individual digit in an adult proximal to flexor digitorum superficialis insertion
  - Prolonged warm ischemia time
  - Severe tissue contamination
- Permissible ischemia time for replant:
  - Proximal to carpus:
    * Warm ischemia time <6 hours
    * Cold ischemia time <12 hours
  - Distal to carpus (eg, digital amputation)
    * Warm ischemia time <12 hours
    * Cold ischemia time <24 hours
- If replantation feasible, prepare patient for operating room or make arrangements for emergent transfer to replant center

- **Infection**
  - General principles
    - Multiple closed spaces and compartments exist in the hand
      * Ideal environment for abscess formation
      * Prevents systemic antibiotics from reaching target
  - Incision and drainage (I&D) generally indicated for abscess formation or deep space infection
    - Most superficial I&D procedures can be performed in the acute care setting
    - Drainage of the deeper spaces in the hand generally performed in the OR

- Management based on type of infection:
  - ◆ Felon (see Chapter 42)
    - ∗ Subcutaneous abscess of the pulp of distal finger or thumb
      - ▲ Pulp composed of multiple small compartments formed by vertical septa
    - ∗ Usually secondary to penetrating injury
      - ▲ May spread contiguously from paronychia
    - ∗ If fluctuance present:
      - ▲ I&D in ED
    - ∗ Can rarely cause secondary infectious flexor tenosynovitis because of proximal extension
  - ◆ Paronychia (see Chapter 43)
    - ∗ Soft tissue infection of proximal or lateral nail fold
      - ▲ Most common infection in the hand
    - ∗ If no fluctuance:
      - ▲ Warm soaks
      - ▲ Oral antibiotics
    - ∗ If fluctuance present:
      - ▲ I&D in ED
      - ▲ Nail removal only indicated if free floating
        - ❖ Indicates tracking of infection under nail
  - ◆ Pyogenic flexor tenosynovitis (see Chapter 44)
    - ∗ Purulent infection within the flexor tendon sheath
      - ▲ Rapid adhesion formation causes severe loss of motion
      - ▲ Destruction of vascular supply results in tendon necrosis
    - ∗ Usually secondary to penetrating injury or hematogenous origin
    - ∗ Kanavel signs of pyogenic flexor tenosynovitis:
      - ▲ Finger held in flexed position
      - ▲ Symmetric enlargement of whole finger (fusiform swelling)
      - ▲ Tenderness to palpation over flexor tendon sheath
      - ▲ Severe pain with passive extension of finger
        - ❖ Often earliest sign
    - ∗ Early discussion with hand specialist recommended
    - ∗ Operative versus nonoperative management
      - ▲ Within 24 hours of onset:
        - ❖ Can consider nonoperative treatment with high-dose intravenous (IV) antibiotics
        - ❖ Immobilization in compressive dressing
        - ❖ Elevation

- ❖ Close observation
- ❖ Low threshold for operative I&D
- ▲ If failure of nonoperative management or >24 hours from onset of symptoms:
  - ❖ Immediate surgical drainage of tendon sheath
- ❖ Septic arthritis (see Chapter 45)
  - ✳ Infection of joint space
    - ▲ Generally secondary to penetrating trauma in the hand
      - ❖ Wound from tooth (fight bite)
      - ❖ MCP joints most commonly involved
    - ▲ Can arise from extension of adjacent soft tissue or bone infection
  - ✳ Presentation of affected joint:
    - ▲ Warmth
    - ▲ Swelling
    - ▲ Tenderness to palpation
    - ▲ Often markedly restricted and painful passive motion
  - ✳ Joint aspiration
    - ▲ Gold standard for diagnosis
    - ▲ Send for culture, Gram stain, cell count, crystal analysis
    - ▲ Criteria for joint sepsis (lower counts may still indicate infection):
      - ❖ White blood cell count >50 000/μL
      - ❖ >50% polymorphonuclear leukocytes
  - ✳ Treatment
    - ▲ Emergent surgical irrigation and debridement in the OR
      - ❖ Can result in irreversible cartilage damage within hours if missed
      - ❖ Better outcomes with earlier operative treatment
    - ▲ Antibiotic therapy
- ❖ Web space and palmar space infections
  - ✳ Web space infection (see Chapter 46)
    - ▲ Also referred to as "collar button" abscess
      - ❖ Related to hourglass configuration with both dorsal and volar components
    - ▲ Presentation
      - ❖ Pain, swelling, and fluctuance in web space
    - ▲ Treatment
      - ❖ I&D
      - ❖ Frequently requires both volar and dorsal incisions
      - ❖ Avoid transverse incision to prevent web space contracture

* Palmar space infection (see Chapter 47)
  ▲ Three potential spaces
    ❖ Thenar space
      ○ Most commonly involved
    ❖ Mid-palmar space
    ❖ Hypothenar space
      ○ Very rarely involved
  ▲ Presentation
    ❖ Pain, swelling, fluctuance over affected space
    ❖ Loss of normal palmar concavity often seen in mid-palmar and thenar space infection
  ▲ Treatment
    ❖ Generally requires open surgical drainage
      ○ More extensive dissection required to access deep spaces of the hand
◆ Bite wounds (see Chapter 49)
  * Human bites
    ▲ Often over MCP joint (fight bite)
      ❖ May communicate with joint
      ❖ Associated with extensor tendon laceration
        ○ Assess for integrity during initial examination
      ❖ Wound frequently appears innocuous on acute presentation
    ▲ Presentation
      ❖ Progressive pain
      ❖ Swelling
      ❖ Erythema
      ❖ Drainage from wound
      ❖ Pain with passive range of motion of involved joint
    ▲ Treatment
      ❖ If joint or tendon sheath involvement:
        ○ Emergent surgical irrigation and debridement
        ○ High risk of progression to septic arthritis or pyogenic flexor tenosynovitis without adequate I&D
      ❖ No joint or tendon involvement
        ○ IV antibiotics
        ○ Close observation
        ○ Consider delayed wound closure
    ▲ Typically a polymicrobial infection
      ❖ Alpha-hemolytic streptococcus (*Streptococcus viridans*)
      ❖ *Staphylococcus aureus*

- *Eikenella corrodens*
- Additional Gram-negative organisms
* Animal bites
  - Incidence
    - Dog bites (90%)
      - Associated with greater soft tissue injury compared to other bites
    - Cat bites (~10%)
      - Small, sharp teeth penetrate bones and joints
      - Higher likelihood of septic arthritis and osteomyelitis compared to dog bite
  - Secondary bacterial infection common
    - Generally polymicrobial
    - Most commonly isolated organisms:
      - *Pasteurella* species (in both dogs and cats)
  - Delayed care and undertreatment common
* Indications for delayed closure:
  - Deep punctures
  - Bites to the hand
  - Extensive crush injury
  - Wounds more than 6 hours old
* Operative indications:
  - Crush injury or devitalized tissue
  - Retained foreign body (eg, tooth fragment)
    - Always obtain radiographs of the injured area
  - Bite to digital pulp space, nail bed, flexor tendon sheath, deep spaces of the palm, or joint penetration
  - Tenosynovitis
  - Septic arthritis
  - Abscess formation
- Osteomyelitis (see Chapter 50)
  * Infection and inflammation of bone
  * Mechanism
    - Hematogenous seeding
    - Contiguous focus
      - Because of trauma with contaminated wounds
    - Direct inoculation into bone (penetrating injury)
  * Diagnosis based on:
    - Imaging

- ❖ Radiographs
- ❖ Computed tomography (best for evaluating bony anatomy)
- ❖ Magnetic resonance imaging (best for evaluation of soft tissues)
  - ▲ Labs
    - ❖ C-reactive protein
    - ❖ Erythrocyte sedimentation rate
    - ❖ Leukocyte count
  - ▲ Gold standard is bone biopsy and culture
- ✳ Initial management generally consists of targeted IV antibiotic therapy for 4 to 6 weeks
- ✳ Indications for operative intervention (rarely emergent):
  - ▲ Abscess formation
  - ▲ Draining sinus
- ■ **High-pressure injection injury** (see Chapter 56)
  - ● Injection of foreign substance under high pressure into the soft tissues
  - ● Entry wound often small, benign in appearance
  - ● Severity of injury dependent on:
    - ❖ Time from injury to treatment
    - ❖ Force of injection
    - ❖ Volume injected
    - ❖ Outcomes related to composition of material injected
      - ✳ Better prognosis
        - ▲ Grease
        - ▲ Chlorofluorocarbons (eg, Freon)
        - ▲ Latex and water-based paints
      - ✳ Worse prognosis
        - ▲ Industrial solvents (eg, paint thinner)
        - ▲ Diesel or jet fuel
        - ▲ Oil-based paints
  - ● Early consultation with hand specialist strongly recommended
  - ● Treatment
    - ❖ Operative
      - ✳ Almost always indicated
      - ✳ Emergent irrigation and debridement followed by broad spectrum IV antibiotics
      - ✳ Higher rates of amputation with greater delay in treatment
        - ▲ Even with appropriate treatment amputation, rates can approach 50%

- ◆ Nonoperative
  - ✳ Generally only appropriate for injection of air or water
  - ✳ IV antibiotics
  - ✳ Elevate extremity
  - ✳ Observe closely for compartment syndrome
- ■ **Vascular injury**
  - ● Findings suggestive of possible arterial injury:
    - ◆ Decreased or absent distal pulse
    - ◆ History of persistent arterial bleeding (bright red, pulsatile)
    - ◆ Large or expanding hematoma
    - ◆ Major hemorrhage with hypotension
    - ◆ Injury to an anatomically related nerve
    - ◆ Anatomic proximity of wound to major artery
  - ● If physical examination is inconclusive and suspicion for arterial injury remains high, consider angiography in the acute setting.
  - ● Methods of hemorrhage control:
    - ◆ Direct manual digital compression
      - ✳ Safe and effective
      - ✳ Apply direct pressure over bleeding artery
      - ✳ Can require up to 15 minutes of uninterrupted pressure for clot formation
    - ◆ Temporary tourniquet application and wound closure
      - ✳ Usually requires pressures of approximately 250 mm Hg in adults and 100 to 200 mm Hg in children
      - ✳ Can use blood pressure cuff if tourniquet not available
      - ✳ Inflate tourniquet, irrigate, debride, close with nonabsorbable suture
      - ✳ Apply overlying compact compressive dressing
      - ✳ Hemostasis attained via tissue tamponade
    - ◆ Avoid blind clamping and ligation in the emergent care setting
      - ✳ High probability of iatrogenic nerve injury because of close anatomic relationship with vascular structures
      - ✳ Should only be performed in the OR with adequate exposure
  - ● Nonoperative management
    - ◆ Isolated radial or ulnar artery laceration with intact palmar arch circulation
      - ✳ In well-perfused nonischemic hand, one intact artery is often sufficient to maintain viability
        - ▲ Because of abundant collateral anastomoses in the hand
      - ✳ Must be able to obtain adequate hemostasis

- Indications for emergent operative intervention:
  - ◆ Failure to obtain hemostasis with conservative methods or progressive hemodynamic instability despite resuscitation
  - ◆ Injury to both radial and ulnar arteries
  - ◆ Presence of critical ischemia with any arterial injury
- Consultation with hand specialist is recommended to aid in decisions regarding need for emergent treatment.

SUGGESTED READINGS

Gillig JD, White SD, Rachel JN. Acute carpal tunnel syndrome: a review of current literature. *Orthop Clin North Am.* 2016;47(3):599-607.

Higgins JP. Replantation and transplantation. In: Wolfe SW, Hotchkiss RN, Pederson WC, Kozin SH, Cohen MS, eds. *Green's Operative Hand Surgery*. Philadelphia, PA: Elsevier; 2017.

Leversedge FJ, Moore TJ, Peterson BC, Seiler JG. Compartment syndrome of the upper extremity. *J Hand Surg Am.* 2011;36(3):544-559.

Osterman M, Draeger R, Stern P. Acute hand infections. *J Hand Surg Am.* 2014;39(8):1628-1635.

Rosenwasser MP, Wei DH. High-pressure injection injuries to the hand. *J Am Acad Orthop Surg.* 2014;22(1):38-45.

Thai JN, Pacheco JA, Margolis DS, et al. Evidence-based comprehensive approach to forearm arterial laceration. *West J Emerg Med.* 2015;16(7):1127-1134.

Tulipan JE, Ilyas AM. Open fractures of the hand: review of pathogenesis and introduction of a new classification system. *Orthop Clin North Am.* 2016;47(1):245-251.

SECTION 2
Bone and Joint Injuries

Section Editor: Christopher Got

CHAPTER

5   Phalanx Fractures

Joseph A. Rosenbaum and Hisham M. Awan

INTRODUCTION

- Pathoanatomy
  - Fractures of the bones of the fingers typically secondary to trauma
  - Force applied to the affected bone exceeds its strength.
- Mechanism of injury
  - Mechanisms of injury include crush; torsional, angular, and axial load; and traction.
  - High-energy mechanisms typically cause comminution.
  - Fracture may be part of a more severe overall injury pattern, including soft tissue injury to ligament, joint capsule, tendon, nerve, and/or vessels.
- Epidemiology
  - Fractures of phalanges and metacarpals are among the most common fractures.
  - Account for approximately 10% of all fractures
  - Common in laborers and athletes
  - Males are affected more than females.

EVALUATION

- History
  - Typically caused by trauma, either direct or indirect
  - Rarely can be pathologic fractures with minimal or no antecedent trauma

- Presentation may be delayed—Patients may dismiss as a "jammed finger" or sprain.
- Often overlooked initially in polytrauma cases
■ Physical examination
  - Assess for edema, angular deformity, rotational deformity, and quality of soft tissues.
  - Assess sensation and capillary refill distally.
  - Assess the other digits as well as the hand and wrist.
  - Test for tendon function individually for each finger (flexor digitorum superficialis, flexor digitorum profundus, extensor digitorum communis).
■ Imaging
  - Obtain finger radiograph initially if fracture is suspected.
  - Proximal, middle, distal phalanx (P1, P2, P3)
  - Open versus closed (Nail bed injury with concomitant P3 fracture is considered an open fracture.)
  - Intra-articular versus extra-articular
  - Stable versus unstable fracture pattern
    ◆ Comminuted versus simple (Simple are generally more stable.)
    ◆ Transverse versus oblique (Transverse are more length-stable.)
  - Angulation (P1 tends to be apex volar, P2 apex dorsal.)
  - Translation
  - Presence or absence of foreign bodies
■ Classification
  - Proximal phalanx
    ◆ Articular fractures
    ◆ Pilon fractures
    ◆ Phalangeal shaft
    ◆ Phalangeal neck
    ◆ Unicondylar fractures
    ◆ Bicondylar fractures
  - Middle phalanx fractures
  - Distal phalanx fractures

ACUTE MANAGEMENT

■ Emergency room management
  - Assess for other injuries.
  - Comfort measures—pain control, elevation, and splinting (Remove splints for radiograph.)

- Remove patient's gloves, rings, and jewelry.
- Elevate, apply ice.
- Radiographs (Order finger radiograph; order hand radiograph if additional injuries are suspected.)

DEFINITIVE TREATMENT

- Principles
  - Proximal interphalangeal (PIP) stiffness is a major concern; early mobilization is beneficial.
  - Extensor mechanism is intimately attached to proximal phalanx, which can lead to adhesions and stiffness with internal fixation.
  - Transverse fractures tend to angulate, whereas long oblique or spiral fractures tend to lead to malrotation.
  - Proximal phalangeal fractures tend to displace with apex volar because of the interossei pulling the proximal fragment into flexion and the central slip pulling the distal fragment into extension.
  - Fracture geometry and stability are often used to help determine stability.
  - Immobilization is generally brief (less than 3 weeks) before transition to buddy taping and restarting range of motion (ROM).
- Proximal phalanx fractures
  - Nonoperative treatment
    - Nondisplaced fractures
    - Closed, displaced, reducible nonarticular fractures that are stable after reduction
      - Reduce with metacarpophalangeal (MCP) joints flexed 70° to 90° and cast with forearm-based dorsal blocking splint with MCP in flexion and interphalangeal joints in full extension.
      - Acceptable reduction features
        - Greater than 50% cortical apposition
        - No malrotation
        - Less than 15° of angulation in any plane
        - Less than 4 mm shortening
        - Full ROM following reduction
  - Surgical indications
    - Open fractures
    - Irreducible or unacceptably reduced fractures

- Unstable fractures
  - Unicondylar fractures or bicondylar fractures
  - Phalangeal neck fractures
  - Long oblique or spiral fractures
- Multiple fractures
- Associated tendon, skin, or soft tissue injuries (relative indication)
- Surgical approach
  - Goal is to allow ROM as early as possible while maintaining reduction.
  - K-wire fixation has the benefit of minimal invasiveness, with least disturbance of extensor mechanism, and therefore, there is theoretical decrease in risk of adhesions.
    - However, fixation is not as robust as with screws/plates.
    - Transmetacarpal pinning—Pin is introduced anterograde through the metacarpal head and the flexed MCP joint.
      - ▲ Applications—phalangeal base, shaft, neck fractures
      - ▲ Keep the pin out of the PIP joint to allow ROM.
    - Intramedullary pinning
    - Crossed pinning
  - Intraosseous wiring
    - Easily available
    - Inexpensive
    - Technically difficult
    - Relatively weak construct
    - Best used in transverse shaft fractures
  - Lag screw fixation
    - Works well in long oblique/spiral fracture patterns
    - Be sure to follow the spiral nature of the fracture—Screws are usually not all inserted in the same plane because they follow the fracture spiral.
  - Plate fixation
    - Rigid fixation
    - Works well for periarticular fractures or those that require bone grafting, or feature comminution
    - However, risk of adhesions and stiffness is increased as there is more required surgical exposure.
    - Soft tissue complications are common.
  - External fixation
    - For open/contaminated/comminuted fractures
    - Associated soft tissue injuries

- Arthroplasty
  - Hemiarthroplasty occasionally indicated for proximal phalangeal base fractures that are not amenable to open reduction internal fixation (ORIF)
- Potential complications
  - Stiffness
  - Infection
  - Painful hardware
  - Malunion
- Specific fracture patterns
  - Phalangeal neck fractures
    - More common in pediatric patients
    - If partially displaced, reduced and closed reduction percutaneous pinning (CRPP)
    - If completely displaced, at risk for avascular necrosis (AVN)
      - ORIF is recommended in these cases, although it does not completely eliminate risk of AVN.
  - Unicondylar fractures
    - Weiss and Hastings classification
      - Type 1—oblique volar
      - Type 2—long sagittal
      - Type 3—dorsal coronal
      - Type 4—volar coronal
  - Highly unstable
    - If nondisplaced, CRPP is recommended.
    - If displaced, CRPP versus ORIF
  - Bicondylar fractures
    - Universally treated operatively
    - Very unstable
    - ORIF indicated, often with dual mini condylar plates
- Middle phalanx fractures
  - For fracture-dislocations (see Chapter 6)
  - Nonoperative treatment
    - Goal of treatment is union without stiffness.
    - Nondisplaced fractures—immobilize for 2 to 3 weeks and monitor with serial radiographs, then transition to buddy taping.
    - Reduction or alignment is acceptable if
      - Less than 10° angulation
      - No malrotation
      - No shortening

- Surgical techniques
  - CRPP versus ORIF
  - Both can lead to stiffness (up to 50% of cases).
  - Fracture geometry and surgeon experience should guide decision on how to proceed operatively.
- Distal phalanx fractures
  - For mallet and jersey finger (see Chapters 7 and 35) respectively.
  - Nonoperative treatment
    - Nondisplaced tuft or shaft fractures
    - If no nail bed injury is present
  - Surgical indications
    - Nail bed injury should be suspected with any displaced tuft fracture or nail avulsion injury.
      - Must be explored by removing the nail under digital block
      - Repair nail bed with 6-0 chromic gut suture.
      - If there are any associated soft tissue injuries (pulp laceration), stabilize it first to allow for easier nail bed repair.
        - Use absorbable suture in children.
      - Replace the nail beneath the eponychial fold if it is available (remove soft tissue from the underside first); if it is unusable, use the foil from suture pack.
      - May stabilize with a single suture through the nail or foil.
      - Eponychial fold should be splinted open for a minimum of 5 to 7 days to allow for new nail growth.
      - Twin "cutback" incisions may be created in the eponychium if more proximal visualization of the germinal matrix is needed.
    - Seymour fractures
      - Pediatric physeal injury with the distal fragment displacing dorsally
      - Nail has appearance of being longer than normal (Figure 5.1).
      - May be overlooked; can lead to osteomyelitis if untreated
      - Administer IV antibiotics, remove nail, perform eponychial cutbacks, irrigate fracture site, reduce, repair any nail bed lacerations, splint eponychial fold open (Figure 5.2A-D)
      - Immobilize with a forearm-based splint or if necessary a cast to keep child from removing dressings.
    - Displaced distal phalanx shaft fractures
      - May be treated with CRPP if unstable pattern

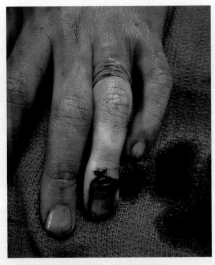

FIGURE 5.1 The "too long" appearance of the nail in a Seymour fracture upon presentation.

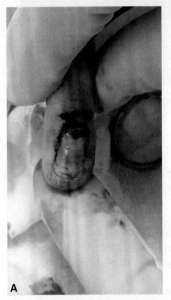
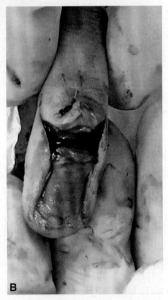

FIGURE 5.2 A-D, Nail removed (A); eponychial cutbacks performed and stabilized with a stay suture, fracture site visualized (B).

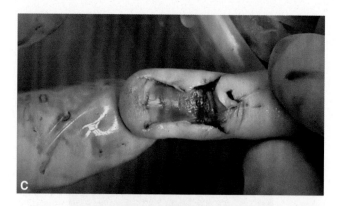

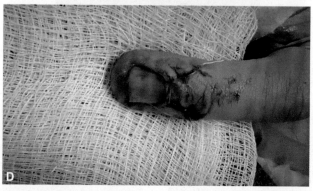

FIGURE 5.2 (*continued*) Nail bed repaired (C); and nail plate replaced to splint open eponychial fold (D).

SUGGESTED READINGS

Baltera RM, Hastings H II. Fractures and dislocations: hand. In: Hammert WC, ed. *ASSH Manual of Hand Surgery*. Philadelphia, PA: Lippincott Williams & Wilkins; 2010:93–110.

Day CS, Stern PJ. Fractures of the metacarpals and phalanges. In: Wolfe SW, Hotchkiss RN, Pederson WC, Kozin SH, eds. *Green's Operative Hand Surgery*. 6th ed. Philadelphia, PA: Churchill Livingstone; 2010.

Dean BJF, Little C. Fractures of the metacarpals and phalanges. *Orthop Trauma*. 2011;23:43–56.

Meals C, Meals M. Hand fractures: a review of current treatment strategies. *J Hand Surg Am*. 2013;38(5):1021–1031.

6   Phalanx Dislocations

Joseph A. Rosenbaum and Hisham M. Awan

INTRODUCTION

- Pathoanatomy
  - Dislocations of the finger joints secondary to trauma
  - Force applied to the joint exceeds the strength of its capsuloligamentous support.
- Mechanism of injury
  - Mechanisms of injury include torsional, angular, and tractional forces across joint.
  - Dislocation may be part of a more severe overall injury pattern including soft tissue injury to ligament, tendon, nerve, and/or vessels.
- Epidemiology/background
  - Dislocations of proximal interphalangeal (PIP) joints are more common than those of distal interphalangeal (DIP) dislocations.
  - PIP injuries are crucial to treat promptly and properly as the PIP joint is highly prone to stiffness once injured.
  - Common in laborers and athletes
  - Males > females

EVALUATION

- History
  - Typically caused by trauma, either direct or indirect
  - Presentation is often acute due to deformity and pain, but may be delayed—patients may initially dismiss injury.
  - May be overlooked initially in polytrauma cases.
- Physical examination
  - Assess for edema, angular deformity, rotational deformity, quality of soft tissues.

- Identify any lacerations, rule out open dislocation.
- Assess sensation and capillary refill distally.
- Assess the other digits as well as the hand and wrist.
- Test for tendon function individually for each finger (flexor digitorum superficialis [FDS], flexor digitorum profundus, extensor digitorum communis).
- Imaging/assessment
  - Obtain finger radiograph initially if PIP joint or DIP joint dislocation is suspected.
  - Identify any fractures if present.
- Classification
  - As with other dislocations, the nomenclature of direction of dislocation is based on which way the distal bone dislocates relative to the proximal bone.
  - PIP dislocations
    - Volar dislocations—the middle phalanx (P2) is dislocated volarly relative to the proximal phalanx (P1).
      * Relatively rare injuries
    - Lateral dislocations
    - Dorsal dislocations—P2 is dislocated dorsally relative to P1.
      * More common than volar
    - Volar fracture-dislocation
    - Dorsal fracture-dislocation
  - DIP dislocations
    - Dorsal dislocations, lateral dislocations
    - Analogous to thumb interphalangeal (IP) joint in anatomical terms

ACUTE MANAGEMENT

- Emergency room management
  - Assess for other injuries.
  - Comfort measures—pain control, elevation, splinting (remove splints for radiograph)
  - Remove patient's gloves, rings, and jewelry.
  - Elevation, ice
  - Radiographs (order finger radiograph; order hand radiograph if additional injuries suspected)
  - Representative image(s)

TREATMENT

- PIP joint dorsal simple dislocations
  - Volar plate may be avulsed, usually from distal insertion.
  - Nonoperative treatment
    - Acute injuries can generally be treated nonsurgically.
    - Reduction maneuver—hyperextension, axial traction, and flexion
    - Volar plate does not typically get entrapped.
    - Ensure concentric reduction on perfect lateral postreduction radiograph.
    - Place into extension-blocking splint in slight flexion for 1 to 2 weeks.
    - Transition to buddy taping and range of motion (ROM) exercises thereafter.
  - Surgical indications
    - Chronic injuries—may present with swan neck deformity or PIP hyperextension
      - Options
        - ▲ Volar plate repair
        - ▲ FDS tenodesis
  - Potential complications
    - Stiffness (especially with immobilization >3 weeks)
    - Chronic pain
    - Posttraumatic osteoarthritis
  - Postoperative care
- PIP joint volar simple dislocations
  - Aka "acute Boutonniere injury"
  - Nonoperative treatment
    - Typically closed management is possible if there is no rotatory component to the dislocation.
      - If rotatory component exists, condyle may buttonhole through the extensor mechanism; attempts at closed reduction will only further tighten and/or entrap soft tissues (commonly lateral band), necessitating open reduction.
    - If no rotational component, closed reduction under digital block via gentle traction with metacarpophalangeal and PIP joints flexed to allow the lateral bands to migrate palmarly.
    - Wrist may be extended slightly to relax the extensor mechanism and facilitate reduction.
    - Check active PIP motion following reduction

- * If patient cannot achieve terminal extension, splint in PIP extension for 6 weeks to treat central slip injury.
  - ◆ Postreduction radiograph of the finger including a perfect lateral to ensure concentric reduction
- Surgical indications
  - ◆ Irreducible by closed means
  - ◆ Rotatory pattern
  - ◆ Open injury
  - ◆ Puckering of skin upon presentation (a sign of interposed soft tissue)
  - ◆ Chronic injuries with Boutonniere deformity
- Surgical approach
  - ◆ Dorsal approach
  - ◆ Identify central slip, which is typically injured
    - * Repair if needed
  - ◆ Identify lateral band, which may be interposed in PIP joint
    - * Repair if needed, excise if irreparable
  - ◆ Reduce, confirm concentric with fluoroscopy
  - ◆ Splint in extension to protect extensor mechanism
- Potential complications
  - ◆ Stiffness
- Postoperative care
  - ◆ If central slip is repaired, zone III extensor tendon protocol is applied.
- Outcomes
  - ◆ Some extensor lag is expected, up to 10° can still be considered a good outcome.
  - ◆ Stiffness of the PIP joint is common.
- ■ PIP joint lateral dislocations
  - ◆ Rare injuries
  - Nonoperative treatment
    - ◆ Closed reduction under digital block
    - ◆ Buddy taping following reduction if stable
  - Surgical indications
    - ◆ Irreducible
    - ◆ Nonconcentric closed reduction
    - ◆ Elite athletes, radial collateral of index finger (for pinch, relative indication)
  - Surgical approach
    - ◆ Lateral approach
    - ◆ Repair collateral ligament to restore stability

- Potential complications
  - Stiffness
- PIP joint dorsal fracture-dislocations
  - Important to consider size of the fragment, comminution, and stability of the reduction (how much flexion is required to maintain reduction).
    - <30% of articular surface is generally stable
    - 30% to 50% is "tenuous"
    - >50% is unstable
  - Nonoperative treatment
    - Smaller fragments with concentric closed reduction "stable" injuries
    - If the joint remains reduced requiring less than 30° of flexion, it is considered stable.
    - If less than 20% of the middle phalanx base is fractured, it can be stable.
    - Splint in slight flexion for no more than 3 weeks, then begin active ROM
  - Surgical indications
    - "Unstable" injuries—based on clinical and radiographic assessment
    - Articular fragments >30% of the surface are generally tenuous, >50% are grossly unstable (Kiefhaber modification of Hastings classification).
    - Nonconcentric closed reduction—dorsal subluxation results in the dorsal "V sign."
  - Surgical approach
    - Options
      * Extension block pinning
      * Joint transfixion with K-wires
      * Open reduction with internal fixation (ORIF) with screw or tension band construct
        ▲ Allows early ROM.
      * Dynamic external fixation for comminuted fractures
        ▲ Allows for ROM during healing.
      * Volar plate arthroplasty
        ▲ Useful when less than 50% to 60% of articular surface involved
        ▲ May be augmented with bone graft
        ▲ PIP joint flexion contractures are common.
      * Hemi-hamate arthroplasty
        ▲ Useful for dorsal fracture-dislocations involving >50% of articular surface or chronic injuries
        ▲ Recreate volar buttress providing stability

- Potential complications
  - ◆ Avoid prominent hardware palmarly into flexor sheath
  - ◆ Stiffness seen with prolonged immobilization
- ■ PIP joint volar fracture-dislocations
  - ◆ Treatment is dictated by size and displacement of the fragment.
  - Nonoperative treatment
    - ◆ Dorsal fragments <20% of articular surface and <2 mm displacement are treated with closed reduction and splinting similar to pure dislocations.
  - Surgical treatment
    - ◆ Indications
      - ∗ Fragment >20%
      - ∗ Displacement >2 mm
      - ∗ Unstable reduction
    - ◆ Options
      - ∗ ORIF with screw fixation
      - ∗ May be augmented with external fixation
      - ∗ Allow early ROM whenever possible
- ■ DIP joint dislocations
  - Rare injuries that can usually be treated nonsurgically
  - Usually dorsal or lateral dislocations
  - Analogous anatomy to thumb IP joint
  - Nonoperative treatment
    - ◆ Closed reduction and splinting
      - ∗ Reduction maneuver
        - ▲ Longitudinal traction
        - ▲ Dorsal pressure on the distal phalanx base
        - ▲ Manipulation into reduced position
      - ∗ Typically stable following reduction
      - ∗ Evaluate postreduction radiograph
      - ∗ Immobilize in slight flexion for 2 to 3 weeks with dorsal blocking splint preventing terminal extension.
  - Surgical treatment
    - ◆ Residual instability
    - ◆ Irreducible (most commonly due to interposed volar plate or flexor tendon)
    - ◆ Large bony fragment from dorsal or volar distal phalanx base
      - ∗ Treat as severe bony mallet or jersey finger, respectively

- Surgical approach
  - Interposed structures may be removed from the joint from a percutaneous approach with a freer elevator.
  - Other option is a volar approach for direct visualization.

SUGGESTED READINGS

Baltera RM, Hastings H II. Fractures and dislocations: hand. In: Hammert WC, ed. *ASSH Manual of Hand Surgery*. Philadelphia, PA: Lippincott Williams & Wilkins; 2010:93-110.

Calfee RP, Sommerkamp TG. Fracture-dislocation about the finger joints. *J Hand Surg Am*. 2009;34(6):1140-1147.

Merrell G, Slade JF. Dislocations and ligament injuries in the digits. In: Wolfe SW, Hotchkiss RN, Pederson WC, Kozin SH, eds. *Green's Operative Hand Surgery*. 6th ed. Philadelphia, PA: Churchill Livingstone; 2010:278-317.

Shah CM, Sommerkamp TG. Fracture dislocation of the finger joints. *J Hand Surg Am*. 2014;39(4):792-802.

7   Mallet Fractures

Andrew D. Sobel

INTRODUCTION

Mallet fractures, or "bony mallets," are common injuries to the fingers. The differentiation from tendinous mallet finger injuries is important to understand so that excellent patient outcomes can result from prompt and effective diagnosis and treatment.

- Pathoanatomy
  - Fracture around the base of the distal phalanx that results in a disruption of the extensor mechanism (Figure 7.1A).
  - Inability to extend at the distal interphalangeal (DIP) joint leads to an extension lag (Figure 7.1B).
  - The lack of force through the terminal slip of the extensor tendon results in overpull through the central slip of the extensor tendon.
  - Chronic pull on the central slip can eventually overpower the flexion forces balancing the proximal interphalangeal (PIP) joint in neutral position, leading to hyperextension at the PIP and a resultant swan-neck deformity.[1]
- Mechanism of injury[2]
  - Begins with axial/compressive force against the distal phalanx
  - The type of mallet fracture depends on the ensuing direction of force.
    - ◆ Forced flexion[3]
      - ∗ Smaller osseous fragment, typically an avulsion at the dorsal aspect of insertion of the terminal slip
    - ◆ Forced hyperextension[4]
      - ∗ Typically results in a larger, intra-articular fragment
- Epidemiology
  - Mallet fracture is less common than tendinous mallet injury in most series.[5,6]
    - ◆ True incidence rates of mallet fracture have not been well defined.
    - ◆ Tendinous mallet finger has an incidence of 9.9/100 000 persons per year.[7]

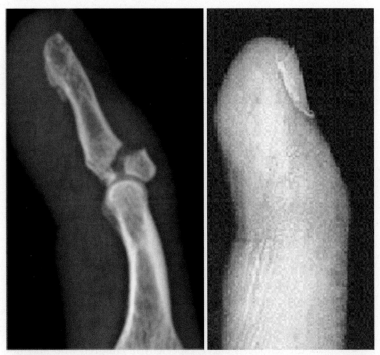

FIGURE 7.1 A, Lateral radiograph of a mallet fracture. From Yoon JO, Baek H, Kim JK. The outcomes of extension block pinning and nonsurgical management for mallet fracture. *J Hand Surg Am.* 2017;42:387.e1-387.e7. B, Clinical appearance of a mallet fracture. Note the extensor lag. From Kalainov DM, Hoepfner PE, Hartigan BJ, Carroll C, Genuario J. Nonsurgical treatment of closed mallet finger fractures. *J Hand Surg Am.* 2005;30:580-586.

- Limited information exists, though the age of patients follows a normal distribution.[5]
- The mechanism of injury is different for different ages of patients.
  - Younger individuals
    - High energy
    - Often sports related (eg, jamming finger on a ball)
  - Older individuals
    - Lower energy
    - Typically occurs from trauma during daily activities or falls
- There may be a suggestion of familial trends with tendinous mallet finger, though this has not been seen with mallet fractures.[8]

- The finger most affected is the middle finger,[5] and injury to the thumb is uncommon.[9]
- The dominant hand is usually affected.[9]

EVALUATION

- History
  - Mechanism
  - Hand dominance
  - Timing of injury. Don't confuse an acute mallet injury with a chronic one!
  - Current functional limitations
  - Occupation
  - Prior injury or surgery to the affected finger
  - If there is a swan-neck deformity, determine that the inciting cause is a mallet injury, not another cause[10] (Table 7.1).
- Physical examination
  - Look for an extension lag at the DIP (Figure 7.1B).
  - Typically, the flexion deformity is passively correctable.
  - Often, there is tenderness over the proximal dorsal distal phalanx.
  - Check the tenodesis effect, especially in children who may not comply with the examination as readily as adults do, to evaluate extension at the DIP.
  - Ensure that there is no subungual hematoma, disruption of the nail plate, or open fracture.
  - Evaluate the PIP and metacarpophalangeal (MCP) joints for evidence of a chronic or alternate problem causing more of a swan-neck deformity.

TABLE 7.1 List of Various Etiologies and Pathophysiologies of Swan-Neck Deformity

Extrinsic	Intrinsic	Articular
Disruption of terminal slip (mallet)	MCP joint volar subluxation	Volar plate attenuation
Flexion contracture of the MCP or wrist	Lateral band translocation/ intrinsic tightness	FDS rupture

Note that flexion of the DIP can be the initial or final step in the development of the swan-neck.

Abbreviations: DIP, distal interphalangeal; FDS, flexor digitorum superficialis; MCP, metacarpophalangeal.

- Imaging
  - Anteroposterior and lateral radiographs should be obtained (Figure 7.1A). A perfect lateral radiograph is very important to determine the true articular involvement, displacement, and subluxation of the fracture (Figure 7.2).[5,11,12]
  - Rule out previous or chronic injury, DIP joint arthritis.
- Classification
  - Doyle (Figure 7.3)[13]
    - Type I—closed tendon injury
    - Type II—open tendon injury
    - Type III—open tendon injury with tissue loss
    - Type IV—mallet fracture
      - Subtype A—transepiphyseal fracture in children
      - Subtype B—fragment size 20% to 50% of the articular surface
      - Subtype C—fragment size >50% of the articular surface
  - Tubiana (Figure 7.4)[14]
    - Type I—tendon rupture (no fracture)
    - Type II—bony avulsion
    - Type III—greater than one-third articular surface with subluxation
    - Type IV—physeal fracture

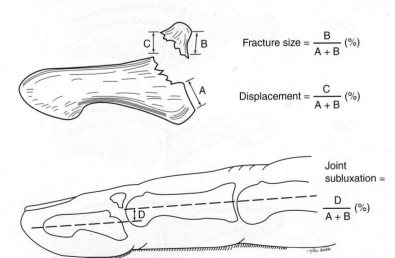

$$\text{Fracture size} = \frac{B}{A + B} \ (\%)$$

$$\text{Displacement} = \frac{C}{A + B} \ (\%)$$

$$\text{Joint subluxation} = \frac{D}{A + B} \ (\%)$$

FIGURE 7.2 Important radiographic parameters to characterize mallet fractures are taken as percentages of the total amount of articular surface. From Bendre AA, Hartigan BJ, Kalainov DM. Mallet finger. *J Am Acad Orthop Surg.* 2005;13:336-344.

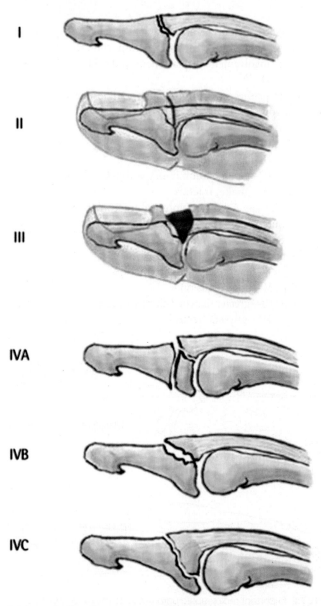

FIGURE 7.3 Doyle classification. From Salazar Botero S, Hidalgo Diaz JJ, Benaïda A, Collon S, Facca S, Liverneaux PA. Review of acute traumatic closed mallet finger injuries in adults. *Arch Plast Surg.* 2016;43:134-144.

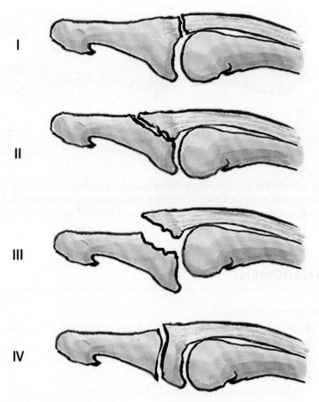

FIGURE 7.4 Tubiana classification. From Salazar Botero S, Hidalgo Diaz JJ, Benaïda A, Collon S, Facca S, Liverneaux PA. Review of acute traumatic closed mallet finger injuries in adults. *Arch Plast Surg.* 2016;43:134-144.

- Wehbé and Schneider (Figure 7.5)[5]
  - Type I—fracture with no volar subluxation of the distal phalanx
  - Type II—fracture with volar subluxation of the distal phalanx
  - Type III—physeal fracture with or without extension into the epiphysis
  - Fracture subtypes
    - A—less than one-third of the articular surface
    - B—one-third to two-thirds of the articular surface
    - C—greater than two-thirds of the articular surface

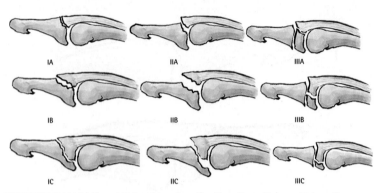

IA   IIA   IIIA

IB   IIB   IIIB

IC   IIC   IIIC

FIGURE 7.5 Webhē and Schneider classification. From Salazar Botero S, Hidalgo Diaz JJ, Benaïda A, Collon S, Facca S, Liverneaux PA. Review of acute traumatic closed mallet finger injuries in adults. *Arch Plast Surg.* 2016;43:134-144.

MANAGEMENT

- Nonoperative treatment
  - There is insufficient evidence to support operative fixation over nonoperative treatment for mallet fractures.[15,16]
  - Splinting the DIP in extension or slight hyperextension is preferred (Figure 7.6).
    - Splint should be maintained at all times for about 6 weeks.
    - Removing the splint at any point during the initial splinting period will "restart the clock" on the 6 weeks.[12]
    - A period of night splinting after the initial splinting period does not change outcomes.[17]
    - Motion at the PIP joint does not result in pulling through the terminal slip of the extensor tendon, and therefore the PIP does not have to be included in the splint.[18]
    - In studies of mallet injuries that included fractures in their cohorts, no difference was found in outcomes after splinting with different types of splints.[19-23]
  - Outcomes of mallet fractures treated with splinting have been good.
    - Many studies only include fractures less than one-third of the joint surface, though those that have included fractures of all sizes and also fractures with volar subluxation have shown good results.[5,24,25]

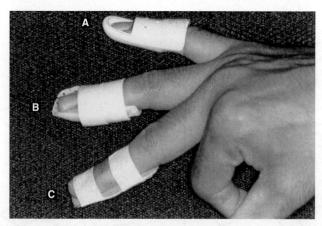

FIGURE 7.6 Extension splinting of a mallet fracture. The DIP is immobilized in extension while the PIP joint is left free. Three commonly used splints are displayed. A, Stack splint. B, Perforated thermoplastic splint. C, Alumafoam splint. DIP, distal interphalangeal; PIP, proximal interphalangeal. From Bendre AA, Hartigan BJ, Kalainov DM. Mallet finger. *J Am Acad Orthop Surg.* 2005;13(5):336-344.

- ◆ More recent data support nonoperative treatment in fractures that are greater than one-third of the joint surface without subluxation.[26]
- ◆ Patients should be counseled about a residual extension lag at the DIP of about 10° and a prominence on the dorsal base of the DIP.
- ◆ Radiographic evidence of arthritis may occur, though clinical outcome commonly does not match the radiographic appearance.[5,24]
- ◆ Outcomes are similar if patients present acutely (<4 weeks) or chronically (>4 weeks) with a mallet fracture.[24,27]
- ■ Surgical indications
  - ● Many have considered that fractures involving greater than one-third of the articular surface or those with volar subluxation should be treated operatively.
  - ● Fractures with increasing articular surface involvement >39% have increasing risks of early and late subluxation.[28]
  - ● A few procedures allow for faster range of motion than does nonoperative treatment, though the overall recovery period is similar.[29-32]

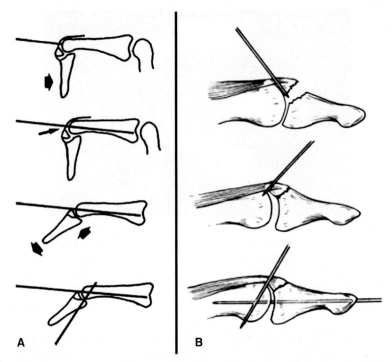

FIGURE 7.7 Extension-block pinning of the mallet fracture aids in the reduction of the fragment, and the transarticular pinning assists in joint stability and preventing volar subluxation during healing. A, Technique by Ishiguro. From Ishiguro T, Itoh Y, Yabe Y, Hashizume N. Extension block with Kirschner wire for fracture dislocation of the distal interphalangeal joint. *Tech Hand Up Extrem Surg.* 1997;1(2):95-102. B, Modified technique. From Bendre AA, Hartigan BJ, Kalainov DM. Mallet finger. *J Am Acad Orthop Surg.* 2005;13(5):336-344.

- Pediatric patients presenting acutely or chronically with dorsal epiphyseal fractures should likely undergo surgery because the outcomes are excellent.[33]
- Surgical approach
  - Transarticular pinning
    - Typically use an 0.045-in pin from the distal tip of the distal phalanx and drive this proximally across the DIP joint.
  - Dorsal blocking pin + transarticular pinning (Figure 7.7)
    - Initial description involves putting the distal phalanx in flexion, driving a pin dorsally through the terminal slip aiming proximally

into the head of the middle phalanx, and then extending the distal phalanx to allow the reduction of the fracture fragment is in contact with the pin.[34]

  ◆ Another option is to place the pin dorsally, just proximal to the fracture, directed distally. Kapandji-style levering of the pin to direct the tip proximally is performed, reducing the fracture fragment distally, and then the pin is driven into the head of the middle phalanx.[35]

- Hook plating[29,36]
- "Umbrella handle"[32] or "fish hook"[31] pinning
- Compression fixation pins[30]
- Open reduction and screw fixation[37]
- Chronic mallet finger with no reparable bone fragment
  ◆ Fowler tenotomy[38]
  ◆ Tenodermodesis[39]
  ◆ Reconstruction of the spiral oblique retinacular ligament[40]
- Arthrodesis can be performed as a salvage option.

■ Potential complications[41,42]
  - Nonoperative
    ◆ Skin irritation from splinting
    ◆ DIP joint stiffness
  - Operative
    ◆ Skin breakdown/necrosis
    ◆ DIP joint stiffness
    ◆ Infection
    ◆ Nail plate deformity
    ◆ Failure of fixation
    ◆ Reoperation

■ Postoperative care
  - With most techniques, patients are placed into a splint and immobilized for 6 weeks to allow for bone-to-bone healing.
  - Some techniques allow for early active range of motion (see Surgical Indications).

SUGGESTED READINGS

Kalainov DM, Hoepfner PE, Hartigan BJ, Carroll C, Genuario J. Nonsurgical treatment of closed mallet finger fractures. *J Hand Surg Am.* 2005;30:580-586.

Salazar Botero S, Hidalgo Diaz JJ, Benaïda A, Collon S, Facca S, Liverneaux PA. Review of acute traumatic closed mallet finger injuries in adults. *Arch Plast Surg.* 2016;43:134-144.

Wehbé MA, Schneider LH. Mallet fractures. *J Bone Joint Surg Am.* 1984;66:658-669.

REFERENCES

1. Stack H. Mallet finger. *Hand.* 1969;1:83-89.
2. Kreuder A, Pennig D, Boese CK, Eysel P, Oppermann J, Dargel J. Mallet finger: a simulation and analysis of hyperflexion versus hyperextension injuries. *Surg Radiol Anat.* 2016;38:403-407.
3. Stark HH, Boyes JH, Wilson JN. Mallet finger. *J Bone Joint Surg Am.* 1962;44–A:1061-1068.
4. Lange RH, Engber WD. Hyperextension mallet finger. *Orthopedics.* 1983;6:1426-1431.
5. Wehbé MA, Schneider LH. Mallet fractures. *J Bone Joint Surg Am.* 1984;66:658-669.
6. Facca S, Nonnenmacher J, Liverneaux P. Treatment of mallet finger with dorsal nail glued splint: retrospective analysis of 270 cases [in French]. *Rev Chir Orthop Reparatrice Appar Mot.* 2007;93:682-689.
7. Clayton RA, Court-Brown CM. The epidemiology of musculoskeletal tendinous and ligamentous injuries. *Injury.* 2008;39:1338-1344.
8. Jones NF, Peterson J. Epidemiologic study of the mallet finger deformity. *J Hand Surg Am.* 1988;13:334-338.
9. Oflazoglu K, Moradi A, Braun Y, Ring D, Chen NC, Eberlin KR. Mallet fractures of the thumb compared with mallet fractures of the fingers. *Hand (N Y).* 2017;12:277-282.
10. Boyer MI, Gelberman RH. Operative correction of swan-neck and boutonniere deformities in the rheumatoid hand. *J Am Acad Orthop Surg.* 1999;7:92-100.
11. Kim JK, Kim DJ. The risk factors associated with subluxation of the distal interphalangeal joint in mallet fracture. *J Hand Surg Eur Vol.* 2015;40:63-67.
12. Bendre AA, Hartigan BJ, Kalainov DM. Mallet finger. *J Am Acad Orthop Surg.* 2005;13:336-344.
13. Doyle JR. Extensor tendons: acute injuries. In: Green DP, Pederson CW, Hotchkiss RN, eds. *Green's Operative Hand Surgery.* 4th ed. New York, NY: Churchill Livingstone; 1999:195-198.
14. Tubiana R. Mallet finger. In: Tubiana R, ed. *Traite de chirurgie de la main.* Paris/New York: Masson; 1986:109-121.
15. Handoll HH, Vaghela MV. Interventions for treating mallet finger injuries. *Cochrane Database Syst Rev.* 2004;CD004574. doi:10.1002/14651858.CD004574.pub2.
16. Geyman JP, Fink K, Sullivan SD. Conservative versus surgical treatment of mallet finger: a pooled quantitative literature evaluation. *J Am Board Fam Pract.* 1998;11(5):382-390.
17. Gruber JS, Bot AG, Ring D. A prospective randomized controlled trial comparing night splinting with no splinting after treatment of mallet finger. *Hand (N Y).* 2014;9:145-150.
18. Katzman BM, Klein DM, Mesa J, Geller J, Caligiuri DA. Immobilization of the mallet finger. Effects on the extensor tendon. *J Hand Surg Br.* 1999;24:80-84.

19. Kinninmonth AW, Holburn F. A comparative controlled trial of a new perforated splint and a traditional splint in the treatment of mallet finger. *J Hand Surg Br.* 1986;11:261-262.

20. Auchincloss JM. Mallet-finger injuries: a prospective, controlled trial of internal and external splintage. *Hand.* 1982;14:168-173.

21. Maitra A, Dorani B. The conservative treatment of mallet finger with a simple splint: a case report. *Arch Emerg Med.* 1993;10:244-248.

22. Richards SD, Kumar G, Booth S, Naqui SZ, Murali SR. A model for the conservative management of mallet finger. *J Hand Surg Br.* 2004;29:61-63.

23. O'Brien LJ, Bailey MJ. Single blind, prospective, randomized controlled trial comparing dorsal aluminum and custom thermoplastic splints to stack splint for acute mallet finger. *Arch Phys Med Rehabil.* 2011;92:191-198.

24. Kalainov DM, Hoepfner PE, Hartigan BJ, Carroll C, Genuario J. Nonsurgical treatment of closed mallet finger fractures. *J Hand Surg Am.* 2005;30:580-586.

25. Okafor B, Mbubaegbu C, Munshi I, Williams DJ. Mallet deformity of the finger. Five-year follow-up of conservative treatment. *J Bone Joint Surg Br.* 1997;79:544-547.

26. Yoon JO, Baek H, Kim JK. The outcomes of extension block pinning and nonsurgical management for mallet fracture. *J Hand Surg Am.* 2017;42:387.e1-387.e7.

27. Garberman SF, Diao E, Peimer CA. Mallet finger: results of early versus delayed closed treatment. *J Hand Surg Am.* 1994;19:850-852.

28. Moradi A, Braun Y, Oflazoglu K, Meijs T, Ring D, Chen N. Factors associated with subluxation in mallet fracture. *J Hand Surg Eur Vol.* 2017;42:176-181.

29. Teoh LC, Lee JY. Mallet fractures: a novel approach to internal fixation using a hook plate. *J Hand Surg Eur Vol.* 2007;32:24-30.

30. Yamanaka K, Sasaki T. Treatment of mallet fractures using compression fixation pins. *J Hand Surg Br.* 1999;24:358-360.

31. Kim DH, Kang HJ, Choi JW. The "Fish Hook" technique for bony mallet finger. *Orthopedics.* 2016;39:295-298.

32. Rocchi L, Genitiempo M, Fanfani F. Percutaneous fixation of mallet fractures by the "umbrella handle" technique. *J Hand Surg Br.* 2006;31:407-412.

33. Reddy M, Ho CA. Comparison of percutaneous reduction and pin fixation in acute and chronic pediatric mallet fractures. *J Pediatr Orthop.* 2016;1.doi:10.1097/BPO.0000000000000896.

34. Ishiguro T, Itoh Y, Yabe Y, Hashizume N. Extension block with Kirschner wire for fracture dislocation of the distal interphalangeal joint. *Tech Hand Up Extrem Surg.* 1997;1:95-102.

35. Tetik C, Gudemez E. Modification of the extension block Kirschner wire technique for mallet fractures. *Clin Orthop Relat Res.* 2002;284-290. http://www.ncbi.nlm.nih.gov/pubmed/12439271. Accessed September 5, 2017.

36. Theivendran K, Mahon A, Rajaratnam V. A novel hook plate fixation technique for the treatment of mallet fractures. *Ann Plast Surg.* 2007;58:112-115.

37. Kronlage S, Faust D. Open reduction and screw fixation of mallet fractures. *J Hand Surg J Br.* 2004;29:135-138.

38. Houpt P, Dijkstra R, Storm van Leeuwen JB. Fowler's tenotomy for mallet deformity. *J Hand Surg Br.* 1993;18:499-500.

39. Iselin F, Levame J, Godoy J. A simplified technique for treating mallet fingers: tenodermodesis. *J Hand Surg Am.* 1977;2:118-121.

40. Thompson JS, Littler JW, Upton J. The spiral oblique retinacular ligament (SORL). *J Hand Surg Am.* 1978;3:482-487.

41. Stern PJ, Kastrup JJ. Complications and prognosis of treatment of mallet finger. *J Hand Surg Am.* 1988;13:329-334.

42. Kang H, Shin SJ, Kang ES. Complications of operative treatment for mallet fractures of the distal phalanx. *J Hand Surg Br.* 2001;26:28-31.

8 Digital Collateral Ligament Injury

Steven T. Lanier and Michael S. Gart

INTRODUCTION

- **Thumb metacarpophalangeal (MP) ulnar collateral ligament (UCL)** (note: thumb radial collateral ligament [RCL] injuries are managed similarly and are far less common, thus they are not discussed separately in this chapter)
  - Mechanism of injury
    - Acute—radial-directed force on abducted thumb, for example, fall with ski pole in hand (Skier's thumb)
    - Chronic—attritional weakening leading to rupture (Gamekeeper's thumb)
  - Normal anatomy
    - Proper collateral ligament (CL)—originates on ulnar aspect of thumb metacarpal (MC) head and inserts onto volar aspect of proximal phalanx
      * Under tension when metacarpophalangeal (MP) joint in 30° of flexion
    - Accessory CL—originates on ulnar aspect of thumb MC head (volar to proper CL) and inserts onto volar plate
      * Under tension when MP in full extension
    - Adductor pollicis (AddP) inserts into thumb MP joint extensor mechanism dorsal (superficial) to the UCL
    - CLs important for MP joint stability—resist valgus stress and volar subluxation of proximal phalanx with respect to MC
      * Tear results in instability, pain, diminished grip and pinch strength, and eventual arthritis
      * Static MP stabilizers—proper and accessory CL, volar plate, dorsal capsule
        ▲ Proper CL and dorsal capsule taught in 30° of flexion
        ▲ Accessory CL and volar plate taught in extension
      * Dynamic stabilizers
        ▲ Thumb extrinsics—extensor pollicis longus (EPL), extensor pollicis brevis (EPB), flexor pollicis longus (FPL)

- ▲ Thumb intrinsics—abductor pollicis longus (APB), flexor pollicis brevis (FPB), AddP
- Pathoanatomy
  - ◆ UCL usually torn from distal insertion onto the proximal phalanx
  - ◆ Stener lesion—distally ruptured UCL retracts proximally and around the AddP insertion onto the extensor mechanism and comes to lie superficial to adductor insertion, making spontaneous healing of the cut ligament ends impossible
- Epidemiology
  - ◆ Incidence is 50 per 100 000
  - ◆ UCL 9× more common than RCL injury
  - ◆ 60% to 90% of complete UCL tears associated with Stener lesion
- Evaluation
  - ◆ History
    - ＊ History of fall onto abducted thumb or other traumatic injury
    - ＊ Acute injuries—pain, swelling, and ecchymosis over ulnar aspect of thumb MP joint
    - ＊ Chronic injuries—instability and resultant weakness of pinch or grip will be more prominent in chronic injuries
  - ◆ Physical examination
    - ＊ Swelling and ecchymosis over ulnar aspect of thumb MP joint
    - ＊ Pain with palpation over site of UCL avulsion, usually at the proximal phalanx insertion
    - ＊ Palpable nodule on ulnar aspect of thumb MC neck/head may represent a Stener lesion
    - ＊ Chronic UCL injuries may present with a supination deformity of the proximal phalanx
    - ＊ Check joint range of motion (ROM)
    - ＊ Obtain imaging before stress testing
      - ▲ Valgus testing contraindicated with thumb MP or proximal phalanx shaft fracture
    - ＊ Valgus stress testing
      - ▲ May require block of joint with local anesthesia to overcome guarding because of pain
      - ▲ Grasp thumb MC neck with one hand and control proximal phalanx rotation with the other hand
      - ▲ Test thumb against valgus stress in both full extension (accessory CL) and in 30° of flexion (proper CL)
      - ▲ Normal valgus laxity—6° in extension and 12° in flexion
      - ▲ Examination findings diagnostic of complete UCL tear:

- No definitive endpoint to mobility under stress
- Greater than 30° of mobility
- Greater than 15° difference in mobility from uninjured side
- If examination is unclear, can perform under fluorography or obtain stress radiographs
  - ▲ Instability in flexion alone—proper collateral ligament tear
  - ▲ Instability in both flexion and extension—proper and accessory collateral ligament tears
- Imaging
  - X-ray (XR) series of thumb
    - ▲ Assess for avulsion fracture at site of UCL insertion onto proximal phalanx, present in 40%
      - Two patterns—avulsion fracture with or without UCL injury
      - If avulsion fracture associated with UCL injury will displace further with valgus stress
    - ▲ Assess for MP joint subluxation with radial and volar translation of the proximal phalanx
    - ▲ Osteoarthritis (OA) may be present in chronic injuries
  - Ultrasound or MRI can diagnose UCL tear and evaluate for Stener lesion if equivocal examination findings
    - ▲ US—sensitivity 76%, specificity 81%, positive predictive value 74%, negative predictive value 87%
    - ▲ MRI—sensitivity and specificity approach 100%
- Classification
  - Grade I—partial UCL tear, no laxity with stress testing
  - Grade II—partial UCL tear, laxity but firm endpoint to stress testing
  - Grade III—complete UCL tear, laxity and no endpoint with stress testing
- Acute management
  - Thumb immobilization with spica splint
  - Nonsteroidal anti-inflammatory drugs for pain relief
- Definitive treatment
  - Nonoperative treatment—Grade I, II, or III without Stener lesion (protocol can be varied by severity of sprain vs partial tear)
    - Weeks 0 to 4—full-time immobilization in thumb spica splint
    - Weeks 4 to 6—therapy working on flexion and extension without valgus stress to joint; immobilization for high-risk activities

* Weeks 6 to 8—begin grip strengthening
* Week 12—return to full activities
- Surgical indications—Grade III with Stener lesion; continued pain and instability following nonoperative management of Grade III injury
  * Contraindications—chronic UCL injuries with thumb MP arthritis are better treated with MP arthrodesis
- Surgical approach
  * Operative technique
    - Regional anesthesia with tourniquet for visualization
    - Mark lazy S incision over dorsoulnar aspect of MP joint
    - Incise skin through dermis with 15 blade
    - Spread longitudinally to identify and protect radial sensory nerve branches, retract radially
    - Identify EPL tendon and the AddP insertion onto extensor mechanism, just ulnar to EPL
      - UCL will be visible superficial to the AddP insertion in cases of a Stenar lesion
    - Incise AddP longitudinally, leaving a 3 mm cuff radially to repair when closing
    - Identify and free UCL from surrounding scar tissue
    - For acute injuries (<6 weeks old) or repairable chronic injuries:
      - Repair proper UCL to its site of insertion using a suture anchor technique
        ○ Insertion site is 3 mm distal to articular surface, 3 mm dorsal to palmar cortex
        ○ Debride insertion site to bleeding bone to aid healing
        ○ If bony avulsion fragment >20% of articular surface repair fragment to bone using K wire
        ○ Thumb held in 15° of flexion and ulnar deviation to tension repair
      - Repair accessory CL with 3-0 nonabsorbable suture
    - For chronic, unrepairable injuries:
      - Resect unrepairable UCL
      - Reconstruct UCL using palmaris longus autograft through drill holes in thumb MP head and base of proximal phalanx
      - Stabilize MP joint with 0.045″ K wire
    - Repair dorsal capsule if torn with 4-0 absorbable suture

▲ Repair AddP insertion with 4-0 absorbable suture
▲ Stress repair in full extension and 30° of flexion
▲ Close skin with interrupted sutures
- Potential complications
  * MP joint stiffness—often improves with motion, not debilitating
  * Radial sensory nerve neuropraxia, laceration, neuroma
  * Recurrent instability
  * Late arthritis
- Postoperative care
  * Thumb spica splint with interphalangeal joint (IP) free for 4 weeks
  * Removable thumb spica splint with protected ROM from 4 to 6 weeks
  * Return to full activities at 12 weeks
- Outcomes
  * Full recovery expected in Grade I and II lesions
  * More than 90% attain good to excellent function after surgical repair of complete tears

■ **Finger proximal interphalangeal (PIP) joint collateral ligaments**
- Mechanism of injury
  - Most common—hyperextension and axial compression of digit
    * Severity ranging from simple sprain to dorsal dislocation or fracture–dislocation of PIP joint
  - Less common—volar dislocation or fracture–dislocation of PIP joint
  - Laterally directed force on border digits—RCL injury of small finger and UCL of index finger
- Normal anatomy
  - PIP joint stabilized by bony configuration of joint and ligamentous "box" spanning from head of proximal phalanx to base of middle phalanx, consisting of the volar plate and proper and accessory collateral ligaments on radial and ulnar aspects of the joint
  - Collateral ligaments primary constraint against radial and ulnar deviation
  - Volar plate resists hyperextension and dorsal dislocation of the PIP joint
  - Checkrein ligaments extend from proximal surface of the volar plate and anchor to the volar surface of the proximal phalanx
- Pathoanatomy
  - Dorsal PIP dislocation ± lateral/rotational forces
    * Avulsion of volar plate from distal insertion onto middle phalanx

* Dorsal dislocation of base of middle phalanx over head of proximal phalanx ± volar lip fracture of base of middle phalanx
* ± Collateral ligament(s) avulsed from proximal origin at head of proximal phalanx because of lateral force component
* Split between proper and accessory collateral ligaments
* Stability of PIP joint after reduction indicates Grade I CL injury
* Lateral PIP dislocation
  * Rupture of one collateral ligament and partial volar plate avulsion from middle phalanx
* Volar PIP dislocation ± lateral/rotational forces
  * Avulsion of volar plate from insertion onto middle phalanx
  * Longitudinal split of the extensor mechanism, separating central slip from ipsilateral lateral band *or* central slip rupture
  * Head of proximal phalanx herniates dorsally through defect and base of middle phalanx dislocates volarly
  * Pure volar dislocation without rotation involves a central slip rupture
  * Collateral ligament(s) avulsed from origin at head of proximal phalanx
  * Stability of PIP joint after reduction indicates Grade I CL injury
* Epidemiology
  * Dorsal dislocation of PIP joint most common
  * Volar dislocation of PIP joint is rare
* Evaluation
  * History
    * History of "jamming finger" with axial and often dorsally directed force
    * History of laterally directed force to finger
    * PIP dislocation
  * Physical examination
    * Swelling, ecchymosis, and tenderness to palpation over area of CL origin or insertion
    * Check joint stability through active range of motion (AROM)—most important determinant of treatment
      * ▲ May require digital block
      * ▲ Note position of redisplacement if occurs
    * Stress testing
      * ▲ Test PIP joint against valgus and varus stress in both full extension (accessory collateral ligaments) and in 30° of flexion (proper collateral ligaments)
      * ▲ Examination findings diagnostic of complete CL tear:

- ❖ No definitive endpoint to mobility under stress
- ❖ Greater than 20° of mobility
- ❖ Greater than 15° difference in mobility from uninjured side
- ❖ Imaging
  - * XR series of finger
    - ▲ Assess for avulsion fracture at site of CL origin and insertion (Figure 8.1)
    - ▲ Evaluate PIP joint for dislocation at baseline and on stress views
    - ▲ After joint reduced findings may be subtle:
      - ❖ Joint space widening on the injured side
      - ❖ Dorsal "V" sign, indicating dorsal subluxation of middle phalanx

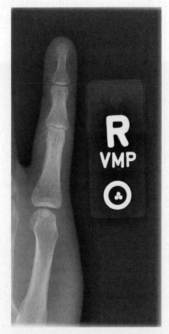

FIGURE 8.1 Anterior-posterior plain film XR of right small finger of a 27-year-old soccer goalie who presented after "jamming" his finger on the goal. He was subsequently unable to extend the finger. Clinical examination was concerning for a central slip injury and PIP radial collateral ligament injury given laxity with ulnarly directed stress testing of the joint. XR demonstrates a small chip fracture of the radial aspect of the proximal phalangeal head.

- ▲ Degenerative joint changes can be seen in chronic untreated CL injuries because of disturbed joint mechanics
  - ✳ Ultrasound or MRI can diagnose CL tear if equivocal examination findings (Figure 8.2)
- Classification
  - ◆ Grade I—partial CL tear, no laxity with stress testing
  - ◆ Grade II—partial CL tear, laxity but firm endpoint to stress testing
  - ◆ Grade III—complete CL tear, laxity and no endpoint with stress testing
- Acute management
  - ◆ Digital block and closed reduction of PIP joint
  - ◆ Extension block splint
  - ◆ Management depends on stability of PIP joint after dislocation
    - ✳ Stable (simple sprain)—buddy taping and immediate AROM

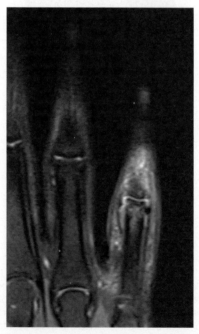

FIGURE 8.2 MRI of the same patient as in Figure 8.1 confirmed a tear of the radial collateral ligament from the radial aspect of the proximal phalangeal head as well as a central slip avulsion.

- ＊ Unstable (ligament tear)—extension block splint in 10° greater flexion than position of joint instability
  - ▲ Places volar plate in anatomic position for healing
- ● Definitive treatment
  - ◆ Nonoperative treatment
    - ＊ Stable (simple sprain)—buddy taping and immediate AROM
    - ＊ Unstable (ligament tear) after dorsal dislocation:
      - ▲ Extension block splint in 10° greater flexion than position of joint instability
      - ▲ Extend splint by 10° each week
      - ▲ Out of splint to buddy tape by week 3—longer period of immobilization results in joint stiffness
    - ＊ Volar dislocation with intact central slip—up to 3 weeks of splinting in extension
    - ＊ If patient unable to extend to neutral (ie, central slip injury) treat for acute boutonniere with 6 weeks immobilization in full extension
    - ＊ Lasting instability of PIP joint after CL injury/tear is relatively uncommon, with stiffness being the more common complication. Most can be managed nonoperatively with good results.
  - ◆ Surgical indications
    - ＊ Unstable PIP joint after dorsal dislocation requiring >30° of flexion for stability
    - ＊ PIP fracture–dislocation with fracture fragment of base of middle phalanx involving >40% of articular surface
      - ▲ CL attached to fracture fragment rather than remaining attached to middle phalanx
    - ＊ Volar PIP fracture–dislocation with large dorsal fracture fragment and central slip injury or that fails closed reduction
    - ＊ Contraindications—advanced arthritis of PIP joint or fixed joint deformity
  - ◆ Surgical approach
    - ＊ Operative techniques
      - ▲ Acute CL injury without articular fracture—exploration via mid-axial incision and direct repair with nonabsorbable suture anchor or
        - ◆ 2 cm mid-axial incision over side of affected CL
        - ◆ Incise transverse retinacular ligament and retract lateral band dorsally

- ◈ Examine proximally for site of CL rupture
- ◈ Repair CL to site of avulsion with suture anchor
- ▲ Acute CL injury with large articular fracture:
  - ◈ One large fragment—open reduction internal fixation (ORIF) via dorsal or volar approach
    - ○ Volar approach—Bruner incision, incise and reflect A3 pulley, retract flexor tendons, PIP capsulotomy between flexor sheath and accessory collateral ligament on one side, elevation and reduction of fracture fragment with lag screw fixation
  - ◈ Multiple fragments
    - ○ Dynamic external traction
    - ○ Volar plate arthroplasty
    - ○ Hemi-hamate arthroplasty
  - ▲ Irreducible—volar approach via Bruner incision, reflect A3 pulley, remove volar plate from joint and direct repair
  - ▲ Chronic CL injury with instability—exploration via mid-axial incision and reconstruction with palmaris tendon graft or distally based slip of flexor digitorum superficialis
- ✳ Range PIP joint under fluoroscopy to determine stability at end of operation
- ◆ Postoperative care
  - ✳ Acute CL injury without articular fracture:
    - ▲ Immobilize in extension for 3 weeks
    - ▲ AROM at 3 weeks with buddy strap
  - ✳ Acute CL injury with articular fracture:
    - ▲ Immediate AROM initiated
    - ▲ PIP splinted in full extension between exercises to prevent flexion contracture
    - ▲ Early passive ROM and dynamic splinting
    - ▲ Graduated return to full activities
- ◆ Potential complications
  - ✳ Extensor lag, persistent pain and swelling, recurrent instability, cold intolerance, nonunion
- ◆ Outcomes
  - ✳ Full recovery expected in Grade I and II lesions
  - ✳ Approximately 10° extensor lag at best is the norm for ORIF of PIP articular fracture

MANAGEMENT ALGORITHM

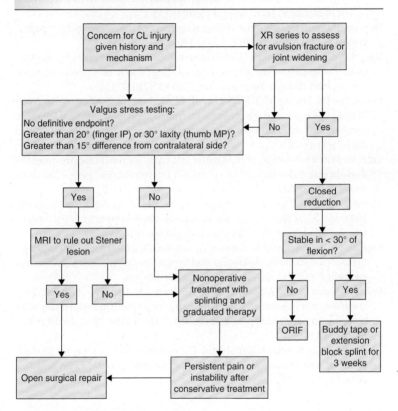

SUGGESTED READINGS

Avery DM III, Caggiano NM, Matullo KS. Ulnar collateral ligament injuries of the thumb: a comprehensive review. *Orthop Clin North Am.* 2015;46(2):281-292.

Caravaggi P, Shamian B, Uko L, Chen L, Melamed E, Capo JT. In vitro kinematics of the proximal interphalangeal joint in the finger after progressive disruption of the main supporting structures. *Hand (N Y).* 2015;10(3):425-432.

Carlo J, Dell PC, Matthias R, Wright TW. Collateral ligament reconstruction of the proximal interphalangeal joint. *J Hand Surg Am.* 2016;41(1):129-132.

Chalmer J, Blakeway M, Adams Z, Milan SJ. Conservative interventions for treating hyperextension injuries of the proximal interphalangeal joints of the fingers. *Cochrane Database Syst Rev.* 2013;(2):CD009030. doi:10.1002/14651858. CD009030.pub2.

Cheung JP, Tse WL, Ho PC. Irreducible volar subluxation of the proximal inter-phalangeal joint due to radial collateral ligament interposition: case report and review of literature. *Hand Surg.* 2015;20(1):153-157.

Heyman P. Injuries to the ulnar collateral ligament of the thumb metacarpopha-langeal joint. *J Am Acad Orthop Surg.* 1997;5(4):224-229.

Kato N, Nemoto K, Nakajima H, Motosuneya T, Fujikawa K. Primary repair of the collateral ligament of the proximal interphalangeal joint using a suture anchor. *Scand J Plast Reconstr Surg Hand Surg.* 2003;37(2):117-120.

Lee SJ, Lee JH, Hwang IC, Kim JK, Lee JI. Clinical outcomes of operative repair of complete rupture of the proximal interphalangeal joint collateral ligament: comparison with non-operative treatment. *Acta Orthop Traumatol Turc.* 2017;51(1):44-48.

Lutz M, Fritz D, Arora R, et al. Anatomical basis for functional treatment of dorsolateral dislocation of the proximal interphalangeal joint. *Clin Anat.* 2004;17(4):303-307.

Merrel G, Slade J. Dislocation and ligament injuries in the digits. In: Wolfe SW, Hotchkiss RN, Pederson WC, Kozin SH, eds. *Green's Operative Hand Surgery.* 6th ed. Philadelphia, PA: Churchill Livingstone; 2010:659-763.

Paschos NK, Abuhemoud K, Gantsos A, Mitsionis GI, Georgoulis AD. Manage-ment of proximal interphalangeal joint hyperextension injuries: a randomized controlled trial. *J Hand Surg Am.* 2014;39(3):449-454.

Roh YH, Koh YD, Go JY, Noh JH, Gong HS, Baek GH. Factors influencing func-tional outcome of proximal interphalangeal joint collateral ligament injury when treated with buddy strapping and exercise. *J Hand Ther.* 2017. doi:10.1016/j.jht.2017.02.010.

Waris E, Mattila S, Sillat T, Karjalainen T. Extension block pinning for unstable proximal interphalangeal joint dorsal fracture dislocations. *J Hand Surg Am.* 2016;41(2):196-202.

9 Base of the Thumb Fractures

Thao Nguyen and Ngozi Mogekwu Akabudike

INTRODUCTION

Base of the thumb metacarpal fractures can be divided into:

- Extra-articular fractures
  - Transverse
  - Oblique patterns
- Intra-articular fractures (Figure 9.1)
  - Bennett—described by E. H. Bennett in 1881 to refer to an avulsion of the palmar-ulnar fragment of the metacarpal base.[1] This fragment remains attached to the trapezium via the anterior oblique ligament (AOL).
  - Rolando—defined by S. Rolando in 1910 as a three-part Y- or T-fracture pattern that includes the shaft, the palmar-ulnar (Bennett) fragment, and the dorsal-radial fragment.[2]

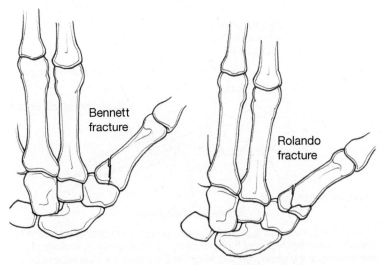

FIGURE 9.1 Classification of intra-articular thumb metacarpal fractures.

- Comminuted—reserved for less than three fragments; however, they are often classified with Rolando fractures.
- **Epidemiology**
  - Fractures involving the thumb metacarpals are common, accounting for 25% of all metacarpal fractures in the hand, with 80% occurring at the base.[3]
  - Bennett fracture is the most common type of metacarpal base fracture of the thumb.[3]
- **Mechanism of injury**
  - Bennett and Rolando fractures typically occur by an axial force on the thumb in flexion.
- **Anatomy**
  - Muscles acting at the first trapeziometacarpal (TM) joint include (Figure 9.2):
    - Abductor pollicis longus (APL)—inserts at the radial base of the metacarpal
    - Adductor pollicis longus (AdPL)—inserts on the ulnar tubercle at the base of the proximal phalanx
    - Flexor pollicis longus (FPL)—inserts on the palmar base of the distal phalanx

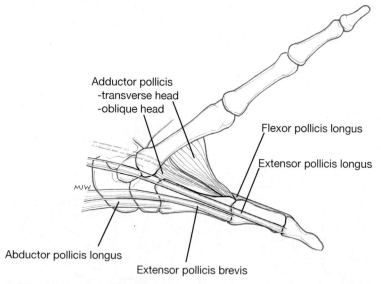

Adductor pollicis
-transverse head
-oblique head

Flexor pollicis longus

Extensor pollicis longus

MJW

Abductor pollicis longus

Extensor pollicis brevis

FIGURE 9.2 Forces acting at the first trapeziometacarpal joint. A, Illustration of the biconcave saddle joint of thumb trapeziometacarpal joint; B, Radiographs demonstrating the biconcave saddle joint of the thumb trapeziometacarpal joint. Courtesy of Thao Nguyen and Ngozi Mogekwu Akabudike.

- ◆ Extensor pollicis longus (EPL)—inserts on the dorsal base of the distal phalanx
- ◆ Extensor pollicis brevis—inserts on the dorsal base of the proximal phalanx
- ● Joint stability is mainly derived from the:
  - ◆ Joint capsule
  - ◆ Bony anatomy
    - ✳ The TM joint is a double or biconcave saddle joint (Figure 9.3) that allows motion in several planes: flexion–extension,

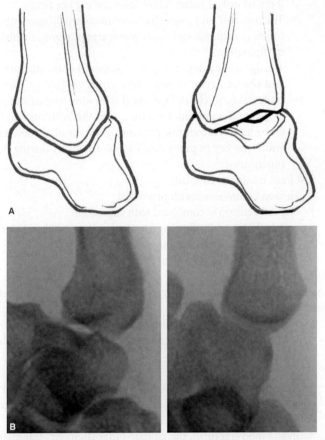

FIGURE 9.3 Bony anatomy of the trapeziometacarpal joint. A, Illustration of the biconcave saddle joint of thumb trapeziometacarpal joint. B, Radiographs demonstrating the biconcave saddle joint of the thumb trapeziometacarpal joint. Courtesy of Thao Nguyen and Ngozi Mogekwu Akabudike.

abduction–adduction, and pronation–supination. Its biconcavity provides nearly 47% of the joint stability in opposition.[4]

- ∗ The palmar beak of the thumb metacarpal interlocks into the recess of the trapezium.
- ◆ Ligaments
  - ∗ The AOL, also known as the palmar beak ligament, originates from the trapezium and inserts at the palmar beak of the thumb metacarpal. The AOL provides 40% of the resistance to pronation.[4] In addition, as the main capsular reinforcement, it resists dorsal radial subluxation during key pinch.
  - ∗ The anterior and posterior intermetacarpal ligaments, between the thumb and index metacarpals, provide resistance to supination.
  - ∗ The dorsal ligament complex, composed of the dorsal radial and the posterior oblique ligaments, originates from the trapezial tubercle and inserts at the radial base of the metacarpal and sometimes partly under the APL insertion.[5] It is the main restraint in preventing dorsoradial subluxation and is the key in providing TM joint stability during power pinch/grasp.[5-7]
- ● TM joint motion is coupled:
  - ◆ Flexion is combined with pronation
  - ◆ Hyperextension is combined with supination
- ● Arc of motion is wide allowing for pinch, grip, and opposition.[8]
  - ◆ Flexion–extension on average is 53°
  - ◆ Abduction–adduction on average is 42°

- ■ **Pathoanatomy**
  The direction of deforming forces is determined by the pull of the musculotendinous attachments.
  - ● Extra-articular fractures occur with apex dorsal angulation because the FPL flexes the distal fragment, whereas the APL extends the metacarpal base.
  - ● Intra-articular fractures
    - ◆ In Bennett fractures, the AdPL pulls the metacarpal shaft into adduction and supination, whereas the APL and thumb extensors displace it proximally.
    - ◆ In Rolando fractures, the palmar-ulnar (Bennett) fragment remains in place, attached to the trapezium via the AOL, whereas the APL displaces the dorsoradial fragment. The metacarpal shaft is adducted because of the pull of the AdPL and EPL.

EVALUATION

- **History and physical examination**
  - Patients will either report a fall on an outstretched hand or a direct axial load on the thumb from contact sports or high-energy trauma.
  - On examination, they will have swelling and ecchymosis at the base of the thumb along with tenderness. The thumb may be angulated with decreased range of motion.
- **Imaging**
  - Standard radiographic imaging should be obtained for complete evaluation.
    - Anteroposterior (AP) view—to obtain a true AP or Robert's view of the TM joint, the hand/forearm is hyperpronated so that the dorsum of the thumb lies flat on the radiographic plate (Figure 9.4A).
    - Lateral view—a true lateral or Bett's view of the thumb requires the palm to be pronated 15° to 35° and the beam angled 20° distally[9] (Figure 9.4B)
    - Oblique view
  - Traction radiographs may be helpful to assess the effect of ligamentotaxis on reduction.

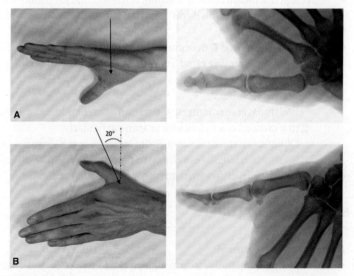

FIGURE 9.4 A, True anterior-posterior or Robert's view of the thumb. B, True lateral or Bett's view of the thumb.

- **Classification**
  Bennett fractures have been categorized into three types by Gedda[10]:
  - Type 1—a large single ulnar fragment and subluxation of the metacarpal base
  - Type 2—an impaction fracture without subluxation of the thumb metacarpal
  - Type 3—a small ulnar avulsion fracture fragment in association with metacarpal dislocation

EXTRA-ARTICULAR FRACTURES

Management of extra-articular thumb metacarpal fractures is similar to those of thumb or finger metacarpal shaft fractures.

- **Nonoperative treatment**
  - Most extra-articular fractures can be treated with closed reduction and thumb spica splint or cast for 3 to 4 weeks.
  - Due to the mobility of the TM and adjacent joints, angulation up to 30° is well tolerated without appreciable functional deficit. Angulation exceeding 30° will result in narrowing of the first webspace and cause compensatory hyperextension of the TM joint.
  - Reduction is achieved through traction, extension, and pronation of the distal metacarpal shaft with direct dorsal pressure at the metacarpal base.
- **Operative treatment**
  - Indications for closed reduction and percutaneous K-wire pinning: vertical oblique fractures that are shortened (because of the pull of the APL) and fractures that exceed acceptable angulation.
    - Operative technique
      - For transverse fractures, the fracture can be pinned directly, in a crossed configuration, or trans-articularly.
      - Oblique fractures may require intermetacarpal K-wire fixation to maintain length in addition to pinning the fracture directly.
  - Extra-articular fractures infrequently require open reduction.

BENNETT FRACTURES

- **Nonoperative treatment**
  - Historically, nonoperative treatment with closed reduction and casting was the recommended treatment for Bennett fractures.[1,11] However, several long-term studies of nonoperative treatment demonstrated continued subluxation resulting in motion loss, weakness, and eventual

symptomatic arthritis.[12,13] Consequently, operative treatment is now the preferred treatment.

- Closed reduction and casting for 4 to 6 weeks is reserved for stable nondisplaced fractures. However, close follow-up is required as these fractures are prone to displacement given the deforming forces at the metacarpal.

- **Operative treatment**
  - Indications for operative fixation include unstable and/or displaced fractures with or without carpometacarpal subluxation, or articular step-off >2 mm.[14,15]
  - Closed reduction percutaneous pinning (CRPP)
    - Closed reduction maneuver can be performed by several techniques:
      - Traction, palmar abduction, and pronation while applying pressure at the dorsoradial metacarpal base.[5,16]
      - Flexing the metacarpophalangeal joint while applying pressure at the metacarpal base.[17]
      - Passive screw home torque reduction technique, popularized by Edmunds, which involves maximally rotating the metacarpal into full opposition. This tightens the dorsal ligament complex to reduce the fracture. In contrast, thumb extension or hitch-hiker position should be avoided as this displaces the fracture.[5]
    - Percutaneous pinning should only be undertaken after successful closed reduction with <2 mm articular step-off. Configurations for K-wire pinning can include any combinations shown in Figure 9.5.
      - An intermetacarpal K-wire from the thumb to index metacarpal.
      - One to two K-wires from the metacarpal to the palmar-ulnar fragment.
      - Alternatively, screw fixation can also be utilized.
  - Open reduction internal fixation (ORIF)
    - If closed treatment does not adequately reduce the TM joint sub-luxation and the articular step-off to within 2 mm, open reduction

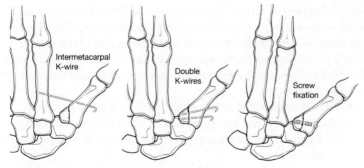

Intermetacarpal K-wire

Double K-wires

Screw fixation

FIGURE 9.5 Fixation configuration for Bennett fractures.

should be considered. The decision between closed reduction versus open reduction of the fracture is debated in the literature. Lutz et al found no difference in radiographic or functional outcomes between ORIF and CRPP.[18] There is no consensus regarding the amount of acceptable articular displacement. Some studies have shown no relationship between the quality of articular restoration with radiographic or clinical outcomes.[19,20] Furthermore, biomechanical studies demonstrate that articular correction within 2 mm is adequate as long as the TM joint is reduced, without increasing the risk of arthritis. In contrast, other studies have demonstrated that anatomic reduction is correlated with better outcomes.[14,21-23]

♦ Open treatment is performed through a Wagner approach. The incision is made over the radial border of the thumb TM joint between the APL and thenar muscles. The incision can be curved palmarly and extended toward the wrist crease. Care should be taken not to injure the branches of the palmar cutaneous branch of the median nerve and the dorsal sensory branch of the radial nerve. The thenar muscles are elevated off the palmar trapezium and the base of the metacarpal and then retracted. Avoid stripping the soft tissue off the palmar-ulnar fragment. A longitudinal capsulotomy is performed to visualize the TM joint. The fragment is then reduced with the help of a clamp or K-wire as a joystick. After articular congruity is obtained, the fragment is fixed with either 0.035 to 0.045″ K-wires or 1.5 to 2.7 mm mini-fragment screws depending on the size of the fragment. An intermetacarpal K-wire from the thumb to the index can be placed for added stability if needed.

ROLANDO FRACTURES

Rolando fractures are more challenging to treat than Bennett fractures because of the number of fragments and/or degree of comminution. Similar to Bennett fractures, some studies demonstrate that the quality of reduction is not correlated with long-term symptoms and development of arthritis, and thus, the authors recommend a more minimal approach with closed treatment.[24-27]

■ **Closed reduction**
  • Closed treatment is indicated for fractures that are minimally displaced or those that have significant comminuted articular fragments.
    ♦ Nondisplaced fractures are pinned with 0.045″ K-wires to prevent displacement.

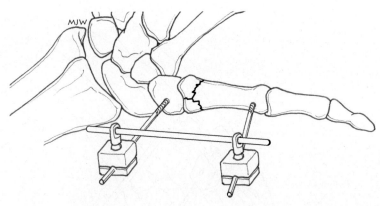

FIGURE 9.6 Thumb spanning external fixator.

- ◆ Fractures with articular fragments too comminuted for anatomic reduction are treated with distraction techniques that rely on capsuloligamentotaxis for reduction. There are several methods to attain distraction:
  - ✳ One option is by placing parallel intermetacarpal K-wires from the base of the thumb to the index metacarpal.[28]
  - ✳ Another method is with the use of external fixation.[29] The external fixator frame is constructed with one rod connecting the half pins in the distal radius with the index metacarpal and another rod connecting the distal radius to the dorsoradial thumb metacarpal. A third rod connects the thumb and index metacarpal half pins (Figure 9.6).
  - ✳ Alternatively, a thumb external fixator system can be applied. It requires 1 to 2 pins each in the metacarpal and trapezium (Figure 9.7).[24,27,30]
- ■ **Open reduction internal fixation**
  - ● Fractures with large fragments are amendable to ORIF through the Wagner approach. Fixation options include K-wires or eccentrically placed 2.0 or 2.4 mm screws in a T- or L-plate.

COMMINUTED INTRA-ARTICULAR FRACTURES

These fractures are treated similar to comminuted Rolando fractures with distraction techniques using K-wires or external fixator.

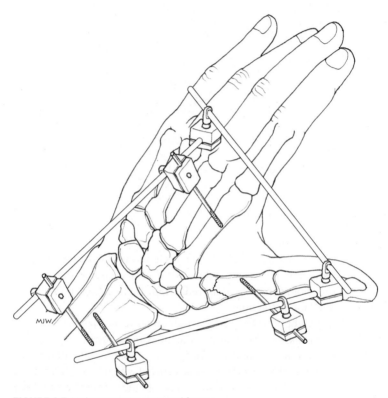

FIGURE 9.7 Wrist spanning external fixator.

POSTOPERATIVE CARE

- After CRPP or ORIF of all base of the thumb metacarpal fractures, the thumb should be placed initially in a thumb spica splint for 2 weeks. The splint is then converted to a thumb spica cast with the interphalangeal joint free for range of motion. The cast and pins can be removed at 4 to 6 weeks postoperatively based on radiographic evidence of healing. The patient is then given a removal thumb spica splint for an additional 3 to 4 weeks when therapy is initiated for active range of motion and strengthening.
- The external fixator is removed when the fracture is consolidated at approximately 6 to 8 weeks. Active finger range of motion is initiated immediately after surgery.

MANAGEMENT ALGORITHM

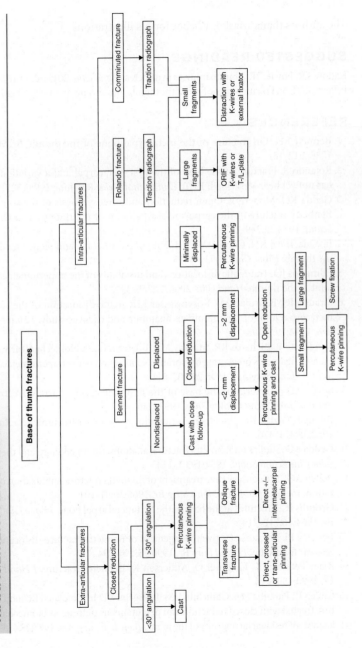

ACKNOWLEDGMENT

The authors thank Mark J. Wieber for his illustrations.

SUGGESTED READINGS

Kadow TR, Fowler JR. Thumb injuries in athletes. *Hand Clin*. 2017;33(1):161-173.
Pellegrini VD Jr. Fractures of the base of the thumb. *J Hand Surg Am*. 1989;4(1):87-102.

REFERENCES

1. Bennett EH. On fracture of the metacarpal bone of the thumb. *Br Med J*. 1886;2:12-13.
2. Rolando S. Fracture of the base of the first metacarpal and a variation that has not yet been described: 1910. *Clin Orthop Relat Res*. June 1996;(327):4-8.
3. Gedda KO, Moberg E. Open reduction and osteosynthesis of the so-called Bennett's fracture in the carpo-metacarpal joint of the thumb. *Acta Orthop Scand*. 1952;22:249-257.
4. Imaeda T, An KN, Cooney WP III. Functional anatomy and biomechanics of the thumb. *Hand Clin*. 1992;8:9-15.
5. Edmunds JO. Traumatic dislocations and instability of the trapeziometacarpal joint of the thumb. *Hand Clin*. 2006;22:365-392.
6. Strauch RJ, Behrman MJ, Rosenwasser MP. Acute dislocation of the carpo-metacarpal joint of the thumb: an anatomic and cadaver study. *J Hand Surg Am*. 1994;19:93-98.
7. Van Brenk B, Richards RR, Mackay MB, Boynton EL. A biomechanical assessment of ligaments preventing dorsoradial subluxation of the trapeziometacarpal joint. *J Hand Surg Am*. 1998;23:607-611.
8. Soyer AD. Fractures of the base of the first metacarpal: current treatment options. *J Am Acad Orthop Surg*. 1999;7:403-412.
9. Billing L, Gedda KO. Roentgen examination of Bennett's fracture. *Acta Radiol*. 1952;38:471-476.
10. Gedda KO. Studies on Bennett's fracture; anatomy, roentgenology, and therapy. *Acta Chir Scand Suppl*. 1954;193:1-114.
11. Pollen AG. The conservative treatment of Bennett's fracture-subluxation of the thumb metacarpal. *J Bone Joint Surg Br*. 1968;50:91-101.
12. Griffiths JC. Fractures at the base of the first metacarpal bone. *J Bone Joint Surg Br*. 1964;46:712-719.
13. Livesley PJ. The conservative management of Bennett's fracture-dislocation: a 26-year follow-up. *J Hand Surg Br*. 1990;15:291-294.
14. Kjaer-Petersen K, Langhoff O, Andersen K. Bennett's fracture. *J Hand Surg Br*. 1990;15:58-61.
15. Cullen JP, Parentis MA, Chinchilli VM, Pellegrini VD Jr. Simulated Bennett fracture treated with closed reduction and percutaneous pinning. A biomechanical analysis of residual incongruity of the joint. *J Bone Joint Surg Am*. 1997;79:413-420.

16. Kahler DM. Fractures and dislocations of the base of the thumb. *J South Orthop Assoc.* 1995;4:69-76.
17. Carlsen BT, Moran SL. Thumb trauma: Bennett fractures, Rolando fractures, and ulnar collateral ligament injuries. *J Hand Surg Am.* 2009;34:945-952.
18. Lutz M, Sailer R, Zimmermann R, Gabl M, Ulmer H, Pechlaner S. Closed reduction transarticular Kirschner wire fixation versus open reduction internal fixation in the treatment of Bennett's fracture dislocation. *J Hand Surg Br.* 2003;28:142-147.
19. Cannon SR, Dowd GS, Williams DH, Scott JM. A long-term study following Bennett's fracture. *J Hand Surg Br.* 1986;11:426-431.
20. Demir E, Unglaub F, Wittemann M, Germann G, Sauerbier M. Surgically treated intraarticular fractures of the trapeziometacarpal joint—a clinical and radiological outcome study. *Unfallchirurg.* 2006;109:13-21.
21. Oosterbos CJ, de Boer HH. Nonoperative treatment of Bennett's fracture: a 13-year follow-up. *J Orthop Trauma.* 1995;9:23-27.
22. Thurston AJ, Dempsey SM. Bennett's fracture: a medium to long-term review. *Aust N Z J Surg.* 1993;63:120-123.
23. Timmenga EJ, Blokhuis TJ, Maas M, Raaijmakers EL. Long-term evaluation of Bennett's fracture. A comparison between open and closed reduction. *J Hand Surg Br.* 1994;19:373-377.
24. Houshian S, Jing SS. Treatment of Rolando fracture by capsuloligamentotaxis using mini external fixator: a report of 16 cases. *Hand Surg.* 2013;18:73-78.
25. Langhoff O, Andersen K, Kjaer-Petersen K. Rolando's fracture. *J Hand Surg Br.* 1991;16:454-459.
26. van Niekerk JL, Ouwens R. Fractures of the base of the first metacarpal bone: results of surgical treatment. *Injury.* 1989;20:359-362.
27. Marsland D, Sanghrajka AP, Goldie B. Static monolateral external fixation for the Rolando fracture: a simple solution for a complex fracture. *Ann R Coll Surg Engl.* 2012;94:112-115.
28. Iselin M, Blanguernon S, Benoist D. First metacarpal base fracture. *Mem Acad Chir (Paris).* 1956;82:771-774.
29. Schuind F, Noorbergen M, Andrianne Y, Burny F. Comminuted fractures of the base of the first metacarpal treated by distraction-external fixation. *J Orthop Trauma.* 1988;2:314-321.
30. Proubasta IR. Rolando's fracture of the first metacarpal. Treatment by external fixation. *J Bone Joint Surg Br.* 1992;74:416-417.

Thumb Collateral Ligament Injury

James Paul Hovis and Ngozi Mogekwu Akabudike

INTRODUCTION

- Pathoanatomy
  - Primary arc of thumb metacarpophalangeal (MCP) joint motion is flexion/extension with minor arcs of abduction/adduction and pronation/supination.
  - The thumb MCP joint has minimal intrinsic stability because of the large radius of curvature of proximal phalanx base.
  - Thumb MCP joint has radial and ulnar collateral ligaments, with each collateral ligament being composed of proper and accessory collateral ligament components.
  - Proper collateral ligaments originate from the condyles of the metacarpal head and travel obliquely to insert on the volar third of the proximal phalanx.
  - Proper collateral ligaments are tight in flexion and loose in extension.
  - Proper ulnar collateral ligament resists radial deviation of thumb in flexion.
  - Proper radial collateral ligament resists ulnar deviation of thumb in flexion.
  - Accessory collateral ligaments originate from an area on the metacarpal head volar to the proper collateral ligament origin and insert on the volar plate and sesamoids.
  - Accessory collateral ligaments are tight in extension and loose in flexion.
  - Accessory ulnar collateral ligament resists radial deviation of thumb in extension.
  - Accessory radial collateral ligament resists ulnar deviation of thumb in extension.
  - Floor of the joint is formed by the volar plate.
  - Dynamic stability is provided to the joint through tendinous attachments of the adductor pollicis, flexor pollicis brevis, and extensor pollicis brevis.

- Mechanism of injury
  - Acute injury because of sudden forced radial deviation (abduction) of the thumb.
  - Acute injury because of sudden forced ulnar deviation (adduction) of the thumb.
  - Chronic instability of the thumb MCP joint from inadequate treatment of an acute ligament tear or progressive attenuation of the ligament.
  - Ligament is commonly torn from the proximal phalanx and still attached to metacarpal. Rarely the ligament can tear proximally from the metacarpal.
  - The most common fracture pattern is an avulsion fracture from the base of the proximal phalanx where the ligament inserts.
  - Associated injuries can include tears of the dorsal capsule and ulnar aspect of the volar plate.
- Epidemiology
  - Acute injury is particularly common in skiers and ball-handling athletes. Falling while gripping the ski pole causes the handle to rapidly abduct the thumb.
  - Chronic injury is also called "gamekeeper's thumb" because of attenuation of the collateral ligament from repetitive breaking of rabbit's necks using the index finger and thumb.
  - Ulnar collateral ligament injury is more common than radial collateral ligament injury.

EVALUATION

- History
  - Fall onto an outstretched hand with the thumb abducted
  - Repetitive abduction activities at the thumb MCP joint
  - Difficulty with pinch or gripping with thumb and index finger
  - Pain worsened by forceful pinch or torsional motions of the hand such as unscrewing jar tops
  - Pain, tenderness, and ecchymosis at the ulnar or radial aspect of the thumb MCP joint
- Physical examination
  - Physical examination is usually sufficient to make the diagnosis.
  - Inspect the resting posture of the thumb for volar subluxation or radial deviation of the MCP joint.
  - Pain with palpation of the ulnar or radial aspect of thumb MCP joint

- Ecchymosis and swelling of the ulnar or radial aspect of thumb MCP joint
- Weakness or pain with power pinch
- Mass at ulnar aspect of thumb MCP joint may represent a Stener lesion.
- Stener lesion—avulsed ligament with or without bony attachment displaced proximal and above the adductor aponeurosis such as that the aponeurosis prevents contact of the injured ligament with the avulsion site.
- There is no potential mass from interposition on the radial side of the MCP joint comparable with the Stener lesion seen on the ulnar side.
- With radial collateral ligament rupture, a dorsoradial prominence of the metacarpal head can be commonly seen.
- Thumb MCP joint range of motion can be limited by pain.
- Similar criteria to assess ulnar collateral ligament stability can be applied to the radial collateral ligament.
- Must stress joint in extension and 30 degrees of flexion
  - Greater than 35 degrees of joint laxity with stress suggests complete ligament tear.
  - Fifteen degrees more joint laxity when compared to contralateral thumb suggests complete ligament tear.
  - Joint opening without resistance or clear endpoint suggests complete tear.
  - Partial torn ligaments usually have a discrete endpoint despite some laxity.
  - Radial deviation of extended thumb tests ulnar accessory collateral ligament.
  - Radial deviation of flexed thumb tests ulnar proper collateral ligament.
  - Ulnar deviation of extended thumb tests radial accessory collateral ligament.
  - Ulnar deviation of flexed thumb tests radial proper collateral ligament.
- Representative image(s)
- Imaging
  - Standard posteroanterior, lateral, and oblique radiographs of hand (Figure 10.1).
  - Inspect for volar subluxation of the MCP joint or radial deviation of the proximal phalanx.
  - Radiographs should be done prior to stressing the joint.
  - Rule out osteoarthritis if consideration is given to ligamentous reconstruction.

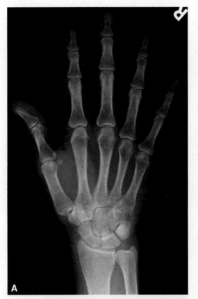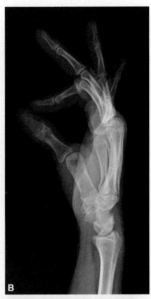

FIGURE 10.1 Anteroposterior (A) and lateral (B) radiographs of the hand demonstrating rupture of the thumb metacarpophalangeal joint ulnar collateral ligament.

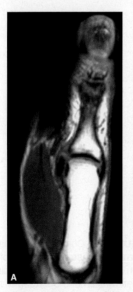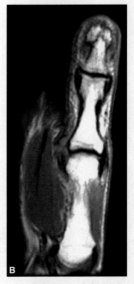

FIGURE 10.2 Coronal T1 images of the hand demonstrating rupture of the thumb metacarpophalangeal joint ulnar collateral ligament. Courtesy of James Paul Hovis and Ngozi Mogekwu Akabudike.

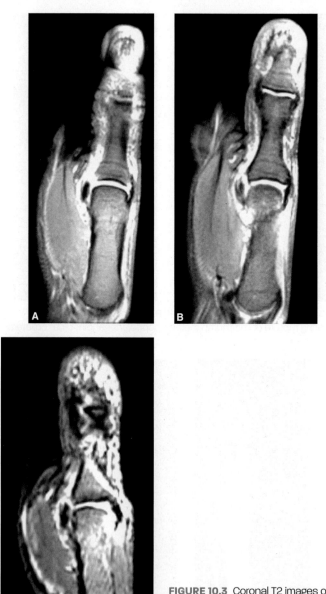

FIGURE 10.3 Coronal T2 images of the thumb demonstrating rupture of the thumb metacarpophalangeal joint ulnar collateral ligament. Courtesy of James Paul Hovis and Ngozi Mogekwu Akabudike.

- MRI and ultrasound can be used to assess the injury but are rarely necessary (Figures 10.2 and 10.3).
- Arthrography is primarily of historical interest.
- Representative image(s)

ACUTE MANAGEMENT

- Acute treatment is usually immobilization in a thumb spica splint or brace with exclusion of the thumb interphalangeal (IP) joint.

DEFINITIVE TREATMENT

- Nonoperative treatment
  - Immobilization of the thumb MCP joint in a thumb spica cast, custom-molded thermoplastic splint, or thumb spica brace for 4 weeks while leaving the IP joint free. Followed by 2 weeks of splint immobilization and active range-of-motion exercises.
    - Indication—acute partial tears—less than 35 degrees laxity with stress, less than a 15 degree differential in laxity compared to the contralateral thumb, and a discrete endpoint to joint opening.
    - Partial acute tears usually heal without significant laxity.
  - Common to have a degree of aching at MCP joint 2 to 3 months after injury despite there being no laxity on examination.
  - Thumb IP joint is left free for range-of-motion exercises to avoid adhesion of flexor and extensor tendons to the injured MCP joint capsule and subsequent IP joint stiffness.
- Operative treatment
  - Primary ligament repair with suture
    - Indication—complete mid-substance tears of the ligament
  - Reapproximation and fixation of the ligamentous avulsion to bone
    - Indication—complete ligament avulsions
  - Fixation with Kirschner wire or mini-fragment screw
    - Indication—avulsion fracture of the ulnar proximal phalanx base
  - Reconstruction with free tendon graft
    - Indication—chronic collateral ligament instability
    - Absolute contraindication—osteoarthritis in the presence of collateral ligament instability

- MCP arthrodesis
  - Indication—chronic collateral ligament instability in the presence of osteoarthritis or failure of ligamentous reconstruction
- Surgical approach
  - Indicated for avulsion of the distal attachment of the ulnar collateral ligament at the base of the proximal phalanx, avulsion fracture of the ulnar base of the proximal phalanx, or reconstruction for chronic instability.
  - A "lazy S"–shaped incision that begins by paralleling the ulnodorsal border of the thumb metacarpal is started about 1 cm proximal to the MCP joint. The incision curves in the volar direction around the ulnar aspect of the MCP joint and extends distally along the ulnar midaxial line.

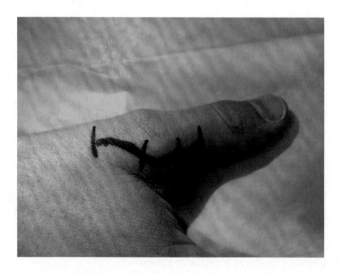

- Dorsal sensory branches of the superficial radial nerve in the sub-cutaneous tissue should be identified and protected.
- The adductor aponeurosis is exposed. If a Stener lesion is present, it can be found at the proximal edge of the adductor aponeurosis. The tendons of the extensor pollicis longus (EPL) and extensor pollicis brevis can also be identified.
- A longitudinal incision is made in the adductor aponeurosis parallel and 3 to 5 mm volar to the ulnar border of the EPL. A 3 to 5 mm fringe of aponeurosis is left attached to the EPL for later repair.

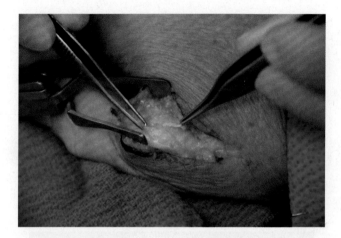

- The aponeurosis is retracted ulnarly and the EPL is retracted dorsally to expose the joint capsule and the injured ligament.
- A longitudinal dorsal capsulotomy is made avoiding disruption of the proximal origin of the ligament.

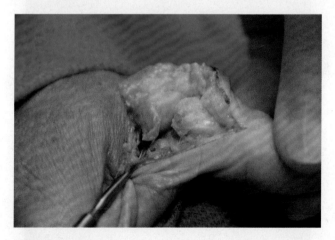

- The MCP joint can then be inspected for intra-articular injury.
- Mid-substance tears can be reapproximated with interrupted figure-of-eight or horizontal mattress sutures using nonabsorbable braided synthetic suture material.
- Ligamentous avulsions can be secured with bone anchors or pull-out suture technique.

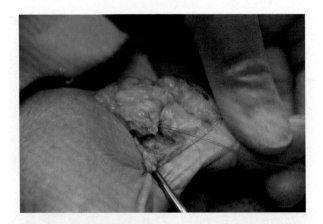

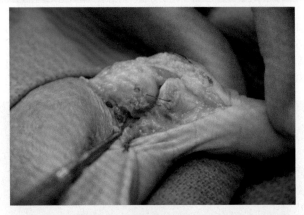

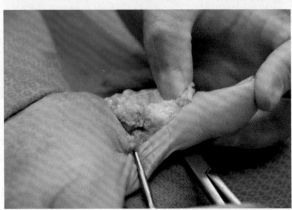

- Bony avulsions can anatomically be reduced with Kirschner wires or mini-fragment screws.
- For ligamentous reconstruction, palmaris longus tendon graft passed through bone tunnels is preferred. If palmaris longus is unavailable, a strip of flexor carpi radialis can be used.

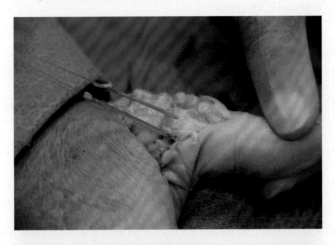

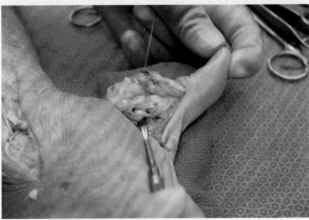

- Additional steps should be considered before closure—suture placed between volar plate and distal volar portion of the repaired ligament, repair of the dorsal ulnar capsule to prevent volar subluxation or rotation of the joint, gentle radial stress to test stability, and the joint may be transfixed with an oblique Kirschner wire to prevent tension on the repair.
- The joint capsule is closed followed by reattachment of the adductor aponeurosis.

- Potential complications
  - Most common complication is injury to the crossing branches of the dorsal sensory branch of the radial nerve.
  - Stiffness can occur because of reattaching the ligament too distally or inserting it in a nonanatomic/nonisometric location.
- Postoperative care
  - Postoperative management is similar for reconstructed collateral ligaments and acute collateral ligament repair.
  - Thumb MCP joint is immobilized in a thumb spica cast for 4 weeks with the IP joint free to prevent adhesions of the extensor mechanism.
  - After 4 weeks, the patient is transitioned to a hand-based custom thermoplastic splint to protect the MCP joint and active range-of-motion exercises are begun.
  - Splint protection is discontinued 6 weeks postoperatively.
  - Vague discomfort and tenderness can be expected and can last for up to 1 year.
  - Stiffness of the MCP joint is expected and can persist for several weeks.
  - Expected range of motion is 80% to 90% of the uninjured thumb.
  - Pinch and grip strength are usually regained to within 5% to 10% of the contralateral thumb.
  - Full athletic participation can be resumed by approximately 4 months postoperatively.

MANAGEMENT ALGORITHM

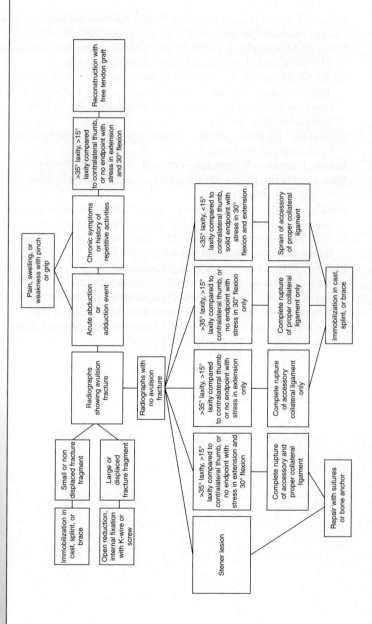

SUGGESTED READINGS

Carlsen BT, Moran SL. Thumb trauma: Bennett fractures, Rolando fractures, and ulnar collateral ligament injuries. *J Hand Surg Am*. 2009;34A:945-952.

Chuter GS, Muwanga CL, Irwin LR. Ulnar collateral ligament injuries of the thumb: 10 years of surgical experience. *Injury*. 2009;40(6):652-656.

Glickel SZ, Barron OA, Catalano LW. Dislocations and ligament injuries in the digits. In: Green DP, Hotchkiss RN, Pederson WC, Wolfe SW, ed. *Green's Operative Hand Surgery*. 5th ed. Vol 1. Philadelphia, PA: Elsevier Churchill Livingstone; 2011:366-379.

Johnson JW, Culp RW. Acute ulnar collateral ligament injury in the athlete. *Hand Clinics*. 2009;25(3):437-442.

Kukadia J, Ashwood N. Gamekeeper's thumb. *Trauma*. 2017;19(1):11-20.

Madan SS, Pai DR, Kaur A, Dixit R. Injury to ulnar collateral ligament of thumb. *Orthop Surg*. 2014;6(1):1-7.

Malik AK, Morris T, Chou D, Sorene E, Taylor E. Clinical testing of ulnar collateral ligament injuries of the thumb. *J Hand Surg*. 2009;34(3):363-366.

McKeon KE, Gelberman RH, Calfee RP. Ulnar collateral ligament injuries of the thumb. *J Bone Joint Surg Am*. 2013;95(10):881-887.

Rhee PC, Jones DB Jr, Sanjeev K. Management of thumb metacarpophalangeal ulnar collateral ligament injuries. *J Bone Joint Surg Am*. 2012;94(21):2005-2012.

Ritting AW, Baldwin PC, Rodner CM. Ulnar collateral ligament injury of the thumb metacarpophalangeal joint. *Clin J Sport Med*. 2010;20(2):106-112.

Tang P. Collateral ligament injuries of the thumb metacarpophalangeal joint. *J Am Acad Orthop Surg*. 2011;19(5):287-296.

11 Metacarpal Fractures

Joseph A. Rosenbaum and Hisham M. Awan

INTRODUCTION

- Pathoanatomy
  - Fractures of the bones of the hand typically secondary to trauma
  - Force applied to the affected bone exceeds its strength.
- Mechanism of injury
  - Mechanisms of injury include crush, torsional, angular, axial load, traction.
  - High-energy mechanisms typically cause comminution.
  - Fracture may be part of a more severe overall injury pattern including soft tissue injury to ligament, joint capsule, tendon, nerve, and/or vessels.
  - Multiple metacarpals may be involved.
- Epidemiology
  - Fractures of phalanges and metacarpals are among the most common fractures.
  - Account for approximately 10% of all fractures
  - Common in laborers and athletes
  - Males are affected more than females.
  - Younger patients are affected more than older patients.

EVALUATION

- History
  - Typically caused by trauma, either direct or indirect
  - Rarely can be pathologic fractures with minimal or no antecedent trauma
  - Presentation may be delayed.
  - Often overlooked initially in polytrauma cases

- Physical examination
  - Assess for edema, angular deformity, rotational deformity, and quality of soft tissues.
    - ◆ Rotational deformity assessment—patient makes a fist, and all fingers should cascade equally and point toward the volar scaphoid tubercle (Figures 11.1 and 11.2).
    - ◆ If patient is unable to flex digits to examine for rotational deformity, examine the nail plates in full extension to see if they are all parallel.
  - Assess sensation and capillary refill distally.
  - Assess the other digits as well as the hand and wrist.
  - Test for tendon function individually for each finger (flexor digitorum superficialis, flexor digitorum profundus, extensor digitorum communis).

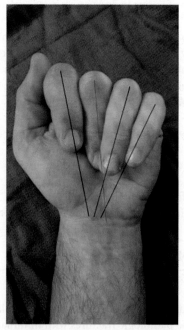

FIGURE 11.1 Digital rotation is assessed with the fingers flexed to 90° at the metacarpophalangeal (MP) and proximal interphalangeal joints, with the distal interphalangeal joints extended. The fingers should all point to the scaphoid tubercle. In this image, the long finger is malrotated, pointing ulnar to the scaphoid.

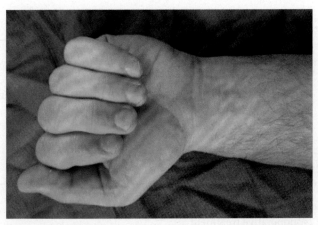

FIGURE 11.2 In this image, the rotation has been corrected, and all digits point toward the scaphoid tubercle.

- Imaging and classification
  - Obtain hand radiograph initially if metacarpal fracture is suspected (posteroanterior, lateral, oblique).
  - Brewerton views (MP flexed 65° with dorsum of fingers lying on plate and tube angled 15° ulnar-to-radial) to assess metacarpal heads
  - Open versus closed
  - Intra-articular versus extra-articular
  - Stable versus unstable fracture pattern
    - ◆ Comminuted versus simple (Simple are generally more stable.)
    - ◆ Transverse versus oblique (transverse more length-stable)
  - Angulation (transverse shaft fractures tend to angulate apex dorsal)
  - Translation
  - Presence or absence of foreign bodies
- Anatomic classification
  - Metacarpal head fractures
  - Neck fractures
    - ◆ Common, especially in ring and small finger ("boxer's fracture")
  - Shaft fractures
    - ◆ Common
  - Base fractures
  - Thumb extra-articular base fractures

ACUTE MANAGEMENT

- Emergency room management
  - Assess for other injuries
  - Comfort measures—pain control, elevation, splinting (remove splints for radiograph)
  - Remove patient's gloves, rings, and jewelry

TREATMENT

- Metacarpal head fractures
  - Nonoperative treatment
    - ◆ Reserved for only nondisplaced fractures
  - Surgical indications
    - ◆ Any articular surface displacement is unacceptable.
  - Surgical approach
    - ◆ Dorsal approach
      - ✳ Screws, headless screw(s), or K-wires can be used for fixation.
      - ✳ External fixation if comminution does not allow for internal fixation.
      - ✳ Stable fixation will allow early motion.
  - Potential complications
    - ◆ Stiffness
- Metacarpal neck fractures
  - Typically will have an apex dorsal deformity
  - Often caused by direct trauma, including punching
  - Nonoperative treatment
    - ◆ Closed injuries
    - ◆ Tolerances vary depending on which metacarpal is involved.
      - ✳ Index and middle—up to 10° to 15° is accepted
      - ✳ Ring—up to 40°
      - ✳ Small ("boxer's fracture")—some authors accept up to 70°
    - ◆ Hand dominance, age, and occupation are also factors to consider.
    - ◆ Malrotation is not accepted if there is any interference with neighboring digits or overall hand function.
    - ◆ Pseudoclawing (metacarpophalangeal [MCP] hyperextension and proximal interphalangeal [PIP] flexion to compensate for the flexed metacarpal neck) is not accepted.

- ◆ Accepting a deformity leads to prominence of the head in the palm as well of loss of dorsal knuckle appearance.
- ◆ Closed reduction may be performed in emergency department.
  - ✻ Median/ulnar nerve block, Bier block, or field block may be used.
  - ✻ Flex MCP and PIP to 90°, apply dorsally directed pressure through the proximal phalanx, and counterpressure on the metacarpal shaft.
- ◆ Cast for 3 to 4 weeks in the "safe position" of James—20° of wrist extension, 70° to 90° of MCP flexion, and full extension of PIP and distal interphalangeal joints—to keep collateral ligaments stretched to prevent contracture.
  - ✻ Some authors advise that immobilizing in the safe position is not essential in pediatric cases.
- Surgical indications
  - ◆ "Fight bite" or other open injuries
    - ✻ For fight bites, perform incision and drainage emergently, but internal fixation is avoided until the wound is clean.
  - ◆ Clinically significant malrotation
  - ◆ Unacceptable angulation
  - ◆ Pseudoclawing
- Surgical technique
  - ◆ Closed reduction percutaneous pinning (CRPP)
    - ✻ Two approaches, anterograde and retrograde
    - ✻ Anterograde
      - ▲ K wire(s) start from metacarpal base
      - ▲ May use multiple wires in "bouquet" technique
    - ✻ Retrograde
      - ▲ Start wires in collateral recess.
      - ▲ Place pins with MCP flexed 70° to 90° to avoid collateral ligament contracture.
    - ✻ Early range of motion is encouraged.
    - ✻ Pins are pulled at 4 weeks post-op.
  - ◆ Open reduction internal fixation (ORIF)
    - ✻ Suboptimal location for plates due to poor distal fixation
    - ✻ May be attempted if fracture is not amenable to CRPP.
- Potential complications
  - ◆ Stiffness
  - ◆ Infection
  - ◆ Recurrence

- Metacarpal shaft fractures
  - Tend to go into apex dorsal deformity
  - Nonoperative treatment
    - Closed injuries
    - Tolerances vary depending on which metacarpal is involved.
      - Index and middle—up to 10°
      - Ring—up to 20°
      - Small—up to 30°
    - Malrotation is unacceptable.
    - Mild shortening is tolerated.
    - Closed reduction under local or regional block and casting in safe position as described earlier
      - Reduction is generally performed with dorsal pressure over the fracture apex while stabilizing metacarpal head or proximal phalanx.
    - Immobilize for 4 weeks
  - Surgical indications
    - Unacceptable angulation (see earlier for tolerances)
    - Malrotation
    - Multiple shaft fractures
    - Open fractures
  - Surgical treatment
    - CRPP with anterograde or retrograde pinning as described earlier
    - ORIF with plates and/or multiple lag screws
      - Operative technique
        - ▲ Dorsal approach
        - ▲ Bury plates under periosteum to avoid extensor tendon adhesion.
    - External fixation for comminuted, bone loss, or contaminated
  - Potential complications
    - Stiffness
    - Tendon adhesions
    - Infection
- Metacarpal base fractures
  - Often seen in association with carpometacarpal (CMC) joint dislocation
  - May require computed tomography to better define articular involvement
  - Nonoperative treatment
    - Nondisplaced fractures only

- ◆ Cast for 4 weeks in safe position.
- Surgical indications
  - ◆ Extra-articular fractures—Follow indications for shaft fractures.
  - ◆ Articular fractures—No displacement or step-off is accepted.
  - ◆ Unstable patterns associated with CMC dislocations
- Surgical technique
  - ◆ K-wires across the CMC joint
  - ◆ ORIF with plate/screw construct
    - ✳ Avoid prominence of hardware into CMC joint
- Potential complications
  - ◆ CMC instability
  - ◆ Tendon adhesions
- Thumb metacarpal base extra-articular fractures
  - Pull of abductor pollicis longus, adductor pollicis, and extensor pollicis longus will bring this fracture into apex dorsal angulation, adduction, flexion, and supination
  - Nonoperative treatment
    - ◆ Closed reduction and casting in thumb spica cast for 4 weeks
      - ✳ Reduction maneuver—axial traction, pronation, extension
      - ✳ Must acquire dedicated thumb radiographs to assess
  - Surgical indications
    - ◆ Residual angulation greater than 30°
    - ◆ Unstable patterns
  - Surgical technique
    - ◆ CRPP with K-wires across CMC joint
      - ✳ Pull pins at 4 to 6 weeks.
    - ◆ ORIF
      - ✳ Rarely used for this fracture

SUGGESTED READINGS

Baltera RM, Hastings H II. Fractures and dislocations: hand. In: Hammert WC, ed. *ASSH Manual of Hand Surgery.* Philadelphia, PA: Lippincott Williams & Wilkins; 2010:93-110.

Day CS, Stern PJ. Fractures of the metacarpals and phalanges. In: Wolfe SW, Hotchkiss RN, Pederson WC, Kozin SH, eds. *Green's Operative Hand Surgery.* 6th ed. Philadelphia, PA: Churchill Livingstone; 2010:239-290.

Dean BJF, Little C. Fractures of the metacarpals and phalanges. *Orthop Trauma.* 2011;23:43-56.

Meals C, Meals R. Hand fractures: a review of current treatment strategies. *J Hand Surg Am.* 2013;38(5):1021-1031.

12 Metacarpophalangeal Dislocations

Joseph A. Rosenbaum and Hisham M. Awan

INTRODUCTION

- Pathoanatomy
  - Dislocation of the metacarpophalangeal (MCP) joint secondary to trauma
  - Force applied to the MCP joint exceeds the strength of its capsuloligamentous support.
- Mechanism of injury
  - Mechanisms of injury include torsional, angular, and tractional forces across joint.
  - Dorsal dislocations may be caused by forced hyperextension.
  - Dislocation may be part of a more severe overall injury pattern including soft tissue injury to ligament, tendon, nerve, and/or vessels.
- Epidemiology/background
  - Dislocations of MCP joints are not very common.
  - Often seen in laborers or athletes
  - Males are affected more than females.

EVALUATION

- History
  - Typically caused by trauma, either direct or indirect
  - Presentation is usually acute due to deformity and pain.
  - May be overlooked initially in polytrauma cases
- Physical examination
  - Digit may be held in extension at the MCP with flexion at proximal interphalangeal and distal interphalangeal.
  - Palmar skin puckering indicates a complex dislocation.

- Assess for edema, angular deformity, rotational deformity, and quality of soft tissues.
- Identify any lacerations, and rule out open dislocation.
- Assess sensation and capillary refill distally.
- Assess the other digits as well as the hand and wrist.
  - Imaging/assessment
    - Obtain hand radiograph if MCP joint dislocation is suspected.
    - Brewerton view may help to identify fractures or joint dislocation.
    - Identify any fractures if present.
  - Classification
    - As with other dislocations, the nomenclature of direction of dislocation is based on which way the distal bone dislocates relative to the proximal bone.
    - Dorsal dislocations—P1 is dislocated dorsally relative to the metacarpal head.
    - Volar dislocations (uncommon)—The proximal phalanx (P1) is dislocated volarly relative to the metacarpal head.

ACUTE MANAGEMENT

- Emergency room management
  - Assess for other injuries
  - Comfort measures—pain control, elevation, splinting (remove splints for radiograph)
  - Remove all gloves, rings, and jewelry.
  - Elevation, ice
  - Radiographs (order hand radiograph, consider wrist or finger radiograph if indicated)

TREATMENT

- Dorsal dislocations
  - Simple subluxation
    - ◆ Closed reduction is possible.
      - ✳ Volar plate draped over metacarpal head, not entrapped within MCP
      - ✳ Reduction maneuver
        - ▲ Flex wrist to relax the flexor tendons

- ▲ Apply distal and volar pressure to the proximal phalanx base to guide it over the metacarpal head.
- ▲ Forearm-based dorsal blocking splint applied, and early motion encouraged
  - ◆ Closed reduction is not possible if the volar plate is displaced into the MCP joint (complex dislocation).
    - ✳ Can occur if axial traction or hyperextension are applied
    - ✳ Palmar skin puckering is pathognomonic.
    - ✳ Sesamoid within the joint is a radiographic sign.
    - ✳ Flexor tendons and lumbricals surround and entrap the metacarpal head.
    - ✳ They are further tightened when more traction is applied.
- Complex dislocation
  - ◆ Metacarpal head is entrapped between the flexor tendons and lumbricals.
  - ◆ Patients will have MCP joint held in extension, unable to flex.
  - ◆ Open reduction is required, generally through a volar, dorsal, or combined approach.
    - ✳ Entrapped structures should always be reduced with a blunt instrument (eg, Freer elevator) to avoid chondral injury.
    - ✳ Volar approach has the advantage of allowing direct visualization of entrapped structures, but puts neurovascular bundle at risk.
      - ▲ A1 pulley can also be released if needed.
      - ▲ Radial digital nerve and artery at risk in volar approach to index MCP dislocations; can be tented over the metacarpal head
      - ▲ Ulnar digital neurovascular bundle similarly at risk in small finger
    - ✳ Dorsal approach has the benefit of visualizing the dislocated phalanx and avoiding neurovascular bundle.
      - ▲ Split the extensor tendon or sagittal band.
      - ▲ If it is preventing reduction, the volar plate may be split longitudinally.
      - ▲ Shearing fractures on the metacarpal head may be identified and treated from dorsal approach.
- Postoperative care
  - ◆ Splint in 30° of flexion for 2 weeks.
  - ◆ Start active range of motion with dorsal block splint at 10° of MCP flexion for 2 weeks, and wean out of splint over the next 4 weeks.

- ◆ Buddy tape for 4 weeks.
- ◆ Advance to unrestricted use at 12 weeks post-op.
- ● Complications
  - ◆ Stiffness
  - ◆ Digital nerve injury
  - ◆ Arthritis
- ■ Volar dislocations
  - ● Rare injury
  - ● Usually reducible with closed means
  - ● Reduction can be blocked by interposed structures.
    - ◆ Volar plate
    - ◆ Collateral ligaments
    - ◆ Dorsal capsule
    - ◆ Juncturae tendinum
  - ● Surgical indications
    - ◆ Irreducible dislocation
  - ● Approach
    - ◆ Dorsal approach is recommended.
- ■ Thumb MCP dislocations
  - ● Usually dorsal
  - ● Usually reducible closed, but may be blocked by volar plate or flexor pollicis longus tendon
  - ● Flexor pollicis longus displaced ulnarly with thenar muscles remaining radial to the metacarpal head
  - ● Reduction maneuver
    - ◆ Avoid axial traction.
    - ◆ Hyperextend the MCP joint and then apply distal pressure to the proximal phalanx base to glide it over the metacarpal head.
  - ● Irreducible dislocations may be approached from a dorsal, volar, or lateral approach.
    - ◆ Volar approach allows visualization of injured volar structures, which may need to be repaired.
    - ◆ Collateral ligaments should be examined for stability following reduction; if grade III instability remains, consider repair or reconstruction.
  - ● Postoperative care
    - ◆ Thumb spica splint positioned in flexion of 10° beyond the point of instability for 2 weeks
    - ◆ Gradually extend 10° per week.

- Complications
  - Stiffness
  - Digital nerve injury
  - Arthritis

SUGGESTED READINGS

Baltera RM, Hastings H II. Fractures and dislocations: hand. In: Hammert WC, ed. *ASSH Manual of Hand Surgery*. Philadelphia, PA: Lippincott Williams & Wilkins; 2010:93-110.

Calfee RP, Sommerkamp TG. Fracture-dislocation about the finger joints. *J Hand Surg Am*. 2009;34(6):1140-1147.

Merrell G, Slade JF. Dislocations and ligament injuries in the digits. In: Wolfe SW, Hotchkiss RN, Pederson WC, Kozin SH, eds. *Green's Operative Hand Surgery*. 6th ed. Philadelphia, PA: Churchill Livingstone; 2010:291-332.

Shah CM, Sommerkamp TG. Fracture dislocation of the finger joints. *J Hand Surg Am*. 2014;39(4):792-802.

Malunion and Nonunion of Fingers and Hand

Tiffany Y. Wu and John R. Fowler

INTRODUCTION

- Pathoanatomy
  - Malunions are usually multiplanar, though one component is predominant.
  - Nonunions are rare (0.2%-0.7% incidence) and mostly atrophic.
  - Nonunions can be due to bone loss, osteomyelitis, inadequate immobilization, or poor fixation.
- Mechanism of injury
  - Angulation—transverse fracture
    - Metacarpal fractures typically have an apex dorsal angulation due to deforming forces of intrinsic muscles and extrinsic flexors.
    - Proximal phalanx fractures typically have an apex volar angulation due to the lumbricals flexing the proximal fragment and the central slip extending distal fragment.
    - Middle phalanx fractures typically have an apex dorsal angulation if the fracture is proximal to the flexor digitorum superficialis insertion and apex volar angulation if the fracture is distal to the flexor digitorum superficialis insertion.
    - If phalanx angulation >15°, then the bone is shortened relative to the extensor tendon. If phalanx angulation >25°, then both flexion and extension are compromised.
  - Rotational—spiral/oblique fracture
    - 5° of malrotation results in 1.5 cm of digital overlap.
  - Shortening—comminuted fracture, crush injury, or open fracture
    - Metacarpal—2 mm of shortening results in 7° of extensor lag and 8% loss of power. 10 mm of shortening results in 45% to 55% loss of power.
    - Proximal phalanx—1 m of shortening results in 12° extensor lag.
  - Intra-articular malunion

EVALUATION

- History
  - Injury, treatment, and duration
  - Location—phalanx versus metacarpal, extra-articular versus intra-articular
  - Complicating factors—infection, pain syndrome
  - Associated injuries—soft tissue defects, neurovascular injuries
  - Patient characteristics—skeletal maturity, hand dominance, occupation, pain, compliance with postoperative protocols
- Physical examination
  - Cosmetic deformity
    - Angular deformity
    - Scissoring—affected finger overlaps adjacent finger. Normally, fingertips should point to scaphoid tuberosity with fingers flexed.
    - Pseudoclawing—Proximal phalanx malunion >25° to 30° results in proximal interphalangeal (PIP) joint extensor lag, which can result in a fixed PIP joint flexion contracture, with resultant hyperextension at metacarpophalangeal joint.
  - Diminished grip and dexterity
  - Stiffness
- Imaging
  - Radiographs—anteroposterior, lateral, oblique
  - Radiographs of contralateral hand can be helpful as preoperative templates for complex malunions.
  - Consider computed tomography for complex malunions.

DEFINITIVE TREATMENT OF MALUNION

- Nonoperative treatment
  - Hand therapy to maximize digit range of motion (ROM), promote tendon excursion, and improve grip strength
  - Angulation—can tolerate up to 10° in index/middle fingers, 20° in ring finger, and 30° in small finger
  - Metacarpal can tolerate up to 5 to 6 mm of shortening.
  - Phalanx can tolerate up to 3 mm of shortening.

- Surgical indications
  - Significant functional or cosmetic problems
  - Osteotomy is rarely indicated for length alone unless it creates a bony block (eg, spiral fractures with a spike protruding into PIP joint or subcondylar fracture malunions), in which case it can be removed through a volar approach.
  - Consider arthrodesis/amputation rather than osteotomy when there is associated joint stiffness, unstable soft tissue coverage, or osteomyelitis.
- Surgical approach
  - Dorsal approach for 2nd through 4th metacarpals
  - Midaxial approach for 5th metacarpal and proximal/middle phalanges
  - Angular deformity—osteotomy at old fracture site allows correction of multiple deformities as well as concurrent tenolysis/capsulotomy.
    - Closing wedge osteotomy (Figure 13.1)
      - Most common; useful in the setting of intrinsic tightness

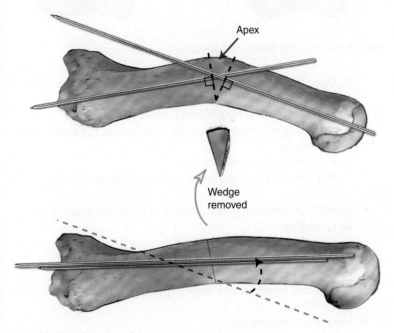

FIGURE 13.1 Closing wedge osteotomy.

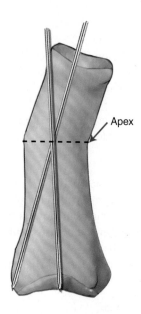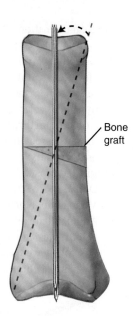

Apex

Bone
graft

FIGURE 13.2 Opening wedge osteotomy.

- ◆ Opening wedge osteotomy with cancellous/corticocancellous bone graft (Figure 13.2)
  - ✳ Useful in the setting of concomitant shortening
- ◆ Surgical pearl—hinge osteotomy through intact opposite cortex
- ◆ Fixation
  - ✳ Dorsal plate for metacarpals
  - ✳ Lateral plate for phalanges and coronal plane correction
  - ✳ K-wires
- Rotational deformity—osteotomy at proximal metaphysis of malunited bone
  - ◆ Complete transverse osteotomy
  - ◆ Step-cut osteotomy with lag screw fixation (Figure 13.3)
  - ◆ Surgical pearl—Place temporary K-wires perpendicular to long axis proximal and distal to osteotomy to assess rotational correction.
- Intra-articular deformity
  - ◆ If fracture line can be visualized and bone quality is satisfactory, can perform osteotomy through fracture
  - ◆ Condylar advancement osteotomy (Figure 13.4)

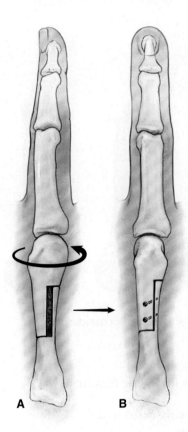

FIGURE 13.3 Step-cut osteotomy. A, Two horizontal cuts are placed in shaft about 2.5 cm apart and a longitudinal wedge cut connecting the two horizontal cuts is made. Derotation of distal fragment opposite the deformity. B, Reduction of the osteotomy and fixation with two interfragmentary screws.

- ◆ For chronic PIP joint fracture/dislocation, can perform hemi-hamate arthroplasty
- ◆ For severe deformities or arthritic joints, consider arthrodesis or arthroplasty.
- ● Nonunion
  - ◆ Resection of pseudoarthrosis, bone grafting, internal fixation
  - ◆ External minifixator and bone grafting
  - ◆ For distal phalanx, can use semistructural bone peg (±K-wire) or compressive screw

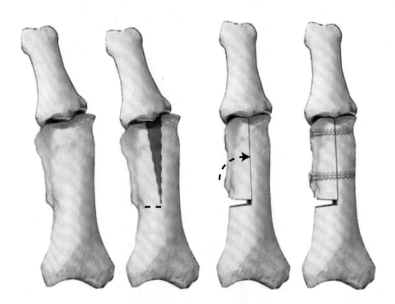

FIGURE 13.4 Condylar advancement osteotomy.

- Potential complications
  - Incomplete or inadequate correction
  - Stiffness
  - Iatrogenic damage to soft tissues
- Postoperative care
  - Forearm-based splint with the wrist mildly extended and the metacarpophalangeal joint immobilized in 60° to 70° of flexion and the interphalangeal joint in full extension
  - Stable fixation allows early active and active-assisted ROM (eg, 3-5 days postoperatively) with progression to passive ROM exercises.
  - When not performing ROM exercises, rest hand in volar splint and elevate.
  - Edema control with elastic garment or compression bandage

SUGGESTED READINGS

Gajendran VK, Gajendran VK, Malone KJ. Management of complications with hand fractures. *Hand Clin.* 2015;31(2):165-177.

Manketlow RT, Mahoney JL. Step osteotomy: a precise rotation osteotomy to correct scissoring deformities of the fingers. *Plast Reconstr Surg.* 1981;68:571-576.

Weckesser EC. Rotational osteotomy of the metacarpal for overlapping fingers. *J Bone Joint Surg Am*. 1965;47:751-756.

Wiesel SW. *Operative Techniques in Orthopaedic Surgery*. Philadelphia, PA: Wolters Kluwer; 2015.

Wolfe SW, Hotchkiss RN, Pederson WC, Kozin SH. *Green's Operative Hand Surgery*. Philadelphia, PA: Elsevier/Churchill Livingstone; 2011.

14 Scaphoid Fractures

Adam S. Martin and Hisham M. Awan

INTRODUCTION

- The scaphoid is the most commonly fractured carpal bone. Although the scaphoid is named for its resemblance to a boat shape (Greek *skafos* = boat), it is often referred to as a twisted peanut shape (Figure 14.1).[1,2] The scaphoid spans both the proximal and distal carpal rows and plays a key role in stability of the carpus. The scaphoid comprises three regions: distal pole (tubercle), waist, and proximal pole. The diagnosis of a scaphoid fracture can be challenging due to delayed patient presentation or the occult nature of the fracture on early radiographs. Malunion or nonunion of scaphoid fractures can lead to altered carpal kinematics, diminished grip strength, and radiocarpal arthritis.

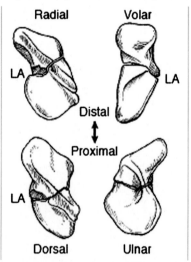
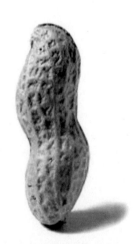

FIGURE 14.1 Bony anatomy of scaphoid. LA, lateral apex. From Ring D, Jupiter JB, Herndon JH. Acute fractures of the scaphoid. *J Am Acad Orthop Surg.* 2000;8:225-231.

- Mechanism of injury—Injury to the scaphoid is typically from a fall on an outstretched hand (35%), which causes extreme wrist extension and compression of the scaphoid against the distal radius. Similar forces can also be generated during athletic competition (59%). High-energy mechanisms such as a fall from height or motor vehicle collision contribute to the remaining scaphoid fractures.
- Epidemiology—The scaphoid is the most frequently fractured bone in the carpus. The most common demographic for this injury are males in their 20s to 30s.[3,4] The reported incidence in the United States is 1.47 per 100 000 person-years, although a study of the U.S. military found a higher incidence of scaphoid fractures with 121 per 100 000 person-years. This injury is relatively rare in children and elderly adults.
- Blood supply—The scaphoid receives blood from two main sources.[5] The proximal pole of the scaphoid is notoriously high risk for avascular necrosis (AVN) because it receives its blood in a retrograde fashion from the dorsal scaphoid branches of the radial artery. These branches supply approximately 80% of the bone and enter the scaphoid via the nonarticular dorsal ridge and distal tubercle. The second source of blood is from the volar scaphoid branches of radial artery, which enter the bone at the scaphoid tubercle and supply the distal 20% of the scaphoid.

EVALUATION

- Presentation—Patients often present with radial-sided wrist pain that localizes to the anatomic snuffbox and is worse with gripping or squeezing. They may recall a specific traumatic event that coincides with the onset of pain. If patients present early, they may report swelling or ecchymosis around the wrist. If the injury is chronic, then the patient may complain of loss of wrist range of motion (ROM), weakness, and difficulty performing push-ups.
- Physical examination—On examination, tenderness to palpation in the anatomic snuffbox or distal tubercle of scaphoid should raise suspicion for a scaphoid fracture (Figure 14.2). In addition, compression of the thumb metacarpal against the scaphoid can be performed to elicit pain. Careful evaluation of remaining wrist and elbow should be performed to rule out any concomitant injuries.
- Imaging—Posteroanterior (PA) in neutral and ulnar deviation (scaphoid), lateral, and 45° oblique radiographs (Figure 14.3) should be obtained.

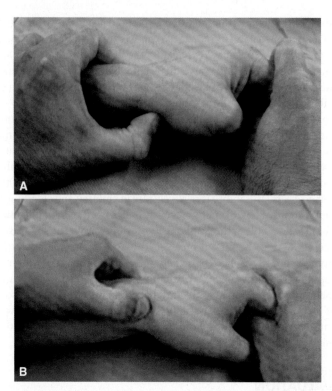

FIGURE 14.2 PE tests for suspected scaphoid fracture. A, palpation of scaphoid tubercle (distal pole); B, palpation of anatomic snuffbox (proximal pole). From Scaphoid fractures. http://morphopedics.wikidot.com/scaphoid-fractures.

Note: Up to 25% of nondisplaced fractures may not be visible on plain radiographs until 7 to 14 days after initial injury.

- A computerized tomography (CT) scan can be a useful adjunct to evaluate fracture displacement or fracture healing. Despite the fact that most acutely treated scaphoid fractures require approximately 3 months to heal, union cannot be easily identified by standard radiographs even at 3 months.
- Magnetic resonance imaging (MRI) can be used to diagnose a fracture when plain radiographs are negative but suspicion remains high. MRI is the most reliable method for early diagnosis of occult fractures.
- Differential diagnosis
  - Distal radius fracture
  - First metacarpal fracture

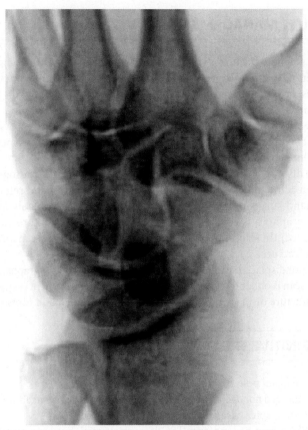

FIGURE 14.3 Scaphoid fracture on radiograph. From Ring D, Jupiter JB, Herndon, JH. Acute fractures of the scaphoid. *J Am Acad Orthop Surg.* 2000;8:225-231.

- Scapholunate ligament injury
- DeQuervain's tenosynovitis
- Carpometacarpal arthritis
- Classification—Scaphoid fractures can be classified by location, chronicity, and stability.[6] The stability has been stratified according to the Herbert's classification system, which divides fractures into four groups: Type A = stable acute, Type B = unstable acute, Type C = delayed union, and Type D = nonunion. Fractures with >1 mm of displacement are considered unstable.

ACUTE MANAGEMENT

- If a scaphoid fracture is suspected but not evident on initial radiographs, then the patient is provisionally treated as if a scaphoid fracture is present and is placed into a thumb spica splint (TSS).[3] At this point, either an early MRI is obtained or radiographs are repeated in 2 weeks. The provisional treatment of a suspected fracture is based on evidence that failure to treat a stable scaphoid fracture within 4 weeks increases the nonunion rate.
- If a displaced scaphoid fracture is identified on initial radiographs, then acute management consists of TSS application and referral to a hand surgeon for fixation. Provided that approximately 80% of the scaphoid is covered in articular cartilage, no fracture callus is formed; therefore, bone healing is contingent on rigid stability of the fracture.
- If a nondisplaced scaphoid fracture is seen on initial radiographs, then a CT scan is obtained to further evaluate for any displacement (Figure 14.4) as fracture displacement is poorly characterized on plain films.

DEFINITIVE TREATMENT

- Stable distal pole fractures
  - Managed nonoperatively via immobilization in a below- or above-elbow thumb spica cast (TSC) for approximately 6 weeks[3,5]
  - Short-arm or long-arm TSC is controversial, but long-arm cast is theorized to decrease time to union by preventing forearm rotation. Several randomized control trials (RCTs) and meta-analyses have been published comparing different types of casts, and, overall, there is insufficient evidence to guide cast selection.
- Stable waist fractures
  - Managed nonoperatively via immobilization in an above-elbow TSC for 6 weeks. Then patient is transitioned into a below-elbow TSC for another 6 weeks or until radiographic union is obtained. May consider early operative fixation for athletes or manual laborers to allow earlier return to activity.
- Stable proximal pole fractures
  - Given the high risk of AVN, up to 40% reported in the literature, any fracture of proximal pole is usually treated operatively.

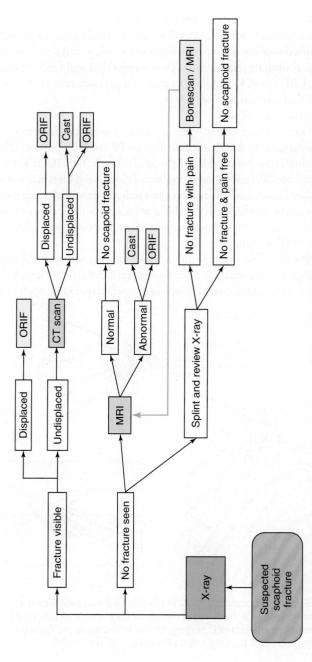

FIGURE 14.4 Management Algorithm of a Suspected Scaphoid Fracture. Abbreviations: CT, computerized tomography; MRI, magnetic resonance imaging; ORIF, open reduction internal fixation.

- ■ Unstable (displaced) distal pole or waist fractures
  - Typically require surgical intervention; commonly a volar approach is utilized to allow better visualization or access to distal pole/waist. Surgical options include volar closed reduction and internal fixation (CRIF) with K-wires or headless compression screws, or open reduction internal fixation (ORIF).
  - Volar CRIF technique
    - ◆ Place wrist in extension with aid of rolled towels; then hold in ulnar deviation with thumb traction; then use IV needle to locate starting point: 2 mm dorsal and ulnar to tip of tubercle, then insert K-wire thru needle; then confirm position of K-wire and then insert centrally in the scaphoid; next, make a stab incision at wire and use a hemostat on wire flush with bone to measure length; then remove IV needle, hand drill over wire, and insert screw (Figure 14.5).
  - Volar ORIF technique
    - ◆ Patient supine on hand table; incision centered over scaphoid tubercle—proximally is same flexor carpi radialis (FCR) approach, distally is angled toward thumb carpometacarpal joint; open FCR

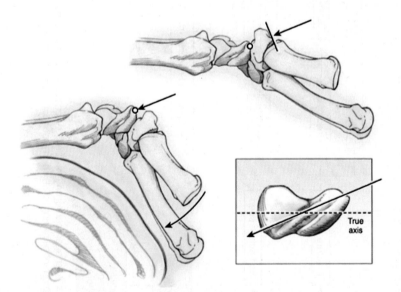

FIGURE 14.5 Volar percutaneous scaphoid fixation starting point. Reprinted from Geissler WB, Slade JF. Fractures of the carpal bones. In: Green DP, Wolfe SW, eds. *Green's Operative Hand Surgery.* 6th ed. Philadelphia, PA: Elsevier/Churchill Livingston; 2011. Copyright © 2011 Elsevier. With permission.

sheath, retract FCR ulnarly, and open FCR subsheath to expose joint capsule; distally develop same interval by splitting thenar muscles off scaphoid and trapezium; place freer in scapulothoracic joint to bluntly expose; then incise joint capsule; proximally: incise long radial lunate (RL) and radioscaphocapitate (RSC) ligaments; reduce fracture via traction ± dental pick ± reduction clamp ± joysticks, and then provisionally fix with 0.045 K-wire from distal to proximal, avoiding central axis (screw path); place central-axis guidewire: ideal starting point is 2 mm dorsal and ulnar to tip of tubercle; then measure length, drill, and place compression screw.

- Unstable (displaced) proximal pole fractures
  - Typically require surgical intervention; commonly a dorsal approach is utilized to allow better exposure or access to proximal pole. Surgical options include dorsal CRIF with K-wires or headless compression screws, or ORIF.
  - Keys to screw fixation include placing the screw along the central axis of the scaphoid and using the longest screw possible while still being sure to countersink the screw deep to articular surface to avoid hardware prominence.
    - Centrally placed screws have been shown to results in significantly shorter union times.
    - Longer screws provide more rigid fixation by reducing forces at the fracture site and distributing bending forces along the length of the screw.
  - Dorsal CRIF technique
    - Patient supine on hand table; to visualize the center axis, pronate wrist until scaphoid looks like cylinder on PA view, then flex wrist to get two poles of scaphoid to overlap like the ring sign; then use 14-gauge angiocath as guide for K-wire insertion: starting point is center of ring on fluoroscopic imaging or 2 mm radial to attachment of scapholunate (SL) ligament; drive K-wire toward scaphoid tubercle; use second guidewire to measure length on central-axis guidewire; in general, subtract 4 mm from measure length to be sure that screw will be countersunk; make skin incision over guidewire; bluntly dissect down to joint capsule; retract extensor pollicus longus (EPL) away; use cannulated reamer to ream 2 mm short of distal scaphoid surface; insert screw (Figure 14.6).
  - Dorsal ORIF technique
    - Patient supine on hand table; make 4 cm longitudinal incision from lister's tubercle to long axis of middle finger metacarpal;

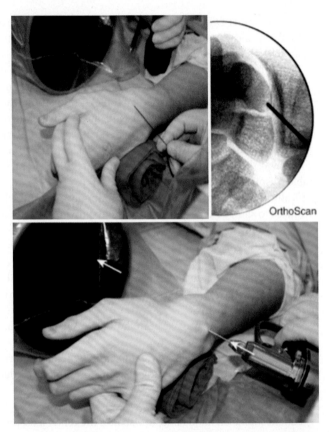

OrthoScan

FIGURE 14.6 Dorsal percutaneous scaphoid fixation starting point. Reprinted from Geissler WB, Slade JF. Fractures of the carpal bones. In: Green DP, Wolfe SW, eds. *Green's Operative Hand Surgery.* 6th ed. Philadelphia, PA: Elsevier/ Churchill Livingston; 2011. Copyright © 2011 Elsevier. With permission.

raise skin flaps at level of extensor retinaculum; incise retinaculum over 3rd dorsal compartment (DC), then release fascia over EPL to retract EPL radially; incise dorsal hand fascia longitudinally, then retract 2nd DC with EPL radially and extensor digitorum communis ulnarly to expose radiocarpal joint; make a "ligament sparing" capsulotomy by splitting the dorsal radiocarpal and dorsal intercarpal ligaments; to achieve reduction and provisional fixation, pull traction on IF, MF, and use K-wire joystick to reduce and then place 1 to 2 K-wires just off central axis;

then place central-axis guidewire with wrist in flexion to access ideal starting point of 2 mm radial to membranous portion of SL ligament; the trajectory of the guidewire is toward the scaphoid tubercle; finally measure, drill wire into trapezium so it doesn't loosen when drilling, ream to within 2 mm of far cortex under fluoroscopy, and place compression screw.

- Late management
  - Scaphoid fractures diagnosed on a delayed basis should be considered for operative fixation regardless of the degree of displacement.[2] This idea is based on several studies that fractures untreated for 4+ weeks are at higher risk for nonunion. The incidence of nonunion in this cohort has been reported to be anywhere from 20% to 80%.
- Postoperative protocol
  - At the first postoperative visit around 10 days after surgery, postop splint is removed, sutures are removed, and a custom, removable below-elbow TSS is used for 3 weeks.[3] In addition, radiographs are obtained to confirm hardware position.
  - Hand therapy may beneficial to work on ROM. Heavy lifting and weight-bearing activity are restricted until radiographic and clinical union is achieved. Once the fracture has united, the splint and activity restrictions are discontinued.
  - A CT can be used to confirm union before return to sport or heavy lifting.
- Management algorithm (Figure 14.7)

Types of Fracture	Treatment
Stable Fracture, Nondisplaced	
Tubercle fracture	Short arm cast for 6 to 8 weeks
Distal third Fracture/incomplete fracture	Short arm cast for 6 to 8 weeks

Waist fracture	Long arm thumb spica cast for 6 weeks, short arm cast for 6 weeks or until CT confirmed healing, especially for
	    Pediatric patients
	    Sedentary or low-demand patients
	    Preference for nonoperative treatment

	Percutaneous or open internal fixation, especially for
	    Active, young, manual worker
	    Athlete, high-demand occupation
	    Preference for early range of motion

FIGURE 14.7 (*Continued*)

Types of Fracture	Treatment
Proximal pole fracture, nondisplaced	Percutaneous or open internal fixation
Unstable Fractures	
Displacement >1 mm Lateral intrascaphoid angle >35° Bone loss or Communication Perilunate fracture-dislocation Dorsal intercalated segmental instability alignment	Dorsal percutaneous/open screw fixation

FIGURE 14.7 Scaphoid fracture management algorithm. Reprinted from Geissler WB, Slade JF. Fractures of the carpal bones. In: Green DP, Wolfe SW, eds. *Green's Operative Hand Surgery*. 6th ed. Philadelphia, PA: Elsevier/Churchill Livingston; 2011. Copyright © 2011 Elsevier. With permission.

COMPLICATIONS

- The reported complications of cast treatment include prolonged periods of immobilization, stiffness, decreased grip strength, delayed return to work or sport, and increased risk of nonunion depending on the fracture location and type.[3,5]
- Untreated scaphoid waist fractures can develop an apex dorsal angulation, commonly known as a "humpback" deformity. Flexion of the distal scaphoid fragment in conjunction with extension of the lunate via its ligamentous attachment to the proximal scaphoid fragment leads to a dorsal intercalated segmental instability deformity.
- Untreated scaphoid nonunion will undergo a predictable pattern of arthritis, otherwise known as scaphoid nonunion advanced collapse. Over 90% of patients with a scaphoid nonunion will demonstrate arthritic changes within 5 years.
- Complications of surgical intervention include nonunion, AVN, hardware failure, hardware prominence, and damage to surrounding tendons and neurovascular structures.

SUGGESTED READINGS

Wolf JM, Dawson L, Mountcastle SB, Owens BD. The incidence of scaphoid fracture in a military population. *Injury*. 2009;40:1316-1319.

Adams BD, Blair WF, Reagan DS, Grunberg AB. Technical factors related to Herbert screw fixation. *J Hand Surg Am.* 1988;13:893-899.

Gelberman RH, Menon J. The vascularity of the scaphoid bone. *J Hand Surg Am.* 1980;5:508-513.

Mack GR, Bosse MJ, Gelberman RH, Yu E. The natural history of scaphoid non-union. *J Bone Joint Surg Am.* 1984;66:504-509.

Trumble TE, Clarke T, Kreder HJ. Non-union of the scaphoid. Treatment with cannulated screws compared with treatment with Herbert screws. *J Bone Joint Surg Am.* 1996;78:1829-1837.

Kang L. Operative treatment of acute scaphoid fracture. *Hand Surg.* 2015;20(2):210-214.

Dias JJ, Wildin CJ, Bhowal B, Thompson JR. Should acute scaphoid fracture be fixed? A randomized controlled trial. *J Bone Joint Surg Am.* 2005;87:2160-2168.

REFERENCES

1. Tada K, Ikeda K, Okamoto S, Hachinota A, Yamamoto D, Tsuchiya H. Scaphoid fracture: overview and operative treatment. *Hand Surg.* 2015;20(2):204-209.

2. Ring D, Jupiter JB, Herndon JH. Acute fractures of the scaphoid. *J Am Acad Orthop Surg.* 2000;8:225-231.

3. Geissler, WB, Slade JF. Fractures of the carpal bones. In: Green DP, Wolfe SW, eds. *Green's Operative Hand Surgery.* Philadelphia, PA: Elsevier/Churchill Livingston; 2011.

4. Van Tassel DC, Owens BD, Wolf JM. Incidence estimates and demographics of scaphoid fracture in the U.S. population. *J Hand Surg Am.* 2010 August; 35(8):1242-1245.

5. Calfee RP, Berger R, Beredjiklian PK, et al. Fractures and dislocations: wrist. In: Hammert WC, Calfee RP, Bozentka DJ, Boyer MI, eds. *ASSH Manual of Hand Surgery.* Philadelphia, PA: Lippincott Williams & Wilkins; 2010.

6. Herbert TJ, Fisher WE. Management of the fractured scaphoid using a new bone screw. *J Bone Joint Surg Br.* 1984;66:114-123.

Michael Moustoukas and Nileshkumar M. Chaudhari

INTRODUCTION

- Overview
  - High-energy injury resulting in dislocation of capitate while lunate remains in lunate fossa.
    - Dorsal dislocation is most common
  - Carpal instability complex
    - Derangement within proximal row and between rows
  - Lesser arc injuries
    - Purely capsuloligamentous
  - Greater arc injuries
    - Concomitant fractures
      - Radial styloid, scaphoid, lunate, capitate, triquetrum, or ulna
- Anatomy[1]
  - Volar extrinsic ligaments
    - Provide primary stabilization of carpus
      - Long radiolunate ligament
      - Radioscapholunate
      - Short radiolunate
      - Ulnolunate
      - Radioscaphocapitate
      - Ulnotriquetrocapitate complex
  - Intrinsic carpal ligaments
    - Scapholunate interosseous ligament (SLIL)
    - Lunotriquetral interosseous ligament
    - Dorsal intercarpal ligament
    - Triquetrum–hamate–capitate complex
    - Dorsolateral scapho-trapezio-trapezoid ligament
    - Scaphocapitate ligament

- Greater arc injuries
  - Transscaphoid perilunate fracture–dislocations
    - Most common perilunate injury
  - Transscaphoid, transcapitate perilunate fracture–dislocations
    - Capitate fracture often missed and results in nonunion, necrosis
  - Transtriquetrum perilunate fracture–dislocations
- Mechanism of injury
  - Axial load with wrist hyperextension, ulnar deviation, midcarpal supination
  - Mayfield classification
    - Predictable pattern of carpal injury
      - Scapholunate dissociation or scaphoid fracture
      - Lunocapitate dislocation
      - Lunotriquetrum dissociation or triquetrum fracture
        - Perilunate dislocation
      - Lunate dislocation
- Epidemiology
  - Less than 10% of all wrist injuries
  - Approximately 60% are trans-scaphoid perilunate dislocations
  - 16% to 25% missed at presentation

EVALUATION

- History
  - Mechanism of injury
- Physical examination
  - Swelling, resistance to motion, tenderness with acute injuries
  - Palpation of carpal bones
  - Thorough neurovascular examination
    - 24% to 45% have median nerve dysfunction
  - Wrist appearance may be benign with chronic injuries
- Imaging
  - Four views of the wrist
    - Posteroanterior (PA), lateral, oblique, and ulnar deviated with clenched fist
    - PA view
      - Scrutinize continuity of Gilula lines
      - SLIL disruption—>2 mm scapholunate (SL) interval or "scaphoid ring sign"

- Lateral view
  - Loss of continuity between radius, lunate, and capitate
- Carpal alignment
  - Scapholunate angle (30°-60°)
  - Radiolunate angle (−15° to 15°)
- CT scan to characterize fractures

ACUTE MANAGEMENT

- Initially treat with 10 minutes of weighted longitudinal traction and finger traps. Elbow at 90°
- Closed reduction with adequate muscle relaxation
  - Stable reduction achieved in 90% of cases
  - Reduces pressure on median nerve
  - Relieves strain on vascular supply to carpal bones
  - Technique
    - Wrist extension + longitudinal traction
    - Volar stabilization of lunate with other thumb
    - Gradual wrist flexion reduces capitate into the concave surface of the lunate.

DEFINITIVE TREATMENT

- Treatment goals
  - Restoration of intercarpal relationships
  - Repair of interosseous ligamentous injuries
  - Stable fixation of fractures
- Nonoperative treatment
  - Closed reduction and casting
    - Associated with poor outcomes and eventual wrist deformity and pain
    - Only used when medical health precludes surgery
- Surgical treatment
  - Closed reduction and percutaneous pinning
  - Open treatment with interosseous ligament repair and fracture fixation
- Operative technique of acute injuries

- Dorsal approach
  - Longitudinal incision ulnar to Lister tubercle
  - Mobilize extensor pollicus longus out of third compartment
  - Wrist capsule usually avulsed from radius
  - Reduce SL, LT joints. Stabilize with K-wires
    - Scaphocapitate and triquetrohamate pinning to support ligamentous repair
  - Fracture fixation with headless, cannulated screws
  - Ligamentous repair with suture anchors
    - SLIL usually avulses from scaphoid
- Dorsal + volar approach
  - Dorsal approach and fixation as above
  - Extended carpal tunnel release
    - Veer ulnarly at proximal wrist crease to avoid palmar cutaneous branch
  - Reliable arciform capsular rent
    - Repair ulnar side of capsule
- Pinning lunate to radius shown to decrease rate of ulnocarpal instability
- Avoid excising comminuted radial styloid fragments
  - Radiocarpal ligaments are attached and can lead to instability.
- Postoperative care
  - Thumb spica splint transitioned to short arm, thumb spica cast at 2 weeks
  - Immobilization for 6 to 8 weeks
  - Pin removal at 8 to 10 weeks post-op
- Potential complications
  - Stiffness
  - Median nerve dysfunction
  - Carpal instability
  - Complex regional pain syndrome
  - Post-traumatic arthritis
  - Loss of grip strength
  - Transient ischemia of lunate may be visible on post-op radiographs.
    - Usually benign and self-limiting
- Outcomes
  - Majority of patients have permanent loss of wrist motion and grip strength.
    - Approximately 70% of contralateral side

- Requires long periods of immobilization
- Risk factors for poor outcome
  - Open injuries
  - Delayed presentation
  - Damage to capitate proximal articular surface
  - Carpal malalignment

REFERENCE

1. Stanbury SJ, Elfar JC. Perilunate dislocation and perilunate fracture-dislocation. *J Am Acad Orthop Surg.* 2011;19(9):554-562.

16 Hook of Hamate Fractures

Katherine M. Dederer and Reid W. Draeger

INTRODUCTION

- Incidence and epidemiology
  - Hook of hamate fractures are estimated at 2% of all carpal fractures[1]
  - Likely underreported due to chronic or low-level symptoms in patients who never present to a hand surgeon or in whom standard radiographs fail to reveal the fracture[2]
  - Most common in athletes involved in racquet or striking sports such as those playing baseball, hockey, golf, and tennis from direct transfer of force during contact or shearing forces associated with ulnar deviation of the wrist during swing[3]
  - Commonly presents in a delayed fashion 5 to 10 months postinjury[4,5]
- Mechanism
  - Typically involves the nondominant hand in golfers and baseball players and the dominant hand in racquet sport athletes
  - May be caused by a sudden direct blow such as striking the ground with a golf club, or an injury from repetitive trauma such as batting[6]
  - Also seen in laborers, construction workers, and others subject to repetitive mechanical trauma to the ulnar hand

ANATOMY

- Located in the ulnar palm radial to the pisiform and ulnar to the transverse carpal ligament
- Ulnar artery is typically found radial or volar to the hook, while the sensory and motor branches of the ulnar nerve may be found ulnar or volar to the hook and are vulnerable to injury during surgery (Figure 16.1).[7]

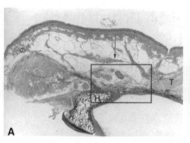 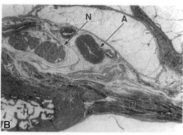

FIGURE 16.1 Cross-sectional anatomy of the volar ulnar wrist. A, ulnar nerve and artery are volar to the hook of the hamate (bottom, labeled H), B, enlargement showing the ulnar nerve (N) and artery (A) volar and radial to the hook of the hamate, respectively. T, thenar musculature; R, flexor retinaculum. Reprinted from Cobb TK, Carmichael SW, Cooney WP. Guyon's canal revisited: an anatomic study of the carpal ulnar neurovascular space. *J Hand Surg.* 1996;21:861-869. Copyright © 1996, with permission from Elsevier.

- Attachments
  - The hamate hook is the site of origin for the flexor digiti minimi muscle, opponens digiti minimi muscle, hypothenar muscles, piso-hamate ligaments, and abuts the distal ulnar extent of the transverse carpal ligament.[8]
    - Hook of the hamate is prominent just radial and distal to the pisiform; total dorsal-volar size averages 26 mm from dorsal cortex to tip of hook.[9]
    - Three anatomic variations from the normal anatomy of the hamate hook: bipartite, hypoplastic, and hook aplastic (Figure 16.2)[10]
    - Fractures may occur at the base, waist, or tip of the hook, although base fractures are most common (Figure 16.3).[11]
    - Blood supply
      - Most of the hook is fed via a basal nutrient artery, which originates from the ulnar artery at the level of Guyon's canal.
      - 71% of patients have a nutrient artery to the tip of the hook, creating a watershed area at the waist of the hook (Figure 16.4).[12]
      - Risk for nonunion and avascular necrosis with waist or tip fractures
- Biomechanics
  - Hook acts as a fulcrum for flexor tendons to the ring and small fingers, increasing grip power.

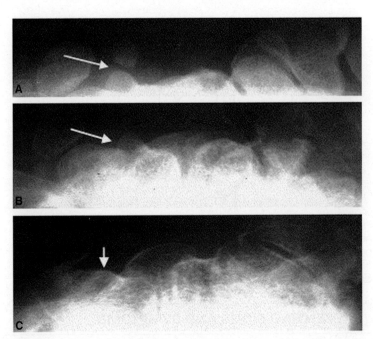

FIGURE 16.2 Types of hamate hooks. A, Bipartite hook (arrow), B, Hypoplastic hook (arrow), C, Aplastic hook (arrow). Reprinted from Chow JC, Weiss MA, Gu Y. Anatomic variations of the hook of hamate and the relationship to carpal tunnel syndrome. *J Hand Surg Am.* 2005;30(6):1242-1247. Copyright © 2005 American Society for Surgery of the Hand. With permission.

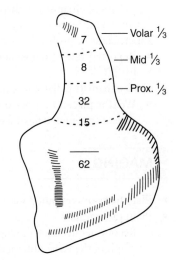

FIGURE 16.3 Of 62 identified hook of hamate fractures, 47 were located in the proximal one-third of the hook. Reprinted with permission from Stark HH, Chao EK, Zemel NP, et al. Fracture of the hook of the hamate. *J Bone Joint Surg Am.* 1989;71(8):1202-1207.

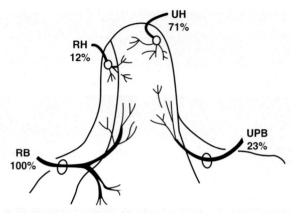

FIGURE 16.4   Presence of various nutrient arteries to the hook of the hamate. RH, radial hook; UH, ulnar hook; RB, radial base; UPB, ulnar palmar branch. Reprinted from Failla J. Hook of hamate vascularity: vulnerability to osteonecrosis and nonunion. *J Hand Surg Am*. 1993;18(6):1075-1079. Copyright © 1993 Elsevier Inc. With permission.

PRESENTING SIGNS AND SYMPTOMS

- Tenderness to palpation in ulnar palm 2 cm distal to and radial to the pisiform, in line with the first metacarpal head
- Presenting complaints may also include weakness in wrist flexion, ulnar digit flexion, and grip along with ulnar nerve paresthesias, or occasionally ulnar artery thrombosis
- Chronic injuries may also present as ruptures of the flexor digitorum superficialis or profundus tendons to the ring or small fingers.[13,14]
  - Reported rate of tenosynovitis, tendon rupture, or fraying in 14% to 25%[13,15]
- Hook of hamate pull test may be used to elicit pain with stress to the hook.
  - Wrist is placed in ulnar deviation and the examiner's hand resists patient's attempted flexion of the ring and small fingers (Figure 16.5).[16]

IMAGING

- Plain films or computed tomography (CT) scan may be used.
- Plain radiographs
  - Recommended views include a carpal tunnel view or oblique radiograph of the wrist obtained in 45° of supination.[17]

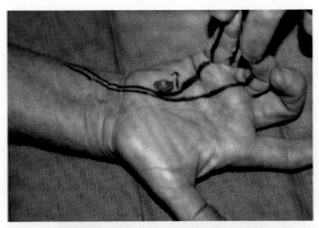

FIGURE 16.5 Location of hook of hamate marked in red. Flexor digitorum profundus tendons to ring and small fingers are drawn in black. Arrow indicates direction of force applied by tendons around hook as the examiner resists the patient's flexion of the ring and small fingers. Reprinted from Wright TW, Moser MW, Sahajpal DT. Hook of hamate pull test. *J Hand Surg Am.* 2010;35(11):1887-1889. Copyright © 2010 American Society for Surgery of the Hand. With permission.

- Look for absence of the hook, sclerosis, or irregularity in the cortex.[18]
- Reported sensitivity of plain radiographs of 31%, and 40% to 50% sensitivity of a carpal tunnel view in identifying hook fractures (Figure 16.6)[5,19]

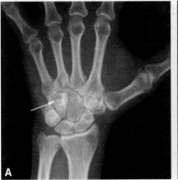
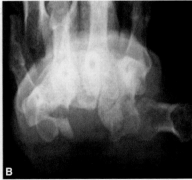

FIGURE 16.6 A, Anteroposterior radiograph and B, carpal tunnel view revealing a displaced hook of hamate fracture. Reprinted from O'Shea K, Weiland AJ. Fractures of the hamate and pisiform bones. *Hand Clin.* 2012;28(3):287-300. Copyright © 2012 Elsevier Inc. With permission.

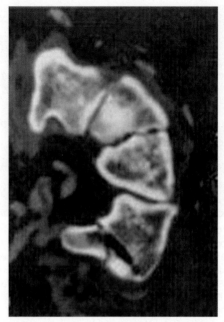

FIGURE 16.7 Axial computed tomography scan revealing fracture through the base of the hamate hook. Reprinted with permission from Andresen R, Radmer S, Sparmann M, et al. Imaging of hamate bone fractures in conventional X-rays and high-resolution computed tomography: an in vitro study. *Invest Radiol.* 1999;34(1):46-50.

- CT scan
  - Greater than 95% sensitivity and specificity in diagnosis; given the low sensitivity of the carpal tunnel radiograph, a CT scan is recommended to confirm the diagnosis when there is a high level of clinical suspicion for a hook of hamate fracture (Figure 16.7).[17]

MANAGEMENT

- Nonoperative treatment
  - More likely to be successful in acute injuries compared with chronic injuries, although a 50% nonunion rate has been reported in acute, nondisplaced fractures treated nonoperatively.[6]
  - Generally not recommended for chronic injuries due to poor success rates

- Method
  - ◆ Immobilization in an ulnar gutter cast for 3 weeks followed by short-arm cast for an additional 3 weeks
  - ◆ Gradual return to activities beginning at 6 weeks
- Complications
  - ◆ 15% rate of flexor tendon rupture, thought to be due to chronic attrition[20]
- Operative treatment
  - Recommended for acute, displaced fractures or chronic fractures
  - Surgical excision versus open reduction and internal fixation (ORIF) (see Controversies)
  - Surgical excision
    - ◆ No adverse effects on grip strength or active wrist range of motion[21]
    - ◆ Care must be taken to protect the ulnar nerve and artery (see Technique Guide: Hook of Hamate Excision).
  - Cast/splint placed at conclusion of procedure to protect wound for 2 weeks
  - Return to play generally guided by scar sensitivity after 2 weeks postoperatively
  - May hasten return to play with use of padded gloves
  - Complications
    - ◆ Reported at a rate of 3%, and most commonly involve injury to the motor branch of the ulnar nerve[22]

CONTROVERSIES

- Decreased finger flexion and grip strength?
  - One study reported 96% of patients with return to normal grip strength and preoperative level of function by 6 months postoperatively.[23]
  - Later cadaveric study reporting 11% to 15% decreased finger flexor strength[24]
- ORIF versus excision?
  - ORIF results in variable rates of healing and is particularly not recommended in athletes in whom a reliable return to play is crucial.[5]
  - Theoretically decreases risk of loss of grip strength associated with excision
  - Can be performed via dorsal percutaneous insertion of a cannulated screw with reports of successful union in a small series of patients[25]

TECHNIQUE GUIDE: HOOK OF HAMATE EXCISION

- Palpate hook 2 cm distal and radial to pisiform on volar hand, and under tourniquet create a 2-to-3-cm curvilinear incision centered over the hook on the radial margin of the hypothenar eminence.
- Bluntly dissect through subcutaneous fat until ulnar artery and nerve are identified proximally, and trace distally past the hook of the hamate. Protect throughout the case.
- Identify and release the distal aspect of the transverse carpal ligament, which abuts the radial margin of the hook.
- Take care to identify and isolate the motor branch of the ulnar nerve, which typically lies near the base of the hook of the hamate.
- Subperiosteally dissect down the hook from palmar to dorsal until the fracture site is identified and remove the free fragment.
- Palpate for any rough bony edges remaining on the hamate body and use a rasp to smooth them as needed.
- Close the retained periosteum over the remaining hamate body to minimize irritation to the surrounding structures.
- Close the skin with interrupted monofilament suture and place a volar splint or soft dressing (Figure 16.8).[6,21]

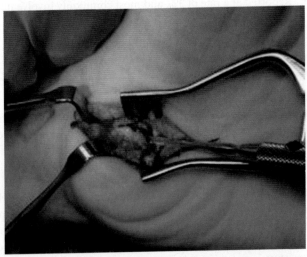

FIGURE 16.8 Subperiosteal excision of the hamate hook. Reprinted with permission from Andresen R, Radmer S, Sparmann M, et al. Imaging of hamate bone fractures in conventional X-rays and high-resolution computed tomography: an in vitro study. *Invest Radiol*. 1999;34(1):46-50.

REFERENCES

1. Andress MR, Peckar VG. Fracture of the hook of the hamate. *Br J Radiol.* 1970;43:141-143.
2. Nisenfield FG, Neviaser RJ. Fractures of the hook of the hamate: a diagnosis easily missed. *J Trauma.* 1974;14:612-616.
3. Urch EY, Lee SK. Carpal fractures other than scaphoid. *Clin Sports Med.* 2015;34(1):51-67.
4. Klausmeyer MA, Mudgal CS. Hook of hamate fractures. *J Hand Surg.* 2013;38;2457-2460.
5. Papp S. Carpal bone fractures. *Hand Clin.* 2010;119-127.
6. Wolfe SW, Cohen MS, Hotchkiss RN, Kozin SH, Pederson WC. *Green's Operative Hand Surgery.* Elsevier Health Sciences. 7th ed. PA: Philadelphia; 2017.
7. Cobb TK, Carmichael SW, Cooney WP. Guyon's canal revisited: an anatomic study of the carpal ulnar neurovascular space. *J Hand Surg [Am].* 1996;21(5):861-869.
8. Bozkurt MC, Tağil SM, Ozçakar L, Ersoy M, Tekdemir I. Anatomical variations as potential risk factors for ulnar tunnel syndrome: a cadaveric study. *Clin Anat.* 2005;18(4):274-280.
9. Criso JJ, Coburn JC, Moore DC, Upal MA. Carpal bone size and scaling in men versus in women. *J Hand Surg.* 2005;30(1):35-42.
10. Chow JC, Weiss MA, Gu Y. Anatomic variations of the hook of hamate and the relationship to carpal tunnel syndrome. *J Hand Surg.* 2005;30(6):1242-1247.
11. O'Shea K, Weiland AJ. Fractures of the hamate and pisiform bones. *Hand Clin.* 2012;287-300, viii.
12. Failla J. Hook of hamate vascularity: vulnerability to osteonecrosis and nonunion. *J Hand Surg [Am].* 1993;18(6):1075-1079.
13. Boulas HJ, Milek MA. Hook of the hamate fractures. Diagnosis, treatment, and complications. *Orthop Rev.* 1990;19(6):518-529.
14. Yamazaki H, Kato H, Nakatsuchi Y, Murakami N, Hata Y. Closed rupture of the flexor tendons of the little finger secondary to non-union of fractures of the hook of the hamate. *J Hand Surg [Br].* 2006;31(3):337-341
15. Bishop AT, Beckenbaugh RD. Fracture of the hamate hook. *J Hand Surg [Am].* 1988;13(1):135-139.
16. Wright TW, Moser MW, Sahajpal DT. Hook of hamate pull test. *J Hand Surg [Am].* 2010;35(11):1887-1889.
17. Andresen R, Radmer S, Sparmann M, Bogusch G, Banzer D. Imaging of hamate bone fractures in conventional X-rays and high-resolution computed tomography: an in vitro study. *Invest Radiol.* 1999;34(1):46-50.
18. Suh N, Ek ET, Wolfe SW. Carpal fractures. *J Hand Surg.* 2014;39(4):785-791.
19. Kato H, Nakamura R, Horii E, Nakao E, Yajima H. Diagnostic imaging for fracture of the hook of the hamate. *Hand Surg.* 2000;5(1):19-24.
20. Milek MA, Boulas HJ. Flexor tendon ruptures secondary to hamate hook fractures. *J Hand Surg.* 1990;15(5):740-744.

21. Devers BN, Douglas KC, Naik RD, Lee DH, Watson JT, Weikert DR. Outcomes of hook of hamate fracture excision in high-level amateur athletes. *J Hand Surg.* 2013;38(1):72-76.

22. Smith P III, Wright TW, Wallace PF, Dell PC. Excision of the hook of the hamate: a retrospective survey and review of the literature. *J Hand Surg Am.* 1988;13:612-615.

23. Demirkan F, Calandruccio JH, Diangelo D. Biomechanical evaluation of flexor tendon function after hamate hook excision. *J Hand Surg [Am].* 2003;28(1):138-143.

24. Ivy AD, Stern PJ. Hamate hook and pisiform fractures. *Oper Tech Sports Med.* 2016;24(2):94-99.

25. Scheufler O, Radmer S, Andresen R. Dorsal percutaneous cannulated mini-screw fixation for fractures of the hamate hook. *Hand Surg.* 2012;17(2):287-293.

17 Hamate Body Fracture

Kenrick C. Lam, Andrew Coskey, and
Niki L. Carayannopoulos

INTRODUCTION

- Pathoanatomy
  - Hamate is a triangular prism-shaped bone in the coronal plane with a large anterior-sided process, the hook of the hamate.
  - Articulates with and bordered by the 4th and 5th metacarpals, pisiform, triquetrum, lunate, and capitate
  - Blood supply
    - Dorsal intercarpal arch—dorsally
    - Branches of the deep palmar arch via retrograde flow—volarly
  - Ligaments
    - Interosseous, dorsal and volar capitohamate ligament
    - Volar and dorsal triquetrohamate ligament
    - Hook of hamate pisiform ligament
    - Three hamatometacarpal ligaments dorsally to the 4th and 5th metacarpals
    - One hamatometacarpal ligament volarly to the 5th metacarpal
  - Extensor carpi ulnaris (ECU) acts as deforming force in fracture or dislocation.
- Mechanism of injury
  - Direct axial load—closed fist punch
    - Dorsal fracture dislocation of carpometacarpal (CMC) joint[1-3]
    - Coronal dorsal hamate fracture[4-7]
  - Blunt force through metacarpal with wrist extended—motorcycle or automobile accident
    - Dorsal fracture dislocation of CMC joint[8-11]
  - Direct trauma to the hamate
    - Sagittal split fracture[12]
    - Nondisplaced with varying comminution[13,14]
  - Fall on outstretched hand
    - Coronal body (ulnar deviated) or sagittal split (radial deviated) fracture[15]

- High-energy injury, crush injury, or perilunate fracture dislocation[13,16-19]
  - Transverse fracture
- Epidemiology
  - Hamate fractures are rare, comprising 1% to 5% of all carpal injuries.[1,20-22]
  - Hook of hamate and coronal body comprise the majority of these fractures.[21,23,24]
  - Associated injury with hamate body fracture:
    - Most common: 4th and 5th CMC joint or fracture dislocation[1,2,7-10,15,25-27]
    - Capitate fracture,[7,18,26,28,29] 3rd metacarpal base fracture, trapezoid fracture,[26,30] triquetral fracture,[31,32] ulnar styloid fracture,[12] scaphoid fracture[25,31,33]
    - Axial carpal instability[22]
    - Hamate dislocation[22,32]
    - Greater arc injury[22]
      * Loss of normal cascade of metacarpal heads and widening of intermetacarpal space between middle and ring metacarpals
    - Compartment syndrome[16]
    - Ulnar nerve palsy[17,34]

EVALUATION

- History
  - Ulnar-sided wrist pain, swelling, and decreased grip strength
  - Often subacute because injuries are radiologically occult
    - Rarely associated with ulnar nerve palsy
  - Recognize compartment syndrome, acute carpal tunnel, or ulnar nerve compression in high-energy injuries
- Physical examination
  - Tenderness over hamate
    - Hamate can be best palpated with a flexed wrist one fingerbreadth distal to the radial edge of the ulnar styloid (Figure 17.1).
  - Pain with axial load applied to the ring and small metacarpal[12]
  - Shortening of 4th and 5th digit may indicate CMC dislocation.
  - Dorsal bony step off or lump may indicate CMC dislocation.
  - Neurovascular status, ulnar and median nerve distribution
- Imaging
  - Anterior-posterior and lateral views of the hand often appear normal.
    - Fracture line—usually oblique, typically radial but also ulnar to radiographic projection of the hook[12]

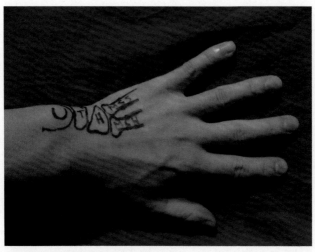

FIGURE 17.1 Relevant bony anatomy.

- Pronation oblique films at 15° and 45° of pronation
  - Look for dorsal fragment on lateral or pronation oblique.[35]
- Observe CMC joint space.
  - Should be contiguous with and of the same width as CMC joint spaces of 2nd and 3rd metacarpals
  - Disruption of this joint space may indicate CMC joint dislocation.[36]
- Obtain a computed tomography (CT) scan when radiographs are negative and mechanism of injury indicates hamate fracture.
- Classification
  - Milch—hamate fracture[12]
    - Type 1—hook of hamate
    - Type 2—sagittal oblique body of hamate fracture
  - Hirano—hamate fracture (Figure 17.2)[21]
    - Type 1—hook of hamate
    - Type 2a—dorsal avulsion
    - Type 2b—coronal body
    - Type 3—transverse body of hamate fracture
  - Ebraheim—coronal body of hamate fracture (Figure 17.3)[6]
    - Type A—center of body
    - Type B—oblique coronal involving the distal articular surface
    - Type C—hamate avulsion in the coronal plane

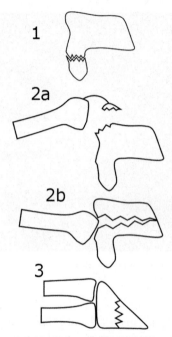

FIGURE 17.2 Hirano's modified Milch classification of hamate body fractures.

- Cain—CMC fracture dislocation (Figure 17.4)[1]
  - Type 1a—subluxation or dislocation of 5th CMC with dorsal ligament disruption and intact hamate
  - Type 1b—dorsal hamate avulsion fracture
  - Type 2—dorsal hamate comminution
  - Type 3—coronal splitting of the hamate

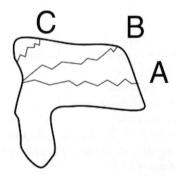

FIGURE 17.3 Ebraheim classification of coronal body fractures.

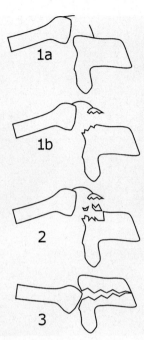

FIGURE 17.4 Cain classification of hamatometacarpal fracture dislocations. All are considered unstable.

ACUTE MANAGEMENT

- Fracture and/or dislocation can be reduced with traction and direct pressure (Figure 17.5).
- Place ulnar gutter in wrist extension and ulnar deviation to minimize pull of ECU (Figure 17.6).
- CT is warranted for surgical planning or negative radiographs.

DEFINITIVE TREATMENT

- Nonoperative treatment
  - Stable injuries can be treated in a ulnar gutter splint or cast for 4 to 6 weeks.[12,14,34,37]
    - Become asymptomatic after treatment even if fibrous union is present

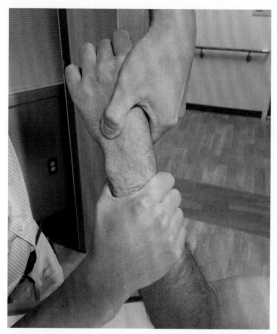

FIGURE 17.5 Reduction maneuver for hematometacarpal fracture dislocation.

* Fracture line is extra-articular or enters CMC joint between facets for articulation of 4th and 5th metacarpals.[22]
* Controversial—nondisplaced or stable Cain types 1 to 3[1,7,24]
* Fracture comminution: Immobilization should include the metacarpal-phalangeal joint of the ring and small finger.

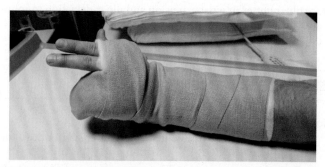

FIGURE 17.6 Hematometacarpal dislocations should be splinted in an ulnar gutter in wrist extension and ulnar deviation.

- Surgical indications
  - Fractures extending through the body of the hamate to the articular surface[21,24]
  - Displaced fractures[7,22]
  - Fracture dislocations of CMC joint[1]
    - Some have effectively treated these closed (Cain types 1b, 2, and 3).[2]
  - Unstable CMC joint dislocations[24]
  - Contraindications
    - Nondisplaced fractures in patients with multiple comorbidities and decreased functional status (author's recommendation)
- Surgical approach
  - Transverse or longitudinal incision should be centered at the intersection of the distal wrist crease and radial edge of ulnar styloid (Figure 17.7).
    - Hamate located under extensor digiti minimi and extensor digitorum communis
      - Must visualize hamate-metacarpal joint to ensure anatomic reduction
    - Consider a volar incision when carpal tunnel or Guyon's canal release is necessary.[16]
  - Fixation with mini-frag, Herbert or Leibinger screws have been described.[4,28,38-41]

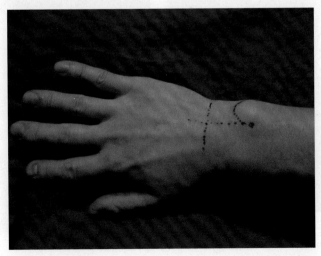

FIGURE 17.7 Skin incision should be centered over the intersection of the ulnar styloid and distal wrist crease.

- K-wires with good results, especially for transverse fractures usually part of a perilunate injury[1,5,8]
  - Shot ulnar to radial using the capitate as a stable point of fixation
  - Lag screw technique—to ensure joint surface reduction and compression of the fracture
- Stress the 4th and 5th CMC
  - If unstable, run K-wires from 4th MC to the capitate and 5th MC K-wire into the hamate[1] (Figure 17.8).
    - Can also K-wire 4th and 5th MC together with the 4th MC wired to the capitate (author's recommendation)
  - Joint spanning plate fixation has been described with mild loss of range of motion upon plate removal at 11 weeks[42]
- Complications
  - Iatrogenic damage to the dorsal ulnar cutaneous branch (theoretical)
  - Loss of reduction with K-wire-only fixation
  - Residual stiffness, pain, and decreased grip strength[6]
  - Nonunion when treated conservatively[30]
  - Avascular necrosis of intra-articular proximal pole in proximal fractures[43]

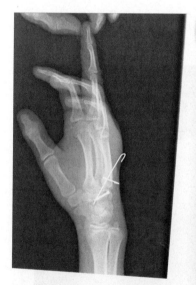 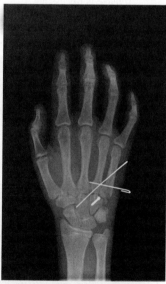

FIGURE 17.8 Post-op radiographs of hamate body fracture and 4th carpometacarpal dislocation treated with open reduction and internal fixation and K-wires.

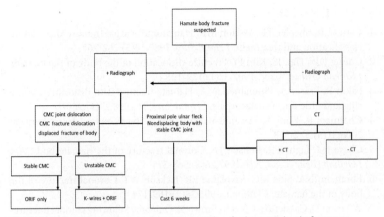

FIGURE 17.9 Proposed management algorithm for hamate body fractures.

- Postoperative care
  - Remove K-wires at 6 weeks
  - Immobilize for 3 weeks followed by functional bracing

MANAGEMENT ALGORITHM

See Figure 17.9.

SUGGESTED READINGS

Amadio PC, Moran SL. Fractures of the carpal bones. In: Green DP, Hotchkiss RN, Pederson WC, Wolfe SW, eds. *Green's Operative Hand Surgery*. 5th ed. Vol 1. Philadelphia, PA: Elsevier; 2005: chap 17:711, 764.

Cain J, Shepler T, Wilson M. Hamatometacarpal fracture-dislocation: classification and treatment. *J Hand Surg*. 1987;12A(2):762-767.

Ebraheim NA, Skie MC, Savolaine ER, Jackson WT. Coronal fracture of the body of the hamate. *J Trauma*. 1995;38(2):169-174.

Hirano K, Inoue G. Classification and treatment of hamate fractures. *J Hand Surg*. 2005;10(2&3):151-157.

O'Shea K, Weiland A. Fracture of the hamate and pisiform bones. *Hand Clin*. 2012;28:287-300.

Seitz WH, Papandrea RF. Fractures and dislocations of the wrist. In: Bucholz, RW, Heckman JD, eds. *Rockwood and Green's Fractures in Adults*. 5th ed. Vol 1. Philadelphia, PA: Lippincott Williams and Wilkins; 2002:chap 19:796-797.

Wharton D, Casaletto J, Choa R, Brown D. Outcome following coronal fractures of the hamate. *J Hand Surg EurVol*. 2010;35(2):146-149.

REFERENCES

1. Cain JE Jr, Shepler TR, Wilson MR. Hamatometacarpal fracture-dislocation: classification and treatment. *J Hand Surg.* 1987;12(5):762-767.
2. Chung DW, Han JS, Kim IY. Fracture-dislocation of the body of the hamate. *J Korean Orthop Assoc.* 1997;32(1):122-125.
3. Fakih R, Fraser A, Pimpalnerkar A. Hamate fracture with dislocation of the ring and little finger metacarpals. *J Hand Surg Br.* 1998;23(1):96-97.
4. Chalmers R, Kong K. An unusual fracture of the hamate. *J Hand Surg Br.* 2006;31(5):577-578.
5. Chase JM, Light TR, Benson LS. Coronal fracture of the hamate body. *Am J Orthop (Belle Mead, NJ).* 1997;26(8):568-571.
6. Ebraheim NA, Skie MC, Savolaine ER, Jackson WT. Coronal fracture of the body of the hamate. *J Trauma.* 1995;38(2):169-174.
7. Wharton D, Casaletto J, Choa R, Brown D. Outcome following coronal fractures of the hamate. *J Hand Surg Eur Vol.* 2010;35(2):146-149.
8. Arora S, Goyal A, Mittal S, Singh A, Sural S, Dhal A. Combined intraarticular fracture of the body and the hook of hamate: an unusual injury pattern. *J Hand Microsurg.* 2013;5(2):92-95.
9. Kaneko K, Ono A, Uta S, et al. Hamatometacarpal fracture-dislocation: distinctive three dimensional computed tomographic appearance. *Chir main.* 2002;21(1):41-45.
10. Takami H, Takahashi S, Hiraki S. Coronal fracture of the body of the hamate: case reports. *J Trauma Acute Care Surg.* 1992;32(1):110-112.
11. Garcia-Elias M, Bishop AT, Dobyns JH, Cooney WP, Linscheid RL. Transcarpal carpometacarpal dislocations, excluding the thumb. *J Hand Surg Am.* 1990;15(4):531-540.
12. Milch H. Fracture of the hamate bone. *J Bone Joint Surg.* 1934(2):459-462.
13. Duckworth A, Ring D. Carpus fractures and dislocations. In: Court-Brown CM, Heckman JD, McQueen MM, Ricci WM, Tornetta P III, McKee MD, eds. *Rockwood and Green's Fractures in Adults.* 8th ed. Vol 8. Philadelphia, PA: Wolters Kluwer Health; 2015.
14. Zoltie N. Fractures of the body of the hamate. *Injury.* 1991;22(6):459-462.
15. Thomas AP, Birch R. An unusual hamate fracture. *Hand.* 1983;15(3):281-286.
16. Ali MA. Fracture of the body of the hamate bone associated with compartment syndrome and dorsal decompression of the carpal tunnel. *J Hand Surgery Br Eur Vol.* 1986;11(2):207-210.
17. Baird DB, Friedenberg Z. Delayed ulnar-nerve palsy following a fracture of the hamate. *J Bone Joint Surg Am.* 1968;50(3):570-572.
18. Møller J, Lybecker H. Simultaneous fracture of the hamate and the capitate bones. *Arch Orthop Trauma Surg.* 1987;106(5):331-332.
19. Ogunro O. Fracture of the body of the hamate bone. *J Hand Surg.* 1983;8(3):353-355.
20. Bizzaro AH. Traumatology of the carpus. *Surg Gynecol Obstet.* 1922;34:574-588.

21. Hirano K, Inoue G. Classification and treatment of hamate fractures. *Hand Surg.* 2005;10(2-3):151-157.

22. Wolfe SW, Hotchkiss RN, Pederson WC, Kozin SH. *Green's Operative Hand Surgery E-Book: Expert Consult: Online and Print.* Elsevier Health Sciences. PA: Philadelphia; 2010.

23. O'Shea K, Weiland AJ. Fractures of the hamate and pisiform bones. *Hand Clin.* 2012;28(3):287-300.

24. Condés JS, Martínez LI, Carrasco MS, Julia FC, Martínez ES. Hamate fractures. *Revista Española de Cirugía Ortopédica y Traumatología (English Edition).* 2015;59(5):299-306.

25. Jones BG, Hems TE. Simultaneous fracture of the body of the hamate and the distal pole of the scaphoid. *J Trauma Acute Care Surg.* 2001;50(3):568-570.

26. Kang S-Y, Song K-S, Lee H-J, Lee J-S, Park Y-B. A case report of coronal fractures through the hamate, the capitate, and the trapezoid. *Arch Orthop Trauma Surg.* 2009;129(7):963-965.

27. Kimura H, Kamura S, Akai M, Ohno T. An unusual coronal fracture of the body of the hamate bone. *J Hand Surg.* 1988;13(5):743-745.

28. Robison JE, Kaye JJ. Simultaneous fractures of the capitate and hamate in the coronal plane: case report. *J Hand Surg.* 2005;30(6):1153-1155.

29. Sabat D, Dabas V, Suri T, Wangchuk T, Sural S, Dhal A. Trans-scaphoid transcapitate transhamate fracture of the wrist: case report. *J Hand Surg.* 2010;35(7):1093-1096.

30. Pruzansky M, Arnold L. Delayed union of fractures of the trapezoid and body of the hamate. *Orthop Rev.* 1987;16(9):624-628.

31. Monteiro E, Torres J, Negrão P, Vidinha V, Silva S, Pinto R. Transscaphoid–transtriquetral–transhamate perilunate fracture–dislocation: case report. *Eur Orthop Traumatol.* 2014;5(2):195-198.

32. Zamfir GD, Arealis G, Ashwood N, Kitsis C. Hand Swelling due to Missed Coronal Fracture of the Body of the Hamate and Hamate-Triquetral Dislocation. Annals of Clinical Case Reports. Department of Trauma and Orthopaedics, Queen's Hospital, UK.

33. Yalcinkaya M, Azar N, Dogan A. A rare wrist injury: simultaneous fractures of the hamate body and scaphoid waist. *Orthopedics.* 2009;32(8). doi: 10.3928/01477447-20090624-23.

34. Howard FM. Ulnar-nerve palsy in wrist fractures. *J Bone Joint Surg Am.* 1961;43(8):1197-1201.

35. Gillespy T III, Stork J, Dell P. Dorsal fracture of the hamate: distinctive radiographic appearance. *Am J Roentgenol.* 1988;151(2):351-353.

36. Fisher MR, Rogers LF, Hendrix RW. Systematic approach to identifying fourth and fifth carpometacarpal joint dislocations. *Am J Roentgenol.* 1983;140(2):319-324.

37. Snoap T, Habeck J, Ruiter T. Hamate fracture. *Eplasty.* 2015;15:ic28.

38. Freeland AE, Finley JS. Displaced dorsal oblique fracture of the hamate treated with a cortical mini lag screw. *J Hand Surg Am.* 1986;11(5):656-658.

39. Loth TS, McMillan MD. Coronal dorsal hamate fractures. *J Hand Surg Am.* 1988;13(4):616-618.
40. Roche S, Lenehan B, Street J, O'Sullivan M. Fourth metacarpal base fracture in association with coronal hamate fracture. *Injury Extra.* 2005;36(8):316-318.
41. Roth JH, de Lorenzi C. Displaced intra-articular coronal fracture of the body of the hamate treated with a Herbert screw. *J Hand Surg.* 1988;13(4):619-621.
42. Marck KW, Klasen HJ. Fracture-dislocation of the hamatometacarpal joint: a case report. *J Hand Surg Am.* 1986;11(1):128-130.
43. Van Demark RE, Parke WW. Avascular necrosis of the hamate: a case report with reference to the hamate blood supply. *J Hand Surg.* 1992;17(6):1086-1090.

Mikael Starecki and James R. Mullen

INTRODUCTION

- Anatomy
  - The pisiform is a pea-shaped sesamoid bone within the tendon of the flexor carpi ulnaris (FCU).
  - Attaches to FCU proximally
  - Distally is attached to the pisohamate, pisometacarpal, and pisotriquetral ligaments
  - Origin of abductor digiti minimi
  - Transverse carpal ligament also has attachments to the pisiform.
  - The ulnar nerve and artery lie radial to the pisiform in Guyon's canal.
- Mechanism of injury
  - Direct impact against a hard surface
  - Forceful contraction of FCU
- Epidemiology
  - 1% to 2% of all carpal fractures
  - Injury is often missed
  - 50% occur in isolation
  - 50% associated with other conditions

EVALUATION

- History
  - Fall on outstretched hand
  - Most commonly produces a transverse pisiform fracture
  - Impact with ground fractures the pisiform at pisotriquetral joint.
  - Forceful contraction of the FCU results in a transverse avulsion fracture.
  - Other patterns include comminuted, parasagittal, and osteochondral impaction fractures.

- Patient will complain of pain with gripping and radioulnar motion.
- Swinging a bat or golf club will be particularly painful.
- Physical examination
  - Hypothenar wrist pain
  - Tenderness over the pisiform
  - Examination should exclude other wrist injuries
  - 50% of the time pisiform fractures occur in conjunction with other injuries.
    - Examples—perilunate dislocation, distal radius or additional carpal fracture
  - Ulnar nerve at risk for injury and requires evaluation
  - Increased risk of ulnar nerve injury/irritation in patients with comminuted fractures and posttraumatic pisotriquetral osteoarthritis.
- Imaging
  - Best seen on the carpal tunnel view and the 30°-to-45° supinated lateral radiograph
  - Potentially seen on lateral view
  - Poorly visualized on anteroposterior and oblique wrist radiographs
  - Rarely diagnosed by computed tomography scan when not seen on radiograph in a patient where there is a high clinical suspicion of injury

MANAGEMENT

- Nonoperative management
  - Acute nondisplaced pisiform fractures can be casted for 3 to 6 weeks.
  - Majority heal by bony or fibrous union.
- Surgical indications
  - Comminuted fractures, displaced transverse fractures, and symptomatic nonunions require excision of the pisiform.
  - An incongruent pisotriquetral joint that results in posttraumatic arthritis with persistent pain is also an indication for surgery.
- Surgery
  - A volar Z-plasty approach to the ulnar side of the wrist is preferred.
  - The transverse limb is centered over distal palmar crease.
  - The ulnar neurovascular bundle must be identified before identifying the pisiform.
  - Once the neurovascular bundle is identified and protected, the pisiform is shelled out of the flexor carpi ulnaris tendon.
  - Care is taken to remove the pisiform without damaging the FCU tendon fibers.

- Potential complications
  - Risk of injury to ulnar nerve
  - Failure to protect FCU can result in FCU rupture.

ULNAR NERVE

- Ulnar nerve injury occurring at time of pisiform fracture are most common neurapraxia.
- Neurapraxias will resolve with observation.
- If symptoms worsen or persist for more than 12 weeks, ulnar nerve exploration in addition to pisiform excision is recommended.
- Exploration of the ulnar nerve is indicated if ulnar nerve dysfunction occurs following pisiformectomy in cases where the nerve was not identified.

Carpal Bone Malunions and Nonunions

Paul C. Baldwin III and John R. Fowler

INTRODUCTION

- Mechanism of injury
  - Scaphoid fractures occur most commonly from a fall onto the outstretched hand, resulting in force transmission of dorsiflexion, ulnar deviation, and intercarpal supination.
- Pathoanatomy
  - Scaphoid nonunions can result in persistent disability, wrist pain, stiffness, and scaphoid nonunion advanced collapse (SNAC).
  - SNAC is a pattern of progressive posttraumatic degenerative arthritis of the radiocarpal and midcarpal joints due to the associated pathomechanics of the scapholunate joint.
  - Fracture location determines vascularity and subsequently risk for nonunion.
    - Vascularity—distal pole > waist > proximal pole
  - Increasing fracture displacement is a risk factor for nonunion and malunion.
- Epidemiology
  - Healing rates of 90% to 95% with cast treatment of distal pole and waist fractures.
  - Frequency of scaphoid nonunion following surgical fixation is unknown.
    - The union rate greatly depends on the location of the fracture (distal, proximal, waist) and other factors such as chronicity and patient factors (smoking, compliance, etc).
  - Proximal pole fractures have higher rates of nonunion due to poor vascularity.

EVALUATION

- History
  - Injury details
    - Mechanism of injury
    - Estimated chronicity
  - Previous treatments
    - Nonoperative
    - Operative
    - Obtain medical records
  - Associated symptoms
    - Pain
    - Loss of motion
    - Loss of function
- Physical examination
  - Inspection—identify for swelling, previous incisions
  - Wrist range of motion
  - Palpation—anatomic snuffbox, proximal pole, distal pole, axial loading of thumb
  - Scaphoid shift test
  - Watson test
- Diagnostic data
  - Plain radiographs:
    - Posteroanterior (Figure 19.1)
    - Lateral
    - 45° pronated and supinated oblique
    - Scaphoid view (posteroanterior in ulnar deviation)
    - Evaluate for sclerosis, cystic formation, bone resorption at the fracture site, hardware loosening, and hardware failure.
    - Evaluate for associated degenerative changes and/or carpal instability.
  - Computed tomography scan (with scanning plane parallel to the longitudinal axis of scaphoid)
    - Evaluate for early degenerative changes of wrist
    - Evaluate for fracture displacement
    - Evaluate for technical errors of previous surgeries
      - Hardware placement
      - Fracture reduction
    - Evaluate for fracture fragment sclerosis (osteonecrosis)

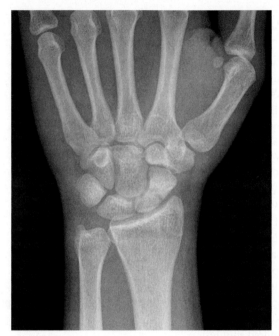

FIGURE 19.1 Posteroanterior radiograph demonstrating scaphoid nonunion.

- Magnetic resonance imaging
  - ◆ Evaluate for vascularity and osteonecrosis.
  - ◆ Evaluate for chondromalacia.
  - ◆ Evaluate for associated ligamentous injury.
- ■ Classifications (radiographic)
  - Mack-Lichtman classification
    - ◆ Type I—nondisplaced, stable, no significant degenerative changes
    - ◆ Type II—unstable, >1 to 2 mm
    - ◆ Type III—unstable, early degenerative changes with radial styloid beaking and joint space narrowing of radioscaphoid joint
    - ◆ Type IV—unstable, midcarpal arthritis present without radiolunate arthritis
    - ◆ Type V—unstable, midcarpal arthritis with radiolunate arthritis
  - Scaphoid nonunion advanced collapse
    - ◆ Stage I—arthrosis localized to radial side of scaphoid and radial styloid

   ◆ Stage II—Stage I findings in addition to scaphocapitate arthrosis
   ◆ Stage III—periscaphoid arthrosis (proximal capitate and lunate can be maintained)

MANAGEMENT

- Thorough history and physical examination (see earlier)
- Plain radiographs and advanced imaging (see earlier)

DEFINITIVE TREATMENT

- Nonoperative treatment
  - ◆ Limited role in the setting of scaphoid nonunion
  - ◆ Continued immobilization can be considered up to 6 months.
  - ◆ Cast immobilization combined with pulsed electromagnetic fields for an average of 4 months can achieve union in up to 69% of cases.
- Open reduction internal fixation surgical indications
  - Any displacement of waist fracture
  - Any proximal pole fracture
  - Unstable fracture patterns
- Contraindications
  - Associated wrist or carpal degenerative arthritis
- Surgical approach
  - Dictated by location of nonunion, previous surgical approaches, surgeon experience, and need for supplemental procedures such as nonvascularized bone grafting (NVBG) and vascularized bone grafting (VBG)
  - Operative technique
    - ◆ Nonvascularized bone grafting
      - ∗ Frequently used for scaphoid nonunions
      - ∗ Graft donor sites commonly include distal radius and iliac crest
      - ∗ Revision screw fixation with NVBG is particularly beneficial in the setting of previous technical errors such as:
        - ▲ Screw malposition
        - ▲ Inappropriate screw diameter/length
        - ▲ Fracture malreduction

* Excise any and all devitalized/necrotic tissue.
* Wedge tricortical iliac crest bone graft
  ▲ Provides solid structural support in setting of scaphoid nonunion with humpback deformity
    ◆ Restores scaphoid length, and alignment in turn improves carpal mechanics.
* Use of NVBG less technically demanding than VBG
* With NVBG, healing occurs via creeping substitution and resorption.
◆ Vascularized bone grafting
  * Utilized in scaphoid nonunions with osteonecrosis
  * More technically demanding than NVBG
  * VBG improves the local biology and healing environment through revascularization.
  * Local rotational VBGs
    ▲ Distal radius VBG
      ◆ Dorsal vascular pedicle based on the 1,2 or 2,3 intracompartmental supraretinacular artery (ICRSA)
        ○ Consider dorsal distal radius VBG in the setting of proximal pole scaphoid nonunions; no significant humpback deformity
        ○ 2,3 ICRSA provides longer pedicle for greater arc of graft rotation.
      ◆ Volar vascular pedicle based on the volar carpal artery
        ○ Useful when deformity correction is needed
        ○ Short pedicle can limit graft excursion.
    ▲ Metacarpal bone graft (MBG)
      ◆ Rotational VBG from 2nd metacarpal
      ◆ Based on 2nd dorsal metacarpal artery or the dorsal intercarpal arch
      ◆ Do not cross mobile wrist joint, and therefore the risk of kinking is theoretically decreased
      ◆ Can be used through single dorsal approach or combined with dorsal and volar approach
  * Medial femoral condyle bone graft (MFCBG)
    ▲ Vascularized corticocancellous bone graft is harvested from the ipsilateral medial femoral condyle
    ▲ Based on pedicle from the descending genicular vessels or the superior medial genicular vessels

- ▲ Provide vascularized structural support to improve deformity correction
- ▲ Requires microsurgical anastomosis
  * Iliac bone graft (IBG)
    - ▲ Vascularized IBG provides structural support and can be used to correct humpback deformity.
    - ▲ Tricortical IBG harvested from iliac crest
    - ▲ Based on pedicle from brances of the deep circumflex iliac vessels
  * Ulnar bone graft
    - ▲ Cortical cancellous graft harvested from distal one-third of the ulna with periosteum
    - ▲ Ulnar artery serves as pedicle
    - ▲ Requires sacrificing ulnar artery with vein interposition reconstruction
    - ▲ Anatomically predictable vascular pedicle
- ◆ Arterialization
  * Direct implantation of local artery into scaphoid
    - ▲ 2nd dorsal intermetacarpal artery or dorsal index artery
    - ▲ Can be useful in the setting of prior VBGs with limited novel VBG options
- ◆ Plate fixation
  * Provides additional torsional stability at nonunion site
  * Consider plate fixation in setting of stable nonunion that failed screw osteosynthesis due to rotational instability.
  * Drawbacks of plate fixation include:
    - ▲ Increased soft-tissue dissection
    - ▲ Potential impingement of the hardware on cartilage
    - ▲ Potential need for hardware removal
    - ▲ Consider primary repair and/or grafting
- ◆ Salvage operations
  * Consider salvage procedures in patients with moderate to advanced radiocarpal or carpal arthritis
  * Salvage operations include:
    - ▲ Proximal row carpectomy
    - ▲ Scaphoid excision and four bone fusion
    - ▲ Radiocarpal fusion
    - ▲ Wrist fusion
- ■ Potential complications
  - ● Infection
  - ● Loss of function

- Stiffness
- Donor site morbidity if grafting utilized
- Need for future surgery
- Postoperative care
  - Wound care
  - Immobilization
  - Frequent plain radiographs for evaluation of healing
  - Consider advanced imaging such as computed tomography to confirm healing.
  - Hand therapy for motion

MANAGEMENT ALGORITHM

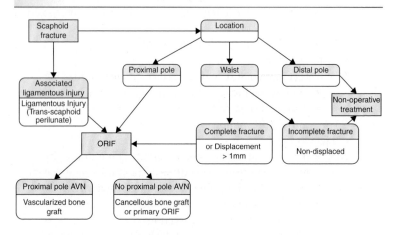

SUGGESTED READINGS

Janowski J, Coady, C, Catalano LW III. Scaphoid fractures: nonunion and malunion. *J Hand Surg Am.* 2016;41(11):1087-1092.

Kazmers NH, Thibaudeau S, Levin S. A scapholunate Ligament-Sparing Technique utilizing the medial femoral condyle corticocancellous free flap to reconstruct scaphoid nonunions with proximal pole avascular necrosis. *J Hand Surg Am.* 2016;41(9):e309-e315.

Moon ES, Dy CJ, Derman P, Vance MC, Carlson MG. Management of nonunion following surgical management of scaphoid fractures: current concepts. *J Am Acad Orthop Surg.* 2013;21:548-557.

Pinder RM, Brkljac M, Rix L, Muir L, Brewster M. Treatment of scaphoid nonunion: a systematic review of the existing evidence. *J Hand Surg Am.* 2015;40(9):1797-1805.

Wolfe S, Hotchkiss R, Pederson W, Kozin S, eds. *Green's Operative Hand Surgery.* Vol 1. 6th ed. Philadelphia, PA: Churchill Livingstone; 2011:chap 18:636-707.

Scapholunate Ligament Injury and Dorsal Intercalated Segment Stability

Mark Henry

INTRODUCTION

- Pathoanatomy
  - Intrinsic scapholunate interosseous ligament (SLIL) begins to fail volarly (1 mm thick, 117 N load to failure), as scaphoid and lunate separate under load, injury propagates around proximal portion of C-shaped ligament to dorsal fibers (3-4 mm thick, 260 N load to failure), completing full disruption.[1,2]
  - Complete rupture of SLIL only will acutely produce normal appearing radiograph when unloaded but loss of carpal relationships when axially loaded (dynamic instability).
  - Scaphoid (and contact area of radioscaphoid interface) translates dorsal and radial, also flexion and pronation; lunate extends and supinates; distal row translates dorsally
  - Additional injury to extrinsic capsular ligaments—secondary stabilizers (radioscaphocapitate, dorsal radiocarpal, dorsal intercarpal) acutely produce abnormal carpal relationships on unloaded radiograph (static instability).
  - Dorsal intercalary segment instability (DISI) can be dynamic or static, measured in sagittal plane on standard radiograph, using lateral SL angle (normal 30°-60°, average 47°) and lateral capitolunate angle >15°
- Mechanism of injury[3]
  - Sudden forceful impact to palm with wrist extended, ulnarly deviated, hand supinated relative to a pronated forearm (particularly if point of impact is over thenar eminence)
  - Low to moderate force and slower rate of application will not cause complete scapholunate disruption (SLD)
- Epidemiology
  - Younger to middle-aged active patients, strong male predominance
  - High-energy falls
  - Collision sports

EVALUATION

- History[4]
  - Mechanism of injury most important
  - Quantify amount of kinetic injury (sufficient to produce true acute SLIL rupture)
  - Angle of wrist and point of impact (increase or decrease likelihood of true SLD), but not every true rupture adheres to the classically described mechanism of injury position
  - Timing of injury—acute <3 weeks, subacute 3 to 6 weeks, chronic >6 weeks
- Physical examination[5]
  - Swelling and tenderness localized over SLIL.
  - Painful scaphoid shift out of fossa over dorsal rim of radius, mechanical clunk when falling back into fossa (Figure 20.1)

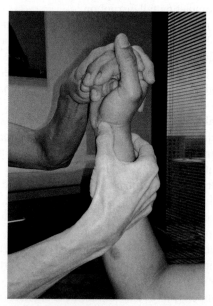

FIGURE 20.1 Scaphoid shift performed with remainder of wrist stabilized by contralateral hand of examiner that also tilts patient's hand radially and ulnarly while ipsilateral examiner's thumb applies dorsally directed force to scaphoid tubercle that will push the dorsal pole of the scaphoid over the dorsal rim of the radius in radial deviation and then allow dorsal pole to drop back into the scaphoid fossa if pressure is removed.

- Reduced range of motion (ROM) acutely; may have normal ROM at more subacute/chronic presentation
- Imaging[6]
  - Normal appearing standard radiographs (as opposed to stress views) if only SLIL ruptured without injury to secondary stabilizers
  - Grip-loaded supinated anteroposterior (AP; Figure 20.2) may show increase in SL diastasis (dynamic instability); diastasis may also show on maximum ulnar deviation view.
  - SL diastasis on unloaded AP, and increased SL angle (Figure 20.3) on lateral (static instability)
  - Axial distraction view shows scaphoid position distal to lunate (Figure 20.4).
  - Magnetic resonance imaging (MRI) arthrogram versus computed tomography (CT) arthrogram, variable accuracy in mid-70% to 90% range dependent on: magnet strength (1.5 vs 3.0 T), surface coils, "superman position," intra-articular contrast, musculoskeletal specialist radiologist.

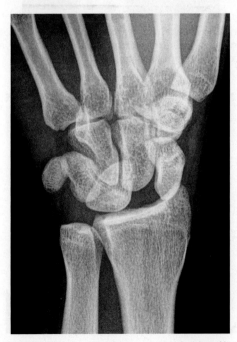

FIGURE 20.2 Coronal plane diastasis between scaphoid and lunate exceeding 3 mm indicates failure of the scapholunate interosseous ligament.

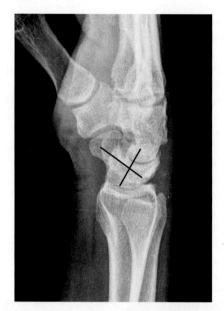

FIGURE 20.3 Increased lateral scapholunate angle >70° indicates static scapholunate interosseous ligament instability (normal 30°-60°, average 47°); also DISI defined by lateral capitolunate angle >15°.

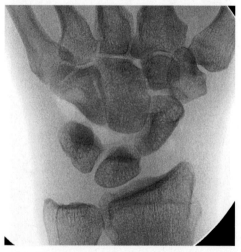

FIGURE 20.4 With axial traction and complete rupture of the scapholunate interosseous ligament, the scaphoid will move distally relative to the more tethered lunate.

TABLE 20.1 Arthroscopic Multidirectional Stress Testing Classification of Perilunate Injuries

	Grade I	Grade II	Grade III
Diastasis	Volar diastasis <2.3 mm; no dorsal diastasis	Volar and dorsal diastasis >2.3 mm	Volar and dorsal diastasis >2.3 mm
Distraction	Scaphoid/triquetrum distracts under arthroscopic traction <10% the height of the SLIL/LTIL interface	Scaphoid/triquetrum distracts under arthroscopic traction 10%-25% the height of the SLIL/LTIL interface	Scaphoid/triquetrum distracts under arthroscopic traction >25% the height of the SLIL/LTIL interface
Translation	Scaphoid/triquetrum translates with probe <10% the PA dimension of the SLIL/LTIL interface	Scaphoid/triquetrum translates with probe 10%-25% the PA dimension of the SLIL/LTIL interface	Scaphoid/triquetrum translates with probe >25% the PA dimension of the SLIL/LTIL interface
Rotation	Scaphoid/triquetrum rotates with probe <10° relative to lunate distal surface	Scaphoid/triquetrum rotates with probe 10°-25° relative to lunate distal surface	Scaphoid/triquetrum rotates with probe >25° relative to lunate distal surface

Abbreviations: LTIL, Lunotriquetral interosseous ligament; SLIL, Scapholunate interosseous ligament.

- Classification[7]
  - By stress radiographs—dynamic (SLIL only injured) versus static DISI (additional failure of secondary stabilizers)
  - By MRI or CT—partial or complete disruption of volar/dorsal portions of ligament viewed on axial images, fluid-sensitive sequences, static carpal malposition
  - By arthroscopic multidirectional stress testing via midcarpal portals—Table 20.1
    - Grade 0—SLIL intact
    - Grade 1—partial tear of volar and/or proximal fibers, dorsal fibers intact
    - Grade 2—complete tear of SLIL, secondary stabilizers intact
    - Grade 3—complete tear of SLIL and secondary stabilizer injury

ACUTE MANAGEMENT

- Clinical evaluation, pain control, immobilization, elevation
  - Determine extent of injury, indications for surgery, and timing
  - Elevate for swelling control, assess for acute median nerve compression
  - Splint in neutral to slight extension for pain control

DEFINITIVE TREATMENT

- Nonoperative treatment
  - Grade 0—as soon as pain and swelling controlled, discontinue removable splint and advance functional status as symptoms permit
  - Grade 1—splint/cast and avoid forceful loading of wrist while retaining hand dexterity for 8 weeks, then advance ROM and strength
- Surgical indications[8]
  - Grade 2/3 complete tears do not heal adequately with immobilization alone.
  - Contraindications—coexisting arthritis already present, low demand older patient not expected to appreciate functional instability, medical comorbidity increasing surgical risk
  - Acute <3 weeks—arthroscopic/limited open incision—reduction and pinning
  - Subacute 3 to 6 weeks—insufficient data to comment on need for reconstruction
  - Chronic >6 weeks—requires reconstruction with new tissue to achieve carpal stability
- Surgical approach[9,10]
  - Begins with arthroscopic evaluation and grading, confirmation that injury is acute not chronic, and survey for associated chondral lesions not previously revealed in workup
  - All arthroscopic repair versus partial open (dorsal)
  - First ensure precise position of lunate (pin to radius fully reduced into lunate fossa—correcting extension, supination, and ulnar translation)
  - Then establish scaphoid relationship to fixed position of lunate—pin scaphoid to lunate—correcting pronation, flexion, dorsal, and radial translation of proximal pole (Figure 20.5)
  - No benefit to suturing short fibrocartilaginous ligament fibers—correct intercarpal reduction places fibers at exact position for healing
  - For reconstruction—intercarpal tenodesis replacing stabilizing function of both volar and dorsal components of original SLIL (10-year disability of the arm, shoulder, hand [DASH] = 9; ROM and grip strength = 85% contralateral)

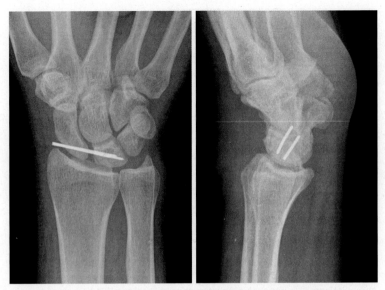

FIGURE 20.5 First lunate is reduced to fossa in radius, then scaphoid is reduced and pinned to lunate, restoring anatomic intercarpal relationships.

■ Potential complications
  ● Injury to superficial radial or lateral antebrachial nerves by pin placement[11,12]
  ● Pin migration beyond skin surface acquires pin tract infection
  ● Avascular necrosis of scaphoid or lunate from excess number of repeated pin passages attempting to establish correct fixation (or drill passages in reconstruction)
  ● Long-term progression of posttraumatic arthritis in 67% to 70% (15-year DASH = 20, ROM and grip strength = 70% contralateral)
■ Postoperative care[1]
  ● Splint/cast for 8 weeks then remove pins
  ● Begin ROM after pin removal, no splint, "dart-thrower's motion" = from extension radial deviation to flexion ulnar deviation
  ● Add progressive strengthening after 3 months of ligament healing

MANAGEMENT ALGORITHM

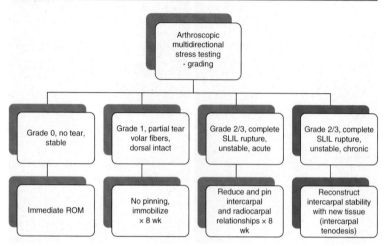

Abbreviations: SLIL, scapholunate interosseous ligament; ROM, range of motion

REFERENCES

1. Kamal RN, Starr A, Akelman E. Carpal kinematics and kinetics. *J Hand Surg Am*. 2016;41:1011-1018.
2. Omori S, Moritomo H, Omokawa S, Murase T, Sugamoto K, Yoshikawa H. In vivo 3-dimensional analysis of dorsal intercalated segment instability deformity secondary to scapholunate dissociation: a preliminary report. *J Hand Surg Am*. 2013;38:1346-1355.
3. Rajan PV, Day CS. Scapholunate interosseous ligament anatomy and biomechanics. *J Hand Surg Am*. 2015;40:1692-1702.
4. Kitay A, Wolfe SW. Scapholunate instability: current concepts in diagnosis and management. *J Hand Surg Am*. 2012;37:2175-2196.
5. Kleinman WB. Physical examination of the wrist: useful provocative maneuvers. *J Hand Surg-Am*. 2015;40:1486-1500.
6. Ringler MD. MRI of wrist ligaments. *J Hand Surg Am*. 2013; 38:2034-2046.
7. Henry M. Reconstruction of both volar and dorsal limbs of the scapholunate interosseous ligament. *J Hand Surg Am*. 2013;38:1625-1634.
8. Rohman EM, Agel J, Putnam MD, Adams JE. Scapholunate interosseous ligament injuries: a retrospective review of treatment and outcomes in 82 wrists. *J Hand Surg Am*. 2014;39:2020-2026
9. Henry MH. Perilunate dislocation and fracture dislocation. In: del Pinal F, ed. *Distal Radius Fractures: Arthroscopic Management*. New York, NY: Springer, 2010:127-149.

10. Nienstedt F. Treatment of static scapholunate instability with modified Brunelli tenodesis: results over 10 years. *J Hand Surg Am.* 2013;38:887-892.
11. Jones DB, Kakar S. Perilunate dislocations and fracture dislocations. *J Hand Surg Am.* 2012;37:2168-2173.
12. Krief E, Appy-Fedida B, Rotari V, David E, Mertl P, Maes-Clavier C. Results of perilunate dislocations and perilunate fracture dislocations with a minimum 15-year follow-up. *J Hand Surg Am.* 2015;40:2191-2197.

Lunotriquetral Ligament Injuries, Midcarpal Instability, and Volar Intercalated Segment Instability

William F. Pientka II, Jonathan D. Boyle,
Timothy R. Niacaris, and David M. Lichtman

LUNOTRIQUETRAL LIGAMENT INJURIES

- Functional anatomy
  - Intrinsic wrist ligaments are thickenings of the wrist capsule, which show organized, stress-oriented alignment of collagen fibers.[1]
  - Lunotriquetral (LT) ligament is composed of three distinct portions: dorsal, membranous, and volar components.
    - Volar aspect of LT ligament is the thickest and biomechanically strongest component.[2-4]
    - Dorsal LT ligament functions as main restraint to rotational deformity.[3,5]
    - Membranous portion is fibrocartilage and functions mainly to permit smooth gliding at the radiocarpal and midcarpal joint surfaces by creating a continuous smooth articulation between the lunate and the triquetrum.
  - Dorsal radiotriquetral (DRT) ligament reinforces LT stability via dorsal anatomic connections to LT ligament.
- Kinematics
  - The lunate and triquetrum are integral parts of the proximal row (PR). Physiologic PR motion is controlled by intercarpal joint reaction forces.
  - With radial deviation, the scaphoid is forced into flexion and the lunate and triquetrum passively follow due to strong scapholunate (SL) and LT ligamentous attachments.
    - This leads to a physiologic VISI (volar intercalated segmental instability; volar-facing lunate).
  - With ulnar deviation, the triquetrum is forced into extension due to its unique helicoid articulation with the hamate.
    - The lunate passively follows leading to a physiologic DISI (dorsal intercalated segment instability; dorsal-facing lunate).

- Pathology and pathomechanics
  - Pathology involves a tear in the membranous, volar, or dorsal components (can be all three).
  - LT instability requires a tear of the membranous portion PLUS a tear in either the dorsal or palmar components.[1]
  - In LT instability, the lunate is abnormally flexed (VISI deformity) as a result of the unresisted flexion moment generated by the scaphoid.[6-8]
    - Lichtman's "ring concept of carpal kinematics" hypothesizes that physiologic wrist "loading" creates a flexion moment at the scaphotrapeziotrapezoid (STT) joint and an extension moment at the triquetrohamate (TH) joint, keeping an intact wrist balanced and motionless.[9]
      - With disruption of the LT ligament, compression through the STT joint leads to scaphoid and lunate flexion while the head of the capitate forces the triquetrum ulnarly and into an extended position.
      - This uncoupling of torque forces at the LT joint leads to a static VISI deformity (Figure 21.1).[7]
  - Complete LT ligament tear may not be sufficient in isolation to cause a VISI deformity, but may show divergence of the LT joint with extreme wrist flexion and radial deviation.[10]
- Etiology
  - Result of a backward fall onto an outstretched hand with the wrist extended and ulnarly deviated
    - Force directed through the hypothenar region drives the pisiform into the triquetrum, forcing it dorsally.
    - LT ligament is injured as the lunate remains in place due to constraint by the long radiolunate ligament and the radiocarpal joint.[6]
    - The force on the ulnar wrist leads to intercarpal pronation, which overloads the LT ligament without disrupting the SL ligament.[10-12]

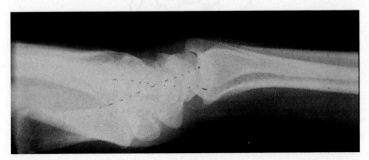

FIGURE 21.1 Lateral wrist radiograph demonstrating a volar intercalated segmental instability deformity.

- Occasionally occurs as a "forme fruste" of perilunate injury or dislocation.[8]
  - Stage III of progressive perilunate instability is LT ligamentous disruption (Figure 21.2).[13]
  - Chronic LT instability can occur after repair of the SL dissociation with failure to recognize LT injury in perilunate dislocations.
- Another proposed mechanism of injury is a fall onto a pronated, radial deviated, and flexed wrist.[14]
- Ulnar positive variance is often associated with acute and attritional (chronic) LT ligament pathology due to increased stress on the triquetrum (and triangular fibrocartilage complex [TFCC] complex) in ulnar deviation.[15,16]
- Isolated LT injuries may also occur with a dorsally applied force with the wrist flexed.[7]
  - This injury pattern causes the interosseous portion of the LT ligament to fail, leaving the volar radiolunotriquetral ligament intact.[7]

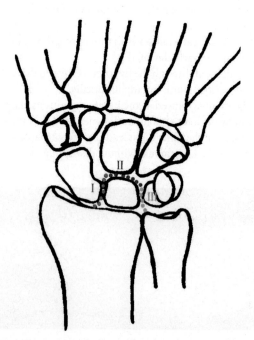

FIGURE 21.2 The stages of perilunate instability.

TABLE 21.1 Viegas Classification of LT Ligament Injuries

Grade 1	Partial or complete LT tear without VISI deformity
Grade 2	Complete LT ligament tear with lesion of palmar ligaments and dynamic VISI deformity
Grade 3	Complete LT ligament tear with lesion of the palmar and dorsal ligaments and static VISI deformity

Abbreviations: LT, Lunotriquetral; VISI, Volar intercalated segmental instability.

- Classification (Table 21-1)
  - The Geissler classification of SL ligament injuries may also be applied to LT ligament injuries.[17]
- Clinical presentation
  - Ulnar wrist pain, weakness, wrist click, loss of range of motion, instability, ulnar sensory deficits, dinner fork deformity
  - Point tenderness at the LT interval
  - Painful click with ulnar deviation and pronation
  - Not specific, as this may also be present in midcarpal instability (MCI)
- LT ballottement test[11]
  - Lunate is grasped between the thumb and index finger of one hand, and the triquetrum is grasped with the other hand and an attempt is made to translate the triquetrum on the stabilized lunate.
  - Test is positive when translation recreates the patient's symptoms.
- Shear test[18,19]
  - With the elbow flexed and the forearm in neutral, the examiner's thumb is used to apply a dorsal force to the triquetrum while their other thumb applies a volar force to the lunate.
  - Laxity of the LT joint compared to the contralateral side, or a recreation of the patient's symptoms is considered positive.
- Radiographic presentation
  - Plain radiography
    - Standard posteroanterior and lateral are the first-line images to be obtained.
    - May be normal or may show disruption of Gilula's lines[20] with LT overlap or proximal triquetral migration (Figure 21.3)[21,22]
    - Static LT injuries may not be evident on standard wrist radiographs; however, radial/ulnar deviation view may reveal an LT disruption.
    - VISI deformity on standard lateral wrist radiographs indicates static instability and is considered a possible sign of "LT dissociation."[21]

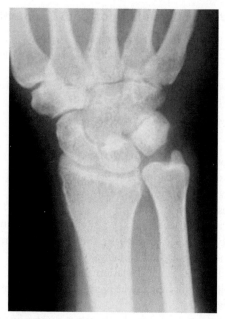

FIGURE 21.3 Anteroposterior radiograph showing lunotriquetral dissociation.

- ◆ Normal radiographic LT angle is 14° dorsal tilt, but in LT dissociation this angle has been shown to be a negative (volar) angle.[10]
- ◆ SL angle less than 30° along with an LT angle greater than 15° indicates LT dissociation.[6]
- ● Radiographic arthrography
  - ◆ Dye leakage within the LT joint may represent LT ligament tear.[23]
  - ◆ High false-positive rate and is now largely of historical interest only[20]
- ● Bone scan
  - ◆ Less specific than arthrography, but may be of use in the diagnosis of acute LT injury[20]
- ● MRI
  - ◆ Improved the capability of diagnosing LT tears
  - ◆ 3T MR arthrography improves the sensitivity and specificity of MRI.
  - ◆ Sensitivities range from 40% to 75% and specificities range from 64% to 100%.[22,24]
- ● Wrist arthroscopy
  - ◆ The gold standard diagnostic tool

TABLE 21.2 Lichtman Classification and Treatment Algorithm of LT Ligament Injury

Classification	Chronicity	Injured Structures	Treatment Recommendation
Stable	Acute or chronic	Membranous portion of LT ligament	Nonoperative/immobilization or arthroscopic debridement
Unstable	Acute unstable	Membranous portion with concurrent volar and/or dorsal LT ligament	Open or arthroscopic reduction and pinning of LT joint with repair of LT ligament
	Chronic unstable	Membranous portion with concurrent volar and/or dorsal LT ligament	LT joint arthrodesis (provided no ulnar positive variance) Ligament reconstruction (alternative)

In addition to the above treatment recommendations, we recommend ulnar shortening osteotomy as well for patients with radiographic evidence of ulnar abutment.

Abbreviation: LT, Lunotriquetral.

- ◆ Allows for diagnosis of ligament tears with the capability for simultaneous debridement or repair.
- ◆ Diagnostic arthroscopic assessment is recommended in the setting of negative MRI with high clinical suspicion of ligament disruption.[21]
- ■ Treatment (Table 21-2)
  - ● Stable/incomplete injuries
  - ● Nonoperative management with splint immobilization extending proximal to the elbow (Reagan, Culver, Butterfield).[1,10,25]
    - ◆ Prevent supination/pronation
    - ◆ Nonsteroidal anti-inflammatory drugs (NSAIDs) or intra-articular corticosteroid injections may be used to decrease symptoms from synovitis during ligamentous healing.[1]
    - ◆ The usual duration of immobilization ranges from 6 to 12 weeks.[1,26]
  - ● Arthroscopic debridement
  - ● Acute unstable injuries
  - ● Arthroscopic evaluation
    - ◆ Best performed through the 4 to 5, 6R, or midcarpal portals
    - ◆ Midcarpal arthroscopy is critical to assessing LT joint stability,[27] with the expectation of no step-off or diastasis with an intact LT ligament.[28]
  - ● Geissler grade II/III lesions
    - ◆ K-wire fixation from the triquetrum to the lunate is performed, with the wrist immobilized for approximately 8 weeks.[21]

- Geissler grade IV lesions—direct repair of the LT ligament
  - Longitudinal curvilinear incision just distal to the dorsal aspect of the ulnocarpal joint. A central longitudinal dorsal incision used when LT repair is being performed as part of a perilunate dislocation.
  - Identify and protect the dorsal branch of the ulnar nerve.
  - The extensor retinaculum is divided; posterior interosseous neurectomy may be performed.
  - Ligament sparing capsulotomy is made on the dorsal wrist, exposing the radiocarpal and midcarpal joint.[21]
  - Direct LT repair may be done in a number of described ways.
  - Prior to ligament repair, the radiocarpal and midcarpal joints should be thoroughly examined for signs of degenerative changes.
    - LT ligamentous complex may be reconstructed using suture anchors (our preference) or through drill holes.
    - Three to four drill holes may be placed through the triquetrum with subsequent passage of nonabsorbable suture through the drill holes into the LT ligament and back through the drill holes and tied over a triquetral bone bridge.[21]
    - K-wires are then placed through the triquetrum into the lunate, which will remain in place while ligament healing takes place.
    - We recommend leaving anchor or repair sutures long and tying them into the dorsal capsule (DRT ligament).
    - Chronic injuries
- LT reconstruction may be performed with tendon autograft or allograft.[10,29,30]
  - Longitudinal dorsal incision is made over the fourth extensor compartment and a ligament-sparing capsulotomy is made.
  - The LT joint is anatomically reduced under direct and fluoroscopic examination and temporarily stabilized with K-wires.
  - 4 to 5 mm bone tunnels are drilled through the lunate and triquetrum.
  - The extensor carpi ulnaris tendon is then harvested 6 cm proximal to the ulnar styloid, splitting the tendon and leaving its distal attachment intact.
  - The split tendon is passed through the drill tunnels and two intra-articular K-wires are used to stabilize the LT joint. The graft is then sutured back to itself.
  - The wrist is immobilized in neutral for 10 to 12 weeks.[31]
  - Allograft may be used for LT ligamentous reconstruction.[32]

- LT arthrodesis
  - ◆ Dorsal two-thirds of adjacent cartilaginous surfaces of the LT joint are denuded of articular cartilage and the arthrodesis may be performed with the use of K-wires, or screws.
- Take care not to change the overall dimensions and alignment of the proximal carpal row.
  - ◆ Wrist is immobilized for 10 to 12 weeks in neutral.[31]
  - ◆ Address ulnar positive variance at time of arthrodesis with ulnar shortening osteotomy.
    - ✳ Associated with higher incidence of failure if left ulnar positive
- Although not routinely performed, LT repair may still be possible in chronic injuries. Posterior interosseous neurectomy is also an option.

PALMAR MIDCARPAL INSTABILITY (PMCI)

- Functional anatomy
  - The DRT ligament is the first component of a series of dorsal stabilizers of the PR.
  - The DRT ligament originates on the distal radius, and crosses obliquely with attachments to the dorsal lunate, dorsal LT ligament, and the dorsal triquetrum.
  - The dorsal radiocarpal ligament (DRCL) acts to resist ulnar translation and excessive flexion of the entire PR.
  - A stable proximal carpal row works in concert with the distal carpal row to allow for the dart-thrower's motion through the midcarpal joint.
- Pathologic anatomy and pathokinematics
  - Disruption or laxity of the DRT ligament results in abnormal flexion (VISI deformity) and hypermobility of the PR when the wrist is relaxed (unloaded) in neutral deviation.[2,33,34]
  - Sectioning of the palmar ulnar arcuate ligament produces a VISI deformity in cadaveric studies.[2,34-36]
  - Excessive PR flexion and hypermobility permit the capitate and distal row to subluxate volarly when wrist compression forces are not engaged (unloaded).
  - The resulting loss of normal midcarpal joint reactive forces permits the distal row to remain in flexion as the wrist moves into ulnar deviation.

- When the wrist reaches full ulnar deviation the TH articulation forces are reengaged and the triquetrum abruptly extends along with the entire PR (with a reduction clunk).
- Etiology
  - Developmental or congenital ligamentous laxity is the most common cause of MCI.[34]
  - May be due to traumatic disruption of the DRT ligament as the result of a distal radius fracture or perilunate dislocation with ulnar translation
- Clinical presentation
  - Typical patient is 20 to 30 years of age with ulnar-sided wrist pain. Frequently occurs in adolescent females[8]
  - Volar sag on the ulnar wrist, which may be confused with dorsal ulnar dislocation[9,34]
  - Painful, audible clunk with active wrist ulnar deviation
  - Positive midcarpal shift test[37]
    - Steady the pronated forearm and apply a palmar directed force on the base of the third metacarpal to accentuate the volar sag of the PR.
    - Move the wrist into ulnar deviation. A positive clunk is experienced as the distal row reduces to an appropriate anatomic location in ulnar deviation.
    - Test is considered positive only when this clunk recreates the patient's symptoms.
  - Lateral wrist radiographs often show a VISI deformity, but may be normal.
    - With equivocal radiographs, consider performing the midcarpal shift test under live fluoroscopy.
    - A positive fluoroscopic shift test will show a characteristic jump from a VISI deformity to a DISI deformity after the elicited clunk in ulnar deviation.[34]
- Classification
  - Palmar MCI
    - Volar sag at the midcarpal joint with history of painful clunk with ulnar deviation[34]
    - Most common form of MCI, described earlier
  - Dorsal MCI
    - Dorsal subluxation of the capitate on the lunate[38,39]
  - Extrinsic (adaptive) MCI
    - Result of a dorsally displaced and malunited distal radius fracture with secondary adaptive changes in the radiocarpal and intercarpal ligaments[40]

- Treatment
  - Palmar MCI
    - NSAIDs and activity modification for all initial encounters, especially in adolescents
    - Custom splints, which apply a dorsally directed force on the pisiform to rotate the proximal carpal row out of flexion, and proprioceptive training are the mainstay of treatment.
      * With activation of selected wrist flexors and extensors, many patients can maintain the reduced position actively.
      * Patients are trained to "set" the wrist prior to active ulnar deviation, preventing a catch-up reduction clunk in ulnar deviation.
    - DRT ligament reefing for those who fail conservative treatment is the author's surgical treatment of choice.
    - Four-corner fusion with or without scaphoidectomy may be required to eliminate the clunk for those who failed prior surgical treatment.
    - Arthroscopic capsular shrinking and radioscapholunate arthrodesis are under investigation.
  - Dorsal MCI
    - Activity modification alone often provides satisfactory clinical outcomes.[38]
    - Reefing of the palmar radiocapitate ligament to the radiotriquetral ligament (closing the space of Poirier)[39]
  - Extrinsic MCI
    - Distal radius osteotomy to realign the carpus over the radius.

SUMMARY

1. LT ligamentous injuries are relatively uncommon and represent one of a number of possible etiologies of ulnar-sided wrist pain.
2. Clinical examination may show a dinner fork deformity or a painful wrist click.
3. LT ballottement test and Kleinman shear test suggest injury to the LT ligamentous complex.
4. Lateral (sagittal) radiographs often reveal a VISI deformity. Coronal views may show a step off at the LT joint with distal translocation of the triquetrum. This may be accentuated by ulnar deviation of the wrist.
5. The gold standard for diagnosis of LT ligament injuries remains wrist arthroscopy, which allows for concurrent diagnosis and treatment of LT ligamentous injuries.

6. Stable injuries have an isolated disruption of the membranous portion of the LT ligament, and may be treated nonoperatively or with arthroscopic debridement.

7. Unstable injuries have disruption of the membranous portion of the ligament with a concurrent disruption of the volar and/or dorsal LT ligament.

8. Acute injuries should be treated with closer reduction percutaneous pinning (CRPP) with ligament repair or reconstruction.

9. Chronic injuries may be treated with LT arthrodesis or LT ligament reconstruction. Ulnar positive variance must be corrected if present, especially with arthrodesis.

10. MCI is due to laxity of the ligaments that stabilize the mobile PR, particularly the DRCL (palmar MCI).
    a. Hypermobility of the PR leads to a VISI deformity in neutral and a "catch up" reduction clunk in ulnar deviation.

11. The DRT ligament is one of the primary stabilizers of the PR. Acute or chronic injury to the DRT ligament (or its bony attachment) seems to be a major cause of PMCI.

12. Most cases of MCI will respond to conservative measures, including splinting.
    a. Midcarpal fusion will eliminate the painful clunk but repair or reefing of the DRT ligament is a promising alternative.
    b. Arthroscopic capsular shrinking and radioscapholunate arthrodesis are under investigation.

REFERENCES

1. Butterfield WL, Joshi AB, Lichtman DM. Lunotriquetral injuries. *J Am Soc Surg Hand.* 2002;2(4):195-203. Web.

2. Viegas SF, Patterson RM, Peterson PD, et al. Ulnar sided perilunate instability: an anatomic and biomechanic study. *J Hand Surg Am.* 1990;15A(2):268-278.

3. Ritt MJ, Bishop AT, Berger RA, Linscheid RL, Berglund LJ, An KN. Lunotriquetral ligament properties: a comparison of three anatomic subregions. *J Hand Surg Am.* 1998;23(3):425-431.

4. Pulos N, Bozentka DJ. Carpal ligament anatomy and biomechanics. *Hand Clin.* 2015;31(3):381-387.

5. Ritt MJ, Linscheid RL, Cooney WP, Berger RA, An KN. The lunotriquetral joint: kinematic effects of sequential ligament sectioning, ligament repair, and arthrodesis. *J Hand Surg Am.* 1998;23(3):432-445.

6. Lee DJ, Elfar JC. Carpal ligament injuries, pathomechanics, and classification. *Hand Clin.* 2015;31(3):389-398.

7. Alexander C, Lichtman D. Triquetrolunate instability. In: Lichtman D, Alexander H, eds. *The Wrist and Its Disorders.* Philadelphia, PA: WB Saunders; 1997:307-316.

8. Niacaris T, Ming BW, Lichtman DM. Midcarpal instability: a comprehensive review and update. *Hand Clin.* 2015;31(3):487-493.

9. Lichtman DM, Schneider JR, Swafford AR, Mack GR. Ulnar midcarpal instability—clinical and laboratory analysis. *J Hand Surg.* 1981;6A:515-523.

10. Reagan DS, Linscheid RL, Dobyns JH. Lunotriquetral sprains. *J Hand Surg Am.* 1984;9(4):502-514.

11. Linscheid RL, Dobyns JH. The unified concept of carpal injuries. *Ann Chir Main.* 1984;3(1):35-42.

12. Murray PM, Palmer CG, Shin AY. The mechanism of ulnar-sided perilunate instability of the wrist: a cadaveric study and 6 clinical cases. *J Hand Surg Am.* 2012;37(4):721-728.

13. Mayfield JK, Johnson RP, Kilcoyne RK. Pathomechanics and progressive perilunar instability. *J Hand Surg.* 1980;5A:226-241.

14. Shin AY, Battaglia MJ, Bishop AT. Lunotriquetral instability: diagnosis and treatment. *J Am Acad Orthop Surg.* 2000;8(3):170-179.

15. Palmer AK. Triangular fibrocartilage complex lesions: a classification. *J Hand Surg Am.* 1989;14:594-606.

16. Palmer AK, Werner FW. Biomechanics of the distal radioulnar joint. *Clin Orthop Relat Res.* 1984;(275):26-35.

17. Geissler WB, Freeland AE, Savoie FH, et al. Intracarpal soft-tissue lesions associated with an intra-articular fracture of the distal end of the radius. *J Bone Joint Surg Am.* 1996;78(3):357-365.

18. Kleinman WB. *Diagnostic Exams for Ligamentous Injuries.* No 51. Rosemont, IL: American Society for Surgery of the Hand, Correspondence Club Newsletter; 1985.

19. Bishop A, Reagan D. Lunotriquetral sprains. In: Cooney W, Linschied R, Dobyns J, eds. *The wrist. Diagnosis and operative treatment.* St. Louis, MO: Mosby, 1998:527-550.

20. Gilula LA, Weeks PM. Post-traumatic ligamentous instabilities of the wrist. *Radiology.* 1978;129:641-651.

21. Nicoson MC, Moran SL. Diagnosis and treatment of acute lunotriquetral ligament injuries. *Hand Clin.* 2015;31(3):467-476.

22. Sachar K. Ulnar-sided wrist pain: evaluation and treatment of triangular fibrocartilage complex tears, ulnocarpal impaction syndrome, and lunotriquetral ligament tears. *J Hand Surg Am.* 2012;37(7):1489-1500.

23. Cantor RM, Stern PJ, Wyrick JD, et al. The relevance of ligament tears or perforations in the diagnosis of wrist pain: an arthrographic study. *J Hand Surg.* 1994;19A(6):945-953.

24. Zanetti M, Saupe N, Nagy L. Role of MR imaging in chronic wrist pain. *Eur Radiol.* 2007;17:927-938.

25. Culver JE. Instabilities of the wrist. *Clin Sports Med.* 1986;5(4):725-740.

26. Ambrose L, Posner M. Lunate-triquetral and midcarpal joint instability. *Hand Clin.* 1992;8:653-658.

27. Hofmeister EP, Moran SL, Shin AY. Anterior and posterior interosseous neurectomy for the treatment of chronic dynamic instability of the wrist. *Hand*. 2006;1:63-70.

28. Hanker GJ. Diagnostic and operative arthroscopy of the wrist. *Clin Orthop Relat Res*. 1991;263:165-174.

29. Shin AY, Bishop AT. Treatment options for lunotriquetral dissociation. *Tech Hand Up Extrem Surg*. 1998;2:2-17.

30. Shahane SA, Trail IA, Takwale VJ, et al. Tenodesis of the extensor carpi ulnaris for chronic, post-traumatic lunotriquetral instability. *J Bone Joint Surg Br*. 2005;87:1512-1515.

31. Wagner ER, Elhassan BT, Rizzo M. Diagnosis and treatment of chronic lunotriquetral ligament injuries. *Hand Clin*. 2015;31(3):477-486.

32. Schweizer A, Steiger R. Long-term results after repair and augmentation ligamentoplasty of rotatory subluxation of the scaphoid. *J Hand Surg Am*. 2002;27:674-684.

33. Lichtman DM, Bruckner JD, Culp RW, Alexander CE. Palmar midcarpal instability: results of surgical reconstruction. *J Hand Surg*. 1993;18A:307-315.

34. Lichtman DM, Wroten ES. Understanding midcarpal instability. *J Hand Surg Am*. 2006;31(3):491-498.

35. Trumble T, Bour CJ, Smith RJ, Edwards GS. Intercarpal arthrodesis for static and dynamic volar intercalated segment instability pattern. *J Hand Surg*. 1988;13A:384-390.

36. Trumble T, Bour CJ, Smith RJ, Glisson RR. Kinematics of the ulnar carpus related to the volar intercalated segment instability pattern. *J Hand Surg*. 1990;15A:384-392.

37. Feinstein WK, Lichtman DM, Noble PC, Alexander JW, Hipp JA. Quantitative assessment of the midcarpal shift test. *J Hand Surg Am*. 1999;24(5):977-983.

38. Louis DS, Hankin FM, Greene TL, et al. Central carpal instability-capitate lunate instability pattern: diagnosis by dynamic displacement. *Orthopedics*. 1984;7:1693-1696.

39. Johnson RP, Carrera GF. Chronic capitolunate instability. *J Bone Joint Surg Am*. 1986;68(8):1164-1176.

40. Taleisnik J, Watson HK. Midcarpal instability caused by malunited fractures of the distal radius. *J Hand Surg Am*. 1984;9(3):350-357.

22 Avascular Necrosis of the Hand and Wrist

Michael Guju, Evan H. Horowitz, and
Francisco A. Schwartz-Fernandes

The article by Gelberman and Gross on the vascularity of the wrist divided the bones of the wrist into three groups based on decreasing risk of avascular necrosis (AVN).[1]

Group	Bones	At-Risk Anatomy
Group 1	Scaphoid, capitate, and 80% of lunate	Supplied by only one vessel or had large areas of bone only supplied by one vessel. Most vulnerable group to avascular necrosis (AVN)
Group 2	Hamate and trapezoid	Do not have internal anastomosis. Minimal risk of AVN
Group 3	Trapezium, triquetrum, pisiform, and 92% of lunates	Have rich internal anastomoses. Least risk for AVN

They further expanded their examination by examining the extent and type of vascular occlusion required to cause AVN (Table 22.1).

AVN DISORDERS

Scaphoid

- Cause of AVN—trauma
  - Epidemiology
    - Osteonecrosis is said to occur in 13% to 50% of cases of fracture of the scaphoid.
    - Incidence of osteonecrosis is even higher in those with involvement of the proximal one-fifth of the scaphoid.[2,3]
- Anatomy
  - The blood supply of the scaphoid is primarily from the radial artery via the artery to the dorsal ridge of the scaphoid.

TABLE 22.1 Risk of Avascular Necrosis According to Gelberman and Gross[1]

Bones	Type of Occlusion Resulting in AVN
Scaphoid and capitate	Intraosseous disruption
Lunates (minority)	Extraosseous disruption
Lunates (majority)	Both extraosseous and intraosseous disruption

AVN, avascular necrosis.

- ♦ The branches enter the scaphoid via foramina at the dorsal ridge at the level of the waist of the scaphoid.[4,5]
  - The proximal pole of the scaphoid relies entirely on this interosseous blood supply.
- Pathophysiology
  - Low-energy falls from a standing height were most common (40.4%).
  - Males are significantly more likely to sustain their fracture after a high-energy injury.[6]
- Clinical history
  - Scaphoid fractures are commonly seen in young, healthy individuals and may occur as a result of a fall on the outstretched arm or a forced dorsiflexion injury of the wrist.[2]
- Physical examination
  - A reliable correlation exists between scaphoid fracture and pain provoked by deep palpation at the volar tubercle of the scaphoid, which is the first bony prominence distal to the volar distal radius. Scaphoid fracture is not very likely when tubercle palpation does not provoke pain in the snuffbox.
- Special provocation maneuvers
  - Watson (scaphoid shift) test—The patient sits with the forearm pronated. The examiner takes the patient's wrist into full ulnar deviation and extension. The examiner presses the patient's thumb with his/her other hand and then begins radial deviation and flexion of the patient's hand.
  - Scaphoid stress test—The patient sits while the examiner holds the patient's wrist with one hand, with the examiner applying pressure with his/her thumb over the patient's distal scaphoid. The patient then attempts radial deviation of the wrist.

TABLE 22.2 Scaphoid Fracture—Herbert Classification

A	Acute, stable	A1	Tubercle
		A2	Nondisplaced crack in the waist
B	Acute, unstable	B1	Oblique, distal third
		B2	Displaced or mobile, waist
		B3	Proximal pole
		B4	Fracture-dislocation
		B5	Comminuted
C	Delayed union		
D	Established nonunion	D1	Fibrous
		D2	Sclerotic
Descriptive			
Special studies		Scaphoid view	
		Kinematic wrist views	

- Classification/imaging
  - A computed tomography bone scan in the long axis of the scaphoid is the best means of differentiating between stable and unstable fractures. Type B fractures should be corrected operatively (Table 22.2).[7]
- Preiser's disease
  - Preiser's disease is a rare condition where ischemia and necrosis of the scaphoid bone occur bilaterally without previous fracture. The lack of perfusion to the proximal pole is often associated with prolonged use of corticosteroids or chemotherapy. X-ray and magnetic resonance imaging (MRI) are used to confirm diagnosis.
- Classification/imaging
  - Staging of Preiser's (Table 22.3)

TABLE 22.3 Preiser Disease Classification[38]

Stage	Radiologic Findings
I	Normal radiograph. Abnormal findings on MRI. Positive bone scan
II	Proximal pole sclerosis of the scaphoid. Generalized osteoporosis
III	Fragmentation of the proximal scaphoid pole with/without pathological fracture
IV	Periscaphoid collapse, fragmentation, and osteoarthritis

Abbreviation: MRI, magnetic resonance imaging.

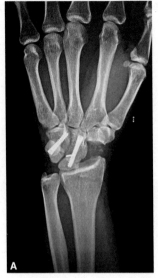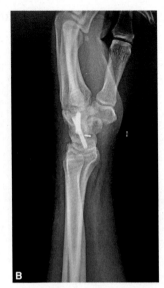

FIGURE 22.1 Four-corner fusion, x-rays on anteroposterior (A) and lateral (B) views.

- Treatment
  - Initial treatment is immobilization
  - There are two surgical procedures to treat Preiser's disease.
    - Proximal row carpectomy (PRC), which is the removal of the proximal row of carpal bones (scaphoid, lunate, and triquetrum)
    - Four-corner fusion with scaphoid excision, which is the removal of the scaphoid bone and fixing of the remaining wrist bones using a "spider plate" or wires (Figure 22.1)[8,9]

LUNATE

- Kienbock's disease
  - Epidemiology
    - This disease most commonly occurs in the dominant hand of males between the ages of 18 and 40 years.
    - A history of manual labor in the affected hand is reported in 95% of cases.[9-11]
  - It is estimated to occur in 2.5% of the population.[8]

- Anatomy
  - 80% of lunates receive their blood supply from both palmar and dorsal sources.
    - The dorsal radiocarpal arch delivers blood from the dorsal aspect of the hand.
    - The palmar radiocarpal and intercarpal arches deliver blood from the palmar aspect of the hand.
    - There are three major intraosseal anastomotic patterns of the lunate, named I, X, Y after their appearance.
      - Each of the patterns has a consistent prevalence in the population (Figure 22.2).
        - I present in 30% population
        - X present in 10% population
        - Y present in 60% population
- 20% of lunates rely solely on the palmar vascular supply from the palmar radiocarpal and intercarpal arches.[4]
  - The lack of a dorsal vascular supply puts these patients at higher risk for AVN during dislocations or hyperextension injuries.[12]
- There are two distinct morphologic classification of the lunate based on its articulation with the other carpal bones.[13]
  - Type I—have a single distal articular facet for the capitate
  - Type II—have a distal articular facet for the capitate and an additional distal articular facet medially for the hamate
- Pathophysiology
  - Disruption along the intraosseous blood supply, via acute or stress fractures, can result in AVN.[4,8-12]
  - An association between negative ulnar variance and increased incidence of lunatomalacia has been described, but the validity is not well established in the literature.[14-22]
    - It is thought that the discrepancy in wrist length increases shearing forces on the lunate, resulting in stress fractures, interrupting the intraosseous blood supply, and leading to AVN.

FIGURE 22.2 Lunate blood supply pattern.

- Lunate phenotype
  - Type I (single distal articular facet for the capitate) have higher incidence of coronal fractures and advanced disease (>stage IIIA) of Kienbock's disease.[23]
- Clinical presentation
  - Unilateral to effected wrist
- Pain in the wrist is dorsal
  - Aggravated by use and relieved by rest
- Physical examination
  - Dorsal wrist swelling, due to radiocarpal synovitis, with tenderness to palpation around dorsal aspect of lunate
  - Limited wrist flexion/extension
  - Diminished grip strength on effected side
  - Pain upon percussion of distal aspect of third metacarpal[11]
- Imaging/classification (Table 22.4 and Figure 22.3)
  Treatment based on classification (Table 22.5)
- Author's preferred procedures for Kienbock's
  - Core decompression
    - Use in stage I, II, and IIIA
    - The core decompression of the lunate takes a dorsal approach to the lunate and removes part of the lunate undergoing AVN. The lunate is identified using a guidewire under fluoroscopic control and a dental burr (2.5 mm) is used to decompress.[13]
      - Most patients who undergo this procedure see no change in Lichtman stage and have no carpal collapse after 5 years.

TABLE 22.4 Lichtman Classification[37]

Stage	Radiographic Findings
I	Normal or linear/stress fracture on MRI/bone scan
II	Lunate sclerosis without collapse
IIIA	Lunate sclerosis and fragmentation with collapse
	Radioscaphoid angle <60°, no scaphoid rotation
IIIB	Lunate sclerosis and fragmentation with carpal collapse
	Radioscaphoid angle >60°
	Fixed scaphoid flexion
IV	Lunate sclerosis and fragmentation with collapse
	Radiocarpal or midcarpal arthritis

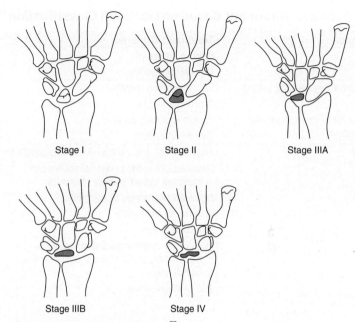

FIGURE 22.3 Lichtman classification.[37]

- Radial shortening osteotomy
  - Use in stage I, II, and IIIA
  - Radial shortening osteotomy is the surgical removal of a distal segment of the radius. The segment is proximal to the head of the ulna. A plate is used to hold the two segments together. The purpose is to reduce pressure on the lunate from the radius.
  - After a 10-year follow-up, there was no advancement in Lichtman staging.[24]
- Proximal row carpectomy
  - Use in stage IIIb and IV (if not osteoarthritic)
  - This procedure removes the scaphoid, lunate, and triquetrum, which comprises the more proximal row of carpal bones.
    - Patients who were over 35 years old at the time of PRC, after long-term follow-up, were satisfied with the results. They reported satisfactory range of motion, grip strength, and pain relief.[25]
- Wrist fusion
  - Use in stage IV or severe osteoarthritis.
  - Four-corner fusion

TABLE 22.5 Treatment Based on Lichtman Classification[37]

Stage	Treatment Options[39]
I	Splint immobilization Core decompression
II or IIIA (negative ulnar variance)	Radial shortening osteotomy Core decompression
II or IIIA (neutral or positive ulnar variance)	Capitate shortening osteotomy Core decompression
IIIB	Scaphocapitate or scaphotrapeziotrapezoid arthrodesis Lunate excision and/or tendon interposition and intercarpal fusion if evidence of synovitis Nickel-titanium memory alloy arthrodesis Proximal row carpectomy Four-corner fusion
IV	Proximal row carpectomy (contraindicated if arthritic changes about head of capitate or lunate facet of radius) Total wrist arthrodesis

- Wrist fusion runs a plate from the radius, over the carpals, and to the metacarpals, locking all in place. This is considered a more radical treatment option as it essentially eliminates wrist range of motion.
  - This procedure is reserved for "advanced Keinbock's disease," although there is no exact definition for this disease classification. Wrist fusion has been compared to lunate replacement, lunate excision, PRC, and limited carpal fusion. There is no strong supporting evidence to select one procedure over the other.[26]

TRIQUETRUM, HAMATE, CAPITATE, TRAPEZOID, PISIFORM, TRAPEZIUM

- Epidemiology
  - AVN of these bones is exceedingly rare.
    - There is scarce literature on the topic.
    - Most literature are single case studies.[27-36]
  - Acute trauma or repeated motion is the most common cause.
  - Multiple steroid injections could also cause AVN

- Clinical presentation
  - AVN of a carpal characteristically presents with wrist pain, stiffness, and weak grip.[34]
- Classification/imaging
  - Planar radiograph is used for diagnosis.[35]
  - T1, T2 MRI is used to confirm diagnosis.[35]
- Treatment
  - No standard of care is established for AVN of these bones.
  - Conservative treatment with splinting and analgesics[34]
  - Surgical debridement or removal of bone has also been explored as a treatment option.[28]

SUGGESTED READINGS

Got J, Cavallasca JA. Bilateral avascular necrosis of the scaphoid (Preiser' disease), a rare cause of wrist pain. *Reumatol Clín* (English Edition). 2014;10(6):418-419. doi:10.1016/j.reumae.2014.04.004.

Streich NA, Martini AK, Daecke W. Proximal row carpectomy: an adequate procedure in carpal collapse. *Int Orthop*. 2008;32(1):85-89.

REFERENCES

1. Gelberman RH, Gross MS. The vascularity of the wrist. Identification of arterial patterns at risk. *Clin Orthop Relat Res*. 1986;202:40-49.
2. Herbert TJ, Fisher WE. Management of the fractured scaphoid using a new bone screw. *J Bone Joint Surg Br*. 1984;66:114-123.
3. Cooney WP, Dobyns JH, Linscheid RL. Fractures of the scaphoid: a rational approach to management. *Clin Orthop*. 1980;149:90-97.
4. Freedman DM, Botte MJ, Gelberman RH. Vascularity of the carpus. *Clin Orthop*. 2001;383:47-59. doi:10.1097/00003086-200102000-00008.
5. Gelberman RH, Menon J. The vascularity of the scaphoid bone. *J Hand Surg Am*. 1980;5:508-513.
6. Duckworth AD, Jenkins PJ, Aitken SA, Clement ND, Court-Brown CM, McQueen MM. Scaphoid fracture epidemiology. *J Trauma Acute Care Surg*. 2012;72(2):E41-E45.
7. Krimmer H, Schmitt R, Herbert T. Scaphoid fractures: diagnosis, classification and therapy. *Unfallchirurg*. 2000;103(10):812-819.
8. Palmer A, Benoit M. Lunate fractures: Kienböck's disease. In: Cooney W, Linscheid R, Dobyns J, eds. *The Wrist: Diagnosis and Operative Treatment*. Philadelphia, PA: Mosby; 1998:431-473.
9. Taniguchi Y, Yoshida M, Iwasaki H, Otakara H, Iwata S. Kienböck's disease in elderly patients. *J Hand Surg Am*. 2003;28(5):779-783.
10. McMurtry RY, Youm Y, Flatt AE, Gillespie TE. Kinematics of the wrist: II. Clinical applications. *J Bone Joint Surg Am*. 1978;60(7):955-961.

11. Szabo RM, Greenspan A. Diagnosis and clinical findings of Kienböck's disease. *Hand Clin.* 1993;9(3):399-408.

12. Gelberman RH, Bauman TD, Menon J, Akeson WH. The vascularity of the lunate bone and Kienböck's disease. *J Hand Surg Am.* 1980;5(3):272-278.

13. Mehrpour SR, Kamrani RS, Aghamirsalim MR, Sorbi R, Kaya A. Treatment of Kienböck disease by lunate core decompression. *J Hand Surg Am.* 2011;36(10):1675-1677.

14. Hulten O. Uber Anatomische Variationen der Hand Gelenkknochen. *Acta Radiol.* 1928;9:155-169.

15. Mirabello SC, Rosenthal DI, Smith RJ. Correlation of clinical and radiographic findings in Kienböck's disease. *J Hand Surg Am.* 1987;12(6):1049-1054.

16. Tsuge S, Nakamura R. Anatomical risk factors for Kienböck's disease. *J Hand Surg Br.* 1993;18(1):70-75.

17. Armistead RB, Linsheid RL, Dobyns JH, Beckenbaugh RD. Ulnar lengthening in the treatment of Kienböck's disease. *J Bone Joint Surg Am.* 1982;64(2):170-178.

18. Beckenbaugh RD, Schieves TC, Dobyns JH, Linsheid RL. Kienböck's disease: the natural history of Kienböck's disease and consideration of lunate fractures. *Clin Orthop Relat Res.* 1980;149:98-106.

19. Chen WS, Shih CH. Ulnar variance and Kienböck's disease: an investigation in Taiwan. *Clin Orthop Relat Res.* 1990;255:124-127.

20. Gelberman RH, Salaman PB, Jurist JM, Posch JL. Ulnar variance in Kienböck's disease. *J Bone Joint Surg Am.* 1975;57(5):674-676.

21. D'Hoore K, DeSmet L, Verellen K, Vral J, Fabry G. Negative ulnar variance is not a risk factor for Kienböck's disease. *J Hand Surg Am.* 1994;19(2):229-231.

22. Nakamura R, Imaeda T, Miura T. Radial shortening for Kienböck's disease: factors affecting the operative result. *J Hand Surg Br.* 1990;15(1):40-45.

23. Rhee PC, Jones DB, Moran SL, Shin AY. The effect of lunate morphology in Kienbock disease. *J Hand Surg Am.* 2015;40(4):738-744.

24. Matsui Y, Funakoshi T, Motomiya M, Urita A, Minami M, Iwasaki N. Radial shortening osteotomy for Kienbock disease: minimum 10-year follow up. *J Hand Surg Am.* 2014;39(4):679-685.

25. Stern PJ, Agabegi SS, Kiefhaber TR, Didonna ML. Proximal row carpectomy. *J Bone Joint Surg Am.* 2005;87(1 suppl 2):166-174. doi:10.2106/JBJS.E.00261.

26. Tambe AD, Trail IA, Stanley JK. Wrist fusion versus limited carpal fusion in advanced Kienbock's disease. *Int Orthop.* 2005;29(6):355-358.

27. Por Y, Chew W, Tsou I. Avascular necrosis of the triquetrum: a case report. *Hand Surg.* 2005;10(1):91-94.

28. Garcia LA, Vaca JB. Avascular necrosis of the pisiform. *J Hand Surg (Edinburgh, Scotland).* 2006;31(4):453-454.

29. Ye BJ, Kim JI, Lee HJ, Jung KY. A case of avascular necrosis of the capitate bone in a pallet car driver. *J Occup Health.* 2009;51:451-453.

30. Whiting J, Rotman MB. Scaphocapitolunate arthrodesis for idiopathic avascular necrosis of the capitate: a case report. *J Hand Surg.* 2002;27A:692-696.

31. Fenton RL. The naviculo-capitate fracture syndrome. *J Bone Joint Surg Am*. 1956;38-A(3):681-684.

32. Vander Grend R, Dell PC, Glowczewskie F, Leslie B, Ruby LK. Intraosseous blood supply of the capitate and its correlation with aseptic necrosis. *J Hand Surg Am*. 1984;9(5):677-683.

33. Bekele W, Escobedo E, Allen R. Avascular necrosis of the capitate. *J Radiol Case Rep*. 2011;5(6):31-36.

34. D'Agostino P, Townley WA, Roulot E. Bilateral Avascular necrosis of the trapezoid. *J Hand Surg*. 2016;36(10):1678-1680. doi:10.1016/j.jhsa.2011.07.022.

35. García-López A, Cardoso Z, Ortega L. Avascular necrosis of trapezium bone: a case report. *J Hand Surg*. 2002;27(4):704-706.

36. Peters SJ, Verstappen C, Degreef I, De Smet LD. Avascular necrosis of the Hamate: three cases and review of the literature. *J Wrist Surg*. 2014;3(4):269-274.

37. Lichtman DM, Mack GR, MacDonald RI, Gunther SF, Wilson JN. Kienböck's disease: the role of silicone replacement arthroplasty. *J Bone Joint Surg Am*. 1977;59(7):899-908.

38. Cha SM, Shin HD, Kim KC. Clinical and radiological outcomes of scaphoidectomy and 4-corner fusion in scapholunate advanced collapse at 5 and 10 years. *Ann Plast Surg*. 2013;71(2):166-169.

39. Bozentka D, Beredjiklan P. Kienbock's disease. *Orthop Knowledge Online J*. 2007;5(1):1-45.

INTRODUCTION

- Definition
  - Dislocation of the radiocarpal joint, with or without
    - ◆ Radial styloid fracture
    - ◆ Dorsal or volar rim avulsion fractures
  - In the category of carpal instability nondissociative
  - This topic does not include articular shear fractures ("Barton" variants), perilunate dislocations, or instability related to distal radius malunion or rheumatoid arthritis.
- Pathoanatomy
  - Proximal carpal row linked to distal radius by the volar (radioscapho-capitate [RSC], short radiolunate [SRL], long radiolunate[LRL]) and dorsal (dorsal radiocarpal [DRC]) extrinsic wrist ligaments
  - Radiocarpal dislocation requires either near-global ligament disruption or a fracture that disrupts the stability of the osseous insertion of the ligaments.
    - ◆ Volar ligaments are typically avulsed from their origin on the distal radius.
      - ∗ One report of avulsion distally from the carpal insertions[1]
    - ◆ If a radial styloid fracture is greater than one-third the width of the scaphoid fossa, the RSC and LRL origins usually remain attached to the fractured fragment.[2]
    - ◆ DRC and capsule may avulse small fragments from the dorsal distal radius.
  - Role of extrinsic wrist ligaments
    - ◆ Palmar structures provide majority of restraint against dorsal (61%) and volar (48%) translation of the carpus.[3]
    - ◆ SRL is the primary stabilizer against volar translation.[4]
    - ◆ RSC is primary stabilizer against ulnar translation,[4,5] but alone is unable to prevent ulnar translation. RSC/LRL together can resist ulnar translation.[6]

- Dorsal intercalated segment instability may predispose to dislocation.[7-9]
- Associated injuries
  - Intercarpal ligament injury
  - Ulnar styloid fracture
  - Distal radioulnar joint (DRUJ) disruption
- Secondary ulnar translation
  - Distal radius osteology (inclination, volar tilt) creates a tendency for ulnar and palmar translation, which is normally restrained by radiocarpal ligaments.[6]
  - Typically develops after wrist immobilization has been discontinued
  - Associated with radiocarpal arthritis and limited range of motion[2]
- Mechanism of injury
  - Typically high-energy injuries
  - Axial load on hyperextended wrist, with aspects of shearing and rotation[10,11]
    - Additional pronation and torsion can lead to DRUJ disruption.[2,12]
    - The radial-based extrinsic ligaments (RSC, SRL, LRL), typically torn during radiocarpal dislocation, tighten with and resist pronation, suggesting that forceful pronation is a part of the injury mechanism.[2]
- Epidemiology
  - Most frequent in young active men[13]
  - Direction of dislocation
    - Dorsal more common, volar quite rare (only 24 reported in literature)[14]
      - Ulnar extremely rare[15,16]
  - Pure ligamentous dislocation without any fractures is uncommon
  - Open injuries are rare, but have high (70%) incidence of neurovascular injury[17]

EVALUATION

- History
  - Mechanism
  - Identification of associated traumatic injuries
- Physical examination
  - Swelling and pain
  - Offset of the hand in the direction of dislocation
  - Obtain a complete neurovascular examination.

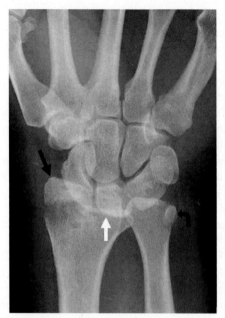

FIGURE 23.1 Posteroanterior radiograph of a dorsal radiocarpal dislocation with radial styloid fracture (black arrow) and ulnar styloid fracture (curved arrow). Note overlap of the proximal row with the shadow of the distal radius, indicating dislocation (white arrow).

- Imaging (Figures 23.1 and 23.2)
  - Radiographs of the elbow, forearm, wrist, and hand
  - In chronic cases or cases with delayed presentation, stress radiographs (distraction, radial deviation, and ulnar deviation) may help establish the diagnosis.
  - Computed tomography (CT) scanning may help with fracture characterization.
- Classification
  - Direction of dislocation (dorsal, volar, radial, and ulnar)[18]
  - Dumontier classification[19]
    - Most useful classification system because it can guide treatment.
    - Type I—radial styloid fracture absent or small (lesser than one-third width of scaphoid fossa)
      - Typically all ligaments are torn.
    - Type II—large (greater than one-third width of scaphoid fossa) radial styloid fracture (Figure 23.3 A and B)

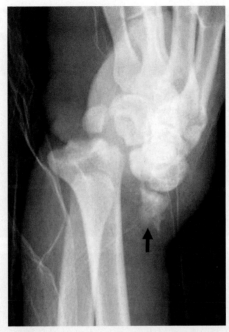

FIGURE 23.2 Lateral radiograph of a dorsal radiocarpal dislocation with radial styloid fracture (arrow).

* Volar extrinsic ligaments intact and attached to radial styloid
  ▲ One report of ligaments avulsed from fractured styloid[13]
- Moneim classification[20]
  ◆ Type I—ligamentous injury limited to the radiocarpal ligaments
  ◆ Type II—addition of intercarpal ligamentous lesion(s)
- Limitations of current classification systems
  ◆ Rely on radiographs, so cannot prove pattern of ligamentous injury[13]
  ◆ Fail to account for postreduction stability and ulnar-sided pathology[13]
- Ulnar translation
  ◆ Measured using carpal-radial distance[21]
    * Distance between the center of the proximal capitate and a line bisecting the radius (mean: 5.7 ± 1.4 mm)
    * Carpal-radial distance ≥ 9 mm represents ulnar carpal translation.
  ◆ Type I—entire carpus (including scaphoid) translates ulnarly[22]
  ◆ Type II—scaphoid stays with radius, remaining carpus translates ulnarly[22]

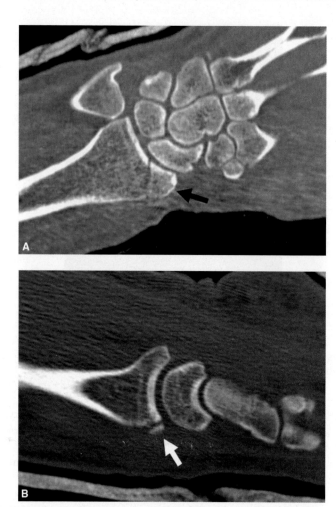

FIGURE 23.3 Postreduction CT images of the patient shown in Fig. 1 demonstrate (A) large radial styloid fracture (black arrow) and (B) dorsal avulsion fracture (white arrow). CT, computed tomography.

ACUTE MANAGEMENT

- Immediate closed reduction
  - Should open irreducible dislocations to remove intervening structures (osteochondral fragments, flexor tendons, median nerve, ulnar neurovascular bundle)[23-25]

DEFINITIVE TREATMENT

- Radiocarpal dislocations are rare and severe injuries, and each must be individually addressed based upon its characteristics and associated injuries.
- Goals of treatment[11]
  - Concentric reduction
  - Treatment of any intercarpal ligament injuries
  - Repair of radiocarpal ligament avulsions
- Nonoperative treatment
  - Closed reduction and casting
    - Several reports of successful treatment[9,10,26,27]
    - Most authors now recommend operative treatment due to reports of failure with closed treatment.[2,9,28,29]
- Surgical indications
  - By Dumontier classification
    - Type I—open reduction and volar ligament repair via volar approach[19]
    - Type II—open reduction and fracture fixation via a dorsal approach[19]
  - Closed reduction and percutaneous pinning (CRPP)
    - Successful treatment with CRPP has been reported by several authors.[8,28,30]
    - CRPP without ligament repair is controversial due to the risk of developing ulnar translation and radiocarpal arthritis.[16,19,29]
    - Success has been reported with arthroscopic reduction and pinning with DRC debridement and reduction of the RSC stump out of the joint.[15,31]
  - Open reduction with internal fixation of fractures
    - Rigid fixation of large radial styloid fractures is recommended.
    - Dorsal or volar fragments large enough to bear fixation are unusual, but may be fixed if encountered.
      - * In particular, a volar lunate facet fracture should be fixed.
    - External fixation may be useful intraoperatively to aid in reduction, and also provides postoperative immobilization.[24]
  - Ligament repair
    - Extrinsic ligament repair has been a subject of some controversy, but most authors recommend it for the prevention of secondary ulnar translation.[11,19]

- Intercarpal ligament injuries
  - Treat as per standard techniques for isolated intercarpal ligament injuries
- Ulnar styloid fractures
  - Fix large ulnar styloid base fractures with tension band or screw.
  - If DRUJ remains unstable, consider repairing ulnocarpal ligaments.
- Secondary ulnar translation
  - Difficult to treat
  - RSC ligament reconstruction
    - Donor options include extensor carpi radialis brevis,[32] flexor carpi radialis,[33] and brachioradialis.[34,35]
    - Outcomes are poor in chronic situations.[32,36]
      - Recurrence in seven of eight patients in one study[32]
    - Negative ulnar variance hypothesized to create a tendency toward recurrent ulnar translation despite repair.[32] No studies have investigated any benefit to creating neutral variance via osteotomy.
  - Radiocarpal fusion
    - For delayed presentation, extreme instability, or advanced arthritis[32,36]
    - Perform radiolunate arthrodesis unless radioscaphoid arthritis is present; in that case, perform radioscapholunate arthrodesis.[37]
- Contraindications
  - Unstable patient
  - Severe soft tissue wounds at the proposed surgical sites
- Operative technique
  - Dumontier type I
    - Volar approach to the wrist via extended carpal tunnel incision
    - Exploration of extrinsic wrist ligaments
    - Percutaneous pinning of the radiocarpal joint in reduced position
    - Ligament repair using suture anchors
  - Dumontier type II (Figure 23.4 A and B)
    - Dorsal approach to the radial side of the wrist
    - Fracture fixation with Kirschner wires, screws, or fragment-specific plates
    - Consider repair of the DRC and capsule using suture anchor

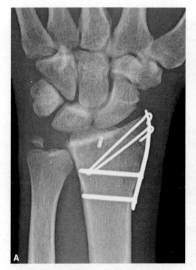 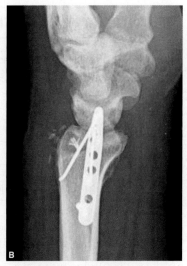

FIGURE 23.4 Postoperative radiographs of the patient shown in Fig. 2 demonstrate (A) fixation of the radial styloid fracture with a fragment-specific plate and (B) dorsal radiocarpal repair with a suture anchor.

- Potential complications
  - Infection
  - Neurovascular injury (including acute carpal tunnel syndrome)
  - Complex regional pain syndrome[38]
  - Loss of strength and range of motion
  - Recurrent instability
  - Ulnar translation of the carpus
  - Posttraumatic osteoarthritis
- Postoperative care
  - Immobilization for 6 to 8 weeks
  - Pin removal (if used) at 6 to 8 weeks post-op
- Outcomes
  - There are no randomized controlled trials—all evidence comes from case series.
  - Delayed presentation, ulnar translation, and the presence of other injuries (particularly DRUJ injury) are associated with poorer outcomes.[19,28,32,39-41]
  - Many patients can return to work (76% in one series).[41]
  - Most nerve injuries improve after reduction.[20]

MANAGEMENT ALGORITHM

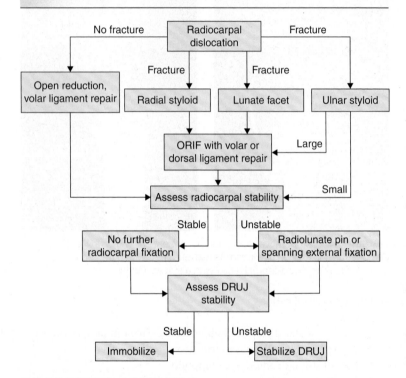

SUGGESTED READINGS

Ilyas AM, Mudgal CS. Radiocarpal fracture-dislocations. *J Am Acad Orthop Surg.* 2008;16:647-655.

REFERENCES

1. Cowley R, Youn A. Pure ligamentous volar radiocarpal dislocation: a case report. *ANZ J Surg.* 2016. doi:10.1111/ans.13503.
2. Freeland AE, Ferguson CA, McCraney WO. Palmar radiocarpal dislocation resulting in ulnar radiocarpal translocation and multidirectional instability. *Orthopedics.* 2006;29:604-608.
3. Katz DA, Green JK, Werner FW, Loftus JB. Capsuloligamentous restraints to dorsal and palmar carpal translation. *J Hand Surg Am.* 2003;28A:610-613.
4. Berger RA, Landsmeer JM. The palmar radiocarpal ligaments: a study of adult and fetal human wrist joints. *J Hand Surg.* 1990;15:847-854.
5. Nakamura T, Cooney WP III, Lui WH, et al. Radial styloidectomy: a biomechanical study on stability of the wrist joint. *J Hand Surg Am.* 2001;26A:85-93.

6. Viegas SF, Patterson RM, Ward K. Extrinsic wrist ligaments in the pathomechanics of ulnar translation instability. *J Hand Surg.* 1995;20A:312-318.

7. Varodompun N, Limpivest P, Prinyaroj P. Isolated dorsal radiocarpal dislocation: case report and literature review. *J Hand Surg.* 1985;10A:708-710.

8. Fennell CW, McMurtry RY, Fairbanks CJ. Multidirectional radiocarpal dislocation without fracture: a case report. *J Hand Surg.* 1992;17A:756-761.

9. De Keating-Hart E, Pidhorz L, Moui Y. Luxation dorsale de l'articulation radiocarpienne chez une femme de 85 ans. *Chir Main.* 2012;31:195-198.

10. Reynolds ISR. Dorsal radiocarpal dislocation. *Injury.* 1980;12:48-49.

11. Ilyas AM, Mudgal CS. Radiocarpal fracture-dislocations. *J Am Acad Orthop Surg.* 2008;16:647-655.

12. Weiss C, Laskin RS, Spinner M. Irreducible radiocarpal dislocation: a case report. *J Bone Joint Surg.* 1970;82-A(3):562-564.

13. Mourikis A, Rebello G, Villafuerte J, Moneim M, Omer GE, Veitch J. Radiocarpal dislocations: review of the literature with case presentations and a proposed treatment algorithm. *Orthopedics.* 2008;31(4):386-392.

14. Jardin E, Pechin C, Rey PB, Gasse N, Obert L. Open volar radiocarpal dislocation with extensive dorsal ligament and extensor tendon damage: a case report and review of the literature. *Hand Surg Rehabil.* 2016;35:127-134.

15. Kamal RN, Bariteau JT, Beutel BG, DaSilva MF. Arthroscopic reduction and percutaneous pinning of a radiocarpal dislocation: a case report. *J Bone Joint Surg.* 2011;93(15):e84.

16. Arslan H, Tokmak M. Isolated ulnar radiocarpal dislocation. *Arch Orthop Trauma Surg.* 2002;122:179-181.

17. Nyquist SR, Stern PJ. Open radiocarpal fracture-dislocations. *J Hand Surg.* 1984;9A:707-710.

18. Bilos ZJ, Pankovich AM, Yelda S. Fracture-dislocation of the radiocarpal joint. *J Bone Joint Surg.* 1977;59-A(2):198-203.

19. Dumontier C, Meyer zu Reckendorf G, Sautet A, Lenoble E, Saffar P, Allieu Y. Radiocarpal dislocations: classification and proposal for treatment. *J Bone Joint Surg.* 2001;83A(2):212-218.

20. Moneim MS, Bolger JT, Omer GE. Radio-carpal dislocation: classification and rationale for management. *Clin Orthop Relat Res.* 1985;192:199-209.

21. DiBenedetto MR, Lubbers LM, Coleman CR. A standardized measurement of ulnar carpal translocation. *J Hand Surg.* 1990;15A(6):1009-1010.

22. Taleisnik J. *The Wrist.* New York, NY: Churchill Livingstone; 1985: 305-306.

23. Songür M, Şahin E, Zehir S, Kalem M. Irreducible dorsal distal radius fracture-dislocation with accompanying dorsal displacement of flexor tendons and median nerve: a rare type of injury. *Int J Surg Case Rep.* 2014;5: 1005-1009.

24. Ayekoloye CI, Shah N, Kumar A, Kurdy N. Irreducible dorsal radiocarpal fracture dislocation with dissociation of the distal radioulnar joint: a case report. *Acta Orthop Belg.* 2002;68(2):171-174.

25. Fernandez DL. Irreducible radiocarpal fracture-dislocation and radioulnar dissociation with entrapment of the ulnar nerve, artery, and flexor profundus II-V: case report. *J Hand Surg.* 1981;6(5):456-461.

26. Tees FJ. Dislocation of the radio-carpal joint. *Can Med Assoc J.* 1935;32(2): 122-127.

27. Moore DP, McMahon BA. Anterior radio-carpal dislocation: an isolated injury. *J Hand Surg Eur.* 1988;13-B(2):215-217.

28. Dahmani O, Elbachiri M, Shimi M, Elibrahimi A, Elmrini A. La luxation radiocarpienne (à propos de neuf cas). *Chir Main.* 2013;32:30-36.

29. Howard RF, Slawski DP, Gilula LA. Isolated palmar radiocarpal dislocation and ulnar translation: a case report and review of the literature. *J Hand Surg.* 1997;22A(1):78-82.

30. Freund LG, Ovesen J. Isolated dorsal dislocation of the radiocarpal joint: a case report. *J Bone Joint Surg.* 1977;59-A(2):277.

31. Hardy P, Welby F, Stromboni M, Blin JL, Lortat-Jacob A, Benoit J. Wrist arthroscopy and dislocation of the radiocarpal joint without fracture. *Arthroscopy.* 1999;15(7):779-783.

32. Rayhack JM, Linscheid RL, Dobyns JH, Smith JH. Posttraumatic ulnar translation of the carpus. *J Hand Surg.* 1987;12A:180-189.

33. Dunn MJ, Johnson C. Static scapholunate dissociation: a new reconstruction technique using a volar and dorsal approach in a cadaver model. *J Hand Surg.* 2001;26A:749-754.

34. Maschke SD, Means KR, Parks BG, Graham TJ. A radiocarpal ligament reconstruction using brachioradialis for secondary ulnar translation of the carpus following radiocarpal dislocation: a cadaver study. *J Hand Surg.* 2010;35A:256-261.

35. Obafemi A, Pensy R. Palmar radiocarpal dislocation: a case report and novel treatment method. *Hand.* 2012;7:114-118.

36. Jebson PJL, Adams BD, Meletiou SD. Ulnar translocation instability of the carpus after a dorsal radiocarpal dislocation: a case report. *Am J Orthop.* 2000;29:462-464.

37. Taleisnik J. Current concepts review. Carpal instability. *J Bone Joint Surg.* 1988;70:1262-1268.

38. Le Nen D, Riot O, Caro P, Le Fevre C, Courtois B. Luxation-fractures de la radio-carpienne: étude clinique de six cas et revue générale. *Ann Chir Main.* 1991;10:5-12.

39. Lahtaoui A, El Bardouni A, Ismael F, et al. Les luxations-fractures radiocarpiennes postérieures (à propos de huit cas). *Chir Main.* 2002;21:252-257.

40. Girard J, Cassagnaud X, Maynou C, Bachour F, Prodhomme G, Mestdagh H. Radiocarpal dislocation: twelve cases and a review of the literature [in French]. *Rev Chir Orthop Reparatrice Appar Mot.* 2004;90:426-433.

41. Yuan BJ, Dennison DG, Elhassan BT, Kakar S. Outcomes after radiocarpal dislocation: a retrospective review. *Hand.* 2015;10:367-373.

24 Acute Triangular Fibrocartilage Complex Tears

Tamara John and Seth D. Dodds

INTRODUCTION

- General considerations
  - Triangular fibrocartilage complex (TFCC) injuries: major cause of *ulnar-sided* wrist pain
  - Important stabilizer of distal radioulnar joint (DRUJ)
  - Absorbs some wrist load from the ulnocarpal (UC) joints[1]
  - Stabilizes forearm rotation—strong connection between distal radius and ulna
  - Supports ulnar carpus[2]
- Blood supply/nerve supply
  - Enters from the periphery (like meniscus in knee)
  - **Peripheral tears** more amenable to healing.[3]
  - **Ulnar artery**—Supplies **ulnar** TFCC through **dorsal** and **palmar** radiocarpal branches
  - **Dorsal and palmar branches of anterior interosseous artery:** supply the radial periphery TFCC
  - **Central TFCC** not amenable to repair; avascular
  - Nerve supply: only to the peripheral aspect of the TFCC, from **posterior interosseus nerve**, **ulnar nerve**, and **dorsal sensory branch** of ulnar nerve.[4,5]
- Components of TFCC (Table 24.1 and Figure 24.1)
  - Articular disk (triangular fibrocartilage)
  - Dorsal and volar distal radioulnar ligaments
  - Ligamentous insertion to the fovea
  - Meniscus homologue
  - UC ligaments
  - Ulnar collateral ligament (UCL)
  - Subsheath of the extensor carpi ulnaris (ECU)
- Articular disk (triangular fibrocartilage)
  - **Base** of articular disk attached to **sigmoid notch** of radius

TABLE 24.1 Structures of the TFCC

TFCC Structure	Origin	Insertion
Articular disk (triangular fibrocartilage)	Radius: sigmoid notch Ulna: fovea/ulnar head	Merges with UCL; triquetrum, hamate, base of fifth MC
Dorsal radioulnar ligament	Sigmoid notch of the radius (dorsal aspect)	Head of ulna (dorsally)
Volar radioulnar ligament	Sigmoid notch of the radius (volar aspect)	Head of ulna (volarly)
Meniscus homologue	TFC	Ulnar styloid
Ulnocarpal ligaments • Ulnolunate • Ulnotriquetral • Ulnocapitate	Triangular fibrocartilage	Respective carpal bones
UCL	Styloid process of the ulna	First fasciculus: medial triquetrum Second fasciculus: pisiform/flexor retinaculum
ECU subsheath	ECU tendon sheath	Ulnar head/TFC

Abbreviations: UCL, ulnar collateral ligament; ECU, extensor carpi ulnaris; MC, metacarpal; TFC, triangular fibrocartilage complex; tfnTFCC, triangular fibrocartilage complex.

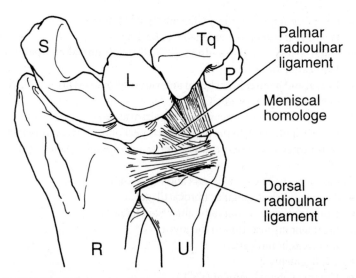

FIGURE 24.1 This line drawing illustrates the triangular fibrocartilage complex and its principal components, the palmar and dorsal radioulnar ligaments, the articular disc, and the meniscal homologue. S, scaphoid; L, lunate; Tq, triquetrum; P, pisiform; R, radius; U, ulna.

- **Apex** of articular disk attached to the dorsal and volar capsule of the UC joint
- Disk continues **ulnarly** and **volarly** to merge with the **UCL**
- Distal: combined ligaments become thickened (**meniscus homologue**)—inserts distally on **triquetrum**, **hamate**, and **base** of the **fifth metacarpal** bone[2,6]
- Definition of **meniscus homologue**: Fibrocartilaginous rim of dense connective tissue that joins with **dorsal** and **volar distal radioulnar ligaments**[7]
  - Superficial dorsal and volar distal radioulnar ligaments (Figure 24.2)
    - Origin—**dorsal** and **volar** aspects of the **radial sigmoid notch**
    - Insertion—**dorsal** ulnar head and **volar** ulnar head, respectively

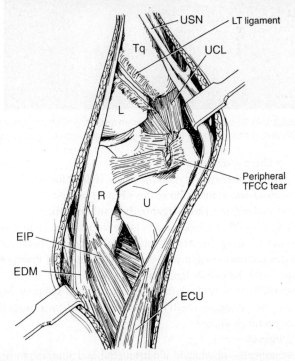

FIGURE 24.2 The illustration demonstrates soft tissue layers overlying the TFCC. There are tears of the palmar and dorsal radioulnar ligaments as well as the lunotriquetral ligaments. ECU, extensor carpi ulnaris; TFCC, triangular fibrocartilage complex; UCL, ulnar collateral ligament; R, radius; U, ulna; L, lunate; Tq, triquetrum; EIP, extensor indicis proprius; EDM, extensor digiti minimi; USN, ulnar sensory nerve.

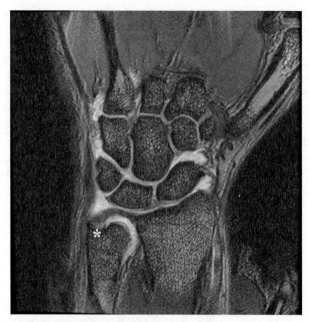

FIGURE 24.3 This T2-weighted MR arthrogram reveals an intact ligamentous, foveal insertion of the triangular fibrocartilage complex, noted by at the asterisk.

- Deep fibers insert onto **ulnar fovea**
- Superficial fibers insert onto the **ulnar styloid fossa**[8]
- Ligamentous foveal insertion of the TFCC (Figure 24.3)
  - Independent structure—**ligamentum subcruentum**
  - Triangular in shape, supported by loose fibrovascular connective tissue
  - Comprises **deep** dorsal and volar distal radioulnar ligaments
  - Shares common origin with superficial ligaments; inserts **deep** to superficial radioulnar ligaments onto **fovea**
  - Intermediate to high signal intensity on fluid-sensitive Magnetic resonance imaging (MRI) sequences should raise suspicion for subcruentum injury[9]
- UC ligaments
  - Components—ulnolunate, ulnotriquetral, and ulnocapitate ligaments
  - Origin—triangular fibrocartilage
  - Insertion—respective carpal bone
- ECU subsheath and UCL
  - **ECU subsheath** more important stabilizer of ulnar wrist compared to UCL

- UCL weaker structure with more laxity[10]
- Major intrinsic stabilizer of DRUJ: **TFCC**
- Major extrinsic stabilizers of DRUJ: **ECU** subsheath, distal fibers of interosseous membrane, pronator quadratus
- Mechanism of injury/epidemiology
  - **Biomechanics**—ulnar side of wrist/TFCC sees **18% to 20% load** across wrist
  - **Ulnar deviation**—increases load across TFCC
  - Increased ulnar variance = increased force across TFCC
  - **Maximal grip** and **pronation** increase ulnar variance, increased force across TFCC[11]
  - **Injury mechanism**—axial load with wrist extended and pronated—for example, falling on outstretched hand
  - Twisting injury—torque to wrist and forearm during racquet sport
  - Idiopathic pain, clicking without known trauma[12]
  - 3% to 9% of all athletic injuries involve the hand/wrist
  - Common in athletes but no specific TFCC epidemiologic data
  - Result of **acute trauma**, **fall**, overuse, repetitive trauma

EVALUATION

- History
  - Wrist axial loading, ulnar deviation, forced extremes of forearm rotation
  - **Specific activities**—rapid twisting of the wrist with ulnar-sided loading, for example, racquet sports/golf
  - Ulnar-sided wrist pain—diffuse, deep, achy/burning; possible radiation
  - May feel clicking in the wrist when forearm rotated/wrist ulnar deviated, for example, lifting a gallon of milk and pouring, turning a steering wheel, playing golf or tennis
- Physical examination
  - **Palpation**—wrist tenderness between ulnar styloid and triquetrum, either dorsally or volarly. Volar tenderness occurs between the distal ulnar head and the pisiform
  - Subtle ulnar-sided wrist swelling compared to the contralateral wrist
  - Click with forearm rotation/wrist ulnar deviation
  - **Test DRUJ**—stabilize ulna, translate radius volarly and dorsally. Note amplitude of firmness in endpoint compared to contralateral. Test with forearm in **neutral**, **pronation**, **supination**

- Additional provocative tests
  - **Hypersupination**—applies load to DRUJ
  - **UC stress test**—axial load, ulnar deviation, wrist extension and/or forearm rotation. Positive test = pain[8]
  - **TFCC compression test**—axial load ulnar side of hand. Positive test = pain[3]
  - **Fovea sign**—Tenderness replicating pain when pressure applied to fovea.[13] Most specific examination finding for TFCC injuries
- Imaging
  - Radiographs
    - Usually normal
    - Assess for ulnar positive variance and evidence of ulnar impaction
    - Rule out associated fracture/dislocation
  - MRI arthrogram (Figures 24.4 and 24.5)
    - **Most commonly used**
    - Tear = ↑ TFCC signal intensity

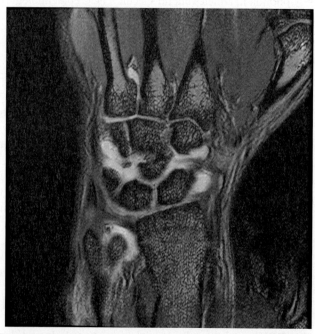

FIGURE 24.4 This T2-weighted MR arthrogram demonstrates an intact peripheral, ulnar-capsular attachment of the triangular fibrocartilage complex to the ulnocarpal ligament.

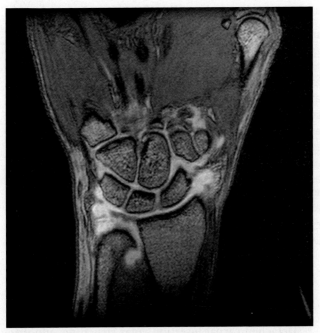

FIGURE 24.5 Here there is disruption of the peripheral, ulnar-capsular attachments of the triangular fibrocartilage complex.

- ◆ Sensitivity 17%, specificity 79%, accuracy 64%[14]
- ◆ Used for **detection** of TFCC tears, not accurate with assessing tear size[15]
- ◆ **High-resolution** MRI increases accuracy of detection of tear to 79%.[16]
- ● Arthroscopic visualization
  - ◆ **Gold standard**
  - ◆ **Trampoline test**—used when TFCC appears intact—probe to depress center of disk. **Good tension**/brisk rebound—disk intact. **Laxity**/no rebound—detachment from fovea or ulnar capsule/ periphery
- ■ Classification
- ■ Proposed by Palmer et al to differentiate traumatic and degenerative lesions—**Palmer classification** (Table 24.2)[17]
  - ● Class 1 type A injuries
    - ◆ Traumatic
    - ◆ Tear at central portion of disk
    - ◆ Do not heal on their own (avascular region)

TABLE 24.2 Palmer Classification of TFCC Injuries

Class 1: Traumatic
• Class 1A: Central disk perforation
• Class 1B: Avulsion of ulnar styloid with or without distal ulnar fracture
• Class 1C: Distal avulsion (carpal detachment)
• Class 1D: Radial avulsion with or without sigmoid notch fracture
Class 2: Degenerative
• Class 2A: TFCC wear without definite perforation
• Class 2B: TFCC wear with lunate and/or ulnar chondromalacia
• Class 2C: TFCC perforation with lunate and/or ulnar chondromalacia
• Class 2D: TFCC perforation with lunate and/or ulnar chondromalacia and lunotriquetral ligament perforation
• Class 2E: TFCC perforation with lunate and/or ulnar chondromalacia, lunotriquetral ligament perforation, and ulnocarpal arthritis

Abbreviation: TFCC, triangular fibrocartilage complex.

- Class I type B injuries
  - Detached ulnar attachment of the TFCC
  - Peripheral/well-vascularized
- Class I type C injuries
  - Detached carpal insertion volar structures, ulnotriquetral ligament, ulnolunate ligament
- Class I type D injuries
  - Detached **triangular disk** at radial attachment: volar and dorsal distal radioulnar ligaments at radial attachment
  - Triangular disk: weaker attachment to radius compared to ulna.[18]
- Class 2 types A to D
  - Class 2 injuries—**degenerative**
  - **Type A**—no chondromalacia
  - **Type B**—chondromalacia
  - **Type C**—looks like 2A/B + definite full thickness tear
  - **Type D**—looks like 2A-C + lunotriquetral ligament disruption
  - **Type E**—looks like 2A-D + UC arthritis[17]

INITIAL MANAGEMENT

- Initial treatment of all suspected isolated TFCC injuries: temporary splint immobilization of wrist/forearm. Sugar tong–type splints can control forearm rotation.

- Unstable/displaced fractures/clearly unstable DRUJ: **acute surgical treatment**
- Stable DRUJ or nondisplaced/no fracture: **nonsurgical**

DEFINITIVE MANAGEMENT

- **Nonsurgical treatment**—temporary long arm cast immobilization wrist/forearm (Munster-type cast), nonsteroidal anti-inflammatory drugs, possible hand therapy after 6 weeks of immobilization (Class 1A tears)
- Arthroscopic repair acute tears: recovery of up to 85% of the contra-lateral grip strength/range of motion[19]
- Indications for operative repair
  - Peripheral TFCC tears (Palmer Class 1B)
  - Horizontal, oblique, vertical tears
  - Proximal split tears
- Contraindications for surgical repair
  - Central/radial TFCC tears generally managed with arthroscopic debridement, as there is poor blood supply and reduced healing potential (although repair techniques are described)
  - Transverse tears
- Treatment considerations with stable DRUJ
  - **Stress examination**—Definitive endpoint with volar/dorsal translation of radius over ulna. Compare with contralateral wrist
  - **Initial treatment**—4 to 6 weeks long arm cast, possible corticosteroid injection
  - **Definitive treatment**—Arthroscopy if fails conservative management. Volar and dorsal radioulnar ligaments intact[9]
  - **Class 1A tears**—Arthroscopic debridement if fails nonoperative treatment
  - **Class IB tears**—Arthroscopically assisted surgical repair of articular disc back to the ulnar or dorsal wrist capsule
- Treatment considerations with unstable DRUJ
  - Tear of the ligamentous insertion at the fovea
  - Repair directly to bone with suture anchors or bone tunnels with an open or arthroscopically assisted approach
  - **Radial-sided tears (Class 1D)**—similar outcomes debridement versus repair[20]

SPECIFIC OPERATIVE TECHNIQUES

- Arthroscopic repair
  - Equivalent outcomes compared with open approach: good-excellent outcomes
  - Arthroscopic: smaller incisions, quicker recovery, possible injury to the dorsal sensory branch of the ulnar nerve
- Contraindications to arthroscopic repair
  - Unstable DRUJ 2/2 fracture/complete ligament disruption
  - Chronic symptomatic DRUJ instability
  - Chronic Essex-Lopresti injuries
  - Concomitant arthritic radiocarpal joint
- Positioning/setup
  - Supine, hand table
  - General/regional anesthesia
  - Upper arm tourniquet
  - Prep/drape operative extremity
  - Appropriate traction setup (with/without tourniquet) with 10 lb traction
  - Wrist in slight flexion and radial deviation (improves portal exposure)
- Portal placement (Figure 24.6)
  - Consider using intraoperative mini-fluoroscopy and 19- or 18-gauge needles to guide portal placement
  - **3-4 portal**—Viewing portal; between extensor pollicis longus and extensor digitorum communis (EDC) tendons[3]
    - 1 cm distal to Lister's tubercle, between scaphoid and lunate
    - 30° 2.3 mm scope in 3-4 portal (distal and ulnar to Lister tubercle)
  - **4-5 portal**—further ulnar: 1 to 1.5 cm distal to Lister's tubercle between EDC and extensor digiti quinti proprius tendons
  - **6R portal**—just radial to ECU—needle localization
  - **6U portal**—just ulnar to ECU tendon—needle localization. Evaluate stability of tear/outflow portal
- Surgical technique
  - Peripheral capsular tears with **a stable DRUJ**
  - 3-4 portal generally portal for the scope; 4-5/6R portals for instrumentation
  - Partial synovectomy with 2.5 mm shaver improves visualization.
  - TFCC trampoline test performed; TFCC injury if redundant/easily deformed (Figure 24.7)
  - Peripheral tear: debride torn TFCC to clean edges

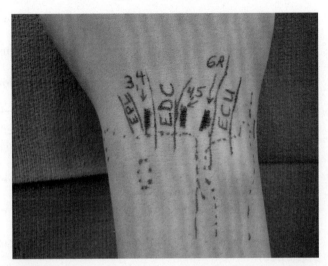

FIGURE 24.6 The surgical markings represent the dorsal compartments of the extensor tendons of the wrist and appropriate wrist arthroscopy portal locations.

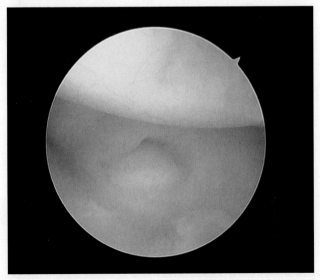

FIGURE 24.7 This arthroscopic image demonstrates a central tear/perforation of the triangular fibrocartilage complex with thinning of the articular disc, commonly seen with ulnar positive variance.

- Place 18- or 19-gauge needle (bevel aligned vertically) into joint at level of tear
- 1 to 1.5 cm longitudinal incision centered at this needle—ensure protection of dorsal sensory branch of ulnar nerve
- Identify dorsal sensory branch of ulnar nerve; blunt dissection to wrist capsule
- Outside in technique
  - Surgeon determines repair suture technique: horizontal versus vertical
  - Wrist capsule/TFCC punctured with 18-gauge needle (25-gauge needle can be used first to localize)[3]
  - Needle passage—horizontal tear—just inferior to torn edge of TFCC; vertical tear—just radial to torn edge of TFCC
  - Repair suture threaded into 18-gauge needle; inserted into wrist via 6U portal
  - Suture retrieval with small blunt-tipped hemostat/suture grasper (Figure 24.8)
    - Can make separate intra-articular puncture; could also work strictly from 6U portal if desired

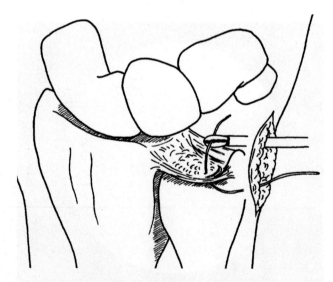

FIGURE 24.8 After being passed beneath the torn edge of the TFCC and through the edge of the articular disc, a small grasper may be used to retrieve the TFCC suture to complete the repair of the peripheral TFCC tear. TFCC, triangular fibrocartilage complex.

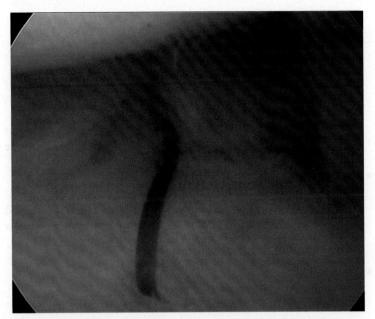

FIGURE 24.9 An arthroscopic closeup view of a peripheral TFCC repair suture stabilizing the peripheral edge of the TFCC. TFCC, triangular fibrocartilage complex

- Protect dorsal sensory branch of the ulnar nerve and then tie knots over the capsule to repair the TFCC cartilage to the dorsal/ulnar wrist capsule (Figure 24.9)
- Tears >5 mm typically require ≥ 2 sutures
- Potential complications of arthroscopic repair[21]
  - Stiffness (forearm rotation or wrist flexion/extension)
  - Dorsal sensory branch of the ulnar nerve injury
  - ECU tendinitis
  - Failure to maintain repair
  - DRUJ instability
- Open repair
  - Positioning/setup
    - Regional block/general
    - Supine, hand table
    - Shoulder abducted 90°, elbow flexed 90°, forearm neutral (a wrist arthroscopy axial traction tower is an ideal positioning device)

EXPOSURE

- Dorsal ulnar incision
- Radial-sided tears—**interval** between fourth and fifth extensor compartments with longitudinal incision in the DRUJ capsule, proximal to TFCC
- **Ulnar-sided tears**—Interval: fifth and sixth extensor compartments or between ECU and FCU extensor retinaculum reflected, capsule incised in line with TFCC or along the UCL. Inspect tear

■ **Surgical technique**
- Suture repair if ECU subsheath or peripheral capsular tear of the TFCC
- Suture anchor fixation, if foveal insertion of the TFCC is disrupted
- Suture fixation through radial drill holes, if repairing a radial sided tear
- Ulnar shortening should be considered if ulnar positive
- Pin DRUJ if the DRUJ is unstable

■ Postoperative care
- Sugar-tong splint in neutral if repair is stable
- **2 weeks post-op**—Munster-style cast to immobilize forearm rotation or custom splint
- **6 weeks post-op**—wrist brace, begin gentle forearm rotation
- **8 weeks post-op**—gentle strengthening exercises
- **12 weeks post-op**—return to activities/sport as tolerated

REFERENCES

1. Abe Y, Moriya A, Tominaga Y, Yoshida K. Dorsal tear of triangular fibrocartilage complex: clinical features and treatment. *J Wrist Surg.* 2016;5(1):42-46.
2. Mathoulin C. *Wrist Arthroscopy Techniques.* Stuttgart/New York: Thieme; 2015.
3. Trumble TE, Dodds SD. Peripheral tears of the TFCC: arthroscopic diagnosis and management. In: Slutsky DJ, Nagle DJ, eds. *Techniques in Wrist and Hand Arthroscopy.* Philadelphia, PA: Churchill Livingstone/Elsevier; 2007:42-53.
4. Nakamura T, Yabe Y. Histological anatomy of the triangular fibrocartilage complex of the human wrist. *Ann Anat.* 2000;182(6):567-572.
5. Bednar MS, Arnoczky SP, Weiland AJ. The microvasculature of the triangular fibrocartilage complex: its clinical significance. *J Hand Surg Am.* 1991;16(6):1101-1105.
6. Palmer AK, Werner FW. The triangular fibrocartilage complex of the wrist: anatomy and function. *J Hand Surg Am.* 1981;6(2):153-162.
7. Benjamin M, Evans EJ, Pemberton DJ. Histological studies on the triangular fibrocartilage complex of the wrist. *J Anat.* 1990;172:59-67.
8. Henry MH. Management of acute triangular fibrocartilage complex injury of the wrist. *J Am Acad Orthop Surg.* 2008;16(6):320-329.

9. Skalski MR, White EA, Patel DB, Schein AJ, RiveraMelo H, Matcuk GR Jr. The traumatized TFCC: an illustrated review of the anatomy and injury patterns of the triangular fibrocartilage complex. *Curr Probl Diagn Radiol.* 2016;45(1):39-50.

10. Ahn AK, Chang D, Plate AM. Triangular fibrocartilage complex tears: a review. *Bull NYU Hosp Jt Dis.* 2006;64(3-4):114-118.

11. Ko JH, Wiedrich TA. Triangular fibrocartilage complex injuries in the elite athlete. *Hand Clin.* 2012;28(3):307-321, viii.

12. Doarn MC, Wysocki RW. Acute TFCC injury. *Oper Tech Sports Med.* 2016;24(2):123-125.

13. Tay SC, Tomita K, Berger RA. The "ulnar fovea sign" for defining ulnar wrist pain: an analysis of sensitivity and specificity. *J Hand Surg Am.* 2007;32(4):438-444.

14. Cody ME, Nakamura DT, Small KM, Yoshioka H. MR imaging of the triangular fibrocartilage complex. *Magn Reson Imaging Clin N Am.* 2015;23(3):393-403.

15. Zanetti M, Bräm J, Hodler J. Triangular fibrocartilage and intercarpal ligaments of the wrist: does MR arthrography improve standard MRI? *J Magn Reson Imaging.* 1997;7(3):590-594.

16. Yoshioka H, Ueno T, Tanaka T, Shindo M, Itai Y. High-resolution MR imaging of triangular fibrocartilage complex (TFCC): comparison of microscopy coils and a conventional small surface coil. *Skeletal Radiol.* 2003;32(10):575-581.

17. Palmer AK. Triangular fibrocartilage complex lesions: a classification. *J Hand Surg Am.* 1989;14(4):594-606.

18. Trumble T. Radial side (1D) tears. *Hand Clin.* 2011;27(3):243-254.

19. Trumble TE, Gilbert M, Vedder N. Isolated tears of the triangular fibrocartilage: management by early arthroscopic repair. *J Hand Surg Am.* 1997;22(1):57-65.

20. Tanaka T, Ogino S, Yoshioka H. Ligamentous injuries of the wrist. *Semin Musculoskelet Radiol.* 2008;12(4):359-377.

21. Leclercq C, Mathoulin C, Member of EWAS. Complications of wrist arthroscopy: a multicenter study based on 10,107 arthroscopies. *J Wrist Surg.* 2016;5(4):320-326.

25 Salvage Procedures of the Wrist

Edward W. Jernigan and Reid W. Draeger

INTRODUCTION

- Primary arthrosis of the radiocarpal and midcarpal joints is uncommon.
- Arthrosis of the wrist may be a result of the sequelae from trauma (bony or ligamentous), crystalline arthropathy, infectious etiology, blood dyscrasias, neoplasm, or infection.
- Goals of treatment include a wrist that is pain-free, functional, and stable.
- Salvage procedures of the wrist can be divided into motion-sparing versus wrist arthrodesis.
  - Functional range of motion of the wrist is approximately 40° of extension, 40° of flexion, and a radial/ulnar deviation arc of motion of 40°.[1]
  - Motion-sparing procedures can be performed with the goal of maintaining functional range of motion of the wrist, with the risks of continued degeneration across preserved articulations.

EVALUATION

- History and physical examination
  - Important to consider patients' age and occupation, which may have implications for preferred treatment methods.
  - Patients with history of inflammatory disease may have polyarticular involvement.
  - Any historic or physical examination findings concerning ongoing infection must be thoroughly evaluated. Any ongoing infection should be eradicated prior to instrumenting the wrist.
- Radiographic evaluation
  - Plain radiographs—In addition to the standard posteroanterior (PA)/lateral/oblique views of the wrist, PA views of the wrist in

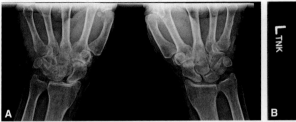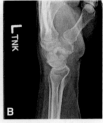

FIGURE 25.1 Clenched pencil (A) and lateral (B) radiographs demonstrating widening of the left scapholunate interval, radioscaphoid arthrosis, extension deformity of the lunate, and preservation of the articular surface of the lunate fossa.

maximum radial and ulnar deviation as well as an AP "clenched pencil" view (see Figure 25.1) can be helpful in determining carpal degenerative changes.[2]

- Cross-sectional imaging
  - Computed tomography (CT)—When considering a motion-sparing procedure, CT can be helpful to evaluate for degenerative changes in joints adjacent to the anticipated site of arthrodesis.
  - Magnetic resonance imaging (MRI)—Can be helpful when assessing vascularity of bone fragments or adjacent soft tissue disease, such as synovitis and tenosynovitis in rheumatoid arthritis.

MOTION-SPARING SURGICAL OPTIONS

- Considerations
  - Must ensure adjacent articulations and resultant articulations are free of degenerative changes when performing motion-sparing surgical options
  - Can be assessed intraoperatively or with the assistance of preoperative imaging
  - Failure to appreciate preexisting arthrosis may result in continued pain or acceleration of degeneration between adjacent and/or resultant joints.
- Scaphoid excision with capitate-lunate-hamate-triquetrum fusion (aka four-corner fusion with scaphoid excision)
- Proximal row carpectomy (PRC)
- Other partial wrist arthrodeses
  - Summarized in Table 25.1

TABLE 25.1 Other Motion-Sparing Arthrodesis Salvage Procedures of the Wrist

Procedure	Common Indications and Etiologies	Contraindications
Radiolunate arthrodesis	Volar and ulnar translation of the carpus related to RA Localized radiolunate arthritis secondary to die punch Failed soft tissue scapholunate ligament reconstruction	Capitolunate arthrosis
Scaphocapitate arthrodesis	Rotatory subluxation of the scaphoid Nonunion of scaphoid Kienböck disease Midcarpal instability	Radioscaphoid arthrosis STT arthrosis
Radioscapholunate arthrodesis	Posttraumatic proximal row degenerative changes Postinfection Inflammatory arthritis	Midcarpal arthrosis
Scapholunate arthrodesis	Scapholunate dissociation Limited indications due to high nonunion rates and unpredictable clinical results	Due to high nonunion rates and unpredictable clinical results, this procedure is not commonly performed
Lunotriquetral arthrodesis	Painful partial coalition of the lunotriquetral joint Symptomatic lunotriquetral dissociative instability	Midcarpal arthritis, nondissociative ulnar midcarpal instability Lunotriquetral dissociation with ulnocarpal impingement
Triquetrohamate arthrodesis	Treatment of painful midcarpal instability (limited indication)	Due to high nonunion rates and unpredictable clinical results, this procedure is not commonly performed
Scaphotrapezio-trapezoidal (STT) arthrodesis	Degenerative arthrosis of STT joint Subluxation of scaphoid Nonunion of scaphoid Kienböck disease Midcarpal instability Congenital synchondrosis of the STT joint	Radioscaphoid degenerative changes; presence of thumb CMC degenerative changes

Abbreviations: CMC, carpometacarpal; RA, rheumatoid arthritis.

Adapted from Rizzo M. Wrist arthrodesis and arthroplasty. In: Wolfe S, Hotchkiss R, Pederson W, Kozin S, Cohen M, eds. *Green's Operative Hand Surgery.* Philadelphia, PA: Elsevier; 2017:373-417.

SCAPHOID EXCISION WITH CAPITATE-LUNATE-HAMATE-TRIQUETRUM FUSION (FOUR-CORNER FUSION)

- Indications
  - Scapholunate advanced collapse (SLAC) wrist (see Figure 25.2)
    - Stage II—Pan-radioscaphoid arthrosis
    - Stage III—Arthrosis of the radioscaphoid and capitolunate joints
  - Scaphoid nonunion advanced collapse (SNAC) wrist
    - Stage II—Radioscaphoid and scaphocapitate arthrosis
    - Stage III—Periscaphoid arthrosis (with sparing of the radiolunate joint)
  - Goal is to stabilize wrist such that lunate transmits load across the preserved radiolunate joint with removal of the scaphoid to minimize persistent pain from the degenerated radioscaphoid articulation.[3]
- Preoperative considerations
  - Radiolunate arthrosis is a contraindication.
  - Cross-sectional imaging can be a helpful modality to evaluate the status of the radiolunate joint; however, this articulation may also be evaluated intraoperatively.

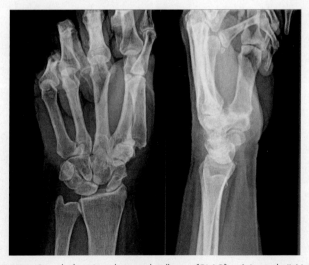

FIGURE 25.2 Scapholunate advanced collapse (SLAC) wrist, grade II. Note the widening of the SL interval and involvement of the entire radioscaphoid joint. The articular surfaces of the radiolunate and capitolunate joints are preserved, making this patient a candidate for either a four-corner fusion or a proximal row carpectomy.

- Fixation techniques (see Figure 25.3)
  - Kirschner wire fixation[4]
  - Circular plate[4,5]
    - May have higher rates of impingement and nonunion[6]
  - Staples[7]
  - Headless compression screws[8]
- Technique pearls[9]
  - The posterior interosseous nerve runs on the floor of the fourth dorsal compartment. Posterior interosseous neurectomy can help prevent postoperative pain.

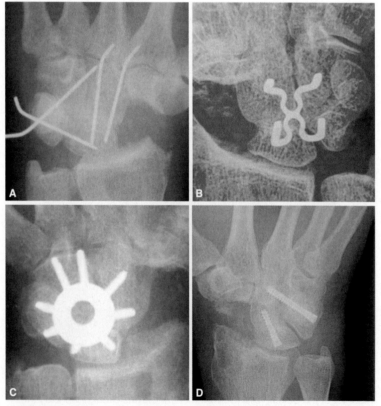

FIGURE 25.3 Fixation techniques of four-corner fusion with scaphoid excision. A, Kirschner wires,[4] B, shape memory staples,[7] C, dorsal circular plate,[5] D, headless compression screws.[8]

- A high-speed bur can be used to facilitate decortication and preparation of the bony surfaces for fusion. The bur can be used to create "craters" on sclerotic bone. Copious irrigation should be used during bur use to prevent thermal necrosis.
- Autogenic cancellous graft can be harvested from the distal radius. The excised scaphoid may also be a source of bone graft.
  - In cases of SNAC wrist, the proximal pole of the scaphoid may be sclerotic and avascular and may be a less optimal graft choice.
- The method of fixation is less important than appropriate preparation of the bone and use of bone grafting.
- Prominent dorsal hardware may lead to impingement in extension.
- Reduction of the radiolunate joint is facilitated by volar translation of the head of the capitate at the capitolunate articulation—best reduced prior to dechondrification of the midcarpal joint in preparation for fusion.
  - Reduction of the radiolunate joint out of extension can be provisionally held with a radiolunate K-wire while midcarpal joint is prepared for fusion.
- Failure to reduce the lunate from its extension deformity may lead to impingement in extension.
- Modifications
  - Scaphoid excision with capitolunate arthrodesis with or without triquetrum excision[10,11]
    - May facilitate easier reduction of the lunate and avoidance of subsequent symptomatic pisotriquetral arthritis[11]
  - Bicolumnar intercarpal arthrodesis of the lunate-capitate joint and the triquetrum-hamate joints[8]
    - Normal lunate-triquetrum and capitate-hamate anatomic relationships preserved and simplified operative technique
- Outcomes
  - See below for comparison with PRC

PROXIMAL ROW CARPECTOMY

- Indications
  - SLAC wrist
  - Kienböck disease (see Figure 25.4)
  - Goal is to resect the proximal row of the carpus (scaphoid, lunate, triquetrum) and allow for transmission of load across the newly formed radiocapitate articulation at the lunate fossa.

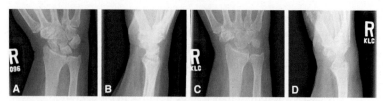

FIGURE 25.4 A 68-year-old female with Kienböck disease. Preoperative posteroanterior (PA) (A) and lateral (B) radiographs demonstrate avascular necrosis of the lunate, with no radiographic evidence of arthrosis of the lunate fossa or the proximal capitate. Intraoperatively, the articular surface of the lunate fossa and capitate was confirmed to be without arthrosis, and a proximal row carpectomy was performed (postoperative PA [C] and lateral [D] radiographs).

- Preoperative considerations
  - Severe wear to the cartilage at the capitate head is a relative contraindication.
  - Incongruity across the radiolunate joint is a contraindication.
- Technique pearls[12]
  - Resection of the terminal division of the posterior interosseous nerve may decrease postoperative pain.
  - Preservation of the radioscaphocapitate ligament is important to prevent ulnar translocation of the carpus.
- Modifications
  - If there is concern about the quality of the cartilage on the proximal pole of the capitate, then the Eaton modification may be performed, which involves a distal-based flap of capsule that is interposed between the proximal pole of the capitate and the radius.[12]
  - Osteochondral resurfacing of the capitate using grafts harvested from the resected carpal bones has also been performed, with outcomes similar to published results of conventional PRC.[13]
- Outcomes
  - See below for comparison with Four-Corner Fusion

COMPARISON OF PROXIMAL ROW CARPECTOMY AND FOUR-CORNER FUSION WITH SCAPHOID EXCISION

- Both procedures result in improvements in pain and subjective outcome scores.[14,15]
- Recent literature with up to 20-year follow-up demonstrates the longevity of both operations.[16,17]

- PRC is associated with radiographic progression or arthrosis; however, many patients with radiographic progression are asymptomatic.[14,16]
- Patients <40 years old have a higher risk of failure (conversion to arthrodesis) of PRC than patients >40 years old.[16]
  - Some advocate four-corner fusion in patients <40 to 45 years old.[9]
- Saltzman et al systematically reviewed 240 patients, 242 wrists[18]
  - No difference was found in radial/ulnar arc of motion.

	Four-Corner Fusion	Proximal Row Carpectomy
Extension	39°	43°*
Flexion	32°	36°*
Flex/ex arc	62°	75°*
Grip strength	74%*	67%

* indicates a significant difference between treatment groups, p < 0.05.

- Complication rate higher in four-corner fusion[18]
  - Four-corner fusion—29%, most common was nonunion (7%)
  - PRC—14%, most common was clinically significant synovitis and edema (3%)

TOTAL WRIST ARTHRODESIS

- Indications
  - Pancarpal arthrosis
  - Failed total joint arthroplasty
  - Progression of arthrosis after prior salvage procedure
  - Reconstruction after extensive trauma or neoplasm-related bone loss
- Rationale
  - Stability and potential pain relief come at the expense of motion across the wrist joint.
- Preoperative considerations
  - Volar subluxation of the lunate across the radiolunate joint may complicate reducing the wrist and may also be associated with a postfusion carpal tunnel syndrome.
    - Therefore, preoperative assessment for mild carpal tunnel syndrome is important, as is counseling patients on the possibility of postoperative symptoms resulting from increased pressure in the carpal canal.
  - Use of a wrist splint prior to surgery may help patients simulate wrist function postfusion, which can be helpful in the decision-making process.

- Fixation techniques
  - Compression wire fixation[19]
  - Dorsal plate fixation[20,21]
    - Several modern systems are available in which the plate is precontoured (see Figure 25.5).
  - Staples[22]
  - Intramedullary fixation[23]
- Technique pearls for dorsal plating[9]
  - Using a system with locking screw capabilities may be helpful in achieving improved fixation in patients with poor bone stock.
  - In patients with prior procedures (such as a PRC or arthroplasty procedure), utilizing a straight plate that can be contoured may afford more flexibility than the precontoured dorsal plates.
  - Five joints should be fused (radiolunate, radioscaphoid, lunocapitate, scaphocapitate, and the 3rd carpometacarpal [CMC] joints).
  - Bone grafting of the fusion sites should be performed using cancellous or cortical autograft (which can be augmented by allograft if needed).
    - Cancellous graft has the advantage of faster incorporation and lower donor site morbidity.[21]
  - Fix plate to the 3rd metacarpal first to allow for compression across the carpus when the plate is fixed to the radius. Ensure drilling of the screw holes in 3rd metacarpal is centralized in the isthmus.

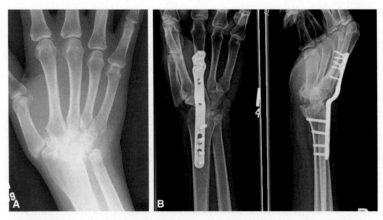

FIGURE 25.5 A) Preoperative radiographs of a 41-year-old female with a history of rheumatoid arthritis and prior proximal row carpectomy with pancarpal arthrosis. B) Post-operative radiographs (AP and lateral) show total wrist fusion with a precontoured dorsal plate. A carpal tunnel release was performed at the time of total wrist fusion.

- The dorsal lip of the distal radius may be resected for improved fit of the plate.
- Modifications
  - Performing PRC prior to placement of the dorsal plate may result in decreased ulnocarpal impingement due to removal of the triquetrum.[24]
    - This modification also decreases the number of joints to be fused, leaving only the radiocapitate and third CMC joints requiring fusion.
- Outcomes/complications
  - High fusion rates (98% according to Hastings et al[21])
  - Most common site of nonunion is third CMC joint.[21]
  - Hardware-related complications necessitating removal of dorsal plate are approximately 16%.[25]
  - Carpal tunnel syndrome (10%-25%), with some authors advocating carpal tunnel release for any total wrist arthrodesis[26]

SUGGESTED READINGS

Green DP, Perreira AC, Longhofer LK. Proximal row carpectomy. *J Hand Surg Am.* 2015;40(8):1672-1676.

Rizzo M. Wrist arthrodesis and arthroplasty. In: Wolfe S, Hotchkiss R, Pederson W, Kozin S, Cohen M, eds. *Green's Operative Hand Surgery*. Philadelphia, PA: Elsevier; 2017:373-417.

Wysocki RW, Cohen MS. Complications of limited and total wrist arthrodesis. *Hand Clin.* 2010;26(2):221-228.

REFERENCES

1. Ryu JY, Cooney WP, Askew LJ, An KN, Chao EY. Functional ranges of motion of the wrist joint. *J Hand Surg Am.* 1991;16(3):409-419.
2. Lee SK, Desai H, Silver B, Dhaliwal G, Paksima N. Comparison of radiographic stress views for scapholunate dynamic instability in a cadaver model. *J Hand Surg Am.* 2011;36(7):1149-1157. doi:10.1016/j.jhsa.2011.05.009.
3. Watson HK, Ballet FL. The SLAC wrist: scapholunate advanced collapse pattern of degenerative arthritis. *J Hand Surg Am.* 1984;9(3):358-365.
4. Rodgers JA, Holt G, Finnerty EP, Miller B. Scaphoid excision and limited wrist fusion: a comparison of K-wire and circular plate fixation. *Hand (N Y).* 2008;3(3):276-281. doi:10.1007/s11552-008-9099-x.
5. Merrell GA, McDermott EM, Weiss A-PC. Four-corner arthrodesis using a circular plate and distal radius bone grafting: a consecutive case series. *J Hand Surg Am.* 2008;33(5):635-642. doi:10.1016/j.jhsa.2008.02.001.
6. Vance MC, Hernandez JD, Didonna ML, Stern PJ. Complications and outcome of four-corner arthrodesis: circular plate fixation versus traditional techniques. *J Hand Surg Am.* 2005;30(6):1122-1127. doi:10.1016/j.jhsa.2005.08.007.

7. Le Corre A, Ardouin L, Loubersac T, Gaisne E, Bellemère P. Retrospective study of two fixation methods for 4-corner fusion: Shape-memory staple vs. dorsal circular plate. *Chir Main.* 2015;34(6):300-306. doi:10.1016/j.main.2015.08.008.

8. Draeger RW, Bynum DK, Schaffer A, Patterson JMM. Bicolumnar intercarpal arthrodesis: minimum 2-year follow-up. *J Hand Surg Am.* 2014;39(5):888-894. doi:10.1016/j.jhsa.2014.01.023.

9. Rizzo M. Wrist arthrodesis and arthroplasty. In: Wolfe S, Hotchkiss R, Pederson W, Kozin S, Cohen M, eds. *Green's Operative Hand Surgery.* Philadelphia, PA: Elsevier; 2017:373-417.

10. Ferreres A, Garcia-Elias M, Plaza R. Long-term results of lunocapitate arthrodesis with scaphoid excision for SLAC and SNAC wrists. *J Hand Surg Eur Vol.* 2009;34(5):603-608. doi:10.1177/1753193409105683.

11. Gaston RG, Greenberg JA, Baltera RM, Mih A, Hastings H. Clinical outcomes of scaphoid and triquetral excision with capitolunate arthrodesis versus scaphoid excision and four-corner arthrodesis. *J Hand Surg Am.* 2009;34(8):1407-1412. doi:10.1016/j.jhsa.2009.05.018.

12. Green DP, Perreira AC, Longhofer LK. Proximal row carpectomy. *J Hand Surg Am.* 2015;40(8):1672-1676. doi:10.1016/j.jhsa.2015.04.033.

13. Tang P, Imbriglia JE. Osteochondral resurfacing (OCRPRC) for capitate chondrosis in proximal row carpectomy. *J Hand Surg Am.* 2007;32(9):1334-1342. doi:10.1016/j.jhsa.2007.07.013.

14. Mulford JS, Ceulemans LJ, Nam D, Axelrod TS. Proximal row carpectomy vs four corner fusion for scapholunate (SLAC) or scaphoid nonunion advanced collapse (SNAC) wrists: a systematic review of outcomes. *J Hand Surg Eur Vol.* 2009;34(2):256-263. doi:10.1177/1753193408100954.

15. Cohen MS, Kozin SH. Degenerative arthritis of the wrist: proximal row carpectomy versus scaphoid excision and four-corner arthrodesis. *J Hand Surg Am.* 2001;26(1):94-104. doi:10.1053/jhsu.2001.20160.

16. Wall LB, Didonna ML, Kiefhaber TR, Stern PJ. Proximal row carpectomy: minimum 20-year follow-up. *J Hand Surg Am.* 2013;38(8):1498-1504. doi:10.1016/j.jhsa.2013.04.028.

17. Berkhout MJ, Bachour Y, Zheng KH, Mullender MG, Strackee SD, Ritt MJ. Four-corner arthrodesis versus proximal row carpectomy: a retrospective study with a mean follow-up of 17 years. *J Hand Surg Am.* 2015;40(7):1349-1354. doi:10.1016/j.jhsa.2014.12.035.

18. Saltzman BM, Frank JM, Slikker W, Fernandez JJ, Cohen MS, Wysocki RW. Clinical outcomes of proximal row carpectomy versus four-corner arthrodesis for post-traumatic wrist arthropathy: a systematic review. *J Hand Surg Eur Vol.* 2015;40(5):450-457. doi:10.1177/1753193414554359.

19. Wood MB. Wrist arthrodesis using dorsal radial bone graft. *J Hand Surg Am.* 1987;12(2):208-212.

20. Larsson SE. Compression arthrodesis of the wrist. A consecutive series of 23 cases. *Clin Orthop Relat Res.* 1974;(99):146-153.

21. Hastings H, Weiss AP, Quenzer D, Wiedeman GP, Hanington KR, Strickland JW. Arthrodesis of the wrist for post-traumatic disorders. *J Bone Joint Surg Am*. 1996;78(6):897-902.
22. Benkeddache Y, Gottesman H, Fourrier P. Multiple stapling for wrist arthrodesis in the nonrheumatoid patient. *J Hand Surg Am*. 1984;9(2):256-260.
23. Kluge S, Schindele S, Henkel T, Herren D. The modified Clayton-Mannerfelt arthrodesis of the wrist in rheumatoid arthritis: operative technique and report on 93 cases. *J Hand Surg Am*. 2013;38(5):999-1005. doi:10.1016/j.jhsa.2013.02.029.
24. Louis DS, Hankin FM, Bowers WH. Capitate-radius arthrodesis: an alternative method of radiocarpal arthrodesis. *J Hand Surg Am*. 1984;9(3):365-369.
25. Berling SE, Kiefhaber TR, Stern PJ. Hardware-related complications following radiocarpal arthrodesis using a dorsal plate. *J Wrist Surg*. 2015;4(1):56-60. doi:10.1055/s-0034-1400069.
26. Wysocki RW, Cohen MS. Complications of limited and total wrist arthrodesis. *Hand Clin*. 2010;26(2):221-228. doi:10.1016/j.hcl.2009.11.003.

26 Distal Radius Fractures

Kathryn Ashley Bentley and
Nileshkumar M. Chaudhari

INTRODUCTION

- Definition
  - Fracture of the distal end of the radius that originates in the metaphyseal region and often extends into the radiocarpal and distal radioulnar joints (DRUJs)
- Epidemiology
  - Most common fracture seen in the emergency department
  - 3% of all upper extremity injuries
  - Incidence of 640 000 annually in the United States[1]
  - Bimodal distribution
    - 5- to 24-year-old high-energy predominantly male
    - Elderly low-energy predominantly female[2]
      - Associated with osteoporosis
      - At 7 years after fracture of the distal radius in the elderly, survival rates were lower than those individuals of the same age and gender in standard population.[2]
- Anatomy
  - Distal radius is the articular surface on which the carpus rests.
  - Metaphysis of the distal radius is primarily cancellous bone.
  - Three articulations
    - Radioscaphoid articulation
    - Radiolunate articulation
    - Sigmoid notch (DRUJ)
  - 80% of axial load is supported by the distal radius and 20% by the ulna and triangular fibrocartilage complex (TFCC).[3]
- Mechanism of injury
  - Younger individuals—falls from height, motor vehicle collisions, injury sustained during athletic participation

- Older individuals—lower energy mechanisms such as falls from standing height
- Pathomechanics
  - Dorsal displacement
    - Fall on an outstretched hand with the wrist in 40° to 90° of dorsiflexion results in a distal radius fracture with dorsal displacement.[4]
    - Volar side of radius initially fails in tension and then the fracture propagates dorsally where bending moment forces cause compression stresses that result in dorsal comminution.
  - Volar displacement
    - Fall on the back of the flexed hand or fall on a forearm in supination followed by pronation around a fixed extended wrist[5]
  - Shearing forces influence injury patterns as well as often resulting in articular surface involvement.[3]
    - Lunate can exert compressive forces on the distal radius, producing a die-punch fracture.[4]
- Associated injuries
  - Up to 68% of distal radius fractures are associated with soft tissue injuries.
    - TFCC injury
    - Scapholunate ligament injury
    - Lunotriquetral ligament injury[6,7]
  - Median nerve injury[8]

EVALUATION

- History
  - Mechanism
  - Identification of associated traumatic injuries
  - Physiologic patient age and comorbidities
  - Lifestyle
  - Occupation
  - Hand dominance
- Physical examination
  - Skin should be inspected for any compromise.

- Swelling, ecchymosis, and tenderness to palpation about the wrist
- Deformity of the wrist is common.
- Careful neurovascular examination should be performed with particular attention to median nerve function.
- Ipsilateral elbow and shoulder should also be examined for associated injuries.
- Imaging
  - Radiographs of the elbow, forearm, wrist, and hand
  - Posteroanterior and lateral views of the wrist should be obtained.
    - ◆ Radiographic measurements
      - ✱ Radial inclination: averages 23° (Figure 26.1)
      - ✱ Radial height: averages 11 mm (Figure 26.2)
      - ✱ Volar tilt: averages 11° to 12° (Figure 26.3)
      - ✱ Ulnar variance: ~2 mm (Figure 26.2)
  - CT scanning may help with fracture characterization.[3]
- Classification
  - Descriptive
    - ◆ Open versus closed, displacement, angulation, comminution, loss of radial length
  - Eponyms
    - ◆ Colles fracture (Figure 26.4A and B)
      - ✱ Extra-articular/intra-articular distal radius fractures demonstrating various combinations of dorsal angulation, dorsal displacement, radial shift, and radial shortening with associated ulnar styloid fracture
      - ✱ "Dinner fork" deformity clinically
      - ✱ More than 90% of distal radius fractures
      - ✱ Mechanism of injury is fall onto hyperextended, radially deviated wrist with the forearm in pronation.
    - ◆ Smith fracture
      - ✱ Reverse Colles fracture
      - ✱ Fracture with volar angulation of the distal radius with volar displacement of the hand and distal radius
      - ✱ Very unstable fracture pattern
      - ✱ Mechanism of injury is a fall onto a flexed wrist with the forearm fixed in supination.
    - ◆ Barton fracture
      - ✱ Fracture—dislocation/subluxation of the wrist in which the dorsal or volar rim of the distal radius is displaced with the hand and carpus.

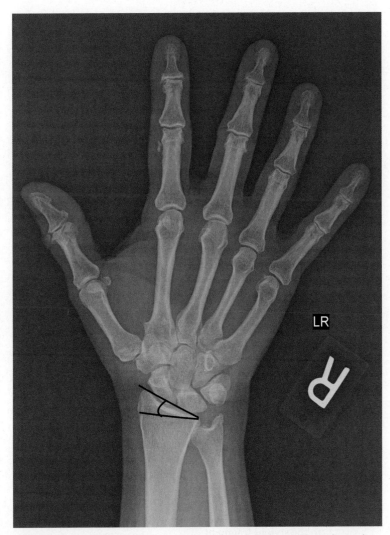

FIGURE 26.1 Radial inclination is measured on an anteroposterior radiograph and is represented by the angle formed by a line from the tip of the radial styloid to the ulnar corner of the distal radial articular surface and a line drawn perpendicular to the longitudinal axis of the radius.

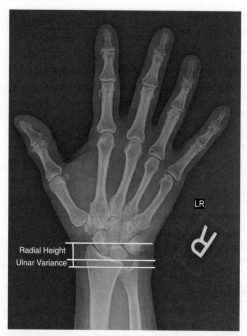

FIGURE 26.2 Radial height is measured on an anteroposterior radiograph of the wrist as the distance between two lines drawn perpendicular to the long axis of the distal radius. The first line intersects the radial styloid and the second line intersects the articular surface of the lunate facet. Ulnar variance is the distance between the ulnar corner of the articular surface of the distal radius and the ulnar head articular surface.

  * Very unstable fracture pattern
  * Mechanism of injury is a fall onto an extended wrist with the forearm fixed in pronation.
 ◆ Chauffeur fracture (radial styloid fracture)
  * Avulsion fracture with extrinsic ligaments remaining attached to the styloid fragment
  * May involve entire styloid or only the dorsal/volar portion
  * Often associated with carpal ligament injury patterns (ie, perilunate dislocations)
  * Mechanism of injury is compression of the scaphoid into the styloid with the wrist in extension and ulnar deviation (ie, chauffeur being struck by the backfire recoil of a starter crank on an early automobile engine)[3,9]

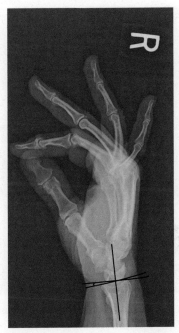

FIGURE 26.3 Volar tilt is measured on a lateral radiograph of the wrist as the angle formed between the articular surface of the distal radius and a line perpendicular to the long axis of the radius.

- Frykman classification of Colles fractures
  - Type I: extra-articular without distal ulna fracture
  - Type II: extra-articular with distal ulna fracture
  - Type III: intra-articular involving radiocarpal joint without distal ulna fracture
  - Type IV: intra-articular involving radiocarpal joint with distal ulna fracture
  - Type V: intra-articular involving DRUJ without distal ulna fracture
  - Type VI: intra-articular involving DRUJ with distal ulna fracture
  - Type VII: intra-articular involving radiocarpal and DRUJ without distal ulna fracture
  - Type VIII: intra-articular involving radiocarpal and DRUJ with distal ulna fracture

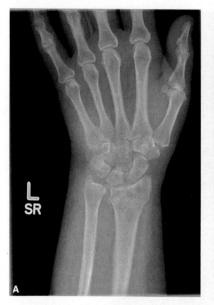 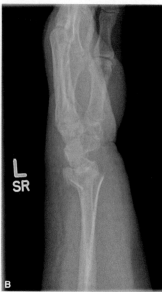

FIGURE 26.4 A and B, Representative radiographs of a classic Colles fracture with an intra-articular split.

- Melone classification of intra-articular fractures (lunate impaction injury)
  - Four major fragments of the distal radius fractures are identified:
    * Shaft
    * Radial styloid
    * Dorsal medial facet
    * Volar medial facet[10]
  - Type I: stable, without comminution
  - Type II: unstable die-punch, dorsal, or volar
    * Type IIA: reducible
    * Type IIB: irreducible
  - Type III: spike fracture; contused volar structures
  - Type IV: split fracture; ulnar column fractured with dorsal and palmar fragments displaced separately
  - Type V: explosion fracture; severe comminution with major soft tissue injury

- Fernandez classification
  - Type I: bending fractures of the metaphysis
    - One cortex fails in tension and the opposite cortex shows comminution.
  - Type II: shearing fractures of the joint surface
  - Type III: compression fractures of the joint surface
    - Impaction of the subchondral and metaphyseal cancellous bone
  - Type IV: avulsion fractures of the ligament attachments
    - Ulnar and radial styloid fractures
  - Type V: high-energy injuries involving bending, compression, shearing, and avulsion mechanisms or bone loss[9]

ACUTE MANAGEMENT

- Immediate closed reduction and splinting
  - Technique of closed reduction
    - Hematoma block
      - Hematoma associated with the fracture is sterilely infiltrated dorsally with 1% lidocaine without epinephrine and allowed to diffuse about the fracture site for about 5 minutes.
    - Arm is suspended with finger traps with 5 to 10 lb of counter-traction across the upper arm.
    - After allowing the arm to hang in the traps for 5 to 10 minutes, pressure is applied with the treating physician's thumb to the distal fracture fragment in a direction that will reduce the displacement.
    - When the distal fragment is translated dorsally and angulated, one may need to distract and hyperextend the fracture first to disimpact the fracture (recreate the deformity) before reducing the deformity with a traction/flexion maneuver.
    - A stable reduced fracture will hold its position with wrist slightly flexed and ulnarly deviated.
    - Sugar tong splint is then applied to hold the reduction.
      - Splint controls forearm rotation and immobilizes the wrist while allowing some elbow flexion.
      - Molding the splint in a three-point mold is helpful to maintain reduction.
        - ▲ Molding over the index metacarpal and proximal forearm dorsally and a countermold at the volar apex of the fracture site[9]

DEFINITIVE TREATMENT

- Goals of treatment
  - Articular congruity
  - Radial alignment and length
  - Motion
  - Stability[9]
- Nonoperative treatment
  - Indications
    - Nondisplaced or minimally displaced fractures
    - Displaced fractures with a stable fracture pattern that can be expected to unite within acceptable radiographic parameters
    - Low-demand elderly patients living a sedentary lifestyle
      - Nonoperative treatment, even in the presence of deformity, yields acceptable outcomes.[11]
  - Acceptable radiographic parameters
    - Radial length: within 2 to 3 mm of the contralateral wrist
    - Palmar tilt: neutral
    - Intra-articular step-off: <2 mm
    - Radial inclination: <5° loss
  - Closed reduction and splinting/casting
    - Initial closed reduction and application of well-molded sugar tong splint with acceptable reduction
    - Weekly radiographs for the first 2 to 3 weeks checking for maintenance of reduction
    - Transition to well-molded short arm cast at 2 to 3 weeks postreduction
    - Short arm cast for 3 to 4 weeks to complete 6 weeks of immobilization or until radiographic healing
  - Risk factors for loss of reduction with closed treatment
    - Dorsal angulation greater than 20°
    - Dorsal comminution
    - Intra-articular fracture
    - Ulna fracture
    - Age older than 60 years
    - >5 mm of radial shortening[11-13]
- Surgical indications
  - High-energy injury
  - Secondary loss of reduction

- Articular comminution or gap >2 mm
- Radial shortening >3 mm
- Dorsal tilt >10° from neutral
- Metaphyseal comminution or bone loss
- Loss of volar buttress with displacement
- DRUJ incongruity[3,14]
- Operative techniques
  - Closed reduction and pinning
    - Percutaneous pinning supplemented by external plaster/fiberglass cast
    - Pins placed through the radial styloid alone, crossed radial styloid and dorsal ulnar corner pins, or radial styloid and DRUJ pins are some of the described methods of pin fixation.
    - Cast and pins are removed at 5 to 6 weeks.
    - Indications
      * Reducible extra-articular fractures and simple intra-articular fractures without metaphyseal comminution[9]
  - External fixation
    - Fracture is closed reduced.
    - Two half-pins are inserted into the 2nd metacarpal and two half-pins are inserted into the radial shaft and then connected by a single bar.
    - Supplemental K-wires are recommended to augment the fixation as there is significant tension decay and loss of reduction with external fixator alone.[15]
    - Indications
      * Damage control orthopedics in the polytraumatized patient
      * Open fractures or fractures with poor soft tissue envelope
      * Used to maintain radial length in fractures with severe comminution
  - Bridge plating
    - Dorsal spanning plate that will bridge the fracture with fixation into 2nd metacarpal and radial shaft
    - Acts as an internal–external fixator and avoids complications associated with external fixation such as hand stiffness and pin site infections
    - More stable than external fixation because decreases the implant to bone distance[16]
    - Indications

- Highly comminuted fractures with metadiaphyseal extension or osteopenic bone
- Distal radius nonunion not amenable to volar fixation
- Stabilization of radiocarpal dislocations
- Early forearm weight bearing desired[17]
- Dorsal plating
  - Dorsal approach
    - Utilizes the interval between the extensor carpi radialis brevis and extensor pollicis longus
    - Allows direct visualization of radial shaft and articular surface
  - Dorsal plates
    - Plate is placed under the extensor tendons, which with older generation dorsal plates has led to extensor tendon irritation and rupture.
    - Newer generation plates are of lower profile and designed to create less extensor tendon irritation.
    - There are also variable angle screw fixation plates that allow for more distal placement of dorsal plates.[18]
  - Indications
    - Dorsal shearing fracture—dislocation
    - Articular fractures requiring direct reduction
    - Grafting of large defects
    - Ipsilateral carpal injuries requiring a dorsal approach[17]
- Volar plating
  - Most common method of fixation of distal radius fractures
  - Volar approach
    - Utilizes interval between flexor carpi radialis subsheath and the radial artery
    - Pronator quadratus is elevated off the radius to expose the fracture.
    - Limit deep distal dissection to avoid disruption of volar radiocarpal ligaments.
  - Volar locking plates
    - Transfer loads from the subchondral surface to the volar cortex and radial shaft.
    - Fixed- and variable-angle distal locking screw options
    - Plates that are designed to fit distal or proximal to the watershed line are available.
    - Allow versatile plate and screw positioning based on the fracture fragments.[19]

- ◆ Indications
  - ✳ Intra-articular or unstable extra-articular distal radius fractures
  - ✳ Dorsally or volarly displaced fractures with comminution
  - ✳ Osteopenic or deficient metaphyseal bone
  - ✳ Early motion desired[20]
- ● Fragment-specific fixation
  - ◆ Stabilizes the major fragments: radial column, volar lunate facet, and dorsal ulnar corner
  - ◆ Plates are designed to stabilize each fragment.
  - ◆ May be used in combination with spanning plates or external fixation to neutralize the longitudinal forces
  - ◆ Indications
    - ✳ Complex articular fracture patterns[17]
- ■ Potential complications
  - ● Carpal tunnel syndrome (CTS)
    - ◆ Acute versus exacerbation of preexisting CTS
  - ● Flexor/extensor tendon irritation/rupture related to hardware
  - ● Spontaneous extensor pollicis longus rupture with conservatively treated nondisplaced distal radius fractures
  - ● Failure of fixation
  - ● Intra-articular placement of hardware[21-23]
  - ● Nonunion or malunion
  - ● Chronic regional pain syndrome[9]
- ■ Postoperative care
  - ● Immobilization for a brief period (~10-14 days) to allow soft tissue healing and decrease swelling
    - ◆ May increase time of immobilization based on fracture complexity/ stability and soft tissues
  - ● Sutures removed at 10 to 14 days
  - ● Begin digital range of motion exercises immediately to prevent stiffness.
  - ● Begin wrist range of motion exercises once immobilization is discontinued.
  - ● Velcro wrist splint can be provided for comfort while participating in gentle activities of daily living.
  - ● Strenuous pushing, pulling, twisting, or lifting should be avoided for 3 months.
  - ● Radiographs are taken at the first postoperative visit at 10 to 14 days and then again at 6 and 12 weeks.

- Outcomes
  - Modern fixation techniques generate successful outcomes in a majority of patients.
    - Restoration of grip strength to 80% to 90% of preinjury values and restoration of range of wrist motion to 80% to 85%
    - 85% to 95% good to excellent results[9]
  - Failure to restore carpal alignment in the sagittal plane is the single most predictive factor of worsening functional outcomes and objective measures of strength.[24]
  - Up to 20% of all patients with a distal radius fracture report persistent symptoms such as pain, nerve symptoms, and disability after 1 year.[25]

REFERENCES

1. Chung KC, Spilson SV. The frequency and epidemiology of hand and forearm fractures in the United States. *J Hand Surg.* 2001;26(5):908-915.
2. Rozental TD, Makhni EC, Day CS, Bouxsein ML. Improving evaluation and treatment for osteoporosis following distal radial fractures: a prospective randomized intervention. *J Bone Joint Surg Am.* 2008;90(5):953-961.
3. Koval KJ, Zuckerman JD. *Handbook of Fractures.* 3rd ed. Philadelphia, PA: Lippincott Williams & Wilkins; 2006:161.
4. Frykman G. Fracture of the distal radius including sequelae-shoulder–hand-finger syndrome, disturbance in the distal radio-ulnar joint and impairment of nerve function: a clinical and experimental study. *Acta Orthop Scand.* 1967;38(suppl 108):1-61.
5. Ellis J. Smith's and Barton's fractures. *J Bone Joint Surg Br.* 1965;47(4):724-727.
6. Geissler WB, Freeland AE, Savoie FH, McIntyre LW, Whipple TL. Intracarpal soft-tissue lesions associated with an intra-articular fracture of the distal end of the radius. *J Bone Joint Surg Am.* 1996;78(3):357-365.
7. Richards RS, Bennett JD, Roth JH, Milne K Jr. Arthroscopic diagnosis of intra-articular soft tissue injuries associated with distal radial fractures. *J Hand Surg Am.* 1997;22(5):772-776.
8. Lindau T. Arthroscopic diagnosis of carpal ligament injuries with distal radius fractures. In: Slutsky D, Osterman A, eds. *Fractures and Injuries to the Distal Radius and Carpus: The Cutting Edge.* Philadelphia, PA: Saunders Elsevier; 2009:443-452.
9. Wolfe SW. Distal radius fractures. In: Wolfe S, Hotchkiss R, Pederson W, Kozin S, eds. *Green's Operative Hand Surgery.* 6th ed. Philadelphia, PA: Elsevier Churchill Livingstone; 2011:561-638.
10. Melone CP Jr. Articular fractures of the distal radius. *Orthop Clin North Am.* 1984;15(2):217-236.
11. Gehrmann SV, Windolf J, Kaufmann RA. Distal radius fracture management in elderly patients: a literature review. *J Hand Surg.* 2008;33(3):421-429.

12. Lafontaine M, Hardy D, Delince PH. Stability assessment of distal radius fractures. *Injury*. 1989;20(4):208-210.
13. Mackenney PJ, McQueen MM, Elton R. Prediction of instability in distal radial fractures. *J Bone Joint Surg Am*. 2006;88(9):1944-1951.
14. Lichtman DM, Bindra RR, Boyer MI, et al. Treatment of distal radius fractures. *J Am Acad Orthop Surg*. 2010;18(3):180-189.
15. Rectenwald JP, Bentley KA, Murray PM, Saha S. Strain as a function of time in extrinsic wrist ligaments tensioned through external fixation. *Hand (N Y)*. 2018;13(1):60-64.
16. Wolf JC, Weil WM, Hanel DP, Trumble TE. A biomechanic comparison of an internal radiocarpal-spanning 2.4-mm locking plate and external fixation in a model of distal radius fractures. *J Hand Surg*. 2006;31(10):1578-1586.
17. Alluri RK, Ryan Hill J, Ghiassi A. Distal radius fractures: approaches, indications, and techniques. *J Hand Surg*. 2016;41(8):845-854.
18. Schneppendahl J, Windolf J, Kaufmann RA. Distal radius fractures: current concepts. *J Hand Surg*. 2012;37(8):1718-1725.
19. Rhee PC, Medoff RJ, Shin AY. Complex distal radius fractures: an anatomic algorithm for surgical management. *J Am Acad Orthop Surg*. 2017;25(2):77-88.
20. Smith DW, Henry MH. Volar fixed-angle plating of the distal radius. *J Am Acad Orthop Surg*. 2005;13(1):28-36.
21. Berglund LM, Messer TM. Complications of volar plate fixation for managing distal radius fractures. *J Am Acad Orthop Surg*. 2009;17(6):369-377.
22. Nana AD, Joshi A, Lichtman DM. Plating of the distal radius. *J Am Acad Orthop Surg*. 2005;13(3):159-171.
23. Asadollahi S, Keith PP. Flexor tendon injuries following plate fixation of distal radius fractures: a systematic review of the literature. *J Orthop Traumatol*. 2013;14(4):227-234.
24. McQueen MM, Hajducka C. Redisplaced unstable fractures of the distal radius. *J Bone Joint Surg Br*. 1996;78(3):404-409.
25. MacDermid JC, Roth JH, Richards RS. Pain and disability reported in the year following a distal radius fracture: a cohort study. *BMC Musculoskelet Disord*. 2003;4(1):24.

Distal Radius Malunion

Anthony LoGiudice and Hisham M. Awan

INTRODUCTION

- Distal radius malunion—an intra-articular or extra-articular distal radius fracture healed in nonanatomic alignment, resulting in wrist pain, degenerative changes, decreased range of motion, altered wrist mechanics, instability, or a combination of these.
- The biomechanical effects of malunion were first described by Rouen in 1919; Campbell detailed treatment with biplanar osteotomies in the 1930s.
- The distal radius may normally bear loads of up to 4000 N, with 80% normally borne by the radius.
- Recent studies showed that increasing ulnar positivity by only 2.5 mm raises the load across the ulna to 42% of the total borne by the wrist.
- Deformity does not correlate well with symptom severity.
- Key measurements—radial inclination, radial length/height, ulnar variance, and radial/volar tilt (Figure 27.1 and Table 27.1)
- Most common deformity is loss of palmar/volar tilt in the sagittal plane and loss of radial length relative to the ulna.
- Malunion is the most common complication of distal radius fracture, with an overall rate as high as 17%.
- Frequently occurs in distal radius fractures managed nonoperatively and in elderly, osteoporotic bone.
- Other causes—inadequate reduction, neglect or delayed presentation, and inadequate fixation or immobilization after operative intervention

EVALUATION

- **History**
  - Ulnar-sided wrist pain is the most common complaint and may be a consequence of altered ulnar variance, incongruity, or malalignment of the sigmoid notch.

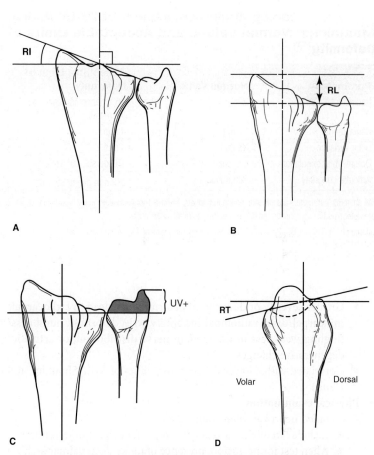

FIGURE 27.1 A, On a posteroanterior radiograph, the radial inclination (RI) is the angle subtended by a line perpendicular to the long axis of the radius and a line reflecting the articular surface of the radius. B, The radial length/height (RL) is the distance between tangents drawn at the radial styloid and the ulnar head, perpendicular to their shaft axes. C, The ulnar variance (UV) reflects the axial relationship between the ulnar head and ulnarmost aspect of the radius (ulnar edge of lunate fossa). The grayed portion of the ulna represents the prominence (positive UV) at the distal radioulnar joint. D, On a lateral radiograph, the radial/volar tilt (RT) is the angle between the articular surface and a line perpendicular to the radial shaft. Adapted from Graham TJ. Surgical correction of malunited fractures of the distal radius. *J Am Acad Orthop Surg.* 1997;5:270-281.

TABLE 27.1 Radiographic Assessment of Distal Radius Malunions: Normal Values and Acceptable Limits of Deformity[14,17]

Parameter	Normal Value[a]	Acceptable Limit of Deformity
Radial inclination	22°	15° change (increase or decrease)
Radial length	11 mm	4 mm
Ulnar variance	Neutral	4 mm
Dorsal–volar angulation	11° volar	15° dorsal, 20° volar
Articular congruity	Congruous	≥2 mm gap or step-off

[a]All anatomic parameters are variable among individuals. The true "normal" values in each particular case are determined by comparison radiographs of the contralateral extremity.

Adapted from Bushnell BD, Bynum DK. Malunion of the distal radius. *J Am Acad Orthop Surg.* 2007;15:27–40.

- Greater severity or duration of deformity may lead to radiocarpal/midcarpal/distal radioulnar instability, wrist deformity, numbness/tingling/weakness in the median nerve distribution, or arthritic/degenerative changes.
- Correlated with a lower DASH (Disabilities of Arm, Shoulder, and Hand) score
- **Physical examination**
  - Detailed neurovascular examination
    - Include careful testing of median nerve for carpal tunnel syndrome.
    - Allen test for perfusion, presence of intact deep palmar arch
  - Decreased range of motion—shifted flexion/extension arc, decreased pronosupination
  - Swelling/edema
  - Dinner fork deformity (Figure 27.2)
  - Prominence of the ulnar head with pronosupination
  - Decreased grip strength ($\downarrow$50%)
  - Prior surgical incisions
  - Focused examination—radiocarpal, ulnocarpal, and distal radioulnar joints (DRUJ). Check for pain, crepitus, and instability.

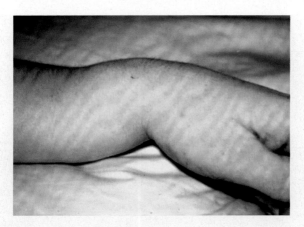

FIGURE 27.2 Dinner fork deformity resulting from loss of radial length, inclination, and palmar tilt.

- **Imaging**
  - Posteroanterior (PA) and lateral wrist radiographs to measure criteria of malunion (Table 27.1)
  - Degenerative changes at the radiocarpal joint, midcarpal joint, and DRUJ should be noted.
  - Check carpal alignment for dorsal subluxation of the carpus (Figures 27.3 and 27.4) or dorsal intercalated segment instability.
- Advanced imaging is not routinely used in initial evaluation. However, it can be useful to evaluate complex and/or intra-articular deformity.
  - Computerized tomography (CT)—shows bony detail of articular incongruity, status of fracture healing, as well as rotational and translational deformities
  - MRI—shows gradient of soft tissue injury at the DRUJ, extrinsic or intrinsic carpal ligaments, and articular cartilage
- **Classification**
  No widely adopted system.
  - Malunions may be described using radiographic parameters (Table 27.1). Alternatively, they may be described using the eponymous fracture pattern from the original injury (Colles fracture, Smith fracture, Barton fracture, etc.).

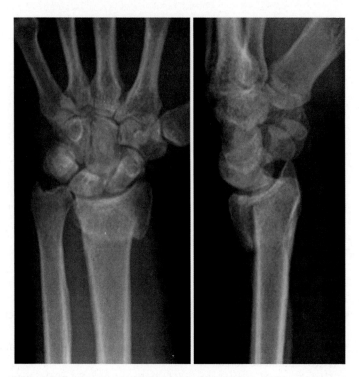

FIGURE 27.3 Posteroanterior and lateral radiographs of a distal radius malunion demonstrating loss of radial inclination and length, increased ulnar variance, and dorsal angulation.

INITIAL TREATMENT

- Patients who present with a distal radius malunion may require extensive workup and multiple visits to determine the best treatment course.

DEFINITIVE TREATMENT

- **Nonoperative treatment** is guided by radiographic criteria as listed in Tables 27.1 and 27.2.
  - Elderly (older than 65 years), low-demand patients may tolerate some deformity and should be allowed to regain function as possible.

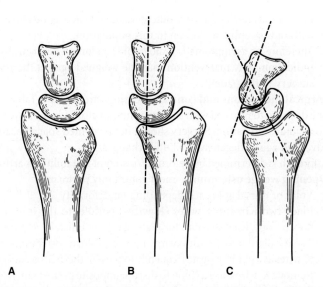

A   **B**   **C**

FIGURE 27.4 Normal anatomy (A) and two patterns of instability caused by dorsal malunion of the distal radius: dorsal radiocarpal subluxation with maintenance of midcarpal alignment (B) and adaptive midcarpal dorsal intercalated segment instability deformity (C). Adapted from Graham TJ. Surgical correction of malunited fractures of the distal radius. *J Am Acad Orthop Surg.* 1997;5:270–281.

TABLE 27.2 **Surgical Indications and Contraindications**

Indications	Contraindications
Pain with motion or activity	Advanced radiocarpal degeneration
Weakness with activity	Advanced intercarpal degeneration
Mechanical symptoms	Fixed intercarpal malalignment
Functional limitations affecting work/lifestyle	Severe osteoporosis
Decreased grip strength	Complex regional pain syndrome
Decreased range of motion	Inability to comply with postoperative therapy
Instability on stress testing	Serious concomitant medical illness
Radiographic evidence of malunion (Table 27.1)	Very low physical demands

Adapted from Bushnell BD, Bynum DK. Malunion of the distal radius. *J Am Acad Orthop Surg.* 2007;15:27-40.

- Functional and/or objective outcomes do not show good correlation with radiographic malunion in this population.
- Therefore, an asymptomatic radiographic malunion is not an absolute indication. Any intervention must be weighed against the risks of surgery to the patient.
- **Surgical indications and contraindications** are listed in Table 27.2.
- The decision to proceed with surgery is multifactorial and elective, with no absolute indication. Surgery should not be denied solely because of advanced age or degenerative DRUJ changes.
- Approach is determined by deformity, resultant instability, or arthrosis.
- **Opening wedge osteotomy**—most commonly performed
  - Volar or dorsal approach depending on deformity
  - Place two Kirschner wires (K-wires) parallel to the joint under fluoroscopy, leaving room for plate placement distally (Figure 27.5).
  - Use oscillating saw with narrow kerf to perform osteotomy, using K-wires as a guide; irrigate frequently to prevent thermal osteonecrosis.
  - Remove K-wires, use a Cobb to disrupt opposite periosteum to allow for distraction/restoration of length/inclination.
  - Select/apply a plate. Volar plates may be applied using a lift-off technique with distal fixation placed first. Fixate distal screws first. Leaving the proximal plate slightly ulnarward will also restore radial inclination upon reduction to the central shaft (Figure 27.6).
  - Dorsal approach/plating may use a lamina spreader or external fixator to maintain correction while applying plate. Structural bone graft may also be used (Figure 27.7).
  - Bone grafting—cancellous equivalent to structural (iliac crest) with appropriate fixation
  - Recent evidence demonstrates that volar plating with palmar cortical contact shows equivalent healing rates even without bone grafting.
  - Advantage—corrects length, tilt, and inclination; also ulnar variance
  - Disadvantage—less stable construct, risk of nonunion if construct is not stable
- **Closing wedge osteotomy**
  - Volar or dorsal approach
  - Complete osteotomy in similar fashion as open; place K-wires parallel to the joint, and proximally perpendicular to the shaft (Figure 27.8).
  - Complete osteotomy, remove bone wedge and reduce
  - Place the plate with K-wires all parallel to each other, or corrected further as needed for volar tilt restoration (Figure 27.8).
  - Advantage—bone-bone contact, stability

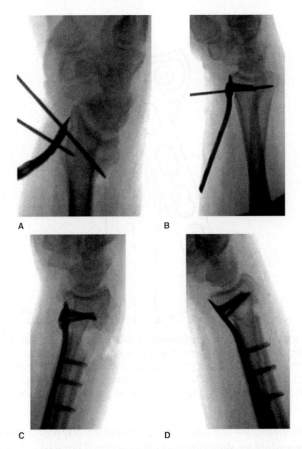

A   B

C   D

FIGURE 27.5 Technique of preliminary distal fixation before osteotomy. A, Case 1, Using a volar plate with a Kirschner wire (K-wire) guide hole that directs the wire parallel to the line of the modular fixed-angle locking pegs, the wire is placed through the plate and parallel to the joint surface. The known, fixed angle of curvature of the plate will ultimately provide the needed anatomic correction when the plate is secured to the radial shaft. The angle of the K wire can be increased to obtain more correction if desired. B, Case 2, The plate's modular locking pegs are predrilled and inserted into the distal fragment. The plate and pegs are then removed to allow the osteotomy cut to be made. C (Case 1) and D (Case 2), The hardware is then reinserted into its preosteotomy position, and the distally fixed plate is used as a joystick to help fine-tune anatomic restoration before proximal fixation to the shaft. Once the plate is fixed, cancellous autograft is packed around the plate to fill the dorsal defect. Adapted from Bushnell BD, Bynum DK. Malunion of the distal radius. *J Am Acad Orthop Surg*. 2007;15(1):27–40.

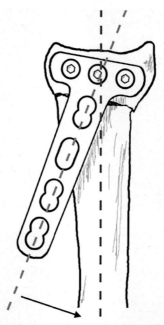

FIGURE 27.6 Technique of distal fixation of volar plate with proximal alignment toward ulna. Realignment of plate over radial shaft restores radial inclination as well as some length. Adapted from Mahmoud M, El Shafie S, Kamal M. Correction of dorsally-malunited extra-articular distal radius fractures using volar locked plates without bone grafting. *J Bone Joint Surg Br.* 2012;94-B(8):1090-1096.

- Disadvantage—shortens radius relative to ulna; may require ulnar-sided procedure for shortening versus resection (Darrach)
- **Sliding osteotomy**—Figure 27.9
- **Trapezoidal osteotomy**—Figure 27.10
- **Distraction osteogenesis**—osteotomy corrected and maintained with external fixator; gradual correction over weeks/months
- **Ulnar-sided procedures**
  - Instability—Adams reconstruction of DRUJ ligaments, triangular fibrocartilage complex repair
  - Impaction—wafer resection, ulnar shortening osteotomy
  - DRUJ/ulnocarpal arthrosis—Darrach procedure, Sauve-Kapandji procedure, arthroplasty
- **Potential complications**
  - Nonunion
  - Persistent pain

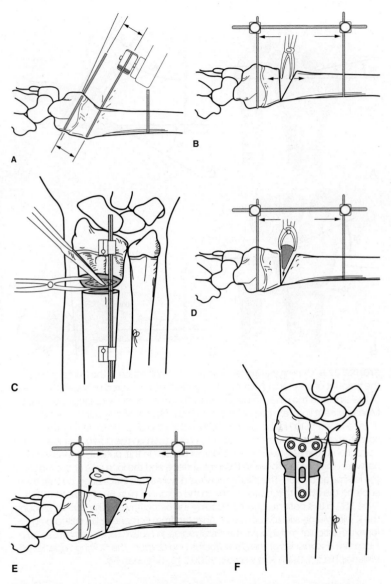

FIGURE 27.7 Distal radius osteotomy technique. A, Saw-cut parallel to joint; B, C, realignment of the radius to corrected position; D, placement of bone graft; E, placement of plate; and F, final plate fixation. Adapted from Weiss APC, Fernandez DL. Osteotomy of the distal radius for malunited Colles' fractures. *Atlas Hand Clin*. 1997;2:159-169.

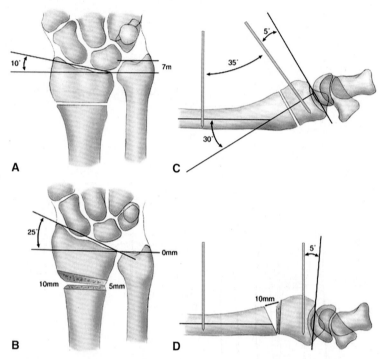

FIGURE 27.8 Closing wedge technique. A, For correction in the frontal plane, the amount of shortening (7 mm in this patient) is measured between the head of the ulna and the ulnar corner of the radius on the anteroposterior radiograph. Measurement lines are perpendicular to the long axis of the radius. The ulnar tilt is reduced to 10° in this patient. B, To restore the ulnar tilt to normal, the osteotomy is opened more on the dorsoradial than on the dorsoulnar side. C, For correction in the sagittal plane, the dorsal tilt (30° in this patient) is measured between the perpendicular to the joint surface and the long axis of the radius on the lateral radiograph. The Kirschner wires (K wires) are introduced, so that they subtend the angle that corresponds to the dorsal tilt plus 5° of volar tilt (30° + 5° = 35° in this patient). D, After opening the osteotomy by the correct amount, the K wires lie parallel to each other. Adapted from Fernandez DL. Osteotomy for extra-articular malunion of the distal radius. In Slutsky D, Osterman L (eds). *Fractures and Injuries of the Distal Radius and Carpus: The Cutting Edge*. 1st ed. Philadelphia, PA: Saunders Elsevier; 2009:529–541; chap 56.

- Hardware irritation
- Nerve injury
- Stiffness
- Persistent instability
- Under correction

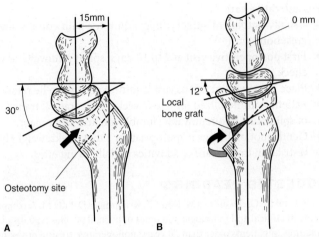

FIGURE 27.9 Sliding osteotomy for Smith fracture malunion. A, Volar deformity of 30°, 15 mm translation. B, Osteotomy performed through prior fracture and anatomically realigned. Adapted from Thivaios GC, McKee MD. Sliding osteotomy for deformity correction following malunion of volarly displaced distal radial fractures. *J Orthop Trauma*. 2003;17:326-333.

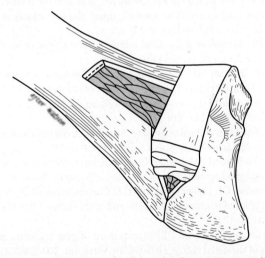

FIGURE 27.10 Trapezoidal osteotomy of dorsal malunion. Fragment is rotated perpendicular to shaft and inset as structural autograft into an opening wedge recipient site. Adapted from Watson HK, Castle TH Jr. Trapezoidal osteotomy of the distal radius for unacceptable articular angulation after Colles' fracture. *J Hand Surg Am*. 1988;13:837-843. Copyright 1998, with permission from the American Society for Surgery of the Hand.

- **Postoperative care**
  - Usually outpatient surgery; may admit for pain control after iliac crest bone graft
  - First postoperative visit at 7 to 10 days; splint removal and wound check
  - Place in new splint versus cast if sutures are able to be removed.
  - Patient is immobilized for 6 to 8 weeks, with gradual transition out of splint/cast into removable durable medical equipment.
  - Gentle motion begins if appropriate at 3 to 4 weeks; weight bearing restriction to self-care or activities of daily living only

SUGGESTED READINGS

Arora R, Gabl M, Gschwentner M, Deml C, Krappinger D, Lutz M. A comparative study of clinical and radiologic outcomes of unstable Colles type distal radius fractures in patients older than 70 years: nonoperative treatment versus volar locking plating. *J Orthop Trauma*. 2009;23(4):237–242.

Bacorn RW, Kurtzke JF. Colles' fracture; a study of two thousand cases from the New York State Workmen's Compensation Board. *J Bone Joint Surg Am*. 1953;35-A:643–658.

Campbell WC. Malunited Colles' fractures. *JAMA*. 1937;109:1105–1108.

Diaz-Garcia RJ, Oda T, Shauver MJ, Chung KC. A systematic review of outcomes and complications of treating unstable distal radius fractures in the elderly. *J Hand Surg Am*. 2011;36(5): 824–835.e2.

Fernandez DL. Malunion of the distal radius: current approach to management. *Instr Course Lect*. 1993;42:99–113.

Gesensway D, Putnam MD, Mente PL, Lewis JL. Design and biomechanics of a plate for the distal radius. *J Hand Surg Am*. 1995;20:1021–1027.

Jupiter JB, Fernandez DL. Complications following distal radial fractures. *Instr Course Lect* 2002;51:203–219.

Lidstrom A. Fractures of the distal end of the radius. A clinical and statistical study of end results. *Acta Orthop Scand Suppl*. 1959;41:1–118.

Posner MA, Ambrose L. Malunited Colles' fractures: correction with a biplanar closing wedge osteotomy. *J Hand Surg Am*. 1991;16:1017–1026.

Shea K, Fernandez DL, Jupiter JB, Martin C Jr. Corrective osteotomy for malunited, volarly displaced fractures of the distal end of the radius. *J Bone Joint Surg Am*. 1997;79:1816–1826.

Slagel BE, Luenam S, Pichora DR. Management of post-traumatic malunion of fractures of the distal radius. *Orthop Clin North Am*. 2007;38:203–216, vi.

Weiss APC, Fernandez DL. Osteotomy of the distal radius for malunited Colles' fractures. *Atlas Hand Clin*. 1997;2:159–169.

Werner FW, Palmer AK, Fortino MD, Short WH. Force transmission through the distal ulna: effect of ulnar variance, lunate fossa angulation, and radial and palmar tilt of the distal radius. *J Hand Surg Am*. 1992;17(3):423–428.

Adam S. Martin and Hisham M. Awan

INTRODUCTION

- Fractures of the distal ulna present in two distinct varieties—isolated distal ulna fractures and distal ulna fractures in association with distal radius (DR) fractures.[1] Isolated distal ulna fractures are relatively rare and can be categorized as distal diaphyseal, aka nightstick, or styloid fractures, whereas distal ulna fractures associated with DR fractures are very common.

- **Mechanism of injury**—Nightstick fractures are the result of a direct blunt trauma to the ulna. Distal ulna fractures in association with DR fractures occur with similar mechanisms as those with isolated DR fractures, such as low-energy falls from standing, high-energy falls from height, or motor vehicle collisions.

- **Epidemiology**—The incidence of DR fractures in the United States is more than 640 000 per year.[2,3] Approximately 50% to 60% of DR fractures have concomitant fractures of the distal ulna. Isolated distal ulna fractures are relatively rare.

- **Anatomy**—The ulnar shaft widens distally to form the ulnar neck.[1] Distal to the neck are the two most distinct structures of the distal ulna: the ulnar head and ulnar styloid (Figure 28.1).[4]

  - The styloid is distal, dorsal, and medial relative to the ulnar head. A groove, called the fovea, lies between the head and styloid and can be palpated on the ulnar side of the wrist between the flexor carpi ulnaris and extensor carpi ulnaris (ECU) tendons; furthermore, the fovea is an important attachment site for the triangular fibrocartilage complex (TFCC).

  - Given that there is little inherent stability provided by the bony structure of the distal radioulnar joint (DRUJ), the TFCC is the main stabilizer of the DRUJ. The TFCC is composed of the palmar and dorsal radioulnar ligaments, articular disk, meniscal homologue, and ECU subsheath.

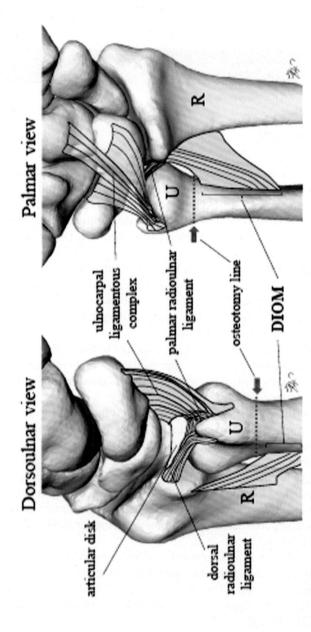

FIGURE 28.1 Distal ulnar anatomy. R, radius; U, ulna; DIOM, distal interosseous membrane. Reprinted from Miyamura S, Shigi A, Kraisarin J, et al. Impact of distal ulnar fracture malunion on distal radioulnar joint instabilitiy: a biomechanical study of the distal interosseous membrane using a cadaver model. *J Hand Surg Am.* 2017;42(3):e185-e191. Copyright © 2017 by the American Society for Surgery of the Hand. With permission.

- The ulnar head articulates with the sigmoid notch of the radius to form the DRUJ. The DRUJ, specifically the ulnar head, is the distal center of rotation for pronation and supination of the forearm.

EVALUATION

- **Presentation**—Patients often present with ulnar-sided wrist pain that localizes to the distal ulna. They may recall a specific traumatic event that coincides with the onset of pain. If patients present early, they may report swelling or ecchymosis around the wrist. If the injury is chronic, then patients may complain of loss of wrist range of motion (ROM) or a sense of instability around the wrist.
- **Physical examination**—On examination, one should have a systematic approach and include inspection, palpation, ROM, and neurovascular status. Inspection may reveal swelling, deformity, and/or ecchymosis. Palpation should include the DR and ulna, specifically the ulnar styloid and fovea. The DRUJ should be assessed for instability via the shuck test.
  - Perform the DRUJ shuck test (Figure 28.2) in neutral and end ranges of pronation/supination and compare with contralateral wrist.

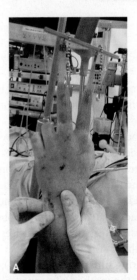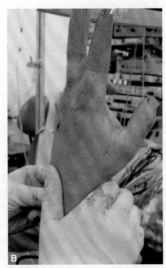

FIGURE 28.2 A-C, Shuck test for distal radioulnar joint instability. Reprinted with permission from Wiesel SW. *Operative Techniques in Orthopaedic Surgery*. 1st ed. Philadelphia, PA: Wolters Kluwer; 2010.

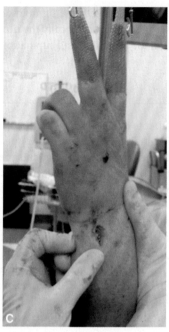

FIGURE 28.2 (continued)

"Shuck" the joint by translating the ulna volarly and dorsally while stabilizing the DR.

- ◆ There should be an equivalent amount of motion in neutral to contralateral wrist and firm endpoints at full supination and pronation.
- ◆ In general, DRUJ is more stable in supination.
- ▪ **Imaging**—Radiographic imaging should consist of a neutral rotation posteroanterior (PA) and true lateral views of the wrist (Figure 28.3). An acceptable PA view is evident when the cortical outline of the concavity of the ECU groove is radial to the long axis of the ulnar styloid. This view is obtained with the shoulder abducted 90°, elbow flexed 90°, and forearm and wrist in neutral. Likewise, an acceptable lateral view is obtained when the volar cortex of the pisiform is between the volar cortices of the scaphoid and capitate, also known as the "SPC lateral."
  - ● Several methods exist for measuring ulnar variance (UV); however, the most commonly used is the method of perpendiculars. A transverse line is drawn through the volar sclerotic line of the lunate fossa of the DR perpendicular to its long axis; the distance

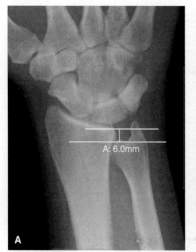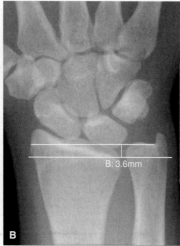

A: 6.0mm

B: 3.6mm

FIGURE 28.3 A,B Proper posteroanterior and lateral radiographs of wrist, ulnar variance measurement. Reprinted with permission from Bridgeforth GM. *Lippincott's Primary Care Musculoskeletal Radiology*. Philadelphia, PA: Lippincott Williams & Wilkins; 2010.

the ulnar head projects proximal or distal to this line is the UV (Figure 28.3).
- ◆ Average UV is approximately 1 mm.
- ◆ With neutral UV, the radius and ulnar receive 80% and 20% of the load, respectively.
- ◆ A 2.5-mm increase in UV will increase load across the ulnocarpal joint approximately from 20% to 40%.
- Computed tomography can be a useful adjunct to better characterize fracture patterns and the degree of DRUJ involvement.
- ■ **Differential diagnosis**
  - DRUJ instability
  - TFCC tear
  - Hook of hamate fracture
  - Ulnocarpal impaction
- ■ **Classification**—Isolated ulnar diaphyseal fractures are typically grouped using descriptive terminology.[3] In particular, those fractures with less than 50% translation and less than 15° angulation are considered stable. For fractures in association with DR fractures, the restoration of the sigmoid notch and the continuity of the dorsal and volar radioulnar ligaments of

	Pathoanatomy of the lesion		Joint surface involvement	Prognosis	Recommended treatment
Type I Stable (following reduction of the radius the distal radioulnar joint is congruous and stable)	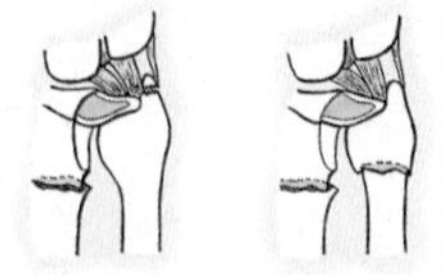 A Fracture of the tip of the ulnar styloid	B Stable fracture of the ulnar neck	None	Good	Stable: Functional aftercare, early forearm rotation exercises Unstable: Assess and correct coronal shift. If still unstable, open reduction internal fixation ulnar neck or shaft.
Type II Unstable (subluxation or dislocation of the ulnar head present)	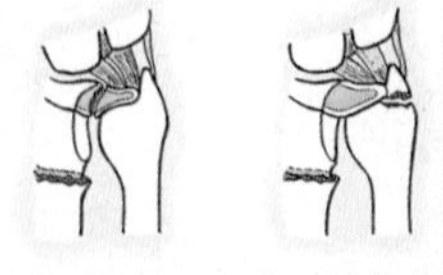 A Tear of the triangular fibrocartilage complex and/or palmar and dorsal capsular ligaments	B Avulsion fracture of the base of the ulnar styloid	None	• Possible chronic instability • Painful limitation of supination if left unreduced • Possible late arthritic changes	Anatomic reduction of radius and sigmoid notch, and *reduced coronal shift.* If still unstable: LAC for four weeks in position of stability, or dual 0.062-in K-wire fixation of radius and ulna, or ulnar styloid fixation, or open or arthroscopic triangular fibrocartilage complex foveal repair
Type III Potentially unstable (subluxation possible)	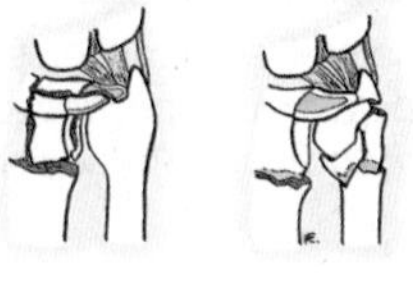 A Intraarticular fracture of the sigmoid notch	B Intraarticular fracture of the ulnar head	Present	• Dorsal subluxation possible together with dorsally displaced die punch or dorsoulnar fragment • Risk of early degenerative changes and severe limitation of forearm rotation if left unreduced	Anatomic reduction of radius and sigmoid notch, and *reduced coronal shift.* Open reduction internal fixation of ulnar head, immediate Darrach (sedentary), or early forearm rotation to enhance remodeling, and late ulnar head resection, arthroplasty, or Sauve-Kapandji if painful Open or arthroscopic triangular fibrocartilage complex repair if still unstable after anatomic fixation.

FIGURE 28.4 Classification of ulnar styloid fractures. Green's distal radius fx chapter. Reprinted from Green DP, Wolfe SW. *Green's Operative Hand Surgery*. 6th ed. Philadelphia, PA, Churchill Livingstone, 2011. Copyright © 2011 Elsevier. With permission.

the TFCC are crucial to maintaining the stability of radioulnar joint.[5] There are three types of distal ulna fractures in association with DR fractures (Figure 28.4). Type I fractures are stable injuries, meaning that with proper reduction of the radius, the DRUJ will be stable and without injury to the articular surface. Type II fractures are unstable injuries, meaning even with adequate reduction of the radius, the ulna remains unstable. Type III fractures are potentially unstable but more importantly they involve comminuted articular injuries that require restoration to prevent arthritis.

ACUTE MANAGEMENT

- For distal ulnar shaft fractures that are displaced less than 50% and angulated less than 15°, the treatment consists of well-fitted forearm immobilization that does not impede wrist or elbow motion.[1] If displaced or angulated more than the aforementioned cutoffs, then closed reduction (CR) should be attempted. If successfully reduced, then patient is placed into a long arm cast for 6 weeks. If CR fails, then patient should be managed surgically with open reduction internal fixation (ORIF) using a 3.5 limited contact dynamic compression plate.

- For distal ulna fractures associated with DR fractures, the acute management is typically dictated by the DR fracture component of the injury, often with reduction, splinting, and referral to a hand surgeon's office for definitive treatment.[6]

DEFINITIVE TREATMENT

- **Stable, extra-articular ulnar styloid fractures**
  - Managed nonoperatively with a removable wrist splint for comfort, return to activity as tolerated, and early forearm rotation exercises[1,3]
- **Unstable, intra-articular ulnar styloid fractures**
  - Treated operatively with anatomic ORIF of the articular fracture fragments
- **Unstable, extra-articular ulnar styloid fractures**
  - Managed operatively with K wires, tension band wiring (TBW), screws, mini fragment plates, or suture anchors
  - Indicated for isolated displaced fractures through the base associated with DRUJ instability or persistent DRUJ instability after satisfactory reduction of a DR fracture
  - Operative technique
    - ◆ A subcutaneous border to the ulna approach is utilized, being careful to protect the dorsal sensory branch of the ulnar nerve.
    - ◆ If using TBW, then 1 to 2 K wires are placed obliquely through the tip of the styloid. A 22- or 24-gauge tension band is wrapped in a figure-of-eight manner around the wire tip and then passed through a drill hole in the ulnar neck (Figure 28.5).
    - ◆ If using a suture anchor construct, then a bone anchor is placed in the fracture site into the ulnar neck. Next the sutures are either passed through the ulnar styloid fragment if large enough or passed around a small fragment. Then, similar to TBW, the sutures are crossed over the subcutaneous border of the ulna and one end is passed through a transverse bone tunnel.
    - ◆ Alternatively, a 2.0-mm ulnar pin plate can be applied over a percutaneous K wire with two proximal screws to rigidly fix unstable styloid base fractures.

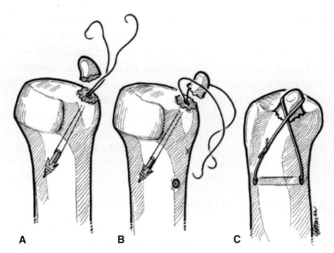

FIGURE 28.5 Suture anchor and tension band fixation techniques. Green's DRUJ instability chapter. A, Insertion of suture anchor at fracture site on distal ulna. B, Capturing the ulnar styloid fragment with sutures. C, Securing the ulnar styloid fragment with sutures passed through a bone tunnel in figure of 8 fashion. Reprinted from Green DP, Wolfe SW. *Green's Operative Hand Surgery*. 6th ed. Philadelphia, PA, Churchill Livingstone, 2011. Copyright © 2011 Elsevier. With permission.

- **Late management[3]**
  - Although usually asymptomatic, ulnar styloid nonunion can be effectively managed with fragment excision. If the removed fragment is large enough to render the TFCC unstable, then the peripheral TFCC can be repaired to the remaining ulna.
  - If the patient develops symptomatic DRUJ arthritis, then surgical options include partial ulnar resection, Sauve-Kapandji, Darrach, or ulnar head prosthetic replacement.
  - If the patient develops chronic DRUJ instability caused by a nonfunctional TFCC, then a ligament reconstruction procedure is indicated.
- **Postoperative protocol[3]**
  - Place in posterior long arm splint with forearm in 45° of supination or pronation based on stability.
  - At 2 weeks post-op, sutures will be removed and patient is transitioned to an above-elbow cast for another 2 weeks. Then patient is converted to below-elbow cast for another 2 weeks, for a total of 6 weeks of immobilization.

- At 6 weeks post-op, patient is transitioned to a removable short arm splint for another 4 weeks while beginning hand therapy to improve ROM.
- Activity restrictions are discontinued once there is an evidence of clinical union, eg, no tenderness to palpation at the fracture site.

MANAGEMENT ALGORITHM[3]

Please refer to Figure 28.4.

COMPLICATIONS

- Potential complications of unstable extra-articular ulnar styloid fractures include chronic DRUJ instability, painful loss of supination, and late arthritis.
- Possible complications of potentially unstable, intra-articular ulnar styloid fractures include DRUJ instability and accelerated arthritis.
- Complications of any surgical intervention include nonunion,[8] hardware failure, hardware prominence, and damage to surrounding tendons and neurovascular structures.

SUGGESTED READINGS

Adams BD. Distal radioulnar joint instability. In: Green DP, Wolfe SW, eds. *Green's Operative Hand Surgery.* Philadelphia, PA: Elsevier/Churchill Livingston; 2011.

Wolfe SW. Distal radius fractures. In: Green DP, Wolfe SW eds. *Green's Operative Hand Surgery.* Philadelphia, PA: Elsevier/Churchill Livingston; 2011.

REFERENCES

1. Calfee RP, Berger R, Beredjiklian PK, et al. Fractures and dislocations: wrist. In: Hammert WC, Calfee RP, Bozentka DJ, Boyer MI, eds. *ASSH Manual of Hand Surgery.* Philadelphia, PA: Lippincott Williams & Wilkins; 2010.
2. Chung KC, Spilson SV: The frequency and epidemiology of hand and forearm fractures in the United States. *J Hand Surg Am.* 2001;26:908-915.
3. Wolfe SW. Distal radius fractures. In: Green DP, Wolfe SW, eds. *Green's Operative Hand Surgery.* Philadelphia, PA: Elsevier/Churchill Livingston; 2011.
4. Miyamura S, Shigi A, Kraisarin J, et al. Impact of distal ulna fracture malunion on distal radioulnar joint instability: a biomechanical study of the distal interosseous membrane using a cadaver model. *J Hand Surg Am.* 2017;42:185-191.

5. Daneshvar P, Chan R, MacDermid J, Grewal R. The effects of ulnar styloid fractures on patients sustaining distal radius fracture. *J Hand Surg Am*. 2014;39(10):1915-1920.

6. Fyrkman G. Fracture of the distal radius including sequelae—shoulder-hand-finger syndrome, disturbance in the distal radioulnar joint and impairment of nerve function. A Clinical and experimental study. *Acta Orthop Scand*. 1967;108:3.

7. Adams, BD. Distal radioulnar joint instability. In: Green DP, Wolfe SW (eds). *Green's Operative Hand Surgery*. Philadelphia, PA: Elsevier/Churchill Livingston; 2011.

8. Hauck RM, Skahen J III, Palmer AK. Classification and treatment of ulnar styloid nonunion. *J Hand Surg Am*. 1996.21:418-422.

29 Distal Radioulnar Joint Injuries

Adam S. Martin and Hisham M. Awan

INTRODUCTION

- The distal radioulnar joint (DRUJ) consists of the concave, cartilage-covered sigmoid notch of the distal radius (DR) and the convex distal ulnar head. The joint has very little inherent stability from the bony architecture, thus the majority of the restraint is from the surrounding soft tissues, in particular the triangular fibrocartilage complex (TFCC). During normal motion, forearm pronation results in dorsal translation of the ulnar head, whereas supination results in volar translation. Given the reliance on soft tissues, DRUJ instability is a relatively common problem. A wide variety of DRUJ injuries and disorders exist (Table 29.1), but this chapter will focus on TFCC tears, DRUJ dislocations, and DRUJ instability.

- **Mechanism of injury**—Injury to the DRUJ is commonly traumatic from a fall on an outstretched hand. Acute, isolated dorsal and volar DRUJ dislocations are because of a fall that results in wrist extension/hyperpronation and supination, respectively. The most common cause of DRUJ instability is from inaccurate reduction of a DR fracture. Other sources of DRUJ instability are unstable ulnar styloid and Galeazzi fractures.

- **Anatomy**—The ulnar head articulates with the sigmoid notch of the radius to form the DRUJ. There is some degree of rotational and sliding motion of the DRUJ given the articular cartilage and radius of curvature mismatch between the ulnar head and sigmoid notch (Figure 29.1).

  - Given that there is little bony stability of the DRUJ, the TFCC is the key stabilizer of the DRUJ. The TFCC is composed of the palmar and dorsal radioulnar ligaments (RULs), articular disk, meniscal homologue, and extensor carpi ulnaris (ECU) subsheath (Figure 29.2).

    - The articular disk, made of fibrocartilage, originates from the lunate fossa of the DR and forms two distinct bundles ulnarly, one that

TABLE 29.1 **Injuries and Disorders of the DRUJ Intra-articular Fractures Without Instability**

Sigmoid notch (intra-articular distal radial fractures)
Ulnar head (including chondral fractures)
Ulnar styloid
TFCC injuries without instability
    Traumatic (some of Palmer Type 1 injuries will be associated with dislocation/instability)
    Degenerative (ulnocarpal impaction syndrome [Palmer Type 2 injuries])
        Idiopathic positive ulnar variance
        Acquired positive ulnar variance
Dislocations and instability
    Acute
        Dorsal with or without fracture
        Palmar with or without fracture
        Multidirectional with or without fracture
        Proximal-distal instability (Essex-Lopresti)
    Chronic (with or without arthritic changes)
        Dorsal with or without malunion or nonunion
        Palmar with or without malunion or nonunion
        Multidirectional with or without malunion or nonunion
        Proximal/distal instability
    Chronic instability after DRUJ resectional arthroplasty
Arthritis (eg, osteo-, posttraumatic, or rheumatoid arthritis, gout, pseudogout)
Other disorders
    Congenital (Madelung deformity)
    Unstable extensor carpi ulnaris tendon
    Fixed forearm rotational contracture
    Tumor (hereditary multiple exostosis involvement of DRUJ)

DRUJ, distal radioulnar joint; TFCC, triangular fibrocartilage complex.

Reprinted with permission from Chidgey LK. The distal radioulnar joint: problems and solutions. *J Am Acad Orthop Surg.* 1995;3(2):95-109.

inserts on the ulnar styloid and the other one on the fovea. The insertion sites are separated by a loose vascular connective tissue called ligamentum subcruentum. The peripheral 20% of the disk is well vascularized and therefore is amenable to healing. Furthermore, vascularity decreases as you move from ulnar to radial.

- The ulnotriquetral and ulnolunate ligaments are technically not part of the TFCC, but nonetheless function as additional stabilizers of the DRUJ.

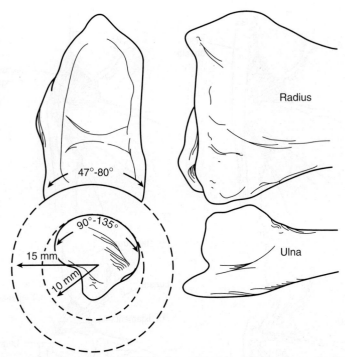

FIGURE 29.1 Distal radioulnar joint bony anatomy. Reprinted with permission from Chidgey LK. The distal radioulnar joint: problems and solutions. *J Am Acad Orthop Surg*. 1995;3(2):95-109.

EVALUATION

- **Presentation**—Patient presentation is highly variable, but patients will likely complain of ulnar-sided wrist pain. They may recall a specific traumatic event that coincides with the onset of pain or report increased pain with certain activities, ie, gripping, twisting doorknobs, open lids on jars. Pain is activity related and may be associated with mechanical symptoms, such as clicking or catching. If the injury is chronic, then patients may complain of loss of wrist range of motion (ROM) or a sense of instability around the wrist.

- **Physical examination**—On examination, one should have a systematic approach, always compare with the contralateral wrist, and include inspection, palpation, ROM, and neurovascular status. Inspection may reveal swelling or deformity. Palpation should include the DR

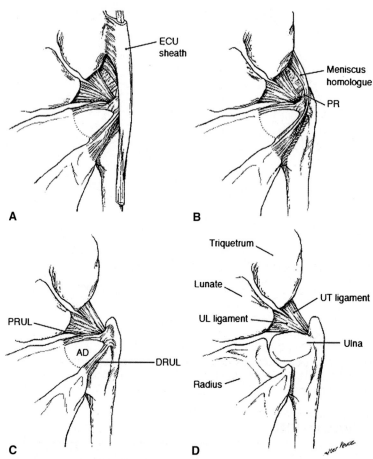

FIGURE 29.2 Triangular fibrocartilage complex anatomy. A, dorsal view of TFCC, B, TFCC with ECU subsheath removed, C, TFCC with meniscal homologue removed, D, TFCC removed. ECU, extensor carpi ulnaris; PR, prestyloid recess; PRUL, palmar radioulnar ligament; AD, articular disc; UT, ulnotriquetral ligament; UL, ulnolunate ligament. Reprinted with permission from Chidgey LK. The distal radioulnar joint: problems and solutions. *J Am Acad Orthop Surg*. 1995;3(2):95-109.

and ulna, specifically the ulnar styloid and fovea. Foveal tenderness, suggestive of TFCC tears, can be elicited by palpation in the soft spot ulnarly between the ECU and flexor carpi ulnaris (FCU) tendons. The ECU synergy test may help rule out ECU tendinitis and is performed by having the patient fully extend all fingers, the examiner then grasps the

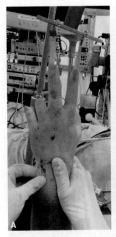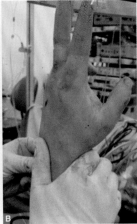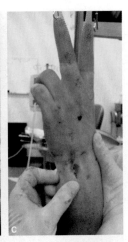

FIGURE 29.3 A–C, Shuck test for distal radioulnar joint instability. Reprinted with permission from Wiesel SW. *Operative Techniques in Orthopaedic Surgery.* 1st ed. Philadelphia, PA: Wolters Kluwer; 2010.

patient's thumb and middle finger and the patient radially abducts the thumb against resistance. The test is positive if this maneuver recreates the dorsal/ulnar wrist pain. The DRUJ should be assessed for instability, crepitus, and pain. Patients may also show decreased grip strength.

- Perform the DRUJ shuck test (Figure 29.3) in neutral and full prona-tion/supination and compare with contralateral wrist. "Shuck" the joint by translating the ulna volarly and dorsally while stabilizing the DR. This maneuver is crucial to determining DRUJ instability.
  - There should be an equivalent amount of motion in neutral to contralateral wrist and firm endpoints at full supination and pronation. In general, DRUJ is more stable in supination.
- **Imaging**—Radiographic imaging should consist of a neutral rotation posteroanterior (PA) and true lateral views of the wrist. An acceptable PA view is evident when the cortical outline of the concavity of the ECU groove is radial to the long axis of the ulnar styloid (Figure 29.4). This view is obtained with the shoulder abducted 90°, the elbow flexed 90°, the forearm in neutral rotation, and the wrist in neutral. Likewise, an acceptable lateral view is obtained when the volar cortex of the pisiform is between the volar cortices of the scaphoid and capitate, also known as the "SPC lateral."

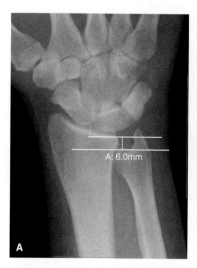
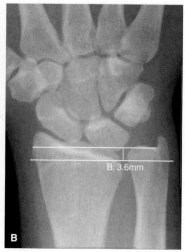

A: 6.0mm

B: 3.6mm

A

B

FIGURE 29.4 A,B, Proper posteroanterior and lateral radiographs of wrist and ulnar variance measurement. Reprinted with permission from Bridgeforth GM. *Lippincott's Primary Care Musculoskeletal Radiology*. Philadelphia: Lippincott Williams & Wilkins; 2010.

- PA radiographs may show widening of the DRUJ, whereas lateral radiographs may show dorsal displacement of the ulnar head (Figure 29.5).
- Several methods exist for measuring ulnar variance (UV); however, the most commonly used is the method of perpendiculars. A transverse line is drawn through the volar sclerotic rim of the DR lunate fossa perpendicular to its long axis; the distance the ulnar head extends distal or proximal to this line is the UV.
  - Average UV is approximately 1 mm, but this changes with motion. Pronation and power grip increase UV, ie, make UV more positive. Supination decreases the UV, ie, makes it more negative.
  - With neutral UV, the radius and ulnar receive 80% and 20% of the load, respectively. A 2.5-mm increase in UV will increase load across the ulnocarpal joint approximately from 20% to 40%.
- Computed tomography (CT) is the imaging modality of choice for evaluating DRUJ instability. The patient is positioned so that the CT scan will capture both wrists to allow direct comparison, from which any gross dislocation will be readily apparent. For more occult subluxation, several methods have been described. The congruent

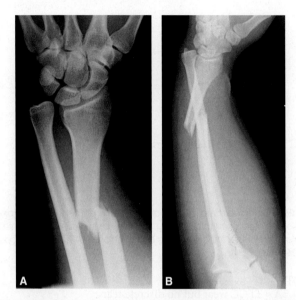

FIGURE 29.5 A,B, Distal radioulnar joint injury on posteroanterior and lateral radiographs. Reprinted with permission from Hunt TR, Wiesel SW. *Operative Techniques in Hand, Wrist, and Forearm Surgery.* 2nd ed. Philadelphia, PA: Lippincott Williams & Wilkins; 2010.

arc method (Figure 29.6) shows that the DRUJ is normal if the arc of the sigmoid notch is congruent with the arc of the ulnar head.
- MRI can be useful to evaluate TFCC tears.
- **Differential diagnosis**
  - DRUJ instability
  - TFCC tear
  - Ulnar styloid/hook of hamate fracture
  - Ulnocarpal impaction
  - ECU/FCU tendinitis
- **Classification**—DRUJ dislocations are classified as volar or dorsal. DRUJ instability is divided into acute and chronic. The Palmer classification is used for TFCC tears and stratifies lesions into traumatic and degenerative tears.
  - Type 1—traumatic (subdivided by location; Figure 29.7)
    - 1A—central tears
    - 1B—peripheral tears (ulnar insertion)
    - 1C—volar tears (near ulnocarpal ligaments)
    - 1D—radial tears (sigmoid notch)

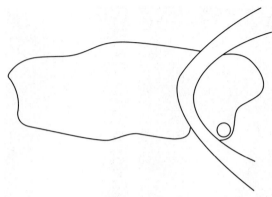

FIGURE 29.6 Congruent arc method of determining distal radioulnar joint subluxation on computed tomography. Reprinted with permission from Chidgey LK. The distal radioulnar joint: problems and solutions. *J Am Acad Orthop Surg.* 1995;3(2):95-109.

- Type 2—degenerative
  - 2A—TFCC wear but no discrete tear
  - 2B—2A + lunate and/or ulnar head chondromalacia
  - 2C—2B + TFCC perforation
  - 2D—2C + ulnocarpal or DRUJ arthritis

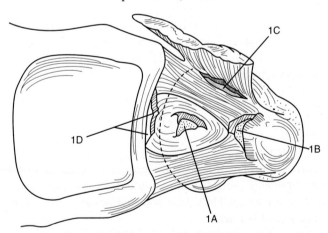

FIGURE 29.7 A to D, Palmer classification for triangular fibrocartilage complex tear subtypes. Reprinted with permission from Calfee RP, Berger R, Beredjiklian PK, et al. Fractures and dislocations: wrist. In: Hammert WC, Calfee RP, Bozentka DJ, et al., eds. *ASSH Manual of Hand Surgery.* 1st ed. Philadelphia, PA: Lippincott Williams & Wilkins; 2010.

DEFINITIVE TREATMENT

- **Stable, traumatic (Type 1) TFCC injuries**
  - Managed nonoperatively initially. Above-elbow splinting with forearm in 45° of supination is performed with repeat physical examination in 6 weeks.
    - If symptoms resolve, then continue nonoperative management with gradual return to full activities
    - If symptoms persist, then operative intervention may be indicated depending on the patient's age, activity level, and goals of care.
      - Type 1A—arthroscopic debridement as central portion is avascular and will not heal.
      - Types 1B to D—arthroscopic versus open repair depending on tear size, with larger tear usually requiring open procedures. Note: Type 1D (radial-sided) tears have poor vascularity, and therefore, debridement should be considered if small.
      - Open approach to TFCC repair is achieved dorsally overlying the fifth extensor compartment (Figure 29.8). A capsular flap is made, and the TFCC is repaired with small bone tunnels or bone anchors.
    - Ulnar positive patients should have their UV treated simultaneously with the TFCC injury. Studies have demonstrated worse outcomes if UV was not improved. Joint leveling procedures include open limited distal ulnar head resection (wafer procedure), arthroscopic wafer procedure, and open diaphyseal shortening.
- **Unstable, traumatic (Type 1) TFCC injuries**
  - Treated nonoperatively with above-elbow casting with forearm in full supination for 6 weeks provided that concentric reduction is obtained and maintained. The initial cast is followed by another 6 weeks in a long arm splint. Patients should be counseled that the need for eventual operative intervention if symptoms persist is higher than if no instability was present.
  - Operative treatment is the same as mentioned earlier for stable traumatic injuries. The most common form to result in instability is an avulsion of the ulnar attachment (Type 1B). Concomitant ulnar positivity should be addressed as stated earlier.
- **Degenerative (Type 2) TFCC injuries**
  - Managed conservatively with symptomatic control until patient elects to proceed with operative intervention

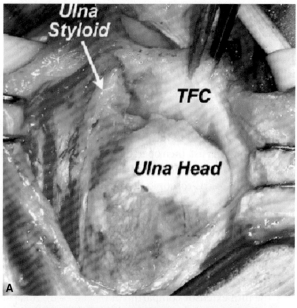

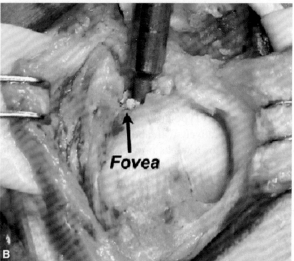

FIGURE 29.8 Dorsal exposure for open triangular fibrocartilage complex repair. A, dorsal exposure of the TFF insertion at ulnar fovea, B, drilling pilot hole at ulnar fovea for later suture anchor placement, C, placement of suture anchor D, passage of suture through the TFCC for repair. Reprinted with permission from Calfee RP, Berger R, Beredjiklian PK, et al. Fractures and dislocations: wrist. In: Hammert WC, Calfee RP, Bozentka DJ, et al., eds. *ASSH Manual of Hand Surgery*. 1st ed. Philadelphia, PA: Lippincott Williams & Wilkins; 2010.

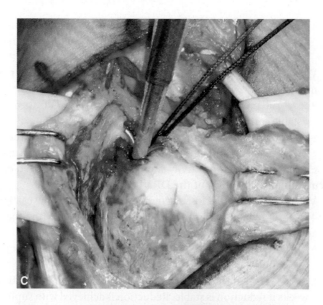

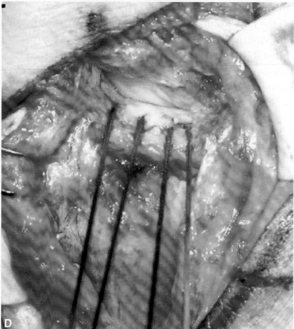

FIGURE 29.8 *(continued)*

- Symptomatic management includes activity modification, long arm splint/compressive wraps, nonsteroidal anti-inflammatory drugs (NSAIDs), and steroid injections.
- Wrist arthroscopy is the procedure of choice once conservative management is unable to provide adequate pain control.
  - Debridement is recommended for central TFCC tears and unstable cartilage lesions.
  - Any other concomitant pathology can be addressed at the same time, ie, removal of loose bodies, debridement/repair of ligaments.
- Concomitant ulnar positivity should be addressed as stated earlier.
- **Acute ulnar dislocation of the DRUJ**
  - Volar—Treated with closed reduction and above-elbow casting for 4 weeks if reduction is stable. Reduction is achieved with pronation and dorsally directed pressure on ulnar head.
    - If DRUJ is unstable, then the TFCC can be repaired as stated previously.
  - Dorsal—Treated with closed reduction and above-elbow casting for 4 weeks if reduction is stable. Reduction is achieved with supination with volarly directed pressure on ulnar head.
    - If the DRUJ is unstable, then the TFCC can be repaired as stated previously.
- **DRUJ instability**
  - Acute—most commonly occurs in association with DR fractures. Any loss of radial height greater than 5 to 7 mm results in tearing of the RULs.
    - No additional treatment is needed if DRUJ is stable after fixation of DR fracture.
      - If unstable after DR fixation, then two operative options exist: open TFCC repair or percutaneous pinning across the radius and ulna.
    - If DRUJ instability is associated with an ulnar styloid base fracture, then open reduction internal fixation of the fracture will stabilize the joint (see chapter 28 for details).
  - Chronic—Secondary to trauma, most often malunited DR fractures that heal in a shortened position. Management varies based on associated pathology, patient activity levels, and presence or absence of arthritis.
    - Nonoperative treatment is rarely beneficial unless the patient is low demand and willing to have limited forearm motion. Nevertheless, the treatment consists of a course of elbow splinting/casting and NSAIDs.

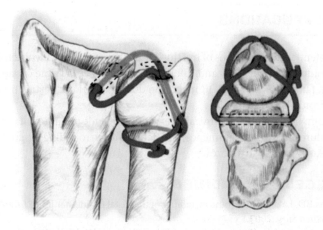

FIGURE 29.9 Example of radioulnar ligament reconstruction. Reprinted from Green DP, Wolfe SW. *Green's Operative Hand Surgery*. 6th ed. Philadelphia, PA, Churchill Livingstone, 2011. Copyright © 2011 Elsevier. With permission.

- ◆ If no arthritis, then the RULs are repaired when able and augmented with tendon graft (Figure 29.9). In conjunction with repair, any bony abnormalities need to be addressed, such as osteotomies for DR malunions, sigmoid notch osteotomies for loss of notch concavity, and/or ulnar shortening. There are various techniques for RUL reconstruction. Graft options include palmaris longus, flexor carpi radialis (FCR), strip of FCU, plantaris, or a toe extensor.
- ◆ If the patient develops symptomatic DRUJ arthritis, then surgical options include partial ulnar resection, Sauve-Kapandji, Darrach, or ulnar head prosthetic replacement.
- ■ **Postoperative protocol**
  - • The details of postoperative management will vary depending on actual procedures performed, given the diversity of DRUJ injuries. Nevertheless, in general, the patient is placed into a long arm splint with forearm in 45° of supination or pronation based on stability.
  - • At first, postoperative visit sutures are removed and patient is put in an above-elbow cast for 4 weeks after surgery. Then patient is converted to below-elbow cast for another 2 weeks.
  - • At 6 weeks post-op, the patient is transitioned to a removable short arm splint for another 4 weeks while beginning hand therapy to improve ROM. Activity restrictions are lifted once painless ROM is achieved.

COMPLICATIONS

- Potential complications of treating DRUJ injuries mostly involve failure to address all the bony and soft tissue pathology at the time of surgery, eg, failure to correct a DR malunion during a RUL reconstruction for chronic DRUJ instability.
- Complications of any surgical intervention include nonunion, hardware failure, hardware prominence, and damage to surrounding tendons and neurovascular structures.

SUGGESTED READINGS

Adams BD, Lawler E. Chronic instability of the distal radioulnar joint. *J Am Acad Orthop Surg.* 2007;15:571-575.

Adams BD. Distal radioulnar joint instability. In: Green DP, Wolfe SW, eds. *Green's Operative Hand Surgery.* Philadelphia, PA: Elsevier/Churchill Livingston; 2011.

Calfee RP, Berger R, Beredjiklian PK, et al. Fractures and dislocations: wrist. In: Hammert WC, Calfee RP, Bozentka DJ, et al, eds. *ASSH Manual of Hand Surgery.* Philadelphia, PA: Lippincott Williams & Wilkins; 2010.

Chidgey LK. The distal radioulnar joint: problems and solutions. *J Am Acad Orthop Surg.* 1995;3:95-109.

Daneshvar P, Willing R, Pahura M, Grewal R, King GJ. Osseous anatomy of the distal radioulnar joint: an assessment using 3-dimensional modeling and clinical implications. *J Hand Surg Am.* 2016;41(11):1071-1079.

Feldon P, Terrono AL, Belsky MR. Wafer distal ulna resection for triangular fibrocartilage tears and/or ulna impaction syndrome. *J Hand Surg Am.* 1992;17:731-737.

Henry MK. Management of acute triangular fibrocartilage complex injury of the wrist. *J Am Acad Orthop Surg.* 2008;16:320-329.

Melone CP Jr, Nathan R. Traumatic disruption of the triangular fibrocartilage complex: pathoanatomy. *Clin Orthop Relat Res.* 1992;275:65-73.

Millard GM, Budoff JE, Paravic V, Noble PC. Functional bracing for distal radioulnar joint instability. *J Hand Surg Am.* 2002;27:972-977.

Ruland RT, Hogan CJ. The ECU synergy test: an aid to diagnose ECU tendonitis. *J Hand Surg.* 2008;33A:1777-1782.

Zimmerman RM, Kim JM, Jupiter JB. Arthritis of the distal radioulnar joint: from Darrach to total joint arthroplasty. *J Am Acad Orthop Surg.* 2012;20:623-632.

30 Galeazzi Fractures

Maharsh K. Patel and Joseph J. King

INTRODUCTION

- Pathoanatomy
  - Galeazzi fractures are defined as a fracture of the distal one-third radial shaft and associated distal radioulnar joint (DRUJ) injury.
    - Variants—fractures anywhere along the radius or fractures of both the radius and ulna with DRUJ disruption
  - DRUJ is the distal articulation of the ulna within the sigmoid notch on the ulnar border of the distal radius.
    - Primarily stabilized by triangular fibrocartilage complex (TFCC)
      * Also has volar and dorsal distal radioulnar ligaments
    - DRUJ is most stable in supination.
  - Incidence of DRUJ instability
    - Unstable in 55% when radius fracture is <7.5 cm from articular surface
    - Unstable in 6% when radius fracture is >7.5 cm from articular surface
  - Major deforming forces
    - Pronator quadratus—insertion pronates the distal radius with proximal and volar displacement
    - Brachioradialis—causes shortening
    - Thumb extensors and abductors—result in shortening and re-laxation of the radial collateral ligament
- Mechanism of injury
  - Indirect trauma such as a fall onto an outstretched hand with the forearm in pronation (Figure 30.1)
    - Forceful axial loading with torsion of forearm
  - Direct trauma to the forearm and/or wrist
    - Motor vehicle accidents, blunt trauma, etc.

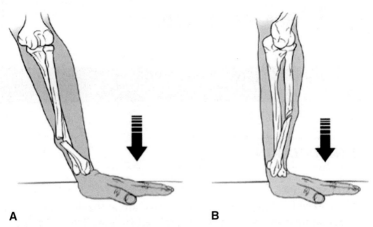

A **B**

FIGURE 30.1 Mechanism of injury. A, a type I fracture (apex volar) that occurs with axial loading with the forearm in supination. B, a type II fracture (apex dorsal) that occurs with axial loading with the forearm in pronation. From Atesok KI, Jupiter JB, Weiss APC. Galeazzi fracture. *J Am Acad Orthop Surg.* 2011;19(10):623-633.

- Epidemiology
  - Incidence
    - ≤3% of all forearm fractures in children
    - ≤7% of all forearm fractures in adults

EVALUATION

- History
  - Symptoms include local pain, swelling, deformity, decreased wrist range of motion after associated history of forearm trauma.
- Physical examination—see Figure 30.2
  - Tenderness and swelling of the distal forearm
  - Limited and painful wrist motion and forearm pronation/supination
  - Prominent distal ulna
  - DRUJ stress causes wrist or forearm pain.
  - Neurovascular examination; however, neurovascular injury is rare
- Imaging—see Figure 30.3
  - Definitive diagnosis typically made with plain radiographs
    - Anteroposterior (AP)/lateral views of the forearm, wrist, and elbow

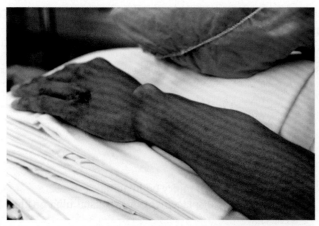

FIGURE 30.2 Clinical picture of Galeazzi fracture with radial deformity and a prominent distal radioulnar joint. Courtesy of Michelle Lin, MD.

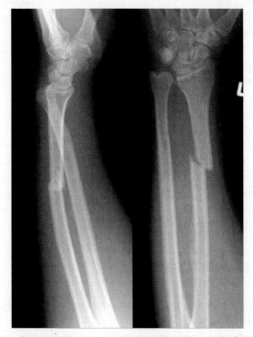

FIGURE 30.3 Radiographs (anteroposterior and lateral views) of Galeazzi fracture (type II). Case courtesy of Radswiki, Radiopaedia.org, rID: 12221.

TABLE 30.1 Orthopaedic Trauma Association (OTA) Classification of Radius and Ulna Fractures

22-A2.3	Simple fracture of radius with dislocation of DRUJ
22-A3.3	Simple fracture of radius and ulna (distal zone radius) with dislocation of DRUJ
22-B2.3	Wedge fracture of radius with dislocation of DRUJ
22-B3.3	Wedge fracture of radius and ulna with dislocation of DRUJ

Abbreviation: DRUJ, distal radioulnar joint.

- Signs of possible DRUJ injury on imaging
  - Dorsal or volar displacement of the distal ulna on the lateral wrist view
  - Widening or incongruity of DRUJ on AP view
  - Ulnar styloid fracture at the base
  - Radial shortening ≥5 mm
  - DRUJ asymmetry compared to contralateral radiographs
- Axial CT wrist recommended for DRUJ assessment when evaluation is difficult on plain radiographs
- It is critical to not miss DRUJ injury with a combination of meticulous assessment of imaging and physical examination.
- Classification
  - OTA classification of radius/ulna (Table 30.1)
  - Fracture classification based on displacement of distal fragment
    - Type I (apex volar)—dorsal displacement of distal fragment of radius with anterior (volar) dislocation of distal ulna
      * Typically occurs due to axial loading with forearm in supination.
    - Type II (apex dorsal)—volar displacement of distal fragment of radius with posterior (dorsal) dislocation of distal ulna
      * Typically occurs due to axial loading with forearm in pronation.

ACUTE MANAGEMENT

- Evaluation for open fracture, neurovascular injury, and any other associated injuries
- Closed reduction and long arm splinting with forearm in supination

DEFINITIVE TREATMENT

- Nonoperative treatment
  - Closed reduction with forearm in supination and long arm, above elbow casting preferred management for children with good outcomes reported.
  - Closed reduction and casting not recommended as definitive treatment in adults due to significant fracture and DRUJ instability. Poor outcome rates of nonoperative treatment in adults have been reported as high as 80%.
- Operative management
  - Open reduction with internal fixation (ORIF) of radius and stabilization of the DRUJ are recommended in adults.
    - Anatomic reduction of radius and DRUJ is required.
  - Surgical treatment is rarely needed in children.
- Surgical indications
  - Galeazzi fracture dislocation in adults (standard of care)
  - Failure to obtain an adequate closed reduction of the radius fracture and/or DRUJ dislocation in children
- Treatment algorithm
  - See management algorithm flowchart in Figure 30.4.
- Surgical approach
  - Operative technique for radius ORIF
    - Volar approach to radius (approach of Henry)
      - Interval between flexor carpi radialis and brachioradialis
    - Anatomic reduction and compression plate fixation
      - Typically 3.5 mm dynamic compression plate
      - Lag screw across the fracture is preferred if possible.
    - Radial bow must be restored.
    - In children, if surgery is needed then can perform ORIF with plate or flexible nails for radial fixation
  - Operative technique for DRUJ reduction
    - If DRUJ stable after ORIF of radius, immobilize in supination for 6 weeks
    - If DRUJ reducible but unstable after ORIF of radius, cross-pin ulna to radius and remove pins after 4 to 6 weeks
      - May also consider TFCC exploration and repair through dorsal approach

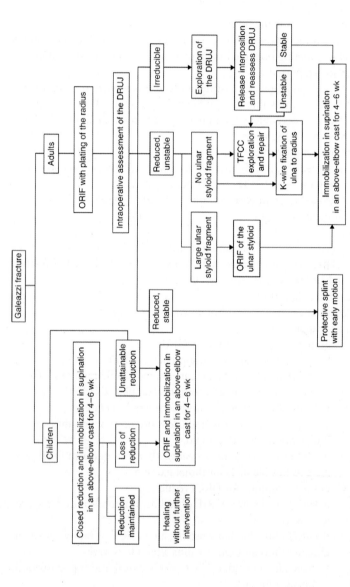

FIGURE 30.4 Management algorithm. ORIF, open reduction with internal fixation; DRUJ, distal radioulnar joint; TFCC, triangular fibrocartilage complex. From Atesok KI, Jupiter JB, Weiss APC. Galeazzi fracture. *J Am Acad Orthop Surg.* 2011;19(10):623-633.

- ◆ If DRUJ reduction is blocked, open reduction is needed (rare).
  - ＊ Most commonly caused by interposition of extensor carpi ulnaris tendon
- ◆ If a large ulnar styloid fragment exists, consider styloid ORIF and immobilize in supination if DRUJ is unstable.
- ■ Potential complications
  - ● Compartment syndrome
    - ◆ Assess volar, dorsal, and mobile wad compartments.
    - ◆ Treat with emergent fasciotomy.
  - ● Neurovascular injury
    - ◆ Usually iatrogenic
    - ◆ Superficial radial nerve at risk with volar approach of Henry
    - ◆ Posterior interosseous nerve at risk with proximal radius approach
    - ◆ If no recovery at 3 months, consider exploration
  - ● DRUJ subluxation
    - ◆ Due to gravity, pronator quadratus, or brachioradialis
    - ◆ May occur due to malreduction of radius fracture
  - ● Refracture after hardware removal
  - ● Nonunion
    - ◆ Uncommon with stable fixation
  - ● Malunion
    - ◆ Nonanatomic reduction of radius fracture or failure to restore radial bow may result in loss of pronation/supination and painful range of motion due to persistent DRUJ instability.
    - ◆ May require osteotomy or distal ulnar shortening in cases of ulnocarpal impaction.
    - ◆ Salvage options include Darrach procedure, Sauve-Kapandji procedure, hemiresection arthroplasty, and implant arthroplasty.
  - ● Radioulnar synostosis
    - ◆ Uncommon—3% to 9% incidence
    - ◆ Worst prognosis is distal synostosis.
    - ◆ Best prognosis is diaphyseal synostosis.
- ■ Postoperative care
  - ● If DRUJ is stable, early motion is recommended.
  - ● If DRUJ is unstable, immobilize forearm in supination for 4 to 6 weeks in long arm splint/cast.
  - ● Supination of forearm decreases rotational forces around the DRUJ.

SUGGESTED READINGS

Atesok KI, Jupiter JB, Weiss APC. Galeazzi fracture. *J Am Acad Orthop Surg.* 2011;19(10):623-633.

Egol KA, Koval KJ, Zuckerman JD. *Handbook of Fractures.* Philadelphia, PA: Lippincott Williams & Wilkins; 2010.

Makhni MC, Makhni EC, Swart EF, Day CS. *Radius and Ulna Shaft Fractures. Orthopedic Emergencies.* New York, NY: Springer International Publishing; 2017:177-179.

Tsismenakis T, Tornetta P. Galeazzi fractures: is DRUJ instability predicted by current guidelines? *Injury.* 2016;47(7):1472-1477.

Tendon Injuries

Section Editor: Craig Rodner

CHAPTER

31 Extensor Tendon Injuries

Mark Henry

INTRODUCTION

- Pathoanatomy
  - Extensor mechanism—multiple origins and multiple insertions
  - Extensor digitorum communis (EDC) and proprius tendons—extrinsic origins
  - Interossei and lumbricals—intrinsic origins
  - Insertions—direct at the base of the distal phalanx (P3) and the middle phalanx (P2) via sagittal bands at the base of the proximal phalanx (P1)
  - Juncturae tendinum transverse connections between EDCs at the metacarpal level.
- Mechanism of injury
  - Closed tensile failure rupture (base of P3, P2, sagittal bands)
  - Open sharp laceration (anywhere)
  - Segmental loss as part of industrial trauma involving adjacent structures
- Epidemiology
  - Active adults of all ages, both sexes, wide spectrum

EVALUATION

- History
  - Mechanism of injury—tensile overload versus sharp laceration versus complex trauma
  - Closed versus open
  - Specific object causing open injury

- Degree of contamination
- Patient demographics/risk factors (diabetes, vascular disease, smoking)
- Physical examination
  - Demonstration of tendon function/lack of function across injury zone (Figure 31.1)
  - Appearance of early central slip avulsion is subtle (flexible boutonniere), but key is hyperextension of distal interphalangeal (DIP) with attempted proximal interphalangeal (PIP) extension (Figure 31.2).
  - Active extension versus resistance from initially flexed PIP joint required to prove insertion at base of P2, simply maintaining extension not sufficient
  - Check for coronal subluxation at metacarpophalangeal joints—ruptured sagittal band
  - Proximal EDC laceration can be partially substituted by juncturae tendinum.
- Imaging
  - Distinguish tendon avulsion at base of P3 from shearing impaction fracture of DIP/PIP joint (Figure 31.3).
  - Not all fracture fragments at the dorsal base of P2 represent loss of central slip continuity (Figure 31.4)—requires physical examination.
- Classification (Table 31.1)

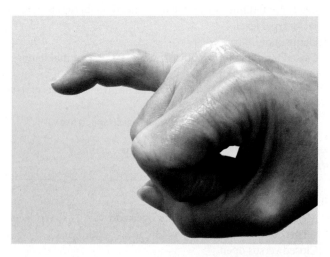

FIGURE 31.1 Terminal tendon avulsion leaves patient unable to actively extend distal interphalangeal joint.

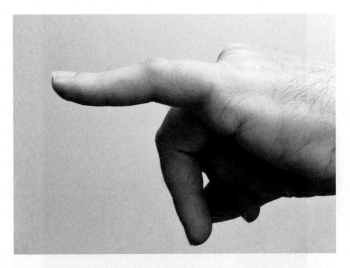

FIGURE 31.2 Early evaluation of a central slip avulsion is subtle, but the hallmark feature is the hyperextension posture of the distal interphalangeal joint while the patient attempts to extend the proximal interphalangeal (further tested by resisted extension from a flexed posture).

ACUTE MANAGEMENT

- Topically clean wound in ER
- Splint in extension of the involved joint.
- Stabilize any associated fractures.

DEFINITIVE TREATMENT

- Nonoperative treatment
  - Zone 1 closed rupture—splint continuously in full extension 8 weeks
  - Zone 3 closed rupture—splint continuously in full extension 6 weeks
  - Zone 5 sagittal band closed rupture—splint continuously in full extension 6 weeks
- Surgical indications
  - Open direct tendon lacerations
  - Late presenting sagittal band ruptures in a high-demand patient.
  - Attritional rupture with uncompensated functional deficit

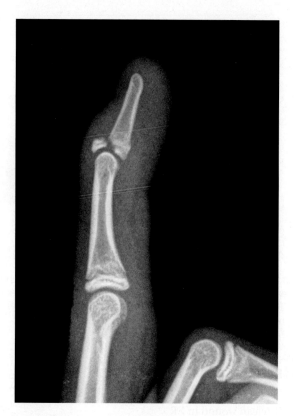

FIGURE 31.3 Shearing impaction fractures of the dorsal base of P3 demonstrate a larger dorsal fragment with the fracture plane perpendicular to the articular surface as opposed to traction avulsion fragments that are smaller with the fracture plane perpendicular to the line of pull of the extensor tendon.

- Contraindications
  - Medical comorbidity precluding safe surgery
  - Patient does not perceive functional deficit and is satisfied.
- Surgical approach
  - Debride irregular borders of trauma wound and any contaminants.
  - Extend trauma wound as needed longitudinally, not directly overlying tendon.
  - Approximate tendon edges with tacking sutures at radial and ulnar borders.

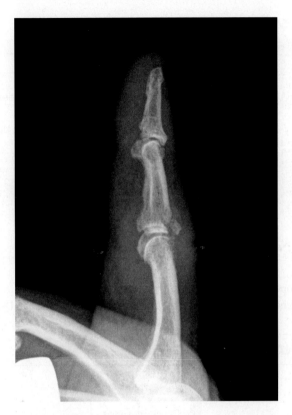

FIGURE 31.4 Dorsal base of P2 fragments does not necessarily indicate loss of continuity of the central slip.

- Perform core suture for longitudinal strength, slow absorbing monofilament.
- Anchor repair of central slip to base of P2 if central slip laceration (Figure 31.5)
- Late sagittal band ruptures and attritional ruptures reconstructed with tendon transfers
■ Potential complications
- Inadequate purchase of longitudinal tendon fibers by suture pattern
- Wound infection in contaminated open trauma cases (particularly with late presentation)
- Patient noncompliance with postoperative splinting—rupture

TABLE 31.1 **Extensor Tendon Zones of Injury**

Zone	Anatomic Level	Typical Injury
1	DIP joint	Closed rupture (mallet finger)
2	P2	Sharp laceration
3	PIP joint	Closed rupture with volar PIP dislocation
4	P1	Sharp laceration
5	MP joint	Closed sagittal band rupture (boxer's knuckle)
		Open sharp laceration
6	Metacarpal	Sharp laceration
7	Wrist	Sharp laceration
		Attritional rupture with long-standing tenosynovitis
8	Distal forearm—tendon	Sharp laceration
9	Proximal forearm—muscle	Sharp laceration

Abbreviations: DIP, distal interphalangeal; MP, metacarpophalangeal; PIP, proximal interphalangeal.

- Postoperative care
  - Rehabilitation according to zone after direct surgical repair (Table 31.2)

MANAGEMENT ALGORITHM

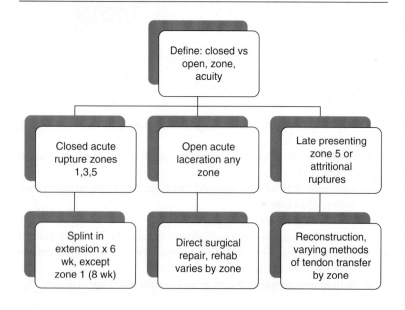

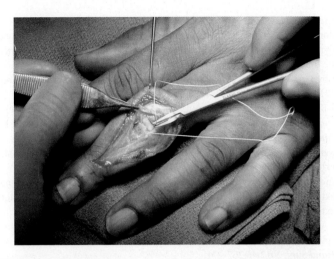

FIGURE 31.5 Central slip avulsions from the base of P2 are repaired with a suture anchor directly to bone.

TABLE 31.2 Rehabilitation by Zone after Direct Surgical Repair

Zone	Rehabilitation Following Direct Surgical Repair
1–2	Splint in continuous extension 8 wk
3–4	Daily sessions of short arc active PIP flexion to 30°, splint in full extension between sessions 6 wk; DIP blocking
5–6	Free daily active extension limited only by relative offset splint; composite extension night splint for greater comfort
7–9	Composite extension splint 4 wk, progressive ROM over next 2 wk

Abbreviations: DIP, distal interphalangeal; MP, metacarpophalangeal; ROM, range of motion.

Data from Hall B, Lee H, Page R, Rosenwax L, Lee AH. Comparing three post-operative treatment protocols for extensor tendon repair in zones V and VI of the hand. *Am J Occup Ther*. 2010;64:682-688.

SUGGESTED READINGS

Altobelli GG, Conneely S, Haufler C, Walsh M, Ruchelsman DE. Outcomes of digital zone IV and V and thumb TI to TIV extensor tendon repairs using a running interlocking horizontal mattress technique. *J Hand Surg Am*. 2013;38:1079-1083.

Bulstrode NW, Burr N, Pratt AL, Grobbelaar AO. Extensor tendon rehabilitation a prospective trial comparing three rehabilitation regimes. *J Hand Surg Br*. 2005;30:175-179.

Catalano LW, Gupta S, Ragland R, Glickel SZ, Johnson C, Barron OA. Closed treatment of nonrheumatoid extensor tendon dislocations at the metacarpophalangeal joint. *J Hand Surg Am*. 2006;31:242-245.

Chester DL, Beale S, Beveridge L, Nancarrow JD, Titley OG. A prospective, randomized trial comparing early active extension with passive extension using a dynamic splint in the rehabilitation of repaired extensor tendons. *J Hand Surg Br*. 2002;27:283-288.

Crosby CA, Wehbé MA. Early protected motion after extensor tendon repair. *J Hand Surg*. 1999;24:1061-1070.

Hall B, Lee H, Page R, Rosenwax L, Lee AH. Comparing three post-operative treatment protocols for extensor tendon repair in zones V and VI of the hand. *Am J Occup Ther*. 2010;64:682-688.

Howard RF, Ondrovic L, Greenwald DP. Biomechanical analysis of four-strand extensor tendon repair techniques. *J Hand Surg Am*. 1997;22:838-842.

Khandwala AR, Webb J, Harris SB, Foster AJ, Elliot D. A comparison of dynamic extension splinting and controlled active mobilization of complete divisions of extensor tendons in zones 5 and 6. *J Hand Surg Br*. 2000;25:140-146.

Kitis A, Ozcan RH, Bagdatli D, Buker N, Kara IG. Comparison of static and dynamic splinting regimens for extensor tendon repairs in zones V to VII. *J Plast Surg Hand Surg*. 2012;46:267-271.

Mowlavi A, Burns M, Brown RE. Dynamic versus static splinting of simple zone V and zone VI extensor tendon repairs: a prospective, randomized, controlled study. *Plast Reconstr Surg*. 2005;115:482-487.

32 Mallet Finger

Steven R. Niedermeier and Hisham M. Awan

INTRODUCTION

- Mallet finger is an injury to the terminal extensor mechanism at the level of the distal interphalangeal (DIP) joint. This can be caused by either tendon rupture in zone 1 or an avulsion fracture of the distal phalanx with a fragment of bone that remains attached to the tendon.
- There are two proposed mechanisms of injury.
  - **Traumatic impaction blow** (Figure 32.1)—the initial step involves an axial force to finger held in extension followed by either one of two steps:
    - ◆ Extreme passive DIP joint hyper*flexion*, which results most commonly in a tendinous mallet finger.
    - ◆ Extreme passive DIP joint hyper*extension*, which results most commonly in a bony mallet finger.
  - **Dorsal laceration**—less common; sharp or crushing laceration to the dorsal DIP joint
- Mallet fingers comprise approximately 9% of all tendinous/ligamentous lesions with an incidence estimated at 5.6% of all tendinous lesions in the hand. The literature does not show any gender difference; however, high-energy injuries are seen in younger, male patients and low-energy mechanisms are seen in the elderly.
- The ulnar three fingers are the most commonly affected digits, and tendinous injuries are more common than bony avulsion injuries.
- With the loss of the terminal extensor tendon insertion, the central slip receives all of the tension; the volar plate and transverse retinacular ligament attenuate; the lateral bands sublux dorsally; and the proximal interphalangeal (PIP) joint may be forced into extension in chronic injures. The inability to extend the DIP joint and the PIP joint extension is referred to as a swan neck deformity of the finger (Figure 32.2).

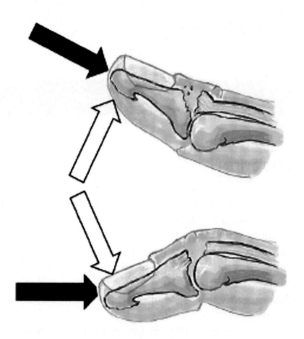

FIGURE 32.1 Mechanisms of injury for mallet finger.

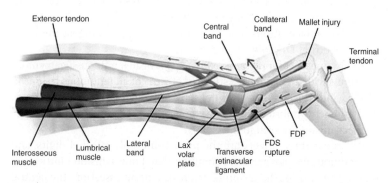

FIGURE 32.2 Mechanism of swan neck deformity in the setting of mallet finger. FDS, flexor digitorum superficialis; FDP, flexor digitorum profundis.

EVALUATION

- Patient's history usually includes mechanism of injury, and the patient will usually present in the acute phase.

- Patients will most commonly endorse painful and/or swollen DIP joint as the primary complaint. In addition, patients will complain of an inability to extend the DIP joint.
- On examination, the patient will have a painful and swollen DIP joint with the joint held in flexion (Figure 32.3). The patient will lack the ability to actively extend the tip of the finger.
  - It can often be difficult to note a DIP joint resting in flexion because of the amount of joint swelling. The examiner can passively (hyper)extend the DIP joint and ask the patient to maintain this position. Patients with a mallet finger will not be able to maintain extension of the fingertip.
- Plain radiographs can reveal a bony avulsion of the dorsal lip of the distal phalanx articular surface (Figure 32.4). If the injury is purely tendinous, the DIP joint will appear to rest in flexion without a bony avulsion (Figure 32.5).
- There are two classification systems that are used most commonly:
  - **Wehbe and Schneider**—describes injury severity (Table 32.1)
  - **Doyle**—describes injury pattern (Table 32.2)

ACUTE MANAGEMENT

- DIP joint splinting is the most common initial treatment for either tendinous or bony mallet fingers.

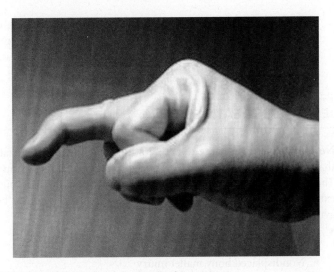

FIGURE 32.3 Clinic photograph of mallet finger injury.

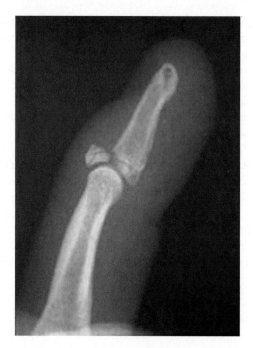

FIGURE 32.4 Lateral plain radiograph of a bony mallet finger injury.

- If there is an open injury, the patient should receive an up-to-date tetanus booster, antibiotics, and thorough irrigation, debridement, and exploration of the wound bed under local anesthesia upon presentation.

DEFINITIVE TREATMENT

- **Nonoperative**—There are many iterations of splint immobilization that are utilized for nonoperative management of mallet finger injuries. The primary goal, regardless of splint type, is to hold the DIP joint in extension to oppose the ruptured terminal extensor tendon or bony avulsion in place.
  - Indications
    - Acute (less than 12 weeks) soft tissue injury
    - Nondisplaced bony mallet injury

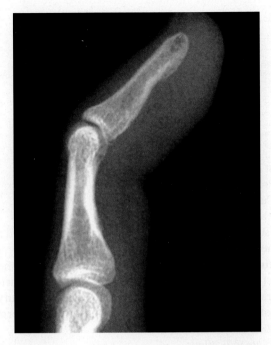

FIGURE 32.5 Lateral plain radiograph of a tendinous mallet finger injury.

- Full-time splinting is recommended for 6 to 8 weeks to avoid gap formation. The PIP joint should be left free to avoid unnecessary joint stiffness.
- This is followed by 2 to 6 weeks of nighttime splinting and splinting during vigorous activities. Progressive flexion exercises can begin at 6 weeks.

TABLE 32.1 Wehbe and Schneider Classification

Types	
1	No distal interphalangeal (DIP) joint subluxation
2	DIP joint subluxation
3	Epiphyseal and physeal injuries
Subtypes	
A	Less than 1/3 of the articular surface
B	1/3– 2/3 of the articular surface
C	More than 2/3 of the articular surface

TABLE 32.2 **Doyle Classification**

Type I	Closed injury with or without small dorsal avulsion fracture
Type II	Open injury (laceration)
Type III	Open injury (deep soft tissue abrasion involving skin and tendon substance)
Type IV	Mallet fracture
	Distal phalanx physeal injury (pediatrics)
	Fracture involving 20–50% of the articular surface
	Fracture involving greater than 50% of the articular surface

- Most commonly used splints include (Figure 32.6)
  - Prefabricated, molded polyethylene (Stack) splint
  - Custom, thermoplastic Stack splint
  - Abouna splint
- A residual extensor lag may persist at cessation of closed treatment (although it is typically less than 10°).
- ■ **Operative**—Most authors agree that the classification of the lesion is the most important indicating factor for surgical management. Patient demographics, history on presentation, time since the injury, and the degree of extension deficit are also commonly used to determine need for surgical intervention.
  - Absolute indications
    - Volar subluxation of the distal phalanx
    - Inability to tolerate splinting
  - Relative indications
    - More than 50% of the articular surface is involved.
    - More than a 2-mm articular gap
  - Contraindications
    - Simple, closed mallet finger injuries

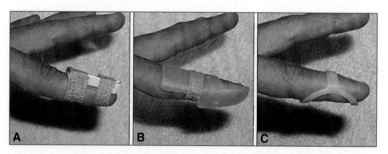

FIGURE 32.6 Different splint types. A, alumifoam extension splint. B, molded plastic stack splint. C, oval-8 finger splint.

- **Closed reduction percutaneous pinning (CRPP) versus open reduction internal fixation (ORIF)**
  - **CRPP**—extension block pinning consists of a Kirschner wire (K-wire) through the extensor tendon dorsally and proximal to the avulsion fragment into the middle phalanx. The DIP joint is then extended, and this K-wire acts as a lever to reduce the avulsion fragment into the distal phalanx. A transarticular K-wire is then placed in a retrograde fashion through the distal phalanx and into the middle phalanx to prevent DIP joint flexion and loss of reduction (Figure 32.7).
    - **Complications**—short-term stiffness, septic arthritis, improper fracture reduction, and posttraumatic osteoarthritis
    - **Postoperative care**—Routinely the DIP joint is immobilized in extension for 6 to 8 weeks to allow the extensor tendon to heal before K-wire removal in clinic. This is followed by nighttime splinting in extension for an additional 2 to 4 weeks. Formal physiotherapy is often helpful to regain DIP joint range of motion and strength.
  - **ORIF**—There are a myriad of different techniques that use K-wires, small screws, hook plates, sutures, tension band, etc. The main advantage of this procedure is the direct access to the extensor tendon. Exposure is routinely made through a dorsal approach overlying the DIP joint.

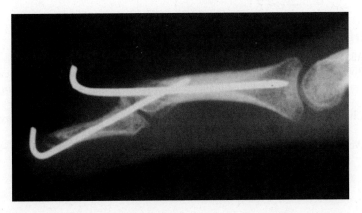

FIGURE 32.7 Lateral radiograph utilizing dorsal block and transarticular closed reduction percutaneous pinning techniques.

- **Acute open mallet finger**—For a purely tendinous mallet, a combination of irrigation and debridement with primary tendinous repair and primary closure is indicated. If primary repair of the extensor tendon cannot be achieved, the tendon may be sutured incorporating the skin (tenodermodesis) or can be reconstructed with tendon graft in a primary or delayed fashion. The patient is then splinted in DIP joint extension postoperatively.

MANAGEMENT ALGORITHM

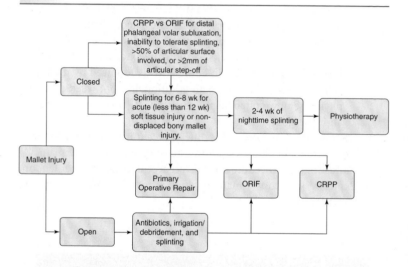

SUGGESTED READINGS

Alla SR, Deal ND, Dempsey IJ. Current concepts: mallet finger. *Hand.* 2014;9:13-44.

Botero SS, Hidalgo Diaz JJ, Benaida A, Collon S, Facca S, Liverneaux PA. Review of acute traumatic closed mallet finger injuries in adults. *Arch Plast Surg.* 2016;43:134-144.

Cheung JPY, Fung B, Ip WY. Review of mallet finger treatment. *Hand Surg.* 2012;17(3):439-447.

Wehbe MA, Schneider LH. Mallet fractures. *J Bone Joint Surg Am.* 1984;66(5): 658-669.

CHAPTER 33

Sagittal Band Rupture (Traumatic Extensor Tendon Dislocation)

Matthew S. Torkington and David J. Warwick

INTRODUCTION

The extensor mechanism to the fingers is a complicated arrangement of structures that contribute to finger extension. At the level of the metacarpophalangeal (MCP) joint, the extensor tendon is held in a central position by the sagittal bands. The sagittal band is part of the extensor retinacular system at the MCP joint and forms a close cylindrical tube around the metacarpal head.[1]

Sagittal band rupture resulting in dislocation of the extensor digitorum communis (EDC) was first described by Legouest; the condition is often referred to as Boxer's knuckle after Gladden published his case report in 1957. While Gladden originally described an injury to the capsule or extensor tendon, his term of boxer's knuckle has become associated with EDC instability over the MCP joint due to a sagittal band injury.[2]

- Pathoanatomy
  - The sagittal bands are separate from, and are superficial to, the collateral ligaments dorsally; as they sweep volarward they approach the accessory collateral ligament and blend with the volar plate.
  - The sagittal band has a thinner superficial layer and a deeper thicker layer containing a tunnel through which the extensor tendon runs.[3]
  - Section experiments[4] show that
    - When the ulnar sagittal bands are completely divided, there is no extensor instability throughout flexion and extension of the digit.
    - If 50% of the proximal radial sagittal band was sectioned, then extensor subluxation occurred.
    - This was worse with increasing wrist and MCP joint flexion.
    - Disruption of the distal 50% of the radial sagittal band did not result in extensor instability.

- With complete division of the ulnar sagittal band in cadaver specimens, EDC tends not to subluxate, although there is a greater tendency if the adjacent juncture tendinum is divided.[5]
- Radial dislocation of the EDC is rarely reported. This is partly because of the normal tendency for EDC to slip ulnarward due to the ulnar inclination of the asymmetric metacarpal heads and soft tissue insertions, as well as the forward descent of the metacarpal heads with flexion.[6]

■ Mechanism of injury
  - The mechanism of injury can be closed or open
  - Closed rupture can occur with forced flexion of the digit and a flexed, ulnar-deviated wrist.
  - Another proposed mechanism in punch injuries is when a punch is landed on the relative narrow dorsal-distal edge of the index or long finger metacarpal rather than the relatively broad area of the dorsum of the flexed proximal phalanges.[7]
  - Atraumatic acute and chronic sagittal band rupture has been reported in the elderly; it is particularly prevalent in rheumatoid arthritis (RA) due to attenuation or even rupture secondary to the pathologic process of RA.[8]
  - The pathology in the atraumatic rupture is different from traumatic ruptures because only the superficial layer originating from its insertion point on the radial aspect is involved, whereas in traumatic ruptures, both the deep and superficial layers, originating a few millimeters radial to the extensor tendon, are affected.[9]

EVALUATION

■ History and physical examination
  - The diagnosis is usually made through history and examination.
  - Presentation is usually with focal pain and swelling over the MCP joint, with the middle finger being most commonly affected.[10]
  - The patient may have a dynamic instability, with obvious extensor tendon dislocation during movement with clicking or crepitus.
  - Although the patient can hold the finger in the extended position, with flexion the tendon dislocates to the ulnar side. The tendon now runs palmar and ulnar to the axis of rotation and so the patient may then not be able to extend the tendon actively. This differentiates a sagittal band rupture from an extensor tendon rupture or radial nerve palsy.[11]
  - The possible differential diagnoses are shown in Table 33.1.

TABLE 33.1 Differential Diagnosis of Sagittal Band Ruptures

Radial nerve palsy
Trigger finger
Collateral ligament injury
Snagging of collateral ligament on osteophyte
Extensor tendon injury

- Imaging
  - **Plain radiographs** are useful to rule out associated fracture or to exclude an osteophyte that snags the collateral ligament in flexion.
  - **Ultrasound and Magnetic resonance imaging** (MRI) are reliable. MRI can assess associated joint capsule injury; if present, the injury will respond more poorly to nonoperative management.[12]
- Classification
  - A classification system has been proposed by Rayan and Murray[13] (Table 33.2).

MANAGEMENT

- Nonoperative management
  - Acute closed injury can be treated operatively but can usually be managed successfully without surgery. There is a limited evidence base.
    - Type 1 and 2 sagittal band injuries (without ulnar-palmar subluxation) can be treated with buddy taping for 4 weeks but patients should be warned that symptoms may persist for up to a year. It is reasonable to offer surgical exploration if symptoms persist for more than 3 months.[14]

TABLE 33.2 Classification of Sagittal Band Injuries

Type 1: Injuries with no instability
Type 2: Tendon subluxation or snapping
Type 3: Frank dislocation

- Ritts et al[15] reported on two closed non-RA traumatic type 3 sagittal band injures, one ulnar and one radial EDC dislocation which they treated with closed reduction and extension splint immobilization with good functional outcomes with no reoccurrence of the injury.
- Catalano et al[16] retrospectively reviewed 10 patients with 11 type 3 sagittal band injures which they treated with a "sagittal band bridge" (Figure 33.1). This custom-made thermoplastic splint differentially holds the injured MCP joint in 25° to 35° of hyperextension relative to the adjacent MCP joints. They report that all had full range of motion and that eight had no pain and three had moderate pain. Five digits had no extensor subluxation, with three having a "barely discernible subluxation." Three had moderate subluxation, which was considered a failure. Only one of these went on to have surgical sagittal band reconstruction.
- In a larger retrospective review, of splinting with either MCP extension or a sagittal band bridge, 92 patients with 68 traumatic and 24 atraumatic were assessed. The subluxation resolved in 77/92 patients. In the traumatic group, EDC tendon subluxation resolved in 95% of acute, 100% of subacute (3-6 weeks), and 67%

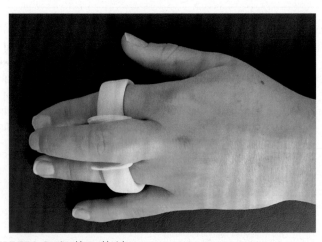

FIGURE 33.1 Sagittal band bridge.

of chronic injuries (>6 weeks). In the atraumatic group, there was 100% resolution in acute presentations, 67% with subacute, and 57% with chronic presentation.[17]

- In the **senior author's practice**, sagittal band injuries diagnosed within 3 to 6 weeks are offered either a sagittal band splint for 6 weeks or surgery followed by the splint for 4 weeks. In chronic presentations (at least 6 weeks after injury), splinting is less predictable and so surgical repair or reconstruction is more likely to give a better result.

■ Surgical management
  - In acute open injuries, exploration and direct surgical repair of the sagittal band would be indicated. Associated injuries such as a metacarpal neck fracture or a penetrating tooth injury to the metacarpal head must be considered.
  - For acute closed injuries, both splinting and surgery are options; as far as we are aware there are no trials comparing the two. Because a splint is needed in either event, the more active patient may prefer the security of a surgical repair as long as the risks of surgical intervention are appreciated.
  - Direct repair with realignment of the extensor tendon with simple sutures (Figure 33.2) for acute injury has been used successfully with good outcomes[18] followed by a postoperative sagittal band bridge splint.

■ **Reconstruction options**
  - For delayed presentations or cases of failed nonoperative management, there are a number of options described.
    ◆ Wheeldon[19] used the ulnar juncturae tendinum from the adjacent tendon and sutured to the palmar radial sagittal band remnant of the deep intermetacarpal ligament.
    ◆ McCoy[20] described taking the radial side of the extensor tendon cut distally and then wrapped around the lumbrical and sutured back onto itself.
    ◆ Carroll[21] used a distally based ulnar slip of EDC which was then looped around the radial collateral ligament and sutured back on to itself with release of the ulnar sagittal band.
    ◆ Eisenbaum[22] described a partial-thickness trapdoor three-sided flap fashioned from the dorsal joint capsule, brought through an incision in the ulnar sagittal band, and sutured back down, which centers the tendon and creates a new, stable tunnel through which it may glide.

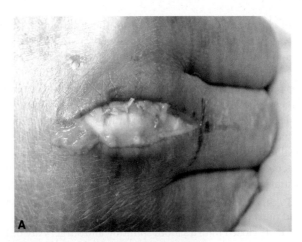

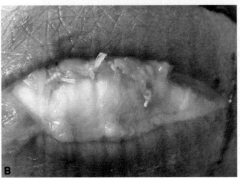

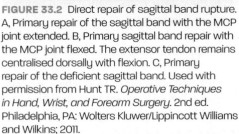

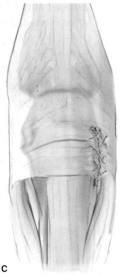

FIGURE 33.2 Direct repair of sagittal band rupture. A, Primary repair of the sagittal band with the MCP joint extended. B, Primary sagittal band repair with the MCP joint flexed. The extensor tendon remains centralised dorsally with flexion. C, Primary repair of the deficient sagittal band. Used with permission from Hunt TR. *Operative Techniques in Hand, Wrist, and Forearm Surgery.* 2nd ed. Philadelphia, PA: Wolters Kluwer/Lippincott Williams and Wilkins; 2011.

- ◆ Watson[23] again used a distally based slip of EDC but this time passed it around the transverse intermetacarpal ligament.
- ■ The **senior author** prefers the anatomical simplicity of the Watson reconstruction (Figure 33.3).

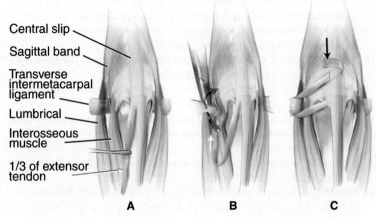

Central slip

Sagittal band

Transverse intermetacarpal ligament

Lumbrical

Interosseous muscle

1/3 of extensor tendon

A   B   C

FIGURE 33.3 Extensor loop for sagittal band reconstruction as described by Watson 1997. A, A distally based slip of extensor tendon constituting no more than one third the width of the tendon is harvested. B, The slip of extensor tendon is rerouted from proximal to distal around the deep intermetacarpal ligament. C, The tendon slip is then attached to the extensor tendon (usually radially) through a weave distal to the MCP joint. Used with permission from Hunt TR, operative techniques in hand, wrist and forearm surgery. 2011 Wolters Kluwer/Lippincott Williams and Wilkins.

REFERENCES

1. Rayan GM, Murray D, Chung KW, Rohrer M. The extensor retinacular system at the metacarpophalangeal joint. Anatomical and histological study. *J Hand Surg Br.* 1997;22(5):585-590.
2. Kleinhenz BP, Adams BD. Closed sagittal band injury of the metacarpophalangeal joint. *J Am Acad Orthop Surg.* 2015;23(7):415-423.
3. Kichouh M, Vanhoenacker F, Jager T, et al. Functional anatomy of the dorsal hood of the hand: correlation if ultrasound and MR findings with cadaveric dissection. *Eur Radiol.* 2009;19(8):1849-1856.
4. Young CM, Rayan GM. The sagittal band: anatomic and biomechanical study. *J Hand Surg Am.* 2000;25(6):1107-1113.
5. Farrar NG, Kundra A. Role of the juncturae tendinum in preventing radial subluxation of the extensor communis tendons after ulnar sagittal band rupture: a cadaveric study. *ISRN Orthop.* 2012:597681. doi:10.5402/2012/597681.
6. Tubiana R, Thomine JM, Mackin E. *Examination of the Hand and Wrist.* 2nd ed. New York, NY: Informa Healthcare; 1998.
7. Stracher M, Posner MA. Boxer's knuckle. *Tech Hand Up Extrem Surg.* 2002;6(4):196-199.

8. Chinchalkar SJ, Pitts S. Dynamic assist splinting for attenuated sagittal bands in the rheumatoid hand. *Tech Hand Up Extrem Surg.* 2006;10(4):206-211.

9. Ishizuki M. Traumatic and spontaneous dislocations of extensor tendon of the long finger. *J Hand Surg Am.* 1990;15(6):967-972.

10. Inoue G, Tamura Y. Dislocation of the extensor tendons over the metacarpophalangeal joints. *J Hand Surg Am.* 1996;21(3):464-469.

11. Lin JD, Robert J, Strach MD. Closed soft tissue extensor mechanism injuries. *J Hand Surg Am.* 2014;39(5):1005-1011.

12. Arai K, Toh S, Nakahara K, Nishikawa S, Harata S. Treatment of soft tissue injuries to the dorsum of the metacarpophalangeal joint (Boxer's knuckle). *J Hand Surg Br.* 2002;27(1):9.

13. Rayan GM, Murray MD. Classification and treatment of closed sagittal band injuries. *J Hand Surg Am.* 1994;19(4):590-594.

14. Strauch RJ. Chapter 5: Extensor tendon injury. In: Wolfe SW, Pederson WC, Hotchkiss RN, Kozin SH, Cohen MS, eds. *Green's Operative Hand Surgery.* 7th ed. Philadelphia, PA: Elsevier; 2017.

15. Ritts GD, Wood MB, Engber WD: Nonoperative treatment of traumatic dislocations of the extensor digitorum tendons in patients without rheumatoid disorders. *J Hand Surg.* 1985;10A:714-716.

16. Catalano LW III, Gupta S, Ragland R III, Glickel SZ, Johnson C, Barron OA. Closed treatment of nonrheumatoid extensor tendon dislocations at the metacarpophalangeal joint. *J Hand Surg Am.* 2006;31(2):242-245.

17. Peelman J, Markiewitz A, Kiefhaber T, Stern P. Splintage in the treatment of sagittal band incompetence and extensor tendon subluxation. *J Hand Surg Eur.* 2015;40(3):287-290.

18. Kettelkamp DB, Flatt AE, Moulds R. Traumatic dislocation of the long-finger extensor tendon: a clinical, anatomical, and biomechanical study. *J Bone Joint Surg Am.* 1971;53(2):229-240.

19. Wheeldon FT. Recurrent dislocation of extensor tendons in the hand. *J Bone Joint Surg.* 1954;36B:612-617.

20. McCoy FJ, Winsky AJ. Lumbrical loop operation for luxation of the extensor tendons of the hand. *Plast Reconstr Surg.* 1969;44(2):142-146.

21. Carroll C, Moore JR, Weiland AJ. Posttraumatic ulnar subluxation of the extensor tendons: a reconstructive technique. *J Hand Surg Am.* 1987;12A:227-231.

22. Eisenbaum SL. Trapdoor pulley repair for chronic subluxation of the digital extensor tendon. *Plast Reconstr Surg.* 1988;82:1081-1082.

23. Watson HK, Weinzweig J, Guidera PM. Sagittal band reconstruction. *J Hand Surg.* 1997;22A:452-456.

34 Flexor Tendon Injuries

Andrew Campbell and Hisham M. Awan

INTRODUCTION

- Anatomy
  - Flexor tendons
    - Flexor carpi ulnaris
    - Flexor carpi radialis (FCR)
    - Flexor pollicis longus (FPL)
    - Flexor digitorum superficialis (FDS)
    - Flexor digitorum profundus (FDP)
  - Important anatomic relationships
    - FCR is the closest tendon to the median nerve in the forearm.
    - There are nine tendons (FDS ×4, FDP ×4, and FPL) and one nerve (median nerve) in the carpal tunnel.
    - FPL is the most radial tendon in the carpal tunnel.
    - In the forearm, wrist, and hand, the FDS tendons lie superficial to FDP. At the level of the metacarpophalangeal (MCP) joints, FDS splits and FDP becomes superficial. FDS slips rejoin at **Camper Chiasm** and insert on the middle phalanx. FDP inserts on the distal phalanx (Figure 34.1).
  - Tendon anatomy
    - Structure
      - Composed of bundles of collagen fascicles surrounded by epitenon, a surface that is crucial for gliding
    - Nutritional supply
      - Arterial supply—vinculae from digital arteries
      - Synovial diffusion
    - Pulley system
      - Prevents bowstringing of flexor tendon
      - A2 and A4 are most important in fingers.
      - Oblique pulley is most important in the thumb.

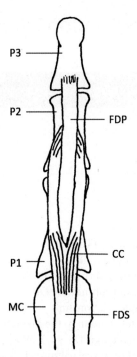

FIGURE 34.1 Relationship of flexor digitorum superficialis (FDS) and flexor digitorum profundus (FDP) on the palmar aspect of a finger. CC, Camper's Chiasm; MC, metacarpal; P1, proximal phalanx; P2, middle phalanx; P3, distal phalanx.

- Mechanism of injury
  - Most commonly results from penetrating trauma or lacerations to the palmar aspect of the hand or volar wrist/forearm
  - Jersey finger (see Chapter 35)—avulsion of FDP insertion on the distal phalanx due to forceful distal interphalangeal (DIP) joint extension during FDP contraction

EVALUATION

- History
  - Penetrating trauma or laceration to palmar hand or volar wrist/forearm
  - Weak or absent flexion of digit

- Physical examination
  - Inspection
    - ◆ Assess wounds for foreign bodies, identify injured structures, evaluate for evidence of arthrotomy.
    - ◆ Assess digital cascade.
      - ✳ Digit with a flexor tendon injury is held extended at rest relative to other fingers.
      - ✳ Persistent extension at proximal interphalangeal (PIP) or DIP joints during passive wrist extension is indicative of flexor tendon injury.
        - ▲ Passive wrist extension normally causes flexion at MCP, PIP, and DIP joints (**tenodesis effect**).
  - Strength/range of motion
    - ◆ Loss of active flexion of digit
    - ◆ **Test FDS and FDP for each finger** (Figure 34.2)
  - Neurovascular examination
    - ◆ Given proximity of nerves and vessels to finger flexor tendons, concomitant neurovascular injuries are common.
    - ◆ **Document a thorough examination at the time of injury.**

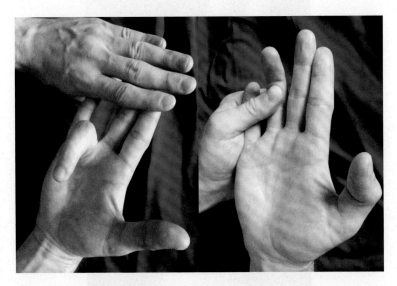

FIGURE 34.2 Demonstration of how to test flexor digitorum superficialis (*left panel*) and flexor digitorum profundus (*right panel*) of the ring finger.

  - ◆ Assess perfusion to each digit (<2-second capillary refill is normal).
  - ◆ Assess two-point discrimination on radial and ulnar aspect of each digit (<6 mm is normal).
- ▪ Imaging
  - ● Radiographs should be obtained to rule out the presence of foreign bodies or bony injury.
  - ● Advanced imaging is not usually required.
- ▪ Classification
  - ● Acute versus chronic
  - ● Traumatic versus atraumatic
  - ● **Zone of injury** (Figure 34.3 and Table 34.1)

ACUTE MANAGEMENT

- ▪ Vascular compromise
  - ● The poorly perfused digit should undergo urgent operative exploration and possibly microvascular repair

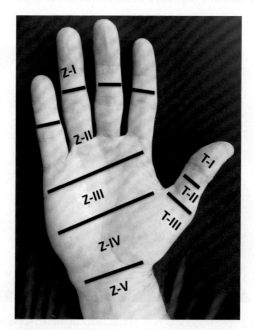

FIGURE 34.3 Flexor tendon zones of injury. Z, zone; T, thumb zone.

TABLE 34.1 **Flexor Tendon Zones of Injury**

Zone of Injury	Anatomic Landmarks	Repair Strategy If Injured
Zone I	Distal to FDS insertion on midpoint of middle phalanx. Only FDP is injured	Tendon to bone repair if <1 cm of distal tendon stump is remaining Direct tendon repair
Zone II	FDS insertion (midpoint of middle phalanx) to level of A1 pulley (distal to palmar crease) FDP is superficial to FDS	Direct tendon repair *Historically poor results after tendon repair ("no man's land"), but results improving with modern rehab protocols*
Zone III	Proximal aspect of A1 pulley (distal palmar crease) to origin of lumbricals from FDP tendons (distal edge of transverse carpal ligament)	Direct tendon repair *Complicated by vicinity of tendons to digital nerves, superficial arch, and lumbrical muscles*
Zone IV	Carpal tunnel	Direct tendon repair *Avoid violation of TCL. Repair TCL if it is lacerated unless median nerve is also injured, then TCL must be completely released*
Zone V	Proximal aspect of transverse carpal ligament to the musculotendinous junction	Direct tendon repair *Often associated with neurovascular injury*
Zone TI	Distal to thumb IP joint	Direct tendon repair
Zone TII	Thumb A1 pulley to IP joint	*Higher rerupture rate than other fingers*
Zone TIII	Thenar eminence	

Abbreviations: FDP, flexor digitorum profundus; FDS, flexor digitorum superficialis; IP, interphalangeal; TCL, transverse carpal ligament.

- Well-perfused digit
  - Copious irrigation
  - Loose closure and/or exploration under local anesthesia with digital block
  - Dorsal blocking splint to prevent flexion and proximal tendon migration

DEFINITIVE TREATMENT

- Nonoperative treatment
  - Wound care and early range of motion is indicated in partial lacerations of <50% tendon width

- Surgical indications
  - <33% tendon width involved—debridement alone to prevent triggering
  - >50% tendon width involved—surgical repair
    - Optimal timing is <2 weeks
- Surgical repair
  - Treatment strategy depends on zone of injury, but typically surgery consists of end-to-end tendon repair (Figure 34.3 and Table 34.1)
  - Approach
    - Brunner incision. Incorporate laceration if possible.
      - Second incision proximally if tendon has retracted
    - Identify, tag, and debride tendon edges.
      - Handle tendon atraumatically to prevent adhesion formation.
    - Provisionally assess tension on repair.
      - If interposition graft is necessary for adequate tendon length, palmaris longus tendon is often used.
      - Release pulleys as necessary to allow the tendon to glide without interference (A2 and A4 are most important and should be preserved).
    - Repair with minimum of four core sutures with 3-0 or 4-0 tapered needle.
      - **Core suture strength is related to suture material, caliber of suture, and most importantly the number of sutures crossing the repair site.**
      - Augment with epitendinous suture which improves gliding and increases repair strength.
  - Pearls
    - Consider repairing one slip of FDS instead of both to decrease volume within flexor sheath.
    - Wide-awake surgery allows the surgeon to test repair integrity and glide.
- Potential complications
  - Tendon adhesions (most common)
  - Stiffness, joint contracture (improved with early active motion protocols)
  - Rerupture
    - Rerepair
    - Two-stage reconstruction
      - Stage 1—pulley reconstruction and placement of temporary silicone grafts (Hunter rod)

⁕ Stage 2—3 months later when the flexor sheath has reformed, the Hunter rods are removed and a tendon graft is repaired to the distal phalanx.
- Postoperative care
  - **Controlled early mobilization is key.**
    ◆ Tendon repairs weaken during the first 3 weeks post-op if immobilized.
    ◆ Tendons with repair site gap <3 mm begin developing increased tensile strength after week 3.
  - Multiple early active and passive motion protocols have been described.

SUGGESTED READINGS

Chang J, Noland S, Adams JE, et al. Tendon. In: Hammert WC, ed. *ASSH Manual of Hand Surgery*. Philadelphia, PA: Lippincott Williams & Wilkins; 2010:93-110.

Gelberman RH, Boyer MI, Brodt MD, Winters SC, Silva MJ. The effect of gap formation at the repair site on the strength and excursion of intrasynovial flexor tendons. An experimental study on the early stages of tendon-healing in dogs. *J Bone Joint Surg Am*. 1999;81(7):975-982.

Kim HM, Nelson G, Thomopoulous S, Silva MJ, Das R, Gelberman RH. Technical and biologic modifications for enhanced flexor tendon repair. *J Hand Surg Am*. 2010;35A:1031-1037.

Seiler JG III. Flexor tendon injury. In: Wolfe SW, Hotchkiss RN, Pederson WC, et al, eds. *Green's Operative Hand Surgery*. 6th ed. Philadelphia, PA: Churchill Livingstone; 2010.

Nisha J. Crouser, Steven R. Niedermeier, and
Hisham M. Awan

INTRODUCTION

- Jersey finger is an injury to the terminal flexor mechanism at the level of the distal interphalangeal (DIP) joint. This can be due to either rupture of the flexor digitorum profundus (FDP) tendon in Zone 1 or an avulsion fracture of the distal phalanx with a fragment of bone that remains attached to the tendon (Figure 35.1). The degree of retraction of the tendon ranges from minimal displacement to retraction into the palm.
- **Mechanism of injury**—Injury occurs when a flexed DIP joint is forcefully hyperextended and the FDP tendon ruptures at its weakest point, which is the insertion site (Figure 35.2). The term "jersey finger" is derived from the classic scenario in which an athlete grabs an opponent's jersey and the DIP joint is hyperextended. Rupture most often occurs at the bony insertion and less often at the musculotendinous junction.
- **Epidemiology**—The injury commonly occurs in athletes who are involved in contact sports, most notably rugby and football, but can occur in nonathletes as well. Musculotendinous rupture is rare and occurs most often in a traumatic distal phalanx amputation injury or in patients with underlying inflammatory conditions. The ring finger is

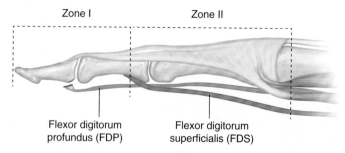

FIGURE 35.1 Anatomic location of injury in jersey finger. FDS, flexor digitorum superficialis; FDP, flexor digitorum profundus.

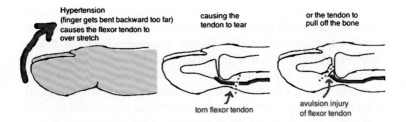

FIGURE 35.2 Mechanism of injury for jersey finger.

involved in 75% of FDP avulsions. The higher susceptibility of the ring finger to this injury is related to several anatomic differences. It has been demonstrated that the ring finger has the least independent motion of all the digits. Also the insertion of the ring finger FDP is weaker than the FDP insertion of the long finger. Finally, the ring finger extends farther than the other digits during full grip and absorbs the most force during pull-away testing, making it prone to avulsion.

EVALUATION

- **Presentation**—Patients often present with acute pain and swelling over the volar surface of the distal finger. The point of maximal tenderness may indicate the location of the avulsed tendon.
- **Physical Examination**—On examination, the affected finger lies in extension relative to other fingers in resting position (Figure 35.3). Patients are unable to actively flex the DIP joint when asked to make a fist. Often

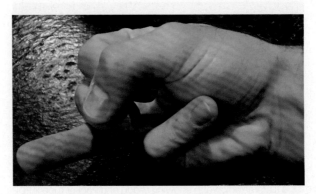

FIGURE 35.3 Clinic photograph of jersey finger injury with ring finger held in extension.

patients will resist flexion of the entire finger as a result of pain, which can obscure the diagnosis. In the acute setting, an FDP avulsion can be misdiagnosed as a "sprained finger." It is essential that the clinician isolates DIP and proximal interphalangeal (PIP) joint motion to prevent a delay in diagnosis. In some cases, the physician may be able to palpate the flexor tendon retracted proximally along the flexor sheath.

- **Imaging**—Anteroposterior, lateral, and oblique radiographs should be obtained to assess for avulsion fractures or articular injuries. A bony avulsion fragment of the volar lip of the distal phalanx articular surface may be present (Figure 35.4). Approximately 50% of FDP avulsions are associated with an osseous fragment. If the injury is purely tendinous, the only radiographic finding will be slight extension of the DIP in resting position. MRI can be used if the diagnosis is unclear or the location of the retracted tendon is unknown.

- **Differential diagnosis**
  - Anterior interosseous nerve paralysis
  - Trigger finger
  - Swan neck deformity

- **Classification**—The Leddy and Packer classification system is used most commonly (Table 35.1). Type I, II, and III injuries are most common.
  - In type I injuries, there is complete tendon rupture with retraction into the palm. The tendon is tethered in the palm by the lumbrical origin and both the vinculum longus profundus (VLP) and brevis profundus (VBP) are ruptured. As a result, there is significant vascular compromise, and expedited surgical intervention is required within 7 to 10 days of the injury.

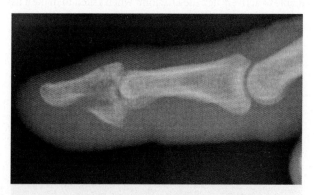

FIGURE 35.4 Lateral radiograph showing Leddy and Packer type III FDP avulsion. FDP, flexor digitorum profundus.

TABLE 35.1 The Leddy and Packer Classification System

Type	Level of Retraction	Vincular System Disrupted	Treatment
I	Palm	VLP and VBP	Primary tendon repair within 7–10 d
II	PIP and/or small volar cortical avulsion	VBP	Primary tendon repair within 10 d (may be delayed)
III	A4 pulley (entrapped large osseous fragment)	None	Repair of fracture fragment within 8–12 wk
IV	Bony avulsion + tendon avulsion with variable retraction	Variable	Fix fracture first then reattach tendon within 12 wk
V	Bony avulsion + comminuted P3 fracture	Variable	Repair within 12 wk

Abbreviations: PIP, proximal interphalangeal; VBP, vinculum brevis profundus; VLP, vinculum longus profundus.

- Type II injuries involve retraction of the FDP tendon to the level of the PIP joint, and there may be a small volar cortical avulsion. The VLP is preserved in this case because it arises at the level of the PIP volar plate, but the VBP is disrupted.
- Type III injuries are defined as FDP retraction to the level of the A4 pulley of the middle phalanx. Retraction to this level is the result of a large bony fragment avulsion. Both vincula are intact with type III injuries permitting a delay in surgical correction, if necessary.
- Type IV injuries are complex and defined as simultaneous osseous distal phalanx avulsion and distal phalanx fracture.
- Type V injuries are similar to type IV with comminution of the distal phalanx.

ACUTE MANAGEMENT

- Splinting is used as initial management prior to surgical intervention. The forearm can be included in the splint to try and limit retraction.

DEFINITIVE TREATMENT

- All cases of jersey finger in which the tendon has completely avulsed from its insertion require surgical intervention. The accepted length of time until surgery and type of procedure are dependent upon the classification of the injury. It is important to determine the extent of injury at the time of diagnosis because certain cases require surgical correction within 7 to 10 days of the injury. Timely management is recommended in all cases, because it can be difficult to determine the degree of retraction of the tendon on physical examination.

■ **Type I/II**

- Surgical options include dorsal button, direct tie around bone, suture anchor, or a combination of techniques.
- An attempt to localize the level of retraction preoperatively should be made using physical examination and imaging modalities. Intraoperatively, the tendon is identified using a Bruner approach, in which a volar zigzag incision is made from the level of tendon retraction proximally to the distal DIP joint. The flexor sheath is then exposed. An incision is made just distal to the A2 pulley to locate the tendon. A suture is passed through the tendon and the tendon is advanced through the flexor tendon pulley system to the distal phalanx. This often requires dilation of the pulley system. A pediatric feeding tube may be helpful in passing the tendon under the pulleys. Attempts should be made to preserve the A2 and A4 pulleys. Overadvancement of the tendon should be avoided to prevent quadriga. In type I injuries, the distal end of the tendon will be avascular as a result of the disrupted vincula and should be trimmed prior to reapproximation. In type II rupture, the vincula remain intact, but fibrosis may develop at the FDS chiasm, which may limit tendon gliding. The fibrotic end should be debrided in these cases.
- **Dorsal button technique** (Figure 35.5)
  - ◆ The bone bed on the distal phalanx should be prepared by removing any soft tissue, while still preserving the palmar plate to promote direct tendon-bone healing. Next, Keith needles are drilled into the distal phalangeal bone bed exiting through the mid portion of the nail plate and paired sutures are passed through the tendon and tied over a button on top of the nail plate via the Keith needles.
  - ◆ Disadvantages—The pull-through button technique may lead to tendon-bone gapping due to the distance between the fixation point of the tendon-bone and the suture knot. This can also damage the nail plate, including deformity and nail fold necrosis, but these complications are rare.
- **Suture anchor technique**
  - ◆ This technique has potential advantages of complete internalization of the suture anchor without disruption of the nail plate or

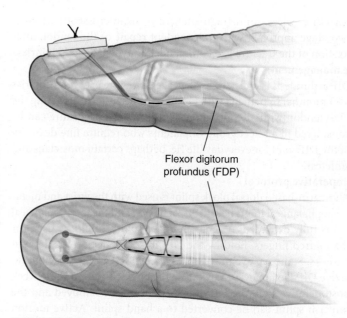

FIGURE 35.5 Dorsal button repair. FDP, flexor digitorum profundus.

dorsal incision. For this technique, holes are drilled at a 45° angle from distal-volar to proximal-dorsal to increase the resistance to pullout of the implant. Intraoperative fluoroscopy is used to ensure that there has been no disruption of the dorsal cortex or the DIP joint. To allow for direct tendon-bone healing, the FDP must be flush with the bone.

- ◆ Disadvantages—This technique is less successful in patients with osteoporotic bone or avulsion fractures. It also has been associated with higher risk of contracture after the procedure.
- Currently, there is not enough literature to the support the use of one technique over another. Future studies are needed to make evidence-based recommendations; the surgical technique used is left to surgeon preference.
- ■ **Type III/IV/V**
  - The presence of an intact vincula system makes type III to V injuries more amenable to later repair. These injuries are repaired with open reduction internal fixation (ORIF) of the fracture. Various techniques have been proposed with successful results, including fixation with

Kirschner wires, mini-fragment screws, or interosseous wires. A two-stage approach with independent repair of the tendon after fixation of the fracture is recommended in type IV and V injuries.

- **Late management**
  - DIP arthrodesis is indicated as a salvage procedure in chronic injuries (>3 months) in patients with chronic stiffness. Reconstructing the FDP tendon with a tendon graft in a two-stage procedure can be considered in a select group of patients who require fine dexterity of the DIP joint for everyday life (ie, perhaps certain musicians and athletes).
- **Postoperative protocol**
  - A forearm-based dorsal block splint is used with the wrist and metacarpophalangeal joints held at 30° of flexion and the interphalangeal joints fully extended. A separate finger splint should be used for the injured fingers, holding the DIP in 45° of flexion for the first 3 weeks. Some passive movement is permitted at this stage but no active DIP flexion, wrist flexion, or finger extension. At the 4-week postoperative visit, the DIP finger splint can be removed and the forearm splint can be converted to a hand splint. Active motion can be initiated at this time. Return to resistive exercises is most commonly allowed at 8 weeks.

COMPLICATIONS

- The main complications after FDP avulsion injury repair are DIP joint stiffness and contracture. Studies estimate an average loss of 10 to 15° of extension after injury. There is also a risk of rerupture or loss of fixation postsurgical intervention. Another complication that can occur is quadriga caused by a functional shortening of the FDP tendon due to overadvancement of the FDP during repair, adhesions, or retraction of the tendon. The result is an inability to fully flex the fingers adjacent to the injured finger, which manifests as decreased grip strength. Additional complications can be seen with associated fractures, including decreased joint stability and arthrodesis.

SUGGESTED READING

Ruchelsman DE, Christoforou D, Wasserman B, Lee SK, Rettig ME. Avulsion injuries of the flexor digitorum profundus. *J Am Acad Orthop Surg.* 2011;19(3):152-162.

CHAPTER

36 Peripheral Nerve Injury and Repair Principles

D. Nicole Deal and Patricia A. Drace

INTRODUCTION

- Pathoanatomy
  - Epineurium[1-3]
    - Circumferentially organized connective tissue layer in between and around fascicles for nourishment and protection
  - Perineurium
    - Circumferentially organized around each fascicle
    - Forms blood–brain barrier and contributes to tensile strength
  - Endoneurium
    - Loose collagen matrix, longitudinally organized within fascicles
    - Protection and nourishment of axons
  - Fascicles
    - Divide and unite to form plexuses[3]
    - Fascicular matching important for repair
  - Blood supply
    - Anastomosis of blood vessels[2]
      * Two major arterial systems
        ▲ Superficial
        ▲ Interfascicular epineurium—microvessels
          ❖ Trauma increases permeability
          ❖ More susceptible to compression trauma than endoneurial vessels, which can lead to intrafasicular edema and secondary nerve injury
      * One longitudinal system
        ▲ Within endoneurium and perineurium[3]
        ▲ Endoneurial capillaries function as blood–brain barrier
          ❖ Disrupted by toxin, ischemia, trauma, histamine, serotonin

- Mechanism of injury
  - Stretch—most common
    - Commonly associated with motor vehicle collision (MVC)
  - Compression/ischemia
  - Transection/laceration—30%[1]
    - Glass, knife, fan, saw, auto metal, long bone fracture
  - Blast—complex injury with soft tissue and often vascular involvement, may involve shrapnel
    - Often necessitates fasciotomy following arterial repair
- Epidemiology
  - Consecutive study of all peripheral nerve injuries in 2006 found 73.5% occurred in upper extremity[4]
    - Ulnar nerve most commonly injured
    - Combined lesions usually involve ulnar and median nerves
    - Most common cause of injury—MVC
  - Crush injury most likely type of limb injury to be associated with peripheral nerve trauma (1.9% of extremity trauma)[5]
  - Limb dislocation confers 1.46% rate of nerve injury[5]
  - Some studies show equal rates of peripheral nerve injury in males and females, whereas others show male predominance of up to 83%[5,6]
  - 83% of peripheral nerve injuries at the time of limb trauma are patients younger than 55 years[5]
  - Upper extremity injury—radial nerve injury most common followed by ulnar and median nerves[6]
  - Traumatic brain injury present in 60% of peripheral nerve injury patients[6]
- Nerve injury physiology[1]
  - Transection of axons results in
    - Cell body edema
    - Shift in metabolism from synthesis of neurotransmitter to production of structural materials
    - Traumatic degeneration—proximal axon stump degenerates to node of Ranvier or even to cell body
    - Wallerian degeneration—distal axon stump and myelin degenerate in a retrograde manner
      - 48 to 96 hours after injury
      - Schwann cells mediate phagocytosis of myelin and axon debris
    - Loss of blood–brain barrier
      - Injured nerve exposed to proteins, which act as antigens and may lead to autoimmune reaction

- Nerve regeneration physiology
  - Schwann cells support axon regeneration[1]
    - Begin to divide within days of injury
    - Cell linings contain nerve growth factor receptors
    - Cytokine-mediated process (interleukin [IL]-1, IL-6, transforming growth factor beta) along with macrophages as part of inflammatory process
  - Axon growth cone makes way for neurite growth
    - Axons that cannot find distal stump grow into surrounding tissues or become disorganized scar/neuroma
    - Axons that reach distal stump have reasonable chance of reaching distal target organ
    - Axon growth average 1 mm/d
  - Distal reinnervation
    - Occurs by three mechanisms[1]
      - Remyelination
      - Collateral sprouting distally from preserved axons
      - Regeneration from site of injury
    - Functional reinnervation needs to reach target organ by 12 to 18 months in order to allow for recovery prior to fibrosis
    - Sensory and motor end organs degenerate over time (1+ years)
      - Earlier reinnervation yields improved functionality

EVALUATION

- History
  - Straightforward wound—laceration, no significant contamination
    - Primary repair is preferred
  - Wound with extensive tissue damage—gunshot wound (GSW), penetrating trauma with extensive soft tissue and/or vascular injury, contaminated wounds
    - Extent of nerve damage cannot immediately be assessed until the wound declares itself.
  - Closed traction injury—can have variable presentation
    - Worse outcomes with situations associated with scapulothoracic dissociation where nerves and vessels can be significantly disrupted and retracted

- Physical examination
  - Sensory examination—altered sensation in the distribution of affected nerve
    - Test sensation to light touch, pain/pinprick, and temperature as best as possible
    - Tinel sign[1]—useful in following patients over time with nerve injury
      - Over area of lesion in first-degree injury
      - Generally moves distal at 1 in/mo during recovery of second-degree lesions
      - Third-degree lesions—weaker Tinel sign that recovers slower than expected
      - Fourth- and fifth-degree lesions—Tinel sign never moves distally
  - Motor examination—weakness, paralysis of muscles innervated by affected nerve
    - Test all muscles distal to the injury site innerved by affected nerve for motor strength
  - Skin changes—skin loses vasomotor tone, anhidrosis
  - May have ischemia in the vicinity of injury/affected nerve if vascular supply is damaged at the time of injury
- Imaging—In the case of nerve injury, electrodiagnostic testing is the most useful adjunctive test available and is basically an extension of the physical examination.
  - Electromyography/nerve conduction velocity (EMG/NCV)—often more sensitive for return of function than physical examination and can contribute significantly to understanding of nerve injury and severity. See Table 36.1 for EMG/NCV findings.
    - EMG—tests muscle response to stimuli by insertion of needle into muscle to record electrical response of neighboring motor units.

TABLE 36.1 Electromyography Findings With Peripheral Nerve Injury

	Insertional Activity	Rest Activity	Biphasic and Triphasic Potentials	Interference
Normal	Normal	Silent	Yes	Complete
Neuropraxia	Normal	Silent	No	None
Axonotmesis	Increased	Fibrillations and sharp waves	No	None
Neurotmesis	Increased	Fibrillations and sharp waves	No	None

* First evidence of recovery is return of motor unit action potentials on needle examination of muscle innervated closest to site of injury.[1]
* Acutely, EMG cannot determine degree of injury except complete versus incomplete lesions.
  ▲ EMG performed at 2 weeks or earlier is useful only for exact localization of injury, not for determination of injury severity.
* Can see recovery response on EMG weeks to months before clinical contraction is visible.
◆ NCV—tests peripheral nerve response to stimuli
  * Confirms clinical examination and useful in localization of lesion
  * Results highly sensitive but can be nonspecific
  * Preserved for 7 days after nerve injury so avoid testing immediately after injury
  * Neuropraxia (see Table 36.1):
    ▲ Compound muscle action potential (CMAP) and nerve action potential (NAP) distal to lesion are maintained indefinitely so *distal stump continues to conduct*
    ▲ Proximal to the injury, may have partial or complete conduction block
  * Axonotmesis and neurotmesis (see Table 36.1):
    ▲ EMG findings depend on timing from injury:
      ◆ Immediately after injury, no changes at neuromuscular junction but conduction block may be present with proximal stimulation
      ◆ 9 to 11 days postinjury will illustrate loss of CMAP and NAP, *distal stump no longer conducts.*
      ◆ Wallerian degeneration complete at 1 to 2 weeks
        ○ Degree of axon loss versus demyelination can be determined at this point.
  * EMG/NCV timing:
    ▲ Study at 7 days can localize lesion and can tell only complete versus incomplete injury
    ▲ Study at 2 weeks can differentiate neuropraxia versus axonotmesis and neurotmesis
    ▲ Study at 3 to 4 weeks after fibrillation potentials have developed provides greatest amount of information[1]
    ▲ Study at 3 to 4 months may detect early reinnervation
● Radiographs—can be useful in certain cases
  ◆ Bony stability required for appropriate nerve treatment

- ◆ Scapulothoracic dissociation concerning for brachial plexus injury
- ● Magnetic resonance imaging (MRI)
  - ◆ Can identify nerve discontinuity at the fascicular level, verifying the need for surgical repair[7]
  - ◆ MRI can be used for early detection of acute axonal nerve lesions
    - ✱ Nerve hyperintensity on T2 MRI is present at 24 hours following denervation, which precedes EMG spontaneous activity by 24 hours.[8]
  - ◆ Can be useful to determine muscle denervation after nerve injury
- ● Ultrasound—Can be used to determine nerve continuity and to some degree extent of injury (accuracy of nerve injury classification 93.2%)[9]
- ■ Nerve injury classification (see Table 36.2)
  - ● Seddon
    - ◆ Neuropraxia
      - ✱ Local myelin damage/segmental demyelination with focal conduction block
      - ✱ Usually caused by compression, thus all continuity of structures (axons) is preserved.
      - ✱ Conduction within the nerve and distal to the lesion remains intact.
      - ✱ No distal degeneration or Wallerian degeneration
      - ✱ After a crush injury, can expect return of function within days to 12 weeks provided there is no ongoing compression or insult
    - ◆ Axonotmesis
      - ✱ Loss of axon continuity with endoneurium damage, perineurium and epineurium remain intact
      - ✱ Crush and stretch injuries with varied connective tissue injury
      - ✱ Wallerian degeneration occurs but NCV often preserved for 7 days after injury
      - ✱ Recovery takes many months—reinnervation depends on degree of injury, distance to muscle target, and surrounding tissue viability.
    - ◆ Neurotmesis
      - ✱ Physiologic disruption or complete nerve transection from sharp laceration, massive trauma, severe traction with nerve rupture
      - ✱ If only physiologic, order of function of failure is as follows—motor, then proprioception, touch, temperature, pain, and sympathetic fails last
      - ✱ Recovery of function does not happen spontaneously, reinnervation does not occur without intervention/repair.

TABLE 36.2 Classification of Nerve Injuries

Seddon	Sunderland	Myelin Intact?	Axon Intact?	Endoneurium Intact?	Perineurium Intact?	Epineurium Intact?	Surgery?	Recovery
Neuropraxia	1	No	Yes	Yes	Yes	Yes	No	Complete (weeks-months)
Axonotmesis	2	No	No	Yes	Yes	Yes	No	Complete (months)
	3	No	No	No	Yes	Yes	Not usually unless neurolysis	Fibrosis, severe retrograde cell body injury and end organ change may preclude full recovery
	4	No	No	No	No	Yes	Excise damaged segment and repair vs reconstruct	Retrograde neuron damage, intrafascicular fibrosis, minimal useful recovery
Neurotmesis	5	No	No	No	No	No	Repair vs reconstruction	No spontaneous recovery

Sunderland S. *Nerve Injuries and Their Repair: A Critical Appraisal* [reprint]. 1st ed. Edinburgh, NY: Churchill Livingstone; 1991.

- Sunderland[3] (see Table 36.2)
  - Type 1—Neuropraxia
    - Complete recovery expected
  - Type 2—Axonotmesis with intact endoneurium
    - Physiologic disruption of axon with endoneurium intact
    - Regenerating axons grow along same path as they occupied before injury
    - Complete recovery expected
  - Type 3—Axonotmesis with damage to endoneurium
    - Retrograde injury to cell bodies leads to intrafascicular fibrosis
    - Longer delay in regrowth—end-organ changes may occur
    - Incomplete recovery
  - Type 4—Axonotmesis with damage to endoneurium and perineurium
    - More significant retrograde cell damage and intrafasicular fibrosis
    - Requires excision of damaged segment with repair or reconstruction
  - Type 5—Neurotmesis
    - No spontaneous recovery, requires surgical intervention
- Factors affecting outcome following nerve injury[10-12]:
  - Time to repair—unfavorable prognosis for delay in repair of greater than 6 to 12 months
  - Age—nerve regeneration potential is best for children, worse in patients older than 50 years[10]
  - Direct repairs have better outcomes than those requiring graft.[10]
  - Length of repair—outcomes worse with each 1-cm increase in defect length[10]
    - Optimal recovery with autologous grafts <5 cm[13] and conduits <3 cm[14]
  - Distance to distal targets—axon regeneration must traverse greater distance for reinnervation of muscle/sensory organ for proximal injury[10,11]
  - Sensory recovery is often better than motor recovery for repair of mixed nerve injuries.[10]
  - The nerve injured matters—Radial nerve has better prognosis for recovery than median and ulnar nerves.[10]
  - Mechanism and associated soft tissue injury—scarring, devascularization of surrounding tissues leads to worse prognosis
  - Gender—female patients have better outcomes than male patients (does not take injury severity into account, women may have milder injuries than men).[10]

ACUTE MANAGEMENT

- Open injury with neurologic deficit (algorithm from Ray and Mackinnon[12])—surgical exploration and either repair or observe if nerve in continuity
  - Sharp injury—direct repair
  - Crush injury—approximate nerve ends if possible to minimize retraction and need for additional graft length
    - Plan for nerve graft in 3 weeks to 3 months so that zone of injury has declared itself
  - GSW—observe for 4 months for recovery
    - Nerve injury most often due to thermal injury or neuropraxia from bullet rather than transection[15]
- Closed injuries
  - Physical examination localizes to area of known entrapment:
    - EMG no earlier than 3 to 4 weeks
      - If no recovery, consider surgery for decompression
      - If partial recovery, consider continued observation versus surgical exploration with nerve conduction studies (NCS)
  - Physical examination does not localize injury:
    - Observe with EMG until 3 months
    - If no recovery, plan for surgery with intra-op NCS and neurolysis versus nerve graft
- Pain control—necessary for neuropathic type pain including burning and dysesthesias
  - Can use selective serotonin reuptake inhibitors, gabapentin, baclofen, and tricyclic antidepressants[1] for reduction of hypersensitivity and nerve excitability
  - Nonsteroidal anti-inflammatory drugs
  - Opioids
  - Topical agents—lidocaine patch, capsaicin

DEFINITIVE TREATMENT

- Nonoperative treatment
  - Observation with serial EMG for first- to third-degree injuries
    - Should recover without intervention
    - EMG will show fibrillations at 4 to 6 weeks
    - Consider surgery if no recovery on EMG by 3 months

- Surgical indications
  - Fourth- and fifth-degree injuries
    - Sharp laceration/transection—immediate reconstruction within 72 hours[1]
      - * Nerve ends not contused so can repair right away
      - * If not repaired acutely, can have retraction of proximal and distal stumps, making graft necessary at time of reconstruction with less optimal results
    - Blunt or avulsion injuries—early reconstruction at several weeks postinjury
      - * Can tack down stumps at time of vascular repair to prohibit retraction
      - * Assess viability of nerve ends prior to repair and resect scar as necessary
    - Delayed reconstruction for uncertain nerve continuity or when natural recovery could be better than surgical intervention
      - * Follow EMG and intervene by 3 to 6 months
  - Contraindications to surgery
    - Delay of surgery longer than 18 to 24 months can lead to irreversible muscle atrophy and fibrosis can occur. Attempting reinnervation after this time does not provide any benefit to the patient.
- Surgical approaches
  - External neurolysis—decompress scar and fibrosis from partially injured nerve[1]
    - Incise epineurium to ensure release of scar
  - Direct (end-to-end) repair
    - Requires skeletal stability, clean wound, appropriate vascularity, no crush
    - Immediate/early primary repair improves outcomes.[16]
    - Direct repair with some tension is better than nerve graft with no tension.[17]
    - Completely resect damaged nerve tissue back to healthy fascicles to avoid repair within the zone of injury (which leads to intraneural scar).[12]
    - Properly realign motor and sensory zones within the nerve for optimal outcomes.[12]
    - Prophylactically release zones of compression such as the carpal and cubital tunnel to avoid nerve regeneration stalling at these areas.[12]
    - No functional difference between fascicular and epineurial repair but studies have shown:

* More accurate axonal alignment with fascicular repair
* Potential for increased scar and blood supply damage with fascicular repair[17]
- Fibrin glue can be used additionally to minimize suture trauma (equal parts of thrombin and fibrinogen)[18]
- For distal forearm and wrist lacerations, take intraneural topography of fascicular groups into account when repairing
  * Three terminal branches of ulnar nerve at proximal palm[19]:
    ▲ Branch to hypothenar musculature and interossei is most ulnar-dorsal
      ◆ Important to align these groups during repair in order to enhance chance of intrinsic muscle recovery
    ▲ Cutaneous branch to fourth web space/common digital nerve
    ▲ Branch to hypothenar skin and ulnar aspect of small finger
  * Three fascicular main groups of the median nerve at the wrist and distal forearm[19]:
    ▲ Two sensory fascicular groups on ulnar aspect become common digital nerves to second and third web spaces
    ▲ One large fascicular group on the radial side that includes sensory and motor to radial digital nerve of index finger, two digital nerves to the thumb. Motor to thenar musculature on volar-radial aspect
- Nerve grafting
  - Required when direct repair has too much tension or is not possible
  - Autograft
    * Scaffold with neurotrophic factors, viable Schwann cells for axonal regeneration
    * Nonimmunogenic
    * Select based on size of nerve gap, location, associated donor site morbidity
    * Common grafts[11]:
      ▲ Medial and lateral antebrachial cutaneous nerves
      ▲ Dorsal cutaneous branch of ulnar nerve
      ▲ Superficial and deep peroneal nerves
      ▲ Intercostal nerves
      ▲ Posterior and lateral cutaneous nerves of thigh
      ▲ Sural nerve
    * Cable graft—multiple small caliber nerves aligned in parallel for size mismatch

* Trunk graft—mixed motor-sensory whole-nerve graft
  ▲ Poor results because of thickness and inability to revascularize
* Vascularized graft—only for long graft in poorly vascularized area
  ▲ Commonly used for brachial plexus injuries
* Techniques
  ▲ Reverse graft to avoid distal branch axonal dispersion
  ▲ Make graft 10% to 20% longer than gap to account for shortening with fibrosis
  ▲ Protect graft by immobilizing for 4 weeks until normal nerve tensile strength is reached.[3]
* Cons—sensory loss at donor site, limited supply of donors, second surgical site, neuroma formation at donor site, inferior to primary tension-free repair[12]

◆ Allograft
  * Current processed nerve allograft techniques yield no tissue rejection, implant complications, or adverse experiences[20]
  * Offers meaningful recovery with grafts[20] of 5 to 50 mm
  * No donor site morbidity
  * Quicker surgical time without graft harvest
  * If grafts are freeze-thawed or treated with detergent, this destroys immunogenicity and grafts can have equivalent outcomes to autograft[21]

◆ Conduit
  * No donor morbidity but no neurotrophic factors or Schwann cells
  * Conduit acts as barrier to scar and prevents neuroma formation by guiding axon growth
  * For gaps shorter than 3 cm or limited to noncritical sensory nerves because of variable results[12,14,22]
  * Caprolactone conduits equivalent to autograft in results
    ▲ Collagen conduits next best, polyglycolic acid conduits functionally inferior[14]
  * Reduced operative time[22]
  * Large nerve diameter may predispose to conduit failure[22]

● Nerve transfer—established for proximal/brachial plexus injury but also reasonable if patient presents delayed, scarring at injury site, segmental loss of nerve function, or if injury is a long distance from target organ.[12] Can provide earlier reinnervation than direct repair if target is very distal.
  ◆ Commonly used nerve transfers[18]:
    * See Table 36.3

TABLE 36.3 Common Upper Extremity Nerve Transfers

Injured Nerve	Missing Function	Donor Nerve	Recipient Nerve	Timing	Reinnervation	Notes
Suprascapular	Shoulder abduction, external rotation	Distal spinal accessory	Suprascapular	Injuries less than 6-9 mo old	EMG shows reinnervation by 6 mo	Transfer only middle and distal branches of spinal accessory
Long thoracic	Scapula stabilization, forward abduction	Medial pectoral, thoracodorsal, intercostal	Long thoracic			
Axillary	Shoulder abduction	Triceps branch of radial nerve, medial pectoral	Axillary	Injuries less than 6-9 mo old	EMG shows reinnervation by 6 mo	Select size-matched branch of nerve for transfer
Musculocutaneous	Elbow flexion	Ulnar nerve fascicle to FCU; median nerve fascicle to FCR, FDS	Brachialis branch; biceps branch			
Musculocutaneous	Elbow flexion	Intercostal	Musculocutaneous	Injuries less than 6-9 mo old	Reinnervation starts 6-9 mo post-op	Technically demanding with potential nerve tension, pleural tear
Spinal accessory	Shoulder elevation and abduction	Medial pectoral, C7 redundant fascicle	Spinal accessory			
Ulnar	Intrinsic hand	Terminal AIN (branch to pronator quadratus)	Ulnar nerve fascicles to deep motor branch			
Median	Thumb opposition	Terminal AIN (branch to pronator quadratus)	Median (recurrent) motor			

(continued)

TABLE 36.3 Common Upper Extremity Nerve Transfers (continued)

Injured Nerve	Missing Function	Donor Nerve	Recipient Nerve	Timing	Reinnervation	Notes
Median	Finger flexion	FCU, brachialis	AIN			
Median	Pronation	ECRB, FCU, FDS	Pronator branch			
Radial	Wrist and finger extension	FCR, FDS ± PL	ECRB and PIN			
Sensory						
Median sensory	Thumb-index key pinch area sensation	Ulnar common sensory branch to fourth web space	Median common sensory branch to first web space			
Median sensory	Thumb-index key pinch area sensation	Dorsal sensory branch of the ulnar nerve	Median common sensory branch to first web space			
Ulnar sensory	Ring and small finger sensation	Median common sensory branch to the third web space	Ulnar common sensory branch to the fourth web space; ulnar digital nerve to the small finger			
Ulnar sensory	Ulnar border of the hand sensation	Lateral antebrachial	Dorsal sensory branch of the ulnar nerve			

Abbreviations: AIN, anterior interosseous nerve; ECRB, extensor carpi radialis brevis; EMG, electromyography; FCR, flexor carpi radialis; FCU, flexor carpi ulnaris; FDS, flexor digitorum superficialis; PIN, posterior interosseous nerve; PL, palmaris longus.

Ray WZ, Mackinnon SE. Management of nerve gaps: autografts, allografts, nerve transfers, and end-to-side neurorrhaphy. *Exp Neurol.* 2010;223:77-85; Green DP, Wolfe SW. *Green's Operative Hand Surgery.* Philadelphia, PA: Elsevier/Churchill Livingstone; 2011.

- ◆ Attempt to size match and match sensory/motor function if possible
- ◆ Con to nerve transfer—donor muscle can no longer be used as a muscle transfer
- Muscular neurotization—for patients with loss of supplying motor nerve, a nerve graft is directly sewn to the target muscle neuromuscular junction.
  - ◆ Neurotization capable of innervating de novo motor end plates in chronically denervated muscle, thus may offer improved outcomes in patients with chronic injury past the point appropriate for nerve grafting[23]
- Potential surgical complications
  - ◆ Often due to delayed referral to surgeon with expertise in treating peripheral nerve injuries—observation for too long prior to surgical intervention leads to less satisfactory outcomes
  - ◆ Severe neurogenic pain may persist after repair.
  - ◆ Recovery after repair or grafting of fourth- and fifth-degree injuries rarely produces a completely normal motor and sensory function.
- ■ Postoperative expectations and care
  - Different nerves have different recovery potentials:
    - ◆ Although sensory recovery is similar between the median, radial, and ulnar nerves, motor recovery is better for radial than ulnar and median high-level repair.[24] Lower-level nerve repairs have more similar outcomes.
  - Therapy and rehabilitation—require reeducation to optimize outcomes after nerve repair or transfer. Motor and somatosensory reorganization depends on patient participation in sensory and motor rehabilitation.[25,26]
    - ◆ Ultrasound applied transcutaneously can accelerate recovery after axonotmesis injury[27]
    - ◆ Transcutaneous electrical nerve stimulation may be useful[1]
    - ◆ Desensitization for pain reduction
    - ◆ Static or dynamic splinting depending on concurrent injuries may protect repair and decrease inflammation

REFERENCES

1. Campbell WW. Evaluation and management of peripheral nerve injury. *Clin Neurophysiol.* 2008;119:1951-1965.
2. Lee SK, Wolfe SW. Peripheral nerve injury and repair. *J Am Acad Orthop Surg.* 2000;8:243-252.
3. Sunderland S. *Nerve Injuries and Their Repair: A Critical Appraisal* [reprint]. 1st ed. Edinburgh, NY: Churchill Livingstone; 1991.

4. Kouyoumdjian JA. Peripheral nerve injuries: a retrospective survey of 456 cases. *Muscle Nerve.* 2006;34:785-788.

5. Taylor CA, Braza D, Rice JB, Dillingham T. The incidence of peripheral nerve injury in extremity trauma. *Am J Phys Med Rehabil.* 2008;87:381-385.

6. Noble J, Munro CA, Prasad VS, Midha R. Analysis of upper and lower extremity peripheral nerve injuries in a population of patients with multiple injuries. *J Trauma.* 1998;45:116-122.

7. Filler AG, Kliot M, Howe FA, et al. Application of magnetic resonance neurography in the evaluation of patients with peripheral nerve pathology. *J Neurosurg.* 1996;85:299-309.

8. Bendszus M, Wessig C, Solymosi L, Reiners K, Koltzenburg M. MRI of peripheral nerve degeneration and regeneration: correlation with electrophysiology and histology. *Exp Neurol.* 2004;188:171-177.

9. Zhu J, Liu F, Li D, Shao J, Hu B. Preliminary study of the types of traumatic peripheral nerve injuries by ultrasound. *Eur Radiol.* 2011;21:1097-1101.

10. He B, Zhu Z, Zhu Q, et al. Factors predicting sensory and motor recovery after the repair of upper limb peripheral nerve injuries. *Neural Regen Res.* 2014;9:661-672.

11. Mackinnon SE, Dellon AL. *Surgery of the Peripheral Nerve.* New York: Stuttgart/Thieme Medical Publishers/G. Thieme Verlag; 1988.

12. Ray WZ, Mackinnon SE. Management of nerve gaps: autografts, allografts, nerve transfers, and end-to-side neurorrhaphy. *Exp Neurol.* 2010;223:77-85.

13. Haase J, Bjerre P, Simesen K. Median and ulnar nerve transections treated with microsurgical interfascicular cable grafting with autogenous sural nerve. *J Neurosurg.* 1980;53:73-84.

14. Deal DN, Griffin JW, Hogan MV. Nerve conduits for nerve repair or reconstruction. *J Am Acad Orthop Surg.* 2012;20:63-68.

15. Kline DG. Timing for brachial plexus injury: a personal experience. *Neurosurg Clin N Am.* 2009;20:24-26, v.

16. Mackinnon SE. New directions in peripheral nerve surgery. *Ann Plast Surg.* 1989;22:257-273.

17. Hentz VR, Rosen JM, Xiao SJ, McGill KC, Abraham G. The nerve gap dilemma: a comparison of nerves repaired end to end under tension with nerve grafts in a primate model. *J Hand Surg.* 1993;18:417-425.

18. Narakas A. The use of fibrin glue in repair of peripheral nerves. *Orthop Clin North Am.* 1988;19:187-199.

19. Chow JA, Van Beek AL, Bilos ZJ, Meyer DL, Johnson MC. Anatomical basis for repair of ulnar and median nerves in the distal part of the forearm by group fascicular suture and nerve-grafting. *J Bone Joint Surg Am.* 1986;68:273-280.

20. Cho MS, Rinker BD, Weber RV, Chao JD, Ingari JV, Brooks D, Buncke GM. Functional outcome following nerve repair in the upper extremity using processed nerve allograft. *J Hand Surg.* 2012;37:2340-2349.

21. Dumont CE, Hentz VR. Enhancement of axon growth by detergent-extracted nerve grafts. *Transplantation.* 1997;63:1210-1215.

22. Moore AM, Kasukurthi R, Magill CK, Farhadi HF, Borschel GH, Mackinnon SE. Limitations of conduits in peripheral nerve repairs. *Hand N Y N.* 2009;4:180-186.

23. Swanson AN, Wolfe SW, Khazzam M, Feinberg J, Ehteshami J, Doty S. Comparison of neurotization versus nerve repair in an animal model of chronically denervated muscle. *J Hand Surg.* 2008;33:1093-1099.

24. Roganovic Z, Pavlicevic G. Difference in recovery potential of peripheral nerves after graft repairs. *Neurosurgery.* 2006;59:621-633.

25. Malessy MJ, Bakker D, Dekker AJ, Van Duk JG, Thomeer RT. Functional magnetic resonance imaging and control over the biceps muscle after intercostal-musculocutaneous nerve transfer. *J Neurosurg.* 2003;98:261-268.

26. Oud T, Beelen A, Eijffinger E, Nollet F. Sensory re-education after nerve injury of the upper limb: a systematic review. *Clin Rehabil.* 2007;21:483-494.

27. Mourad PD, Lazar DA, Curra FP, et al. Ultrasound accelerates functional recovery after peripheral nerve damage. *Neurosurgery.* 2001;48:1136-1141.

Rachel Michael, Roy E. Schneider, and Margaret Jain

INTRODUCTION

- **Pathoanatomy**
  - Nerve layers (from deep to superficial)[1]
    - Endoneurium—Connective tissue that surrounds each axon or nerve fiber
    - Perineurium—Strong layer of connective tissue that surrounds each fascicle and can withstand high pressures
    - Epineurium—Outer layer that covers the entire nerve, allows for nerve gliding and protection
  - **Median nerve** (C5-T1) traverses the forearm and runs through the carpal tunnel. Proximal to the carpal tunnel, the *palmar cutaneous branch* divides from the median nerve proximal to the wrist and provides sensation to the radial palm. The *recurrent motor branch* divides from the median nerve at or around the level of the carpal tunnel and supplies most of the thenar muscles. The median nerve divides into the *common digital nerves,* which subsequently divide into *proper digital nerves.* Proper digital nerves supply the radial three digits and the radial side of the ring finger. Dorsal sensory nerves branch from the proper digital nerves just proximal to the proximal interphalangeal joint and travel dorsal to supply sensation to the dorsal, distal fingers.
  - **Ulnar nerve** (C7-T1) traverses the forearm deep to the flexor carpi ulnaris muscle belly and tendon. Five centimeters proximal to the wrist crease, the *dorsal cutaneous branch* splits from the ulnar nerve to provide sensory innervation of the dorsal, ulnar hand, whereas a *palmar cutaneous branch* provides sensation to the ulnar palm via branching *dorsal digital nerves.* The ulnar nerve proper continues through Guyon canal, distal to which it divides into a *sensory branch* and a *(deep) motor branch.* The sensory branch divides in the mid-palm into common and proper digital nerves, which supply sensation

to the ulnar side of the ring finger and the small finger. The deep motor branch innervates the intrinsic muscles of the hand.
- At the finger level, the digital nerves run volar to the digital arteries.
- **Mechanism of injury**
  - Seddon classification
    - I—Neurapraxia[1] (first-degree injury)
      - Temporary loss of nerve conduction without axonal disruption
    - II—Axonotmesis[1]
      - Axons are cut though Schwann cells and surrounding nerve layers remain intact.
      - Usually a result of a crush or traction injury
      - Wallerian degeneration occurs distal to injury.
    - III—Neurotmesis[1]
      - Complete nerve disruption
      - Requires surgical intervention for recovery
      - Wallerian degeneration occurs distal to injury.

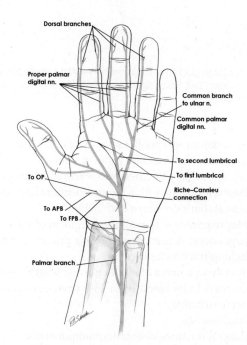

FIGURE 37.1 Anatomic course of the median nerve. APB, abductor pollicis brevis; FPB, flexor pollicis brevis; OP, opponens pollicis.

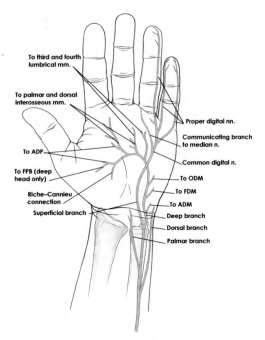

FIGURE 37.2 Anatomic course of the ulnar nerve. ADM, abductor digiti minimi; ADP, adductor pollicis; FDM, flexor digiti minimi; FPB, flexor pollicis brevis; ODM, opponens digiti minimi.

- Injury mechanism will predict severity of injury and recovery
  - Sharp injuries have smaller zones of injury.
  - Crush injuries are associated with severe and diffuse tissue injury.
    - Edema formation within the endoneurium leads to diminished axonal transport/nerve dysfunction.
    - May require resection of larger segment of nerve, resulting in larger nerve deficits, may preclude primary repair
  - Stretching/traction injuries
    - Stretching a nerve 8% of its normal length results in a 50% decrease in its blood flow; 15% stretch results in complete nerve ischemia.[2]
- Associated injuries
  - Phalangeal fractures/dislocations/amputations
  - Digital artery injury
  - Flexor tendon injuries

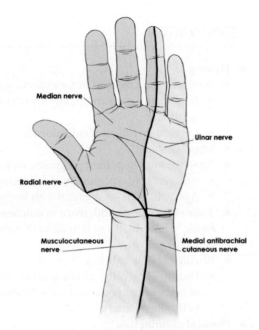

FIGURE 37.3 Sensory distribution of the volar surface of the distal forearm, wrist, and hand.

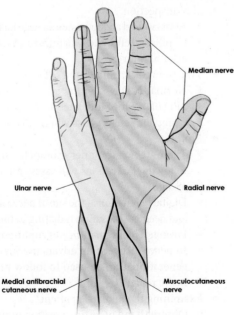

FIGURE 37.4 Sensory distribution of the dorsal distal forearm, wrist, and hand.

EVALUATION

- **History**
  - Significant past medical history affecting nerve function:
    - Neuropathy, most commonly diabetes mellitus or cubital tunnel syndrome
    - Cervical myelopathy/radiculopathy
  - Smoking status
  - Age—the most important prognostic factor for recovery after repair
    - <12 years old—possibility of full recovery
    - Age > 40 years—associated with worse sensory recovery
  - Time of injury—no difference in outcomes from time of injury to repair.[1] However, delay in treatment influences type or feasibility of primary repair.
  - Bleeding at time of injury
    - History of excessive bleeding at time of injury highly indicative of nerve injury because of volar location of the nerve in relation to the digital artery.
- **Physical examination**
  - Skin inspection
    - Assess wound and soft tissue damage for possible need for flap coverage
    - Capillary refill and warmth to assess perfusion and potential arterial injury
  - Two-point discrimination (2PD)
    - Normal 2PD is ≤6 mm
    - 2PD of ≥8 mm indicates loss of protective sensation
    - Complete sensory loss when 2PD is >25 mm
  - Motor
    - There are no motor nerve branches in digits. Motor examination following lacerations will assess for associated tendon injury.
  - Tinel sign[3]
    - Digital percussion at the site of nerve injury produces pain or "pins and needles" sensation radiating in the sensory nerve distribution.
    - Positive Tinel sign indicates ruptured axons of the affected nerve.
    - In nerve recovery, an advancing Tinel move indicates nerve re-generation. Can be used to follow progression of recovery after nerve repair.
  - Examining the pediatric patient[4]
    - Observe hand in resting position noting any obvious deformities, injuries, and spontaneous movements.

- ◆ Sensory examination—observe trophic changes, color, and presence of sweat. Ask parents' opinion about sensation.
  - ✳ Skin wrinkle test—used to identify nerve injury in a noncooperative patient. When submerged in water, a finger with a digital nerve injury will not demonstrate normal skin wrinkling.[5]
- **Imaging**
  - Plain films are necessary only where there is concern for a retained foreign body or to rule out associated fractures.

ACUTE MANAGEMENT

- Patients should receive antibiotics for dirty wounds
  - First-generation cephalosporin (Cefazolin) in most patients
  - Add penicillin for farm injuries
  - If patient has a beta-lactam allergy—vancomycin or clindamycin
- Tetanus if indicated
- Bedside irrigation to clean wound, repair of lacerations if delayed repair is planned
- Educate patient on the expectations of recovery

DEFINITIVE TREATMENT

- Nonoperative
  - Neurapraxia usually recovers spontaneously. Treated with reassurance, monitoring patient's sensory recovery.
- Surgical indications
  - Open wound with distal sensory loss is assumed to represent nerve laceration.
  - Goal of surgery—improve sensation and prevent neuroma formation
- Operative techniques
  - Primary nerve repair (neurorrhaphy)[6]
    - ◆ Indications—acute injury, clean nerve transection with gapping only secondary to elastic retraction. Repair must be tension-free. Best utilized within 10 to 14 days of injury.
    - ◆ Contraindications—if nerve gap is large, or if there is tension on repair
  - Nerve grafting (autograft or allograft)[6]
    - ◆ Indications—inability to repair nerves in a tension-free manner because of

  * Traditional "gold standard" treatment when primary nerve repair is not possible
- Autograft options:
  * Lateral antebrachial cutaneous nerve—best size match for digital nerve injuries between metacarpophalangeal and distal interphalangeal.
  * Sural nerve—best size match for injuries near common digital bifurcation
  * Others—anterior interosseous nerve, posterior interosseous nerve, medial antebrachial cutaneous nerves
- Allograft (cadaveric decellularized tissue)[7]
  * Advantages
    - Unlimited supply of graft material without loss of sensation from a donor site
    - Ideal for larger nerve gaps (>3 cm)
    - Reported improved sensory function relative to conduits[8]
  * Disadvantages—cost
- Nerve conduits
  - Synthetic (polyglycolic acid or collagen conduits)[9]
    * Degradable conduits (collagen, chitin, polyglycolic acid)
      - Similar outcomes to autologous nerve grafts with short nerve gap (1 cm or less) without donor sensory loss[9]
      - Disadvantage—cost, possibility of being inferior to allograft
  - Autologous venous nerve conduits
    * Advantage—less cost compared to synthetic conduits, and no cutaneous sensory loss compared to autologous nerve grafting
    * Disadvantage—poorer results in delayed nerve repair, technically difficult
  - Indications
    * <3 cm gap for sensory nerves only. Can also be used in conjunction with digital reimplantation. Also indicated with concurrent zone II flexor tendon injuries. Also used to bridge nerve gaps after resection of tumors or neuromas
  - Contraindications—nonviable nerve ends, infection/sepsis, or poor soft tissue coverage
- Surgical approaches[10]
  - Midlateral
    * A longitudinal incision on the lateral side of the digit. Start at the most dorsal portion of the volar skin crease at the proximal

phalangeal joint and extend distally, staying slightly dorsal, just past the distal phalangeal joint skin crease.

◆ Volar Brunner incision
  ✳ Zigzag incisions in diagonal fashion through the volar phalangeal pads. Note—the digital nerve and vessel are separated from the volar subcutaneous tissue by Grayson ligament.

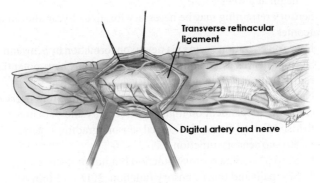

FIGURE 37.5 Midlateral approach.

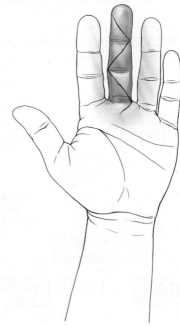

FIGURE 37.6 Brunner incision.

- Postoperative care
  - Immobilization—for 3 to 10 days in intrinsic plus position
  - Early range of motion[11]
    - For isolated nerve injuries, immediate immobilization protects the repair; however, early joint range of motion is needed for nerve gliding and to prevent stiffness. Strength exercises can begin at 6 weeks.
  - Sensory retraining may be necessary for up to 1 year after injury.
- Outcomes
  - Nerve regeneration occurs via new axon formation by Schwann cells. Sensory nerves lack a motor end plate and thus have potential for reinnervation even long after injury.
  - Nerves regenerate at a rate of approximately 1 to 2 mm every day.
  - Outcomes dependent on injury type/severity and patient age.
  - British Medical Research Council sensory grading system:
    - S0—no sensory function
    - S1 to S2—some sensory function but not protective
    - S3—pain and touch sensory function, 2PD >15 mm
    - S3+—2PD 7 to 15 mm
    - S4—normal sensory function

MANAGEMENT ALGORITHM

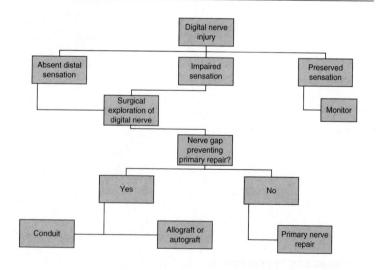

REFERENCES

1. Brunton LM. Nerve injuries and nerve transfers. In: Boyer MI, ed. *AAOS Comprehensive Orthopaedic Review*. Rosemont, IL: American Academy of Orthopaedic Surgeons; 2014.
2. Slutsky DJ. The management of digital nerve injuries. *J Hand Surg*. 2014;39(6):1208-1215.
3. Green DP. *Green's Operative Hand Surgery*. Philadelphia, PA: Elsevier/Churchill Livingstone; 2005.
4. Staheli LT. Upper limb. In: Staheli LT, ed. *Fundamentals of Pediatric Orthopedics*. Philadelphia, PA: Wolters Kluwer Health/Lippincott Williams & Wilkins; 2008:chap 13.
5. Phelps PE, Walker E. Comparison of the finger wrinkling test results to established sensory tests in peripheral nerve injury. *Am J Occup Ther*. 1977;31(9):565-572.
6. Isaacs J. Nerve repair: primary, autograft, allograft, conduits, and transfers. In: Murray P, Hammert W, eds. *Hand Surgery Update VI*. Chicago, IL: American Society for Surgery of the Hand; 2016:287-292.
7. Karabekmez FE, Duymaz A, Moran SL. Early clinical outcomes with the use of decellularized nerve allograft for repair of sensory defects within the hand. *Hand*. 2009;4(3):245-249.
8. Means KR, Rinker BD, Higgins JP, Payne SH Jr, Merrell GA, Wilgis EF. A multicenter, prospective, randomized, pilot study of outcomes for digital nerve repair in the hand using hollow conduit compared with processed allograft nerve. *Hand*. 2016;11(2):144-151.
9. Muheremu A, Ao Q. Past, present, and future of nerve conduits in the treatment of peripheral nerve injury. *BioMed Res Int*. 2015; 2015:1-6.
10. Hoppenfeld S, DeBoer P. The wrist and hand. In: Hoppenfeld S, DeBoer P, eds. *Surgical Exposures in Orthopaedics: The Anatomic Approach*. 4th ed. Philadelphia, PA: Lippincott Williams & Wilkins; 2003:184-255:chap 5.
11. Yu RS, Catalano LW III, Barron OA, Johnson C, Glickel SZ. Limited, protected postsurgical motion does not affect the results of digital nerve repair. *J Hand Surg*. 2004;29(2):302-306.

38 Median Nerve Injuries

Sohaib K. Malik and Alan R. Koester

INTRODUCTION

- Pathoanatomy
  - Median nerve derived from medial and lateral cords of brachial plexus contains fibers from all five nerve roots (C5-T1).
  - Median nerve runs down the medial aspect of the arm in the anterior compartment, medial to the biceps and brachialis (initially lateral to brachial artery), then crosses over brachial artery, and becomes medial to it just before the antecubital fossa.
  - Enters forearm between pronator teres and under the bicipital aponeurosis (lacertus fibrosus).
    - Median nerve gives motor branches to pronator teres, flexor carpi radialis (FCR), palmaris longus, and flexor digitorum superficialis (FDS).
  - Median nerve then travels between flexor digitorum profundus (FDP) and FDS and emerges between FDP and flexor pollicis longus (FPL).
    - Anterior interosseous nerve branches proximally, runs along the interosseous membrane between FPL and FDP, gives sensory innervation to volar wrist capsule, and motor to FDP to 2nd/3rd digits, FPL, and pronator quadratus.
    - The palmar cutaneous branch divides 5 cm proximal to wrist and runs between the FCR and palmaris longus, supplying sensation to lateral hand and palm.
  - The nerve then enters the hand via the carpal tunnel, along with the tendons of FDS, FDP, and FPL.
    - Motor recurrent branch divides after (50%), under (30%), or through (20%) the transverse carpal ligament and innervates abductor pollicis brevis, opponens pollicis, and flexor pollicis brevis (superficial head only).
    - Palmar digital branches and proper palmar digital branch supplies sensory to the volar aspects of the thumb, index, middle and radial aspect of the ring finger, as well as the dorsal/distal aspects of these fingers.

- ◆ The radial two lumbricals are also supplied by the median nerve.
- ■ Mechanism of injury
  - ● Etiologies include penetrating trauma, crush, traction, ischemia, and less common mechanisms such as thermal and electric shock, radiation, percussion, and vibration.[1]
  - ● Lacerations
    - ◆ Usually because of penetrating trauma, fractures, gunshot wound (GSW)
  - ● Stretching/compression/crush
    - ◆ Blunt trauma, fracture malunion, iatrogenic with prolonged tourniquet use or retraction
    - ◆ 8% elongation will diminish nerve's microcirculation, 15% elongation will disrupt axons.
- ■ Epidemiology
  - ● Estimated 2% to 3% of patients admitted to trauma centers have peripheral nerve injuries, and this percentage is higher if plexus and root injuries are included.[2]
  - ● Traumatic median nerve injury is the second most common isolated nerve injury behind ulnar nerve injury.[3,4]
  - ● 2700 admissions in 2006 for median nerve injuries costing in the range of 28 000 dollars[3]

EVALUATION

- ■ History
  - ● Paresthesia and numbness of palm, volar thumb, index, long, and radial ring finger, as well as dorsal/distal tips of these digits
  - ● History of blunt or penetrating trauma, fractures, traction injuries to shoulder
- ■ Physical examination
  - ● Inspection of any open wounds if acute injuries. If long-term nerve injury, thenar atrophy as well as hand deformities apparent
  - ● Injury to median nerve at different levels causes different syndromes.
    - ◆ Above the elbow (eg, a supracondylar humerus fracture vs GSW/ stab wound)
      - ✳ Loss of pronation of forearm, weakness in flexion of the hand at the wrist, loss of flexion of radial half of digits and thumb, loss of abduction and opposition of thumb[5]
      - ✳ Presence of ape hand deformity when hand is at rest because of hyperextension of index finger and thumb, and an adducted thumb
        - ▲ See Figure 38.1

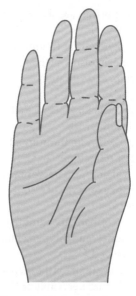

FIGURE 38.1 Ape hand.

- ❋ Presence of benediction sign when attempting to form a fist because of loss of flexion of radial half of digits[5]
  - ▲ See Figure 38.2
- ❋ Sensory deficit: loss of volar sensation in thumb, index, long, and radial ring finger, as well as distal/dorsal aspect of these digits, and loss of sensation to the palm[5]
- ◆ In proximal forearm (eg, tight cast/splint or forearm fracture)
  - ❋ Anterior interosseous nerve syndrome
  - ❋ Loss of pronation of forearm, loss of flexion of radial half of digits and thumb
- ◆ At the wrist (ie, wrist laceration)
  - ❋ Loss of abduction and opposition of thumb
  - ❋ Presence of ape hand deformity when hand is at rest may be likely secondary to denervation of the thenar muscles
- ● Sensory examination can reveal impaired sensation of the thumb, index, long, and ring finger using two-point discrimination or Semmes-Weinstein monofilament testing.
- ● Patients with a nerve injury will often develop Tinel's sign over the site of nerve injury. This is performed by gently tapping along the nerve to discern the level of injury, which causes the patient to experience an electrical sensation that propagates distally along the nerve distribution.[5]
  - ◆ After nerve is repaired, this sign should propagate distally along the nerve as axons regenerate.[5]

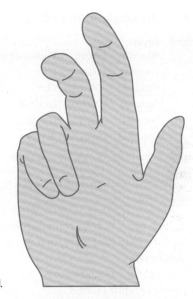

FIGURE 38.2 Benedict hand.

TABLE 38.1 Seddon Type Classification for Nerve Injury

Seddon Type	Degree	Myelin Intact	Axon Intact	Endoneurium Intact	Wallerian Degeneration	Reversible
Neurapraxia	1st	No	Yes	Yes	No	Reversible
Axonotmesis	2nd	No	No	Yes	Yes	Reversible
Neurotmesis	3rd	No	No	No	Yes	Irreversible

From Birch R. Compound nerve injury. In: Birch R, ed. *Surgical Disorders of the Peripheral Nerves.* 2nd ed. Edinburgh, Scotland: Churchill Livingstone; 1975:89-111; Menorca RMG, Fussell TS, Elfar JC. Peripheral nerve trauma: mechanisms of injury and recovery. *Hand Clin.* 2013;29(3):317-330; Dahlin LB, Wiberg M. Nerve injuries of the upper extremity and hand. *EFORT Open Rev.* 2017;2(5):158-170.

- Classification
  - See Tables 38.1 and 38.2

ACUTE MANAGEMENT

- After initial evaluation, neurapraxia/axonotmesis versus neurotmesis needs to be determined as this will likely guide surgical intervention.[6]
- Workup
  - Plain radiographs
    - Upper extremity fractures associated with paresthesias need to be reduced to decrease tension on the nerve. In particular, the

AQ7   **TABLE 38.2** **Sunderland Type Classification for Nerve Injury**

Sunderland Grade	Myelin Sheath	Axon	Endoneurium	Perineurium	Epineurium
I	Disrupted	Intact	Intact	Intact	Intact
II	Disrupted	Disrupted	Intact	Intact	Intact
III	Disrupted	Disrupted	Disrupted	Intact	Intact
IV	Disrupted	Disrupted	Disrupted	Disrupted	Intact
V	Disrupted	Disrupted	Disrupted	Disrupted	Disrupted

From Menorca RMG, Fussell TS, Elfar JC. Peripheral nerve trauma: mechanisms of injury and recovery. *Hand Clin.* 2013;29(3):317-330; Dahlin LB, Wiberg M. Nerve injuries of the upper extremity and hand. *EFORT Open Rev.* 2017;2(5):158-170; Sunderland S. *Nerves and Nerve Injuries.* 2nd ed. New York, NY: Churchill Livingstone; 1978:133-138.

median nerve may be compromised in supracondylar humerus fracture, both bone forearm fracture, and distal radius fractures.

- CT angiogram
  - Concern for vascular injury
- Electromyography (EMG)
  - Can be performed 3-6 months following nerve injury to establish a baseline
    - Can be helpful to distinguish between neurapraxia, axonotmesis, and neurotmesis as well as to follow progression after treatment[7]
- Ultrasound (US)
  - Examine nerve continuity[8]
- MRI/CT myelography
  - Can be used to view muscle denervation, sites of compression, nerve disruption, as well as more proximal injuries, such as nerve root avulsions[9]
- Intraoperative nerve action potentials
  - Can be used to assess status of injury to a nerve that is in continuity as well as determining whether a lesion is nonfunctioning (eg, neuroma)[10]

DEFINITIVE TREATMENT

- Operative indications
  - Neurotmesis with sharp transection of the nerve
  - Nerve injury with associated vascular injury
  - Median nerve injury with gross contamination of wound
  - Distal radius fracture with acute carpal tunnel syndrome

- Neurapraxia or axonotmesis with no spontaneous recovery within a 6-month period
■ Indications to observe
  - Neurapraxia injuries
  - Axonotmesis injuries
■ Considerations for early explorations
  - Primarily dependent on mechanism of injury, time to presentation, and wound contamination
  - History of clean stab wound yields most amenable situation to early repair.
    - Acute repair within 7 days has superior outcomes to delayed repair.
    - Delayed repair may be necessary if soft tissue is grossly contaminated; however, this could result in fibrosis around nerve and increase in the likelihood for requiring a nerve graft.
■ Surgical technique
  - Approach to the median nerve depends upon where traumatic injury is located.
  - Key points
    - Nerve must be mobilized, tension free, and able to rotate 180° freely after completion of repair.
  - Nerve repair
    - Adventitial tissue is pushed back from each end of the neural stump to expose true epineurium. Bundles are then matched and drawn together using 10-0 nylon sutures. For median nerve, between 6 and 8 key bundles should be sutured together.[7]
    - 9-0 nylon sutures are passed through the perineurium and epineurium.
    - Epineurial repair is then performed with 9-0 nylon sutures. Number of sutures needed is dependent upon diameter of nerve fiber.[7]
  - Fibrin clot glue
    - Can use fibrin clot glue when repairing nerves, which lets surgeon use fewer sutures. Important to have the larger bundles in correct position before applying glue.
  - Nerve grafting
    - Indications
      * >3 cm gap
      * Sural nerve continues to be the autologous graft of choice for median nerve injuries.[5]
      * Can also use nerve conduits that are synthetic and biologic polymers used to bridge gaps up to 1cm

  * Decellularized allografts can also be used to assist with nerve repairs and has shown some promise.[5,11]
- Postoperative care
  - Forearm splinting with wrist in 30° of flexion for 3 weeks
  - Thumbs and fingers should be free. Wrist should be blocked beyond 30° but should allow full flexion.
  - Can start occupational therapy with vigorous, active flexion against resistance with gentle passive stretching exercises.[7]
- Complications
  - Early rupture of repair can be associated with pain and neuroma formation.
  - Failure to recover after primary nerve repair or nerve grafting necessitates reexploration and revision of repair.

REFERENCES

1. Robinson LR. Traumatic injury to peripheral nerves. *Suppl Clin Neurophysiol.* 2004;57:273-286.
2. Noble J, Munro CA, Prasad VS, Midha R. Analysis of upper and lower extremity peripheral nerve injuries in a population of patients with multiple injuries. *J Trauma.* 1998;45:116-122.
3. Lad SP, Nathan JK, Schubert RD, Boakye M. Trends in median, ulnar, radial, and brachioplexus nerve injuries in the United States. *Neurosurgery.* 2010;66(5):953-960.
4. Eser F, Aktekin LA, Bodur H, Atan C. Etiological factors of traumatic peripheral nerve injuries. *Neurol India.* 2009;57(4):434-437.
5. Pederson WC. Median nerve injury and repair. *J Hand Surg Am.* 2014;39:1216-1222.
6. Campbell WW. Evaluation and management of peripheral nerve injury. *Clin Neurophysiol.* 2008;119:1951-1965.
7. Birch R, Quick T. Nerve injury and repair. In: Wolff SW, Hotchkiss RN, Pederson WC, Kozin SH, Cohen MS, eds. *Green's Operative Hand Surgery.* 7th ed. Philadelphia, PA: Elsevier; 2017:979-1022.
8. Zhu J, Liu F, Li D, Shao J, Hu B. Preliminary study of the types of traumatic peripheral nerve injuries by ultrasound. *Eur Radiol.* 2011;21:1097-1101.
9. Grant GA, Goodkin R, Maravilla KR, Kliot M. MR neurography: diagnostic utility in the surgical treatment of peripheral nerve disorders. *Neuroimaging Clin N Am.* 2004;14(1):115-133. doi:10.1016/j.nic.2004.02.003.
10. Murovic JA. Upper-extremity peripheral nerve injuries: a Louisiana State University Health Sciences Center literature review with comparison of the operative outcomes of 1837 Louisiana State University Health Sciences Center median, radial, and ulnar nerve lesions. *Neurosurgery.* 2009;65(4 suppl):A11-A17. doi:10.1227/01.NEU.0000339130.90379.89.
11. Buncke GM, Ko JH, Thayer WP, Safa B. Comparison of outcomes from processed nerve allograft, hollow tube conduits, and autograft in peripheral nerve repair: level 3 evidence. *J Hand Surg.* 2014;39:e14.

39 Ulnar Nerve Injuries

Vishavpreet Singh, Ardalan Sayan,
and Alan R. Koester

INTRODUCTION

- Epidemiology
  - Ulnar nerve compression is the second most common upper extremity compressive neuropathy (only secondary to median nerve compression neuropathy), with an incidence of 25 and 19 cases per 10 000 person-years in men and women, respectively.[3]
  - Approximately 70% involve entrapments at the elbow level, 12% lacerations, 8% stretches/contusions, and 10% other (ie, gunshot wounds [GSW], fractures, tumors.)[2]
  - Typically affects males in working age group (18-45 years) with a median income of $36 000[1]
  - From 1993 to 2006, ulnar nerve injury was the most frequent major upper extremity peripheral nerve injury resulting in hospital admission when compared with median, radial, and brachial plexus injuries.[1]
  - Healthcare costs associated with ulnar nerve injuries range from $10 563 to $42 000 per individual.[1]
  - Recovery and functional results are inferior with repairs after ulnar nerve injuries when compared to those achieved following median and radial nerve repairs.[1,4,5]
- Mechanism of injury
  - Entrapment/compression (most common cause of ulnar nerve injury)
    - Multiple causes (intrinsic versus extrinsic) and sites of compression in the upper extremity (Table 39.1)
  - Lacerations
    - Usually because of penetrating trauma, GSW, fractures
  - Stretching/contusion
    - Blunt trauma, iatrogenic (ie, instrument positioning, prolonged tourniquet use), heterotrophic ossification, fractures, fracture malunion

TABLE 39.1 Sites of Ulnar Nerve Compression in the Upper Extremity

Around the neck and axilla
1. Cervical root impingement due to disc herniation, facet arthropathy, etc.
2. Masses (ie, Pancoast tumor, enlarged lymph nodes, hematomas)
3. Vascular lesions (ie, aneurysms)
Around the elbow
1. Most common sites
a. Between the two heads of FCU/aponeurosis
b. Within arcade of Struthers (hiatus in medial intermuscular septum)
c. Between Osborne ligament and MCL (cubital tunnel)
2. Less common sites
a. Medial intermuscular septum
b. Medial epicondyle
c. Fascial bands within FCU
d. Anconeus epitrochlearis
e. Fascia of FDS
f. Fractures and medial epicondyle nonunions
g. Heterotrophic ossification
h. Masses/cysts
i. Osteophytes
Around the wrist
1. Guyon canal: three zones
a. Zone 1: Proximal to bifurcation of the nerve, usually secondary to ganglia and hook of hamate fractures, and presents with mixed motor and sensory symptoms
b. Zone 2: Surrounds deep motor branch, usually secondary to ganglia and hook of hamate fractures, and presents with motor symptoms only
c. Zone 3: Surrounds superficial sensory branch, usually secondary to ulnar artery thrombosis or aneurysm, and presents with sensory symptoms only

Abbreviations: FCU, flexor carpi ulnaris; FDS, flexor digitorum superficialis; MCL, medial collateral ligament.

- Pathoanatomy
  - Anatomic course of the ulnar nerve throughout the upper extremity predisposes the nerve for injury as it passes through constricting areas of the elbow and wrist and becomes very superficial at other areas along its course.
  - Basic understanding of ulnar nerve anatomy and innervation patterns guides identification of the source of pathology.
    - Ulnar nerve consists of nerve fibers from C7 to T1 nerve roots and lies medial to brachial artery in the upper arm and exits the

posterior compartment as it descends down the humerus to enter the anterior compartment through the medial intermuscular septum.

◆ Enters the cubital tunnel posterior to medial epicondyle, medial to elbow joint capsule and medial collateral ligament

◆ After exiting the cubital tunnel, it gives off muscular branches to flexor carpi ulnaris (FCU) and enters volar aspect of the forearm through heads of FCU, supplying ulnar half of flexor digitorum profundus (FDP).

◆ In the forearm, it continues its course between FDP and flexor digitorum superficialis (FDS) and gives off the dorsal cutaneous branch (DCB) approximately 8 cm proximal to the pisiform bone. The DCB provides sensory innervation to small finger, ulnar aspect of ring finger, and ulnar aspect of carpus and hand.

◆ At the level of the wrist, the nerve bifurcates into superficial sensory and deep motor branches at the distal aspect of Guyon canal. Deep motor branch innervates the intrinsic and thumb adductor muscles and superficial sensory gives off the fourth common digital nerve and ulnar proper digital nerve to the small finger.

EVALUATION

■ History

● Paresthesias and numbness of the volar and dorsal sides of the small finger and the ulnar half of the ring finger

● Hand weakness secondary to intrinsic muscle weakness, which leads to reduced grip and pinch strength, difficulty opening bottles, or a loss of coordination during fine manipulation

● Occasionally, patients might complain of pain along the course of ulnar nerve from elbow into the ulnar forearm or hand

● Chronicity of the symptoms should be ascertained along with exacerbating and alleviating factors, comorbidities (ie, diabetes, hemophilia), and occupation (ie, person working with vibrating tools).

◆ Positions of the shoulder, elbow, and wrist that cause or exacerbate symptoms should be recorded.

＊ Elbow flexion—compression of cubital tunnel

＊ Overhead elevation—thoracic outlet syndrome

＊ Wrist flexion—entrapment in Guyon canal

- Physical examination
  - A systematic approach from the proximal origin of the nerve to the most distal aspect is required along with a through sensory and motor examination.
  - Inspection of the upper extremity may reveal cysts/masses along the course of ulnar nerve, deformities about the elbow joint (ie, carrying angle), atrophy of muscles of the hand.
    - Atrophy is most readily appreciated in the first dorsal interosseous muscle in the first web space.
  - Sensory examination reveals impaired sensation in little and ring fingers as quantified by two-point discrimination or Semmes–Weinstein monofilament testing.
    - Note—ulnar nerve injury distal to branching of DCB may present with normal sensation along the dorsal aspects of little and ulnar side of ring finger. Injuries at Guyon canal may also have varying presentation depending on zone of injury (see Table 39.1 for details).
  - Motor examination findings vary depending on the exact nature and chronicity of the injury, as motor function is usually not associated with mild compression. Moderate to severe or prolonged compression can cause muscle weakness and atrophy, whereas a complete transection presents with paralysis.
    - Resistive testing of FDS to the ring and little finger as well as ulnar nerve innervated small muscles in the hand must be performed.
    - Examiner should be aware of anomalous innervation patterns as seen in Martin–Gruber communication (seen in 7.5% of the population) or Riche–Cannieu anastomosis that may blur the clinical presentation.[6-8]
      - Loss of intrinsic muscles of hand leads to inability to flex at metacarpal joints and extend at interphalangeal (IP) joints.
        - Leads to intrinsic minus or claw posture of ring and little finger with hyperextension of metacarpophalangeal (MCP) and flexion at IP joints (Figure 39.1).
        - Note—development of clawing does require intact intrinsic extensor and flexor tendon function and, therefore, ulnar nerve injury at a point proximal to innervation of FDP results in less claw hand deformity because of loss of FDP.[9]
      - Intrinsic muscle weakness also leads to decreased pinch and grip strength

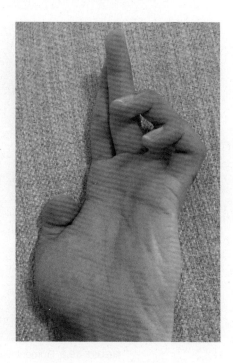

FIGURE 39.1 Ulnar claw posture of ring and little finger with hyperextension of metacarpophalangeal and flexion at interphalangeal joints.

- ▲ Paralysis of the adductor pollicis, deep head of flexor pollicis brevis, and first dorsal interosseus muscles leads to pinch strength decrease by 80%
- ▲ Froment sign—indicates loss of MCP flexion and adduction by adductor pollicis. Thumb IP flexion compensates for loss of thumb adduction when attempting to hold a piece of paper (Figure 39.2).
- ▲ Jeanne sign—a compensatory thumb MCP hyperextension and thumb adduction by extensor pollicis longus. Compensates for loss of IP extension and thumb adduction by adductor pollicis (Figure 39.3).
- * Crossed finger test evaluates the function of first palmar and second dorsal interossei.
- * Wartenberg sign (Figure 39.4)
  - ▲ Characterized by persistent small finger abduction and extension during attempted adduction secondary to weak

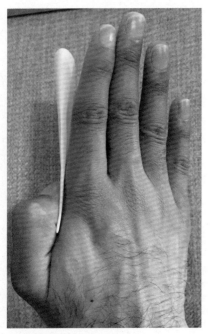

FIGURE 39.2 Froment sign.

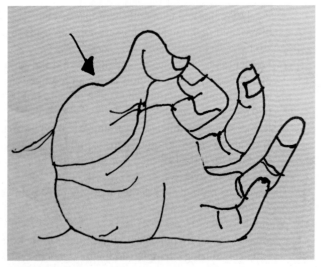

FIGURE 39.3 Jeanne sign.

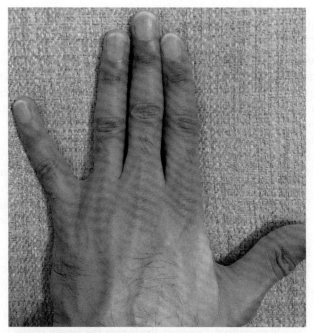

FIGURE 39.4 Wartenberg sign.

third palmar interosseous and small finger lumbrical and unopposed pull of extensor digiti minimi

- Provocative maneuvers
  - Spurling test—radicular symptoms resulting from turning patient's head to the affected side, whereas extending the neck and applying a downward pressure may indicate cervical root compression.
  - Adson maneuver—loss of the radial pulse in the arm by rotating head to the ipsilateral side with extended neck following deep inspiration is associated with thoracic outlet syndrome.
  - Assessment of ulnar nerve stability (ie, subluxation) throughout the range of motion of the elbow
  - Reproduction of symptoms with tapping (Tinel sign) or manual compression over ulnar nerve at the cubital tunnel or with sustained flexion of elbow
- Imaging
  - See Figures 39.1 to 39.4

ACUTE MANAGEMENT

After obtaining a thorough history, performing a physical examination, and ascertaining the mechanism of injury, it is essential to differentiate between neurapraxia/axonotmesis and neurotmesis. Neurapraxias/axonotmesis are stretch injuries that can be treated with observation, whereas neurotmesis are complete transections that require surgical intervention.[9]

- Workup
  - Plain radiographs
    - Fractures associated with paresthesias often require fracture reduction and stabilization.
  - Doppler ultrasound (US) or computed tomography (CT) angiogram
    - If concern for vascular injury on physical examination (ie, absent or diminished pulses)
  - Electromyelography (EMG)
    - Of little use from 0 to 7 days after ulnar nerve injury because Wallerian degeneration must first occur to completion, which takes between 1 and 4 weeks
      - Wallerian degeneration is also dependent on the length of nerve fiber injured, therefore the longer the length of the injured axon, the longer Wallerian degeneration will take.
    - After approximately 2 to 3 weeks following a nerve injury, a baseline EMG can be obtained.
      - At this time point fibrillations may be apparent on needle EMG.
      - May differentiate from significant axonal injury, neurapraxia conduction block
      - Early findings can help to localize the site of injury and to some extent the degree of injury.
      - Baseline EMG can be used to compare with subsequent EMG to help determine if recovery is taking place.
  - High-resolution US
    - One of the newer diagnostic modalities in peripheral ulnar nerve disruption
    - US imaging can now show individual nerve fascicules and can be used to follow nerve continuity.[10]
    - US can reveal discontinuity of the nerve, scar tissue around nerve stump and course, and presence of a neuroma with an accuracy of up to 93%.[11]
    - US is portable and economic and can be performed during surgery.

- Magnetic resonance imaging (MRI)/CT myelography
  - Advanced imaging MRI or CT myelogram may also aid in determining level of lesion, especially higher up, that is, nerve root avulsion injuries.
  - Also can be used to view muscle denervation, nerve edema, sites of compression, and nerve disruption.[12]
- Intraoperative nerve action potentials (NAPs)
  - Intraoperative testing of NAPs can be a helpful modality in determining the status of injuries where the nerve is in continuity.[13]
  - Stimulating and recording electrodes are placed on the nerve proximal to the lesion to assess the normal NAP. The recording electrodes are then moved into the region of injury and then distal to the lesion.
  - Present NAPs indicate the nerve is in continuity; therefore, a neurolysis alone can be performed.[2]
  - When no NAP is recorded across a lesion, this may represent a nonfunctioning nerve or neuroma; in these cases, resection of neuroma and repair of the injured nerve are indicated.
- Treatment
  - Operative indications
    - Neurotmesis with sharp transection of the nerve
    - Humerus fracture or floating shoulder with high ulnar nerve injury
    - Nerve injury with concomitant vascular injury
    - Ulnar nerve injury with gross contamination of wound
    - Neurapraxia or axonotmesis with no spontaneous recovery by 6 months
  - Indications to observe:
    - Neurapraxia injuries
    - Axonotmesis injuries
  - Considerations for early exploration:
    - The first decision the surgeon must make is whether the injury requires early exploration and repair.
      - This is primarily dependent on the mechanism of injury, contamination of the wound and soft tissues, and time to presentation.
      - A history of stab wound with sharp transection of the nerve (neurotmesis).
        - Lacerations of the nerve with acute presentation are most amenable to repair.
        - Immediate exploration and repair has superior outcomes to delayed repair.

- ▲ Acute repair can be up to 7 days without negatively influencing outcome.
- ▲ Delayed repair may be necessary if debridement of soft tissues is required for a grossly contaminated wound to reduce the chance of infection.
- ▲ Delays in repair increase the likelihood for nerve grafting, neuron loss, and fibrosis of the nerve stump and formation of scar tissue, making nerve difficult to mobilize and repair.
- ▲ The two ends of the injured nerve must be resected and the nerve mobilized without undue tension to reduce traction on the repair and aid in excursion.
- ▲ The wound must be properly debrided and the wound bed made suitable for nerve repair.
- ▲ Excessive mobilization may lead to distal stump ischemia and compromise recovery.
- ▲ Repair with wrist in flexed position has been shown to lower tension and reduce gap for nerve repairs in the distal fore.
- Surgical techniques
  - Epineural repair
    - ◆ Approach is determined by level of lesion, and accompanied fracture or vascular injury
    - ◆ Wound bed is debrided and nerve lesion exposed
    - ◆ The proximal neuroma and distal glioma are resected
    - ◆ The nerve must be mobilized to make up for resected ends
    - ◆ The epineurium is repaired in tension-free fashion
    - ◆ The epineurium is repaired using simple interrupted suture
    - ◆ Initially two sutures spaced 180° apart are inserted
    - ◆ Number of sutures needed is dependent on diameter of nerve fiber at the level of the lesion.
    - ◆ The nerve should be free of undue tension and should be able to be rotated 180° after completion of repair.
  - Fascicular repair
    - ◆ Technique includes repair of individual fascicles and placing sutures through the perineurium of each.
    - ◆ Has not demonstrated superiority over epineural repair
    - ◆ Complications of this technique include trauma to the nerve in dissecting out each fascicle and adhesions from extra handling and suture placement in nerve.
  - Autologous nerve graft
    - ◆ Indications

* ≥3 cm gap
* The anterior branch of the medial antebrachial cutaneous nerve provides an ideal donor for ulnar nerve reconstruction.
* This technique limits scarring and donor-site morbidity to the same extremity as the injured nerve.
* Other nerve autograft options include sural nerve, the medial and lateral cutaneous nerves of the forearm, superficial and deep peroneal nerves, intercostal nerves, and the posterior and lateral cutaneous nerves of the thigh.
* Drawbacks include donor site morbidity, the potential of infection, and formation of painful neuroma.

- Nerve conduits:
  - Biologic and synthetic polymers used to bridge gaps
  - May be used in place of autograft. Pros include loss of donor site morbidity for autograft.
  - Complications of this technique include trauma to the nerve in dissecting out each fascicle and fibrosis that develops because of the dissections and numerous sutures placed.
- Nonoperative treatment:
  - Stretch injuries or neurapraxias have a good prognosis for spontaneous recovery.
  - Baseline EMG may be obtained at 2 to 4 weeks and repeat EMG must be obtained in conjunction with serial clinical examinations to document recovery.
  - Acute management—peripheral nerve blocks or indwelling catheter
  - Manage neuropathic pain characterized by burning and dysesthesias.
    * Can be done with topical, oral medication or nerve blockade in the acute setting.
      ▲ First-line agents include gabapentin, amitriptyline, and venlafaxine.
      ▲ Second-line medications include pregabalin, carbamazepine, phenytoin, and lamotrigine, baclofen, and others.
      ▲ Topical agents include lidocaine patches and capsaicin cream.
- Postoperative care:
  - Static and dynamic splinting
  - Early range of motion to prevent nerve adhesions and gliding, encourage joint motion
  - Occupational therapy
  - EMG may be used in conjunction with clinical examinations to follow recovery.

REFERENCES

1. Lad SP, Nathan JK, Schubert RD, Boakye M. Trends in median, ulnar, radial, and brachioplexus nerve injuries in the United States. *Neurosurgery.* 2010;66(5):953-960.
2. Kim DH, Han K, Tiel RL, Murovic JA, Kline DG. Surgical outcomes of 654 ulnar nerve lesions. *J Neurosurg.* 2003;98(5):993-1004. doi:10.3171/jns.2003.98.5.0993.
3. Staples JR, Calfee R. Cubital tunnel syndrome: current concepts. *J Am Acad Orthop Surg.* 2017;25(10):e215-e224. doi:10.5435/JAAOS-D-15-00261.
4. Elhassan B, Steinmann S. Entrapment neuropathy of the ulnar nerve. *J Am Acad Orthop Surg.* 2007;15(11):672-681.
5. Vordemvenne T, Langer M, Ochman S, Raschke M, Schult M. Long-term results after primary microsurgical repair of ulnar and median nerve injuries. A comparison of common score systems. *Clin Neurol Neurosurg.* 2007;109(3):263-271. doi:10.1016/j.clineuro.2006.11.006.
6. Eversmann WJ. Entrapment and compressive neuropathies. In: Green DP, ed. *Operative Hand Surgery.* 3rd ed. New York, NY: Churchill Livingstone; 1993:1341-1389.
7. Norkus SA, Meyers MC. Ulnar neuropathy of the elbow. *Sports Med Auckl NZ.* 1994;17(3):189-199.
8. Taleisnik J, Szabo R. Compression neuropathies of the upper extremity. In: *Operative Orthopaedics.* Vol 2. 2nd ed. Philadelphia, PA: Lippincott; 1993:1419-1465.
9. Woo A, Bakri K, Moran SL. Management of ulnar nerve injuries. *J Hand Surg.* 2015;40(1):173-181. doi:10.1016/j.jhsa.2014.04.038.
10. Koenig RW, Pedro MT, Heinen CPG, et al. High-resolution ultrasonography in evaluating peripheral nerve entrapment and trauma. *Neurosurg Focus.* 2009;26(2):E13. doi:10.3171/FOC.2009.26.2.E13.
11. Lee FC, Singh H, Nazarian LN, Ratliff JK. High-resolution ultrasonography in the diagnosis and intraoperative management of peripheral nerve lesions. *J Neurosurg.* 2011;114(1):206-211. doi:10.3171/2010.2.JNS091324.
12. Grant GA, Goodkin R, Maravilla KR, Kliot M. MR neurography: diagnostic utility in the surgical treatment of peripheral nerve disorders. *Neuroimaging Clin N Am.* 2004;14(1):115-133. doi:10.1016/j.nic.2004.02.003.
13. Murovic JA. Upper-extremity peripheral nerve injuries: a Louisiana State University Health Sciences Center literature review with comparison of the operative outcomes of 1837 Louisiana State University Health Sciences Center median, radial, and ulnar nerve lesions. *Neurosurgery.* 2009;65(4 suppl):A11-A17. doi:10.1227/01.NEU.0000339130.90379.89.

Lisa M. Kruse and Bryan Loeffler

INTRODUCTION

- Anatomy[1]
  - Arises from the posterior cord of the brachial plexus (C5-C8 and/or T1)
  - Traverses the triangular interval (teres major, long head of triceps, humerus) to enter the posterior compartment of the arm
    - Innervates long head of triceps (7 cm from acromion), medial head of triceps (9 cm from acromion)
  - Runs along posterior humerus medial to lateral between medial and lateral heads of triceps
  - Travels adjacent to spiral groove
    - Innervates medial and lateral heads of triceps and anconeus
  - Pierces lateral intermuscular septum
    - Gerwin et al[2]: 20.7 cm proximal to medial epicondyle and 14.2 cm proximal to lateral epicondyle
    - Guse and Ostrum[3]: laterally nerve located on average 12.6 cm proximal to lateral epicondyle and never closer than 10 cm
    - Bono[4]: pierces lateral intermuscular septum 16.0 cm from distal humerus
  - Innervates lateral brachialis muscle
  - Between brachialis and brachioradialis (BR) and then between brachialis and extensor carpi radialis longus (ECRL)
    - Innervates BR and ECRL
  - Divides into superficial branch of the radial nerve (SBRN) and posterior interosseous nerve (PIN) (approximately 3.6 cm proximal to leading edge of supinator) (Figure 40.1)

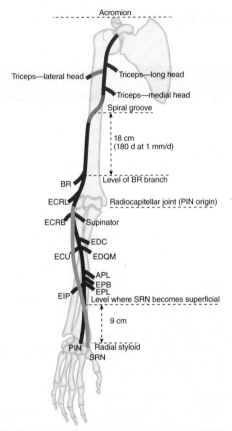

FIGURE 40.1 Anatomic course of the radial nerve and its branches. APL, abductor pollicis longus; BR, brachioradialis; ECRB, extensor carpi radialis brevis; ECRL, extensor carpi radialis longus; ECU, extensor carpi ulnaris; EDC, extensor digitorum communis; EDQM, extensor digiti quinti minimi; EIP, extensor indicis proprius; EPB, extensor pollicis brevis; EPL, extensor pollicis longus; PIN, posterior interosseous nerve; SRN, superficial branch of radial nerve. Redrawn with permission from Cheah A, Etcheson J, Yao J. Radial nerve tendon transfers. *Hand Clin.* 2016;32:323-338.

- Extensor carpi radialis brevis (ECRB) innervated by radial nerve, SBRN, or PIN
- Supinator innervated by radial nerve or PIN
- SBRN descends deep to BR
  - 9 cm proximal to radial styloid emerges superficial to abductor pollicis longus (APL) and extensor pollicis brevis (EPB)
  - Branches to provide sensation to dorsum of hand

- PIN passes beneath the arcade of Frohse and then between deep and superficial heads of supinator
  - Runs between APL/extensor carpi ulnaris (ECU) and extensor digiti minimi (EDM)/extensor digitorum communis (EDC)
  - Innervates in order: ECU, EDC, EDM, APL, extensor pollicis longus (EPL), EPB, extensor indicis proprius (EIP)
  - Terminates in the floor of the fourth dorsal compartment, giving sensation and proprioception to the wrist joint
- Mechanisms of injury
  - Compression neuropathies
    - Compression from C-spine
      - Diagnosis and physical examination findings
        - C6: weakness of wrist extensors, decreased sensation thumb, BR reflex
        - C7: weakness of triceps, decreased sensation in dorsal hand, triceps weakness
      - Imaging
        - C-spine radiographs
        - C-spine MRI
  - Proximal compression sites
    - Compression in axilla by anomalous muscle: accessory subscapularis-teres-latissimus[5]
    - Penetration of nerve by subscapular artery forming a neural loop[6]
    - Lateral head of triceps[7]
  - Radial tunnel syndrome
    - Diagnosis: aching pain in forearm
      - Pain with palpation over radial tunnel (dorsal and volar) 6 cm distal to lateral epicondyle
      - Most prominent with elbow extended, forearm pronated, and wrist flexed[8]
      - Pain with long finger extension
      - Pain with resisted supination
      - Electrodiagnostic evaluation usually negative
      - May occur along with lateral epicondylitis
    - Sites of compression (FREAS)[8]
      - Fascia adjacent to radiocapitellar joint
      - Radial recurrent artery and veins (leash of Henry)
      - ECRB tendinous margin
      - Arcade of Frohse
      - Supinator (including distal edge)

- Treatment
  - Immobilization
  - Anti-inflammatory medications
  - Wrist cock-up splint
  - Corticosteroid injections
  - Radial tunnel decompression
    - ▲ No long-term studies comparing operative and nonoperative treatments[9]
    - ▲ Lister et al improvement in 19 of 20 patients: outcome dependent on correct diagnosis[8] and 51% success rate for surgery[10]
- PIN syndrome
  - Pressure on the nerve with loss of motor function
    - May result from elbow synovitis in rheumatoid arthritis, ganglion cysts, or lipomas[9]
  - Diagnosis: weakness or paralysis of wrist and digital extensors
  - Physical examination findings
    - Weakness of finger extension (EDC/EIP), weakness of thumb extension (EPL/EPB) and abduction (APL)
    - Electrodiagnostic studies demonstrate compression.
    - Advanced imaging to evaluate mass effect
    - May occur along with lateral epicondylitis
  - Treatment
    - Initial nonoperative treatment similar to radial tunnel syndrome
    - No improvement in 90 days surgical decompression
  - Outcome
    - After 18 months muscle fibrosis occurs with irreversible changes.[11]
    - If no return of function after 18 months, consider tendon transfers[9]
- Wartenberg syndrome (cheiralgia paresthetica)
  - Compression of SBRN between fascia of BR and ECRL
  - Worse with pronation and ulnar deviation
  - Causes
    - Compression around wrist (watch band, handcuffs, cast)
    - Associated with De Quervain disease in 50% of cases[12]
  - Treatment
    - Conservative management and injection: 71% successful[12]
    - Surgical decompression: 74% success[12]

- Traction injuries
  - Associated with humeral shaft fracture
    - Incidence
      - 8% to 15% radial nerve palsy in closed fractures
      - 65% to 75% of open fractures
      - Most common in fractures in middle or middle to distal humerus
    - Diagnosis
      - Electrodiagnostic studies at 3 to 4 months
      - Ultrasound can be used to detect nerve entrapment.[13]
    - Treatment (Figure 40.2)
      - 85% to 90% improve with observation over 3 months and an additional 5% to 10% by 6 months (mean time to recovery onset 7.3 weeks, mean time to full recovery 6.1 months)[14]
      - Spontaneous recovery unlikely if no improvement by 7 months
      - Nonoperative treatment
        - Maintain passive range of motion of wrist and digits
        - Splint to maintain wrist in extension
        - EMG at 3 to 4 months
        - Migrating Tinel sign can be used to monitor progress.[15]
      - Surgical exploration indications[15]
        - Open fractures
        - Fractures with associated vascular injury
        - Fractures requiring open reduction and internal fixation
        - Onset after manipulation (controversial)
        - After 4 to 6 months if no recovery
  - Radial sensory nerve (RSN) irritation (traction injury during surgery)
    - Diagnosis: pain and paresthesias in RSN distribution
    - Treatment
      - Conservative management: desensitization therapy
      - Repair if transected as it results in painful neuroma.
- Laceration
  - Iatrogenic or traumatic laceration of radial nerve
  - Diagnosis
    - Loss of function distal to laceration
    - Electrodiagnostics: denervation potential at 10 to 14 days
  - Treatment
    - Initial surgical exploration and microsurgical repair of the nerve epineurium; grouped fascicular repair is not performed
    - Grafting when end-to-end repair not possible for tension-free repair. When associated with open humeral shaft fracture large

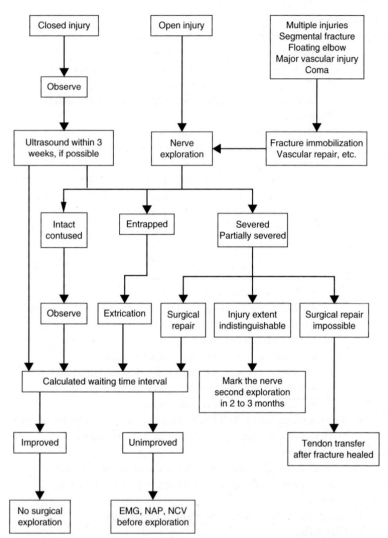

FIGURE 40.2 Algorithm for radial nerve palsy associated with fracture of the humeral shaft. EMG, electromyogram; NAP, nerve action potential; NCV, nerve conduction velocity. Redrawn with permission from Shao YC, Harwood P, Grotz MRW, Limb D, Giannoudis PV. Radial nerve palsy associated with fractures of the shaft of the humerus. *J Bone Joint Surg.* 2005;87B:1647-1652.

zone of injury and should be managed with resection of damaged portion and nerve grafting as secondary procedure[16]

- Prognosis
  - Low-level PIN injuries: 89% good results[17]
  - Mid-level injuries
    * None of 5 repaired radial nerves recovered associated with humerus fracture[18]
    * 88.8% excellent recovery and average recovery time 6.1 months[19]
    * Associated with humerus fracture; 52.9% good recovery[14]

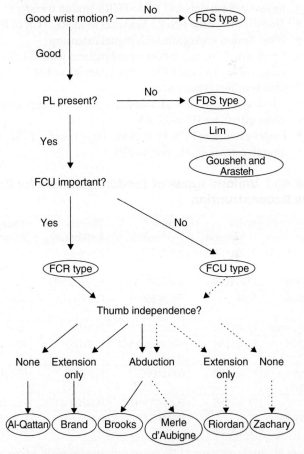

FIGURE 40.3 Suggested algorithm for choice of tendon transfer. FDS, flexor digitorum superficialis; PL, palmaris longus; FCU, flexor carpi ulnaris; FCR, flexor carpi radialis. From Cheah A, Etcheson J, Yao J. Radial nerve tendon transfers. *Hand Clin.* 2016;32:323-338.

* Shergill 30% good, 42% failure[17]
* Kline and Hudson better outcomes in lacerated nerves than those injured in fractures or gunshot wounds[20]

- Late reconstruction: following late presentation or failure of direct nerve repair
  - Nerve transfers
    - Median nerve (redundant fascicles to flexor digitorum superficialis [FDS] and flexor carpi radialis [FCR]) to radial nerve (ECRB and PIN, respectively) 12 patients with good to excellent recovery (Medical Research Council 4 or 5); 7 patients with fair to poor recovery (9 patients had PT to ECRB tendon transfer)[21]
    - Transfer one of the two PT branches to ECRL, FCR to PIN[22]
    - Wrist flexion synergistic with digital extension
    - 6 patients, 20-month follow-up, all patients with M4 recovery of ECRL, EPL; EDC and ECU M4 in 4 patients and M3 in 2 patients
  - Tendon transfers (Figure 40.3)
    - Elbow extension: deltoid, latissimus dorsi, or biceps to triceps
    - Wrist extension: PT to ECRB
    - Finger extension: FDS, FCR, flexor carpi ulnaris (FCU) to EDC
    - Thumb extension: PL, FDS to EPL

TABLE 40.1 Various Types of Tendon Transfers for Radial Nerve Reconstruction

Author	Wrist Extension	Finger Extension	Thumb Extension	Thumb Abduction
Boyes (FDS type)	PT to ECRB/ECRL	FDS to EDC	FDS to EPL	FCR to EPB/APL
Lim (FCR type)	PT to ECRB	Split FCR to EDC	Split FCR to EPL	None
Gousheh and Arasteh	None	FCU to EDC	FCU to EPL	None
Brand (FCR type)	PT to ECRB	FCR to EDC	PL to EPL	None
Tsuge (FCR type)	PT to ECRB	FCR through IOM to EDC	PL to EPL	None
Al-Qattan (FCR type)	PT to ECRB	FCR to EDC	FCR to EPL	FCR to APL
Brooks	PT to ECRB	FCU/FCR to EDC	FCU/FCR to EPL	PL to EPB
Merle d'Aubigne	PT to ECRL/ECRB	FCU to EDC	FCU to EPL	PL/FDS to EPB/APL

Abbreviations: APL, abductor pollicis longus; ECRB, extensor carpi radialis brevis; ECRL, extensor carpi radialis longus; EDC, extensor digitorum communis; EPB, extensor pollicis brevis; EPL, extensor pollicis longus; FCR, flexor carpi radialis; FCU, flexor carpi ulnaris; FDS, flexor digitorum superficialis; IOM, interosseous membrane; PL, palmaris longus; PT, pronator teres.

- ◆ Outcomes[23]
  - ∗ Wrist extension ranged from 30° to 54°
  - ∗ MCP joint extension ranged from 4° to 8°
  - ∗ Thumb abduction ranged from 36° to 55°
- ◆ Complications[23]
  - ∗ Limited wrist flexion
  - ∗ Bowstringing of PL to EPL transfer
  - ∗ PIP joint flexion contracture
  - ∗ Stretch out of transfer
  - ∗ Adhesions
- Radial nerve tendon transfers (Table 40.1)

REFERENCES

1. Leversedge FJ, Boyer MI, Goldfarb CA. *A Pocketbook Manual of Hand and Upper Extremity Anatomy: Primus Manus*. Philadelphia, PA: Lippincott Williams & Wilkins; 2010.
2. Gerwin M, Hotchkiss RN, Weiland AJ. Alternative operative exposures of the posterior aspect of the humeral diaphysis with reference to the radial nerve. *J Bone Joint Surg Am*. 1996;78(11):1690-1695.
3. Guse TR, Ostrum RF. The surgical anatomy of the radial nerve around the humerus. *Clin Orthop Relat Res*. 1995;320:149-153.
4. Bono CM, Grossman MG, Hochwald N, Tornetta P. Radial and axillary nerves Anatomic considerations for humeral fixation. *Clin Orthop Relat Res*. 2000;373:259-264.
5. Kameda Y. An anomalous muscle (accessory subscapularis-teres-latissimus muscle) in the axilla penetrating the brachial plexus in man. *Acta Anat*. 1976;96:513-533.
6. Spinner M. Management of nerve compression lesion of the upper extremity. In: Omer GE, Spinner M, eds. *Management of Peripheral Nerve Problems*. Philadelphia, PA: WB Saunders; 1980:569-587.
7. Lotem M, Fried A, Levy M, Solzi P, Najenson T, Nathan H. Radialpalsy following muscular effort: a nerve compression syndrome possibly related to a fibrous arch of the lateral head of the triceps. *J Bone Joint Surg Br*. 1971;53:500-506.
8. Lister GD, Belsole RB, Kleinert HE. The radial tunnel syndrome. *J Hand Surg*. 1979;4:52-59.
9. Lubahn JD, Cermak MB. Uncommon nerve compression syndromes of the upper extremity. *J Am Acad Orthop Surg*. 1998;6:378-386.
10. Ritts GD, Wood MB, Linscheid RL. Radial tunnel syndrome: a ten-year surgical experience. *Clin Orthop*. 1987;219:201-205.
11. Spinner M. *Injuries to the Major Branches of Peripheral Nerves of the Forearm*. 2nd ed. Philadelphia, PA: WB Saunders; 1978:234.
12. Lanzetta M, Foucher G. Entrapment of the superficial branch of the radial nerve (Wartenberg's syndrome). A report of 52 cases. *Int Orthop*. 1993;17(6):342-345.

13. Bodner G, Buchberger W, Schocke M, et al. Radial nerve palsy associated with humeral shaft fracture: evaluation with US: initial experience. *Radiology.* 2001;219(3):811-816.

14. Shao YC, Harwood P, Grotz MRW, Limb D, Giannoudis PV. Radial nerve palsy associated with fractures of the shaft of the humerus. *J Bone Joint Surg.* 2005;87B:1647-1652.

15. Ljungquist KL, Martineau P, Allan C. Radial nerve injuries. *J Hand Surg Am.* 2015;40:166-172.

16. Shah A, Jebson PJ. Current treatment of radial nerve palsy following fracture of the humeral shaft. *J Hand Surg.* 2008;33(8):1433-1434.

17. Shergill G, Bonney G, Munshi P, Birch R. The radial and posterior interosseous nerves. Results of 260 repairs. *J Bone Joint Surg Br.* 2001;83(5):646-649

18. Ring D, Chin K, Jupiter J. Radial nerve palsy associated with high-energy humeral shaft fractures. *J Hand Surg Am.* 2004;29A:144-147.

19. Gurbuz Y, Kayalar M, Bal E, Sugun TS, Ozaksar K, Ademoglu Y. Long term functional results after radial nerve repair. *Acta Orthop Traumatol Turc.* 2011;45(6):387-392.

20. Kline DGH. Results: radial nerve. In: Hudson AR, ed. *Nerve Injuries.* Philadelphia, PA: WB Saunders; 1995:167-185.

21. Ray WZ, Mackinnon SE. Clinical outcomes following median to radial nerve transfers. *J Hand Surg Am.* 2011;36A:201-208.

22. Garcia-Lopez A, Navarro R, Martinez F, Rojas A. Nerve transfers from branches to the flexor carpi radialis and pronator teres to reconstruct the radial nerve. *J Hand Surg Am.* 2014;39(1):50-56.

23. Cheah, A, Etcheson J, Yao J. Radial nerve tendon transfers. *Hand Clin.* 2016;32:323-338.

CHAPTER

41 Gustilo Classification

Tiffany J. Pan and John R. Fowler

INTRODUCTION

- Classification system for open fractures proposed by Dr Ramon Gustilo and Dr John Anderson in 1976[1]
- Primary study aim was the treatment and prevention of infection in open fractures.
- Classification system was developed for the prospective study arm.

EVALUATION

- History
  - Mechanism of injury (high vs low energy)
  - Environment to which the bone was exposed (clean vs contaminated or farm injury)
- Physical examination (Figure 41.1)
  - Size of traumatic wound
  - Exposed bone
  - Degree of soft tissue damage
  - Vascular injury
  - Neurologic examination
- Imaging
  - Plain films to assess fracture pattern
  - May require advanced imaging for periarticular fractures or suspected vascular injury

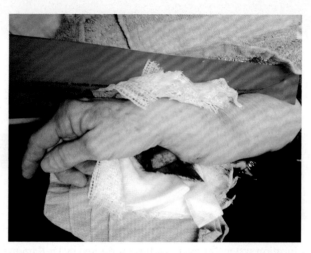

FIGURE 41.1 Type IIIA open distal radius fracture with periosteal stripping.

- Classification
  - Original classification described by Gustilo and Anderson[1] in 1976
    - Type I—clean wound less than 1 cm long
    - Type II—wound longer than 1 cm without significant soft tissue injury
    - Type III—open segmental fracture or open fracture with significant soft tissue injury including traumatic amputation with special categories as follows:
      - Gunshot injuries
      - Farm injuries
      - Vascular injury requiring repair
  - Current complete classification (Table 41.1)

ACUTE MANAGEMENT

- Initiate antibiotics as soon as possible
  - Infection rate increases if antibiotics are delayed >3 hours from the time of injury.
  - Continue antibiotics until 3 to 5 days after the final surgical procedure.
  - Types I and II
    - Gram-positive organism coverage
    - First-generation cephalosporin
    - Fluoroquinolone if allergic

TABLE 41.1 Current Classification

	Type I	Type II	Type III		
			A	B[a]	C[b]
Energy	Low	Moderate	High	High	High
Soft tissue injury	Minimal	Moderate	Extensive	Extensive	Variable
Periosteal stripping	No	No	Yes	Yes	Yes
Fracture pattern	Simple with minimal comminution	Moderate comminution	Severely comminuted, unstable, or segmental	Severely comminuted, unstable, or segmental	Variable but typically as characteristic of other type III fractures
Wound	<1 cm	>1 cm	Variable	Variable, typically >10 cm	Variable
Contamination	Clean or moderately clean	Moderate	Variable	Severe	Variable
Soft tissue coverage	Primary closure or local coverage	Primary closure or local coverage	Primary closure or local coverage	Requires free tissue flap or rotational flap	May require free or rotational flap
Vascular Injury	No	No	No	No	Arterial injury requiring repair

[a]Type IIIB, by definition, requires free or rotation tissue coverage regardless and is not defined by wound size

[b]Type IIIC, by definition, has a concomitant arterial injury requiring repair regardless of other factors but will nearly always share characteristics common to type III high-energy fractures.

- Type III
  - Gram-positive and Gram-negative organism coverage
  - First-generation cephalosporin + aminoglycoside
- Farm injury or bowel contamination
  - Gram-positive, Gram-negative, anaerobic organism coverage
  - First-generation cephalosporin + aminoglycoside + penicillin
- Aquatic environment exposure
  - Fresh water—fluoroquinolone or third-/fourth-generation cephalosporin
  - Salt water—doxycycline and ceftazidime or fluoroquinolone
- Transfer to definitive care center as soon as possible
- Ensure tetanus booster is up to date

DEFINITIVE TREATMENT

- Irrigation and debridement of wound
  - Time to debridement has not been shown to correlate with infection rate, although highly contaminated type III injuries should be addressed urgently.
  - No consensus on high- versus low-pressure irrigation, volume, or whether or not antibiotics should be used.
    - 9L commonly recommended for type III open fractures
    - Antibiotics in solution not clinically proven to improve outcomes
- Surgical debridement
  - Must thoroughly debride all nonviable tissue and foreign material
  - Debridement without a tourniquet can improve identification of viable tissue.
  - Four Cs of muscle viability are as follows:
    - Color
    - Consistency
    - Contractility
    - Circulation
  - Cortical bone fragments without soft tissue attachments must be removed, though large free articular fragments should be retained.
  - Repeat debridements may be necessary at 24 to 48 hours.
- Wound closure
  - Primary closure does not increase risk of complications if a thorough debridement has been performed.

- Multiple debridements over 3 to 7 days are recommended for severe soft tissue injury or highly contaminated wounds.
- Soft tissue reconstruction may be necessary.
- Fracture fixation
  - Method of fracture fixation depends on fracture pattern, location of fracture, and extent of soft tissue damage.
  - Internal fixation with intramedullary or plate fixation
    - Open humeral shaft fractures may be treated with intramedullary fixation, but exploration and open reduction are recommended if there is a concurrent radial nerve palsy.
    - Majority of upper extremity fractures are amenable to plate fixation.
  - External fixation
    - Can be useful in the setting of severe soft tissue injury
    - Advantages—decreased surgical time, preserves blood supply, avoids deep implants
    - Disadvantages—risk for pin-tract infection and fracture malalignment
  - Bone grafting
    - Optimally 2 to 6 weeks after definitive soft tissue coverage
    - Autograft remains the gold standard
- Postoperative care
  - Continue antibiotics for 3 to 5 days after final surgical procedure/ wound closure
  - Activities and weight-bearing status based on fracture pattern and extent of soft tissue damage
  - Nonunion
    - No callus formation at 8 to 12 weeks
    - Early bone grafting with autogenous bone graft
    - Rule out indolent infection

SUGGESTED READINGS

Gustilo RB, Merkow RL, Templeman D. Current concepts review: the management of open fractures. *J Bone Joint Surg Am*. 1990;72-A(2):299-304.

Holtom PD. Antibiotic prophylaxis: current recommendations. *J Am Acad Orthop Surg*. 2006;14:S98-S100.

Noonburg GE. Management of extremity trauma and related infections occurring in the aquatic environment. *J Am Acad Orthop Surg*. 2005;13:243-253.

Zalavras CG, Patzakis MJ. Open fractures: evaluation and management. *J Am Acad Orthop Surg*. 2003;11:212-219.

REFERENCES

1. Gustilo RB, Anderson JT. Prevention of infection in the treatment of one thousand and twenty-five open fractures of long bones: retrospective and prospective analyses. *J Bone Joint Surg Am*. 1976;58-A(4):453-458.

42 Pulp Space Infections

Omri Ayalon and Matthew B. Cantlon

INTRODUCTION

- Definition—Infection contained in the closed and unyielding septal spaces of the distal volar pad of the finger or thumb. Also referred to as a "**felon**."
- Epidemiology—Represents up to 20% of all hand infections[1] and 6% of all incision and drainage procedures performed on the hand.[2]
- Mechanism of injury
  - Vast majority of injuries arise from prior lacerations or penetrating trauma such as wooden or metal splinters or glass (Figure 42.1). Injuries can occur in diabetics from repeated glucose finger-stick testing.
  - Eccrine sweat glands may become colonized with bacteria that occasionally lead to a pulp space infection.
  - Local inoculation from underlying osteomyelitis may also occur.

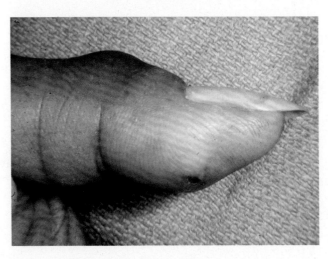

FIGURE 42.1 Pulp space infection from a penetrating trauma.

- Microbiology
  - *Staphylococcus aureus* is the most common (75% of all hand infections). Methicillin-resistant *S. aureus* (MRSA) is now more common than methicillin-susceptible *S. aureus* in most urban centers.[2] Risk factors for MRSA include immunocompromised status, HIV infection, diabetes, intravenous drug use, and being a health care worker.[3,4]
  - Polymicrobial infection is the next most common, followed by *Streptococcal* species.[2]
  - Gram-negative species may occur in diabetics and immunocompromised individuals.

PATHOANATOMY

- Glabrous skin of the volar fingertip is tethered to the periosteum of the distal phalanx and to the flexor sheath more proximally in the finger via **vertical fibrous septa**. Adipose tissue and eccrine sweat glands occupy the closed spaces created by these septae[5] (Figure 42.2).
- Cellulitis or local swelling leads to vascular congestion and swelling within the rigid and unyielding septae, which produces pressure necrosis, acting as a mini "compartment syndrome" of the pulp, usually within 24 to 48 hours of symptom onset.[6]

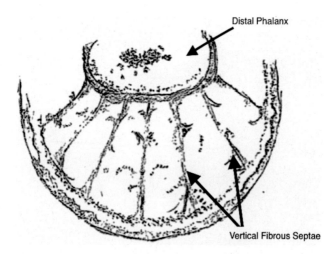

Distal Phalanx

Vertical Fibrous Septae

FIGURE 42.2 Cross section of the distal segment of the finger.

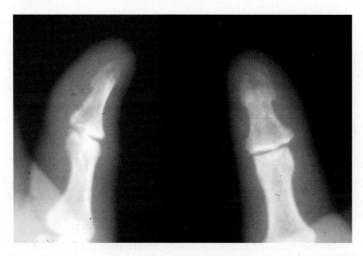

FIGURE 42.3 Anteroposterior and lateral radiographs of a distal phalangeal osteomyelitis from an untreated felon.

- The distal fingertip has high innervation density, and this elevated local pressure leads to pain.
- If left untreated, it can lead to osteomyelitis of the distal phalanx shaft (Figure 42.3). The epiphysis is preserved due to richer vascular supply directly from the distal transverse palmar arch, whereas the pulp tissue is supplied by smaller longitudinal artery branches, which makes the shaft more susceptible to infection.[6]

EVALUATION

- History—Assess duration of symptoms, history and circumstances of penetrating trauma, recent illnesses, immunocompromised status, diabetes, intravenous drug use, medical allergies
- Physical examination
  - Localized or proximally streaking erythema, warmth, tenderness, and swelling in the distal segment volar pulp
  - Assess for discrete collection of purulence amenable for drainage.
  - Spontaneous sinus tract can occur if left untreated.
  - Evaluate for signs of progression to pyogenic flexor tenosynovitis (Kanavel signs including circumferential dactylitis, resting flexed

posture, pain with isolated passive extension of the interphalangeal joints, and volar tenderness to palpation along the flexor sheath).

- Imaging
  - Plain films to establish presence of foreign body
  - MRI if concern of bony involvement in the form of osteomyelitis

MANAGEMENT

- Nonoperative treatment
  - Oral antibiotic treatment alone can be attempted if the process is caught in the cellulitic phase before fluctuance has occurred, usually within the first 24 to 48 hours.
  - Intravenous antibiotics can be considered if there is a concern for osteomyelitis or other associated severe infection such as flexor tenosynovitis or deep space infection.
  - In all cases, strict elevation and active and passive digital motion should be encouraged throughout the course of the treatment.
- Surgical drainage is indicated if any fluctuance is appreciated. It is vital to address expeditiously in order to prevent spread of infection and long-term sequelae.
  - Most can be treated in the emergency room setting, otherwise proceed to the operating room if there is concern of more serious involvement such as potential need for decompression of the flexor sheath.
  - Goals of the procedure
    - Complete decompression of the collection
    - Disrupt the vertical septae in the volar pulp, thus releasing all the micro-"compartments." This can be done both with a scalpel and with a blunt hemostat clamp.
    - Avoid neurovascular bundles.
    - Utilize an incision that won't leave a disabling scar.
    - Keep exploration distal enough to avoid violating the flexor tendon sheath.
    - Take cultures to guide antibiotic therapy.
    - Leave incision open with a wick of gauze or wound packing to allow further egress and healing by secondary intention.
  - Incision options
    - Midaxial is the preferred approach. It can be used for virtually all pulp space infections. It maintains the neurovascular bundle

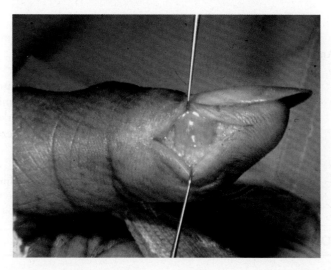

FIGURE 42.4 Midaxial incision for the surgical drainage of pulp space infection.

in the volar section. Scar heals along the axis of motion, thus preventing symptomatic motion contracture.

* When possible, place on the radial side of the thumb and small finger and ulnar side of index, middle, and ring to avoid scar tenderness with pinch (Figure 42.4).

◆ Midline volar is used if most of the fluctuance is central or if a volar sinus tract needs excision. This avoids neurovascular bundles completely. Incision should not cross the distal interphalangeal flexion crease to prevent scar contracture.

◆ Fish mouth—AVOID. It may result in serious complications, including destabilization of the volar fingertip pad, vascular compromise to the pulp, and unsightly scar.

● Surgical aftercare

◆ A gauze wick should be left at the conclusion of surgery. The first dressing change should be performed between 12 and 24 hours. A wick should be maintained for at least 72 hours to allow drainage.

◆ Dressings are changed 2 to 3 times per day and the wick may be discontinued between 3 and 5 days.

◆ Soak the finger in dilute povidone-iodine for 5 to 10 minutes at each dressing change. Simple hand hygiene at dressing changes is also appropriate.

- ◆ Early motion is encouraged to prevent digital stiffness.
- ◆ Majority recover in 3 to 4 weeks with appropriate management.
- ■ Antibiotic options and duration[7]
  - Simple felon with low suspicion for MRSA
    - ◆ Cephalexin or Amoxicillin-Clavulanate (Augmentin) for 7 to 10 days
  - Simple felon with high suspicion for MRSA (immunocompromised status, HIV, diabetics, intravenous drug users, health care workers)
    - ◆ Trimethoprim-sulfamethoxazole (Bactrim) orally or Linezolid (orally or IV) for 10 to 14 days
  - If penicillin or sulfa allergy
    - ◆ Clindamycin or Doxycycline (orally or IV depending on clinical scenario)

COMPLICATIONS

- ■ Fingertip compartment syndrome
- ■ Flexor tenosynovitis
- ■ Osteomyelitis
- ■ Digital tip necrosis
- ■ Pulp deformity. Typically pulp atrophy and is often permanent.
- ■ Pulp instability from infection that involves all the septae. Often resolves with time but can take 6 months to 1 year.

REFERENCES

1. Linscheid RL, Dobyns JH. Common and uncommon infections of the hand. *Orthop Clin North Am*. 1975;6(4):1063-1104.
2. Fowler JR, Ilyas AM. Epidemiology of adult acute hand infections at an urban medical center. *J Hand Surg Am*. 2013;38(6):1189-1193.
3. Wilson PC, Rinker B. The incidence of methicillin-resistant *Staphylococcus aureus* in community-acquired hand infections. *Ann Plast Surg*. 2009;62(5):513-516.
4. Imahara SD, Friedrich JB. Community-acquired methicillin-resistant *Staphylococcus aureus* in surgically treated hand infections. *J Hand Surg Am*. 2010;35(1):97-103.
5. Bolton H, Fowler PJ, Jepson RP. Natural history and treatment of pulp space infection and osteomyelitis of the terminal phalanx. *J Bone Joint Surg Br*. 1949;31B(4):499-504.
6. Yu HL, Chase RA, Strauch B. *Atlas of Hand Anatomy and Clinical Implications*. St. Louis, MO: Mosby; 2004:599.
7. Osterman M, Draeger R, Stern P. Acute hand infections. *J Hand Surg Am*. 2014;39(8):1628-1635; quiz 1635.

Timothy P. Crowley and Susan Stevenson

INTRODUCTION

- Pathoanatomy
  - A paronychia is an infection of the soft tissue structures surrounding the proximal and lateral nail plate (perionychium).
  - The proximal nail fold (eponychium) and lateral nail folds (paronychium) normally provide a watertight seal around the border of the nail plate.
- Mechanism
  - A paronychia develops with the introduction of microbes between the nail plate and the surrounding perionychium. This is often as a result of minor trauma that disrupts the seal between the nail plate and the nail folds. Commonly this is secondary to a hangnail, nail biting, or instrumentation of the perionychium following manicure.
  - Inflammation of the nail fold with erythema, pain, and swelling may progress to abscess formation.
  - If untreated, the abscess can spread and separate the nail plate from the nail bed or it can extend volarly into the pulp space of the finger tip.
  - Chronic paronychia occurs when repeated episodes of inflammation and drainage result in separation of the nail plate and the dorsal soft tissues of the nail fold. Chronic inflammation leads to thickening of the nail fold with resultant reduction in blood flow and thus susceptibility to recurrent episodes of infection (*J Hand Surg Am* 1991;16:314-317).
- Epidemiology
  - Paronychial infection is the most commonly seen hand infection.
  - Mixed bacterial infections are commonly seen, with *Staphylococcus aureus* the most frequently implicated organism.
  - Anaerobic infections are also seen, possibly due to contamination of the initial wound with the oral cavity (*J Hand Surg* 1993; 18:358-359 & *Br J Surg* 1981;68:420).
  - Chronic paronychia is often associated with more atypical bacteria, including Gram-negative organisms, mycobacterial

species, and fungal infections primarily *Candida* (*J Hand Surg* 1993; 18:358-359 & *J Clin Microbiol* 1988;26:950-953).

EVALUATION

- History
  - Initially there is erythema, swelling, and discomfort at the nail fold. This may then progress to abscess formation with fluctuance and visible pus at the nail fold.
  - Discomfort generally worsens as the abscess develops, resulting in a severe throbbing pain that can often disrupt sleep.
  - Duration of symptoms and any preceding treatment should be identified.
  - Factors that may lead to atypical microorganisms or resistance to standard treatment such as immunosuppression, diabetes, or chronicity of infection should be assessed.
  - Risk factors such as nail biting, frequent hand washing, and immersion of the hands in water, as well as tobacco smoking should be elicited.
- Physical examination
  - Examination aims to identify the extent of the infection and the need for surgical drainage of any abscess.
- Imaging
  - Radiographs are not routinely indicated in uncomplicated cases of short clinical duration.
  - Patients who have not responded to initial treatment, who have had chronic symptoms, or those who present with significant abscess and swelling should have radiographs to exclude underlying osteomyelitis or foreign body.
- Classification
  - Acute—associated minor trauma
  - Chronic—associated fungal infection, atypical bacteria, and prolonged exposure to moisture or chemical irritants

ACUTE MANAGEMENT

- In the early stages, preceding abscess formation, the infection can be successfully treated with warm saline soaks, systemic oral antibiotics, and elevation.
- Once fluctuance and/or pus is present at the nail fold, formal decompression of the abscess is indicated (Figure 43.1).

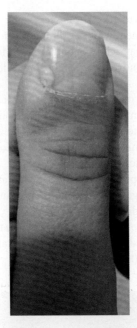

FIGURE 43.1 Paronychia with pus, swelling, and inflammation at the lateral nail fold without evidence of separation of the nail plate from the nail bed.

DEFINITIVE TREATMENT

- Surgical approach
  - Treatment is individualized based on the size and location of the abscess.
  - The vast majority of cases can be dealt with under local anesthesia in the form of a digital ring block.
  - A superficial abscess can be drained by deroofing the overlying skin and application of a dressing.
  - Elevation of the paronychium and eponychium allows drainage of abscess superficial to the nail plate. Care must be taken to splint open the abscess cavity with dressings after washout to prevent premature closure and recollection of the abscess.
  - An abscess that extends beneath the nail plate requires removal of the nail plate either in part or in its entirety, depending on the extent of separation of the nail plate from the nail bed.

- If initial attempts to drain the abscess while preserving the nail plate fail, then subsequent washout should include removal of the entire nail plate as it may act as a contaminated foreign body within the wound. Once removed, the nail plate should not be replaced in the nail fold.
- More proximal collections can require incision of the dorsal nail fold to allow complete elevation of the eponychium exposing the proximal nail plate/nail bed. One or two incisions are placed at right angles to the corners of the proximal nail fold.

- Potential complications
  - Failure to release pus between the nail plate and nail bed can result in permanent damage to the germinal matrix and subsequent abnormal nail growth and deformity.
  - Neglected infections can proceed to involve the pulp space, destruction of the nail bed, osteomyelitis of the distal phalanx, and/or flexor sheath infection (Figure 43.2.)

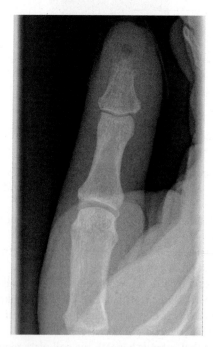

FIGURE 43.2 Plain radiograph showing osteomyelitis of the thumb distal phalanx secondary to neglected paronychia and pulp space infection.

- Damage to the nail bed during drainage can lead to abnormal nail growth and deformity.
- Misdiagnosis of a herpetic whitlow as a paronychia. Drainage of herpetic whitlows is not indicated and can result in bacterial superinfection or systemic viral infection (*Nail Surgery: A Text and Atlas*, Philadelphia, Lippincott Williams & Wilkins, 2001: 201-205).
- Postoperative care
  - Oral antibiotics to complete a 7- to 10-day course.
  - Change of dressings at 24 hours with removal and replacement of any packing as indicated.
  - Early active mobilization to avoid stiffness.
  - If the infection has failed to resolve following adequate decompression, radiographs should be obtained to exclude osteomyelitis, infectious disease advice may be sought, and further formal debridement and washout considered.

MANAGEMENT ALGORITHM

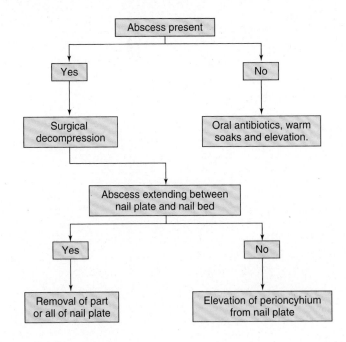

SUGGESTED READINGS

Bednar MS, Lane LB. Eponychial marsupialization and nail removal for surgical treatment of chronic paronychia. *J Hand Surg Am*. 1991;16:314-317.

Brook I. Paronychia: a mixed infection. Microbiology and management. *J Hand Surg Br*. 1993;18(3):358-359.

Jebsen P. Infections of the fingertip: paronychias and felons. *Hand Clin*. 1998;5:547.

Krull EA, Zook EG, Baran R, Haneke E. *Nail Surgery: A Text and Atlas*. Philadelphia, PA: Lippincott Williams & Wilkins; 2001:201-205.

Masson JA. Hand I: fingernails, infections, tumours and soft-tissue reconstruction. *Select Read Plast Surg*. 2002;9(32).

McGinley KJ, Larson EL, Leyden JJ. Composition and density of microflora in the subungual space of the hand. *J Clin Microbiol*. 1988;26(5):950-953.

Reardon CM, McArthur PA, Survana SK, Brotherston TM. The surface anatomy of the germinal matrix of the nail bed in the finger. *J Hand Surg*. 1999;24B:531.

Whitehead SM, Eykyn SJ, Phillips I. Anaerobic paroncyhia. *Br J Surg*. 1981;68(6):420-422

Wolfe SW, Hotchkiss RN, Kozin SH, et al. *Greens Operative Hand Surgery*. 7th ed. Philadelphia, PA: Elseiver; 2017.

Zook EG. Anatomy and physiology of the perionychium. *Hand Clin*. 1990;6(1):1.

Pyogenic Flexor Tenosynovitis

Emily E. Jewell and Reid W. Draeger

INTRODUCTION

- Flexor tendon sheath infections are a surgical urgency because they can have devastating outcomes such as loss of motion, deformity, and loss of digit if treatment is delayed.
- Kanavel originally described the physical presentation of pyogenic flexor tenosynovitis (PFT) in 1912.[1]
- Despite improving antibiotic and surgical treatments, it continues to be crucial to have early detection and treatment of PFT to minimize long-term complications.

ANATOMY

- The flexor tendon sheath is a two-layered structure.
  - Visceral layer adheres closely to the tendon, forming the epitenon.[2]
  - Parietal layer abuts the pulley mechanism.[2]
- These layers connect both proximally and distally to create a closed system. The portion of the tendon that is within the sheath receives its nutrients and blood supply through diffusion of the synovial fluid. The portion of the tendon outside of the sheath receives its blood supply through a direct system through the vinculae.[3]
- Index, middle, and ring finger sheaths extend from the A1 pulley at the level of the distal palmar crease proximally to the level of the distal interphalangeal joint distally.[2,4]
- Thumb tendon sheath is situated around the flexor pollicis longus tendon. This typically communicates with the radial bursa at the level of the metacarpophalangeal (MCP) joint, which then extends proximally past the transverse carpal ligament.
- Small finger tendon sheath extends and typically communicates with the ulnar bursa, which extends proximal to the transverse carpal ligament as well.

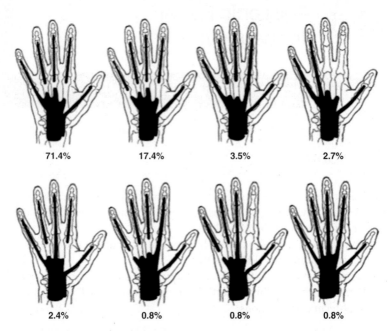

FIGURE 44.1 Illustration demonstrating the anatomic variations of the flexor tendon sheath and bursa patterns of the hand as well as their relative frequency. Reproduced with permission from Doyle JR, Botte MJ. Hand. In: Doyle JR, Botte MJ, eds. *Surgical Anatomy of the Hand and Upper Extremity.* Philadelphia, PA: Lippincott Williams & Wilkins; 2003:605.

- Radial and ulnar bursae frequently communicate (33%–100%) through the space of Parona, which can lead to the formation of a horseshoe abscess.[5,6]
- Anatomic variation of tendon sheath connections exists in approximately 15% to 30% of the population (Figure 44.1).[7-9]

PATHOGENESIS

- Bacteria infect the nutrient-rich synovial fluid of the tendon sheath between the visceral epitenon layer and the parietal layer.[10,11]
- Infection in this closed space leads to tendon damage through multiple pathways.
  - Increased pressure within this closed space is detrimental because the tendon itself receives its nutrients through diffusion from the

synovial fluid. If the synovial space becomes distended with purulent fluid, the tendon will be denied vital nutrients as well as blood supply. This can lead to ischemia and ultimately tendon rupture.[3]

- The tendon sheath itself acts like a barrier and limits the ability of the host's immune system to defend against bacterial proliferation and invasion.[12]
- Anatomic borders of the tendon sheath compound effects of inflammatory response to the infection, leading to stiffness and adhesion formation.[10]
- Owing to the body's poor ability to fight this infection, it has the ability to spread to other flexor tendon sheaths or into the midpalmar, thenar, or lumbrical compartments.[2]

EPIDEMIOLOGY

- PFT represents 2.5% to 9.4% of all hand infections.[11]
- Goal is for early antibiotic therapy directed at the likely causative organism.
- Approximately 20% to 30% of cultures are negative, which is likely due to preoperative antibiotic administration.[13]

Acute Infection

- Direct inoculation is the most likely etiology, which is most likely to be a puncture injury.[4]
- For penetrating injury, skin flora is the likely causative organism, with *Staphylococcus* present in 50% to 80% of cases.[4,14]
- Methicillin-resistant *Staphylococcus aureus* is found in up to 29% of cases.[15]
- Diabetes mellitus and being in a rural area are risk factors for polymicrobial infections.[13]
- Animal bites increase the risk of *Pasteurella* infection.
- Human bites increase the risk of alpha hemolytic *Streptococcus* or *Eikenella*.

Chronic Infection

- An indolent course/chronic infection is more consistent with mycobacterial or fungal infection.
- Musculoskeletal involvement makes up 1% to 5% of extrapulmonary tuberculosis (TB).
- Tuberculous tenosynovitis makes up approximately 5% of bone and joint TB.[16]
- If there is concern for TB, then a synovial biopsy should be sent for Ziehl–Neelsen staining or intradermal tuberculin reaction test should be pursued.[17]

EVALUATION

History

- Direct inoculation through penetrating injury is the most likely cause of PFT.[4]
- 70% of patients with PFT have a recent history of penetrating trauma.[11]
- May also undergo direct spread from adjacent infection such as a felon, septic joint, or deep space infection
- Hematogenous spread is most common with gonococcal infections.[4]

Physical Examination

- Kanavel signs (Table 44.1, Figure 44.2)
  - Excessive tenderness to palpation over the flexor tendon sheath
  - The finger rests in a flexed position.
  - Excruciating pain with passive extension of the finger, which is most marked at the proximal end of the sheath
  - Fusiform swelling of the digit[1]
- All four Kanavel signs are present in 54% of the cases.[13]
- Kanavel signs are 91.4% to 97.1% sensitive but only 51.3% to 69.2% specific to PFT.[18]
- Pain over the tendon sheath has been found to be most sensitive of the four signs, with painful passive extension of the digit being the second most sensitive.[13,18]
- Flexed posture of the digit and fusiform swelling are not independent risk factors for PFT.
- It has been found that tenderness along the tendon sheath, pain with passive extension of the digit, and duration of symptoms less than 5 days correlates to a 87.9% likelihood of being positive for PFT.[19]

TABLE 44.1 Kanavel Signs

1. Tenderness over flexor tendon sheath
2. Pain with passive extension of the digit
3. Digit resting in flexed position
4. Fusiform swelling of involved digit

From Kanavel AB. The symptoms, signs, and diagnosis of tenosynovitis and fascial-space abscesses. In: *Infections of the Hand*. 1st ed. Philadelphia, PA: Lea & Febiger; 1912:201–226.

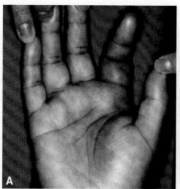 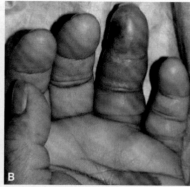

FIGURE 44.2 A, Clinical photograph of the right hand demonstrating pyogenic flexor tenosynovitis (PFT) of the index finger. Note the fusiform swelling and partially flexed posture of the digit. B, Clinical photograph of the left hand of a patient with advanced PFT demonstrating subcutaneous purulence and local ischemia in addition to fusiform digital swelling. Courtesy of Robert Strauch, MD, New York, NY.

Special Cases

- Pediatric cases are less likely to present with classic signs, and pediatric patients are less likely to allow a full and adequate examination.[20]
- Consider further diagnostic testing such as ultrasound of the involved digit.[21]
- Diabetic and immune-compromised individuals may also not have the classic examination because of leukocyte dysfunction, wound-healing deficiency, late presentation due to peripheral and autonomic neuropathies, and diabetic angiopathy leading to decreased inflammatory response.[22]
- Thumb and small finger involvement may be more subtle because they both have auto-decompression mechanisms through their communication with the radial and ulnar bursae, respectively.[19]

Labs/Imaging

- In the setting of PFT, the sensitivity of white blood cell is 39%, erythrocyte sedimentation rate 41%, and C-reactive protein 76%.[23]
- These markers are not always elevated even in the setting of PFT, so they are not predictive of PFT versus other infections of the hand.[19]
- Although diagnosis is primarily based on clinical examination, ultrasound of the affected digit may show thickening of the tendon sheath as well as an increased fluid collection within the sheath itself.[9]

TABLE 44.2 **Michon Classification of Flexor Tenosynovitis**

Infection Stage	Characteristic Findings	Treatment
Stage 1	Serous exudate	Catheter irrigation
Stage 2	Purulent exudate	Minimally invasive drainage ± CCI
Stage 3	Necrosis	Open debridement vs possible amputation

CCI, continuous catheter irrigation.

From Michon J. Phlegmon of the tendon sheaths. *Ann Chir*. 1974;28:277-280.

Classification

- Michon classification system (Table 44.2)[22,24-26]
  - Stage 1: increased fluid in the sheath, but mainly a serous exudate
    - Catheter irrigation alone is sufficient.
  - Stage 2: purulent fluid and granulomatous synovium
    - Minimally invasive drainage ± continuous catheter irrigation (CCI) is sufficient.
  - Stage 3: necrosis of the tendons, pulleys, or tendon sheath
    - Extensive open debridement and possible amputation are needed for these cases.

ANTIBIOTIC TREATMENT

- When Kanavel signs were initially described, antibiotics had yet to be discovered, but now they are a mainstay of treatment.
- Adding antibiotics to treatment improves self-reported outcomes as well as long-term range of motion.[27]
- In patients without a concerning history (immune suppression, farm or animal injury, diabetes), antibiotics should be presumptively initiated to cover likely causative organisms, which include gram-positive organisms.[13]
  - First-generation cephalosporin or first-generation cephalosporin plus a penicillin
- If the patient does have a concerning history, then broad-spectrum antibiotics should be initiated to cover gram-positive and gram-negative rods and anaerobic bacteria.[4]
- IV antibiotics should be continued until there is clinical improvement allowing transition to oral antibiotics, which can be further narrowed on the basis of culture results.

ANTIBIOTICS ALONE

- There has not been a randomized control trial to study the outcomes of antibiotic treatment alone in PFT.
- It has been proposed that patients presenting within 24 hours of onset of symptoms may be treated with antibiotics, splinting, and elevation.[4]
- Administer IV antibiotics for 12 to 24 hours with close monitoring of clinical condition and proceed to surgical intervention if any decline is noted.[28]

LOCAL TREATMENT

- Locally administered corticosteroid has significantly decreased the loss of range of motion in an animal model.[10]
- It has been proposed but not yet studied that local administration of antibiotics would have similar improvement in outcomes of PFT.[10]

OPERATIVE TREATMENT

- The general treatment approach to PFT has been irrigation and debridement, IV antibiotics for 2 to 4 days, with subsequent 2 weeks of oral antibiotics.[19]
- The method of irrigation and debridement, however, is still a controversial topic.

OPEN IRRIGATION AND DEBRIDEMENT

- Open treatment of PFT is the method of treatment initially described in the literature.[29]
- Approach
  - Midaxial incision (Figure 44.3)
  - Bruner incision along the course of the tendon sheath
    - The risk of exposed tendon and tendon sheath if wound breaks down
    - Despite this, it has been shown that this incision with primary closure can result in excellent return to function, range of motion, scar healing, and pain.[11]
- Open treatment remains the mainstay for complicated and advanced cases of PFT.[30]

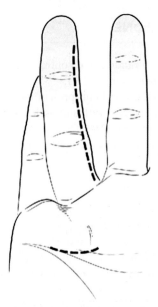

FIGURE 44.3 Illustration demonstrating placement of a midaxial incision for open drainage of pyogenic flexor tenosynovitis. This approach may be combined with a transverse incision at the level of the distal palmar crease to gain proximal access to the tendon sheath for drainage or to obtain a culture. Redrawn from Green DP, Wolfe SW. *Green's Operative Hand Surgery*. 6th ed. Philadelphia, PA, Churchill Livingstone, 2011. Copyright © 2011 Elsevier. With permission.

MINIMALLY INVASIVE IRRIGATION AND DEBRIDEMENT

- Two smaller incisions
  - First incision is made over the A1 pulley of the affected finger at the level of the MCP joint, which is typically a Brunner incision.
  - Second incision is made at the level of the A5 pulley, which is typically a midaxial incision.[13]
- Some form of catheter is then threaded into the tendon sheath from the proximal incision, and the sheath is flushed with irrigant (Figure 44.4).
  - Different catheter techniques have been described, including metal ear suction catheter because it would not buckle upon insertion, 18-gauge angiocatheter, infant feeding tube, and fenestrated catheters.[31-33]

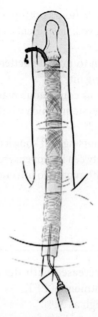

FIGURE 44.4 Illustration demonstrating Neviaser technique for closed tendon sheath irrigation. The technique consists of a proximal zigzag incision for exposure of the tendon sheath, introduction of irrigant into the sheath through a catheter, and a distal counterincision into which a Penrose drain is placed to allow irrigant drainage. Redrawn from Green DP, Wolfe SW. *Green's Operative Hand Surgery*. 6th ed. Philadelphia, PA, Churchill Livingstone, 2011. Copyright © 2011 Elsevier. With permission.

- Limited incision approaches may have improved range of motion postoperatively compared with the open approach.[30,34,35]
- Open debridement and closed catheter irrigation have similar outcomes in terms of clearing the infection.[34]

CONTINUOUS CATHETER IRRIGATION

- CCI is when a catheter is left in the tendon sheath after surgery.
- This will allow for either low continuous irrigation or bolus irrigation.
  - An accepted rate of continuous irrigation is 25 mL/h.
    - Lower rate of infusion may cause less pressure and less discomfort.[28]
  - Bolus irrigation may be 50 mL at a time every 2 hours.

- These systems stay 24 to 48 hours postoperatively.[31,36]
- After the catheter is removed, the patient can progress to 3-times-a-day soaks.[4]
- CCI has not been shown to provide better outcomes with the use of antibiotics within the irrigant.[27]
- Other medications such as continuous marcaine can be used in conjunction with the closed system, which would allow for early aggressive range-of-motion therapy.[6]
- This system does require nursing staff knowledge for appropriate function.
- No statistical difference between intraoperative irrigation and postoperative continuous irrigation with regard to infection resolution or functional outcomes[37]

COMPLICATIONS

- Complications have decreased with the advent of antibiotics and appropriate surgical treatment of PFT.
- Complication rates as high as 38%[13]
  - Possible complications include finger stiffness, decreased range of motion, boutonniere deformity, deep space infection, tendon necrosis or rupture, persistent infection, or need for amputation.[25]
- Loss of range of motion is the most common complication.[2]
  - Due to edema and tendon sheath destruction leading to scarring and decreased excursion of the tendon within the sheath[38]
- Tendon necrosis is one of the more devastating complications, and it is caused by increased pressure within the sheath due to purulent fluid collection, loss of blood supply, necrosis, and eventual tendon rupture.[2]
- Diabetic patients are more likely to have delayed presentation for evaluation and have increased complication rates.
  - Increased time to presentation increases risk of complications and increased time for infection resolution.[7]
  - Likely due to peripheral and autonomic neuropathies and diabetic angiopathy leading to a decreased inflammatory response[22]
  - Diabetics with PFT have an amputation rate of 48% compared with 5% of nondiabetics.[12]
- Patient factors causing increased risk of complication as described by Pang[30]
  - Age over 43

- Medical history including diabetes, peripheral vascular disease, or renal failure
- Initial physical examination upon presentation
  - ◆ No subcutaneous purulence and no ischemia found to have zero amputations and 80% return to total active motion.
  - ◆ Subcutaneous purulence and no ischemia found to have 8% amputation and 72% return to total active motion.
  - ◆ Subcutaneous purulence and necrosis found to have 59% amputation and 49% return to total active motion.

MANAGEMENT ALGORITHM

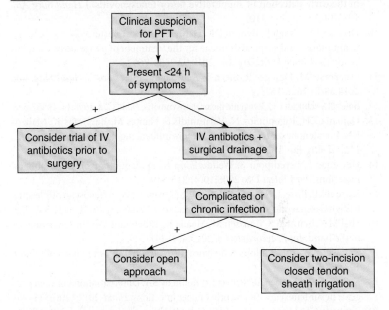

REFERENCES

1. Kanavel AB. The symptoms, signs, and diagnosis of tenosynovitis and fascial-space abscesses. In: Kanavel AB, ed. *Infections of the Hand.* 1st ed. Philadelphia, PA: Lea & Febiger; 1912:201-226.
2. Patel DB, Emmanuel NB, Stevanovic MV. Hand infections: anatomy, types and spread of infection, imaging and findings, and treatment options. *Radiographics.* 2014;34:1968-1986.
3. Scheldrup EW. Tendon sheath patterns in the hand: an anatomical study based on 367 hand dissections. *Surg Gynecol Obstet.* 1951;93(1):16-22.

4. Abrams RA, Botte MJ. Hand infections: treatment recommendations for specific types. *J Am Acad Orthop Surg.* 1996;4:219-230.

5. Aguiar RO, Gasparetto EL, Escuissato DL, et al. Radial and ulnar bursae of the wrist: cadaveric investigation of regional anatomy with ultrasonographic-guided tenography and MR imaging. *Skeletal Radiol.* 2006;35(11):828-832.

6. Gaston RG, Greenberg JA. Use of continuous marcaine irrigation in the management of suppurative flexor tenosynovitis. *Tech Hand Up Extrem Surg.* 2009;13:182-186.

7. Draeger RW, Bynum DK Jr. Flexor tendon sheath infections of the hand. *J Am Acad Orthop Surg.* 2012;20:373-382.

8. Fussey JM, Chin KF, Gogi N, Gella S, Deshmukh SC. An anatomic study of flexor tendon sheaths: a cadaveric study. *J Hand Surg Eur Vol.* 2009;34(6):762-765.

9. Schecter WP, Markison RE, Jeffrey RB, Barton RM, Laing F. Use of sonography in the early detection of suppurative flexor tenosynovitis. *J Hand Surg Am.* 1989;14(2 pt 1):307-310.

10. Draeger RW, Singh B, Bynum DK, Dahners LE. Corticosteroids as an adjunct to antibiotics and surgical drainage for the treatment of pyogenic flexor tenosynovitis. *J Bone Joint Surg Am.* 2010;92:2653-2662.

11. Osterman M, Draeger R, Stern P. Acute hand infections. *J Hand Surg Am.* 2014;39(8):1628-1635.

12. Boles SD, Schmidt CC. Pyogenic flexor tenosynovitis. *Hand Clin.* 1998;14(4):567-578.

13. Dailiana ZH, Rigopoulos N, Varitimidis S, Hantes M, Bargiotas K, Malizos KN. Purulent flexor tenosynovitis: factors influencing the functional outcome. *J Hand Surg Eur Vol.* 2008;33:280-285.

14. Houshian S, Seyedipour S, Wedderkopp N. Epidemiology of bacterial hand infections. *Int J Infect Dis.* 2006;10(4):315-319.

15. Katsoulis E, Bissel I, Hargreaves DG. MRSA pyogenic flexor tenosynovitis leading to digital ischaemic necrosis and amputation. *J Hand Surg Br.* 2006;31:350-352.

16. Sbai MA, Benzarti S, Boussen M, Maalla R. Tuberculous flexor tenosynovitis of the hand. *Int J Mycobacteriol.* 2015;4(4):347-349.

17. Kanavel AB. Tuberculous tenosynovitis of the hand. *Surg Gynecol Obstet.* 1923;37:635.

18. Kennedy CD, Lauder AS, Pribaz JR, Kennedy SA. Differentiation between pyogenic flexor tenosynovitis and other finger infections. *Hand.* 2017;12(6):585-590.

19. Kennedy CD, Huang JI, Hanel DP. In brief: Kanavel's signs and pyogenic flexor tenosynovitis. *Clin Orthop Relat Res.* 2016;474(1):280-284.

20. Luria S, Haze A. Pyogenic flexor tenosynovitis in children. *Pediatr Emerg Care.* 2011;27:740-741.

21. Cohen SG. Point-of-care ultrasound in the evaluation of pyogenic flexor tenosynovitis. *Pediatr Emerg Care.* 2011;27(8):740-741.

22. Flynn JE. Modern considerations of major hand infections. *N Engl J Med.* 1955;252:605-612.

23. Bishop GB, Born T, Kakar S, Jawa A. The diagnostic accuracy of inflammatory blood markers for purulent flexor tenosynovitis. *J Hand Surg.* 2013;38(11):2208-2211.

24. Boyes JH. *Bunnell's Surgery of the Hand*. 5th ed. Philadelphia, PA: JB Lippin-cott; 1970:613-642.

25. Entin MA. Infections of the hand. *Surg Clin North Am*. 1964;44:981-993.

26. Michon J. Phlegmon of the tendon sheaths [in French]. *Ann Chir*. 1974;28:277-280.

27. Giladi AM. Management of acute pyogenic flexor tenosynovitis: literature review and current trends. *J Hand Surg Eur Vol*. 2015;40(7):720-728.

28. Henry M. Septic flexor tenosynovitis. *J Hand Surg Am*. 2011;36(2):322-323.

29. Kanavel AB. The treatment of acute suppurative tenosynovitis—discussion of technique. In: Kanavel AB, ed. *Infections of the Hand. A Guide to the Surgical Treatment of Acute and Chronic Suppurative Processes in the Fingers, Hand, and Forearm*. 5th ed. Philadelphia, PA: Lea & Febiger; 1925:985-990.

30. Pang HN, Teoh LC, Yam AK, Lee JY, Puhaindran ME, Tan AB. Factors af-fecting the prognosis of pyogenic flexor tenosynovitis. *J Bone Joint Surg Am*. 2007;89:1742-1748.

31. Agarwal R, Shah S, Haywood R. Flexor sheath irrigation collection system: the way we do it. *Plast Reconstr Surg*. 2006;117(4):1253-1254.

32. Chung SR, Foo TL. Modifications to simplify intrathecal irrigation for pyogenic flexor tenosynovitis. *Hand*. 2014;9(2);258-259.

33. Jing SS, Iyer S. Simplifying irrigation in flexor tenosynovitis. *J Hand Surg Eur Vol*. 2015;40(3):321.

34. Giladi AM, Malay S, Chung KC. A systematic review of the management of acute pyogenic flexor tenosynovitis. *J Hand Surg Eur Vol*. 2015;40(7):720-728. doi:10.1177/1753193415570248.

35. Neviaser RJ. Closed tendon sheath irrigation for pyogenic flexor tenosynovitis. *J Hand Surg Am*. 1978;3:462-466.

36. Gutowski KA, Ochoa O, Adams WP Jr. Closed-catheter irrigation is as effect-ive as open drainage for treatment of pyogenic flexor tenosynovitis. *Ann Plast Surg*. 2002;49:350-354.

37. Lille S, Hayakawa T, Neumeister MW, Brown RE, Zook EG, Murray K. Continuous postoperative catheter irrigation is not necessary for the treat-ment of suppurative flexor tenosynovitis. *J Hand Surg Br*. 2000;25B:304-307.

38. Schnall SB, Vu-Rose T, Holtom PD, Doyle B, Stevanovic M. Tissue pressures in pyogenic flexor tenosynovitis of the finger: compartment syndrome and its management. *J Bone Joint Surg Br*. 1996;78(5):792-795.

45 Septic Arthritis

Alan R. Blackburn II and John R. Fowler

INTRODUCTION

Pathoanatomy

- Septic arthritis is an infection of the joint space resulting from traumatic inoculation, hematogenous seeding, or contiguous spread.
- Cartilage destruction is rapid by the action of proteolytic enzymes and bacterial toxins, necessitating prompt diagnosis and management to prevent eventual osteomyelitis.

Mechanism of Injury

- Small joints of hand—Most commonly due to traumatic inoculation
- Wrist—Most commonly due to bacteremia with hematogenous seeding

Epidemiology

- *Staphylococcus aureus* and *Streptococcus* are the most common causative organisms, accounting for 91% of septic arthritis cases, regardless of site, although *Gonococcus* should always be high on the differential. If a clenched fist injury has occurred, polymicrobial infections are typical, and *Eikenella corrodens* may be involved in up to 30% of cases.

EVALUATION

History

- Patients often present with a history of penetrating trauma or direct inoculation as with a clenched fist injury, and the source of injury is important in selecting appropriate empiric antibiotic therapy.
- Less commonly, contiguous spread from an adjacent infection may occur, such as with a felon, paronychia, or purulent flexor tenosynovitis.

Physical Examination

- Signs and symptoms include erythema, edema, warmth, and painful range of motion both actively and passively.
- Fluctuance may be present.
- Systemic signs such as fever, chills, or tachycardia may be present; however, these systemic signs may be absent when small joints are affected.

Laboratory Evaluation

- White blood cell count, ESR, and CRP should always be obtained; however, these studies may or may not be elevated when dealing with small joints of the hand.
- Blood cultures should always be sent, especially when systemic symptoms are present.
- Definitive diagnosis is made with synovial fluid analysis; however, aspiration of small joints can be challenging and may yield only minimal amounts of fluid.
  - Aspirate should be sent for Gram stain, aerobic and anaerobic culture, and crystal analysis.
  - Additional fluid may be sent for cell count, fluid protein and glucose levels, and fungal and mycobacterial cultures.
- A diagnosis of joint sepsis is supported by a synovial fluid WBC count of higher than 50 000/mL (>75% neutrophils), glucose 40 mg less than fasting blood glucose, and a positive Gram stain or culture.
- The presence of crystals does not exclude the possibility of coexisting infection.

Imaging

- Radiographs should be obtained to evaluate for a retained foreign body, the presence of gas in the soft tissues, or osteomyelitis.
  - Early in the course of infection, soft tissue swelling and joint capsular distension may be seen.
  - Later, joint space narrowing is demonstrated as cartilage has been destroyed.

MANAGEMENT

- In general, septic arthritis should be treated as a surgical urgency as articular destruction by proteolytic enzymes and toxins begins within the first 24 hours.

- After an aspirate has been obtained to tailor definitive antibiotics, successful conservative management with initial broad-spectrum IV antibiotics and serial joint aspiration has been reported, although this remains controversial and therapeutically unpredictable.
  - Initial antibiotic choice remains controversial. In most cases, we prefer broad-spectrum coverage with Vancomycin and Unasyn, which allows coverage of both methicillin-sensitive *Staphylococcus* and methicillin-resistant *Staphylococcus*, as well as *Eikenella*.
- Superior results are reported with formal arthrotomy and copious irrigation
- When approaches involve the small joints of the hand, the joint capsule and wounds are left open and covered with a moist gauze dressing.
- **Surgical approach to wrist**
  - The wrist joints (radio- and ulnocarpal joints, midcarpal joints, and the distal radioulnar joint) may be accessed via a standard dorsal approach to the wrist between the 3rd and 4th extensor compartments.
  - Transverse incisions may be used separately to open radiocarpal and midcarpal joints.
  - Capsular windows may be used to allow continued drainage.
  - Joints should be distracted, irrigated, and taken through a range of motion to maximize removal of purulent material.
  - Excise inflammatory synovium and necrotic debris.
  - The joint capsule may be left open with placement of a gauze wick, or closed over a drain for continued drainage. (Although some surgeons prefer to close the joint capsule to prevent a direct route to the joint for skin flora.)
  - Retraction of skin edges can be prevented with one or two loosely placed sutures.
- **Surgical approach to metacarpophalangeal joints** (Figure 45.1)
  - Commonly approached dorsally, oftentimes incorporating an overlying wound and allowing for excision of wound edges.
  - The joint capsule is exposed and entered through longitudinal splitting of the extensor tendon hood or through the sagittal band adjacent to the tendon.
  - Apply longitudinal traction, irrigate, and examine for retained foreign body.
- **Surgical approach to proximal interphalangeal joints** (Figure 45.2)
  - A midaxial incision is preferred to avoid injury to the central extensor tendon slip.

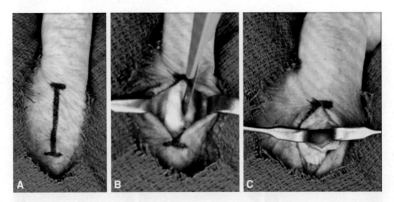

FIGURE 45.1 A, A longitudinal incision is planned over the joint. B, The skin is retracted and extensor tendon split. C, The joint is exposed and irrigated.

- The digital nerves should lie volar to the incision, though dorsal sensory branches may be visualized.
- The transverse retinacular ligament is incised and the joint is entered by excising a portion of the accessory collateral ligament and joint capsule.
- **Surgical approach to distal interphalangeal joints** (Figure 45.3)
    - Approach is through a dorsal "H" or "reverse Y" incision.
    - Skin flaps are created, and the capsule is opened adjacent to a retracted terminal tendon.
    - Protect the insertion to avoid creation of an iatrogenic mallet finger.
- **Postoperative management**
    - Dressing changes three times a day and soaks in dilute povidone-iodine solution with early and aggressive range of motion.
    - Initial intravenous antibiotics with transition to culture-appropriate oral therapy following acceptable response to equivalent IV form.

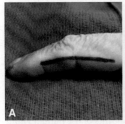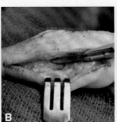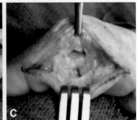

FIGURE 45.2 A, A midaxial incision is planned. B, The neurovascular bundles are retracted volarly. C, The joint is exposed and irrigated.

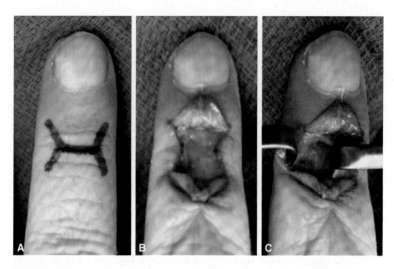

FIGURE 45.3 A, An "H"-shaped incision is planned. B, The skin is retracted and terminal tendon exposed. C, The terminal tendon is retracted to expose the joint.

- Typically, oral antibiotics may be started at 10 to 14 days and continued for 4 to 6 additional weeks.
- If improvement is absent at 24 to 48 hours following surgical intervention, a repeat washout may be indicated.
- **Postoperative complications (worsened outcomes are seen with delay in treatment)**
  - Joint stiffness, joint space narrowing, and possible arthrosis and ankylosis
  - Tendon adhesions
  - Osteomyelitis of adjacent bones

SUGGESTED READINGS

Abrams RA, Botte MJ. Hand infections: treatment recommendations for specific types. *J Am Acad Orthop Surg.* 1996;4:219-230.

Mathews CJ, Kingsley G, Field M, et al. Management of septic arthritis: a systematic review. *Ann Rheum Dis.* 2007;66:440-445.

McDonald LS, Bavaro MF, Hofmeister EP, Kroonen LT. Hand infections. *J Hand Surg.* 2011;36A:1403-1412.

Sinha M, Jain S, Woods DA. Septic arthritis of the small joints of the hand. *J Hand Surg.* 2006;31B:665-672.

46 Web Space Infections

Tiffany J. Pan and John R. Fowler

INTRODUCTION

- Definition
  - A deep infection of the hand that occurs in the webspace between two fingers
  - It is also known as a collar-button abscess in reference to the dumbbell shape reminiscent of collar buttons from the early 20th century
- Pathoanatomy
  - Deep subfascial spaces
    - ◆ Dorsal subcutaneous space
    - ◆ Dorsal subaponeurotic space
      - ✳ Dorsal limit—dense aponeurosis of extensor tendons
      - ✳ Volar limit—metacarpal periosteum and dorsal fascia of interossei muscles
      - ✳ Medial and lateral borders—confluence of aponeurotic sheet and deep fascia over dorsal interossei as well as metacarpal bones and metacarpophalangeal joint capsules
    - ◆ Interdigital webspace
      - ✳ Loose connective tissue between the metacarpal heads
      - ✳ Skin is intimately attached to the palmar fascia volarly but is relatively mobile dorsally
  - Dorsal spread is most common due to the dense attachment of the volar skin to the palmar fascia limiting formation of the abscess
  - Infections are able to track through the loosely organized tissue of the interdigital webspace
- Mechanism of injury
  - Superficial skin fissure in the webspace
  - Palmar callus
  - Penetrating injury, frequently of the volar surface
  - Attempted injection of IV drugs
  - Extension of infection from adjacent fingers

- Epidemiology
  - 5% to 15% of hand infections are deep space infections
  - *Staphylococcus aureus* and group A beta-hemolytic *Streptococcus* are the most common organisms identified
  - Human bites likely to cause polymicrobial infection

EVALUATION

- History
  - Complaints of pain and swelling of both the volar and dorsal aspects of a webspace
  - Penetrating injury to the webspace, frequently on the volar aspect
  - Concurrent infection of other fingers
  - IV drug use
- Physical examination
  - Examine for skin fissures, calluses, or breaks in the skin
  - Swelling, fluctuance, and erythema in the webspace
  - Dorsal swelling can be significant
  - Abduction of fingers adjacent to affected webspace (Figure 46.1)
  - Rule out flexor tendon sheath infection (Kanavel signs)
    - Fusiform swelling
    - Pain with passive extension

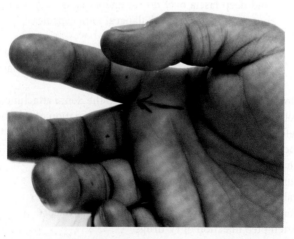

FIGURE 46.1 Collar-button abscess in webspace between index and long fingers with fingers in abducted position.

- ◆ Holds finger in flexed position
- ◆ Tenderness to palpation along the flexor tendon sheath
- ■ Imaging
  - Plain films show soft tissue swelling
  - MRI or CT with contrast can define extent of abscess formation but is often unnecessary if clinical examination is consistent with a collar-button abscess

DEFINITIVE TREATMENT

- ■ Nonoperative treatment
  - No role for nonoperative treatment if an abscess is present
  - If abscess is not present, treat the cellulitis or other superficial infection as appropriate
- ■ Surgical approach
  - Volar and dorsal incisions preferred to ensure complete drainage of both aspects of the abscess
    - ◆ Dorsal longitudinal incision between the digits from just proximal to the metacarpal head to the base of the involved web
    - ◆ Volar incision (Figure 46.2)
      - * Curved longitudinal—from the radial side of the webspace distally to the ulnar side proximally, stopping just distal to the midpalmar crease
      - * "Z" or zigzag—from just proximal to the web to just distal to the midpalmar crease
  - Tract should be opened between the volar and dorsal extensions of the abscess
  - Volar incision and excision of the fascia may be used, but may not adequately drain the dorsal aspect
  - Avoid incisions crossing the webspace as a contracture can develop
  - Allow incision to close by secondary intention
  - May place a Penrose drain or wick
- ■ Potential complications
  - Webspace contracture
  - Incomplete drainage of abscess
- ■ Postoperative care
  - Remove drain at 24 to 48 hours
  - Culture-specific antibiotics
  - Hand soaks
  - Wound healing by secondary intention

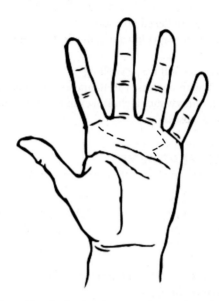

FIGURE 46.2 Curved longitudinal and zigzag volar incisions depicted.

MANAGEMENT ALGORITHM

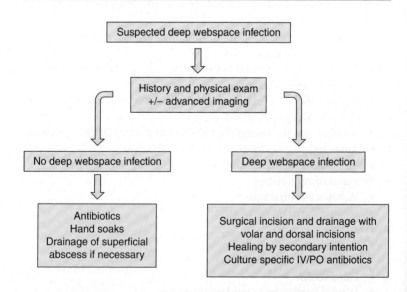

SUGGESTED READINGS

Abrams RA, Botte MJ. Hand infections: treatment recommendations for specific types. *J Am Acad Orthop Surg.* 1996;4:219-230.

Green DP, Wolfe SW. *Green's Operative Hand Surgery.* Philadelphia, PA: Elsevier/ Churchill Livingstone; 2011.

Jebson PJ. Deep subfascial space infections. *Hand Clin.* 1998;14(4):557-566, viii.

McDonald LS, Bavaro MF, Hofmeister EP, Kroonen LT. Hand infections. *J Hand Surg Am.* 2011;36A:1403-1412.

Osterman M, Draeger R, Sern P. Acute hand infections. *J Hand Surg.* 2014;39(8):1628-1635.

Patel DB, Emmanuel NB, Stevanovic MV, et al. Hand infections: anatomy, types and spread of infection, imaging findings, and treatment options. *Radiographics.* 2014;34:1968-1986.

Hannah A. Dineen and Reid W. Draeger

INTRODUCTION

- Hand infections, which include cellulitis, paronychia and felons, flexor tenosynovitis, and deep palmar space infections, are frequently encountered by primary care and emergency physicians in addition to orthopedic surgeons. Early diagnosis and treatment is key to optimal outcomes.
- Epidemiology
  - Occur from direct inoculation from penetrating trauma, or from untreated infections elsewhere in the hand that spread contiguously into the deep spaces of the hand.[1]
  - Approximately 2% to 15% of hand infections involve the deep spaces of the hand.[2,3]
- Pathoanatomy
  - Deep spaces of the hand include the thenar, midpalmar, Parona's quadrilateral, dorsal subaponeurotic, and interdigital subfascial web space (Figure 47.1 and Table 47.1)[1,3-6]
- Mechanism of injury
  - Infection can occur from inoculation such as penetrating trauma or bites.[1]
  - Untreated infections in surrounding regions may spread through adjacent spread.
  - More rarely hematogenous spread may occur to any of the palmar spaces.[7] Knowledge of anatomy of these regions and their boundaries can help identify and predict spread of deep infection.
  - Untreated flexor tenosynovitis can cause infection within the palmar spaces
    - ◆ The radial bursa is contiguous with the flexor pollicis longus (FPL) tendon sheath while the ulnar bursa communicates with the small finger flexor tendon sheath.
    - ◆ Approximately 50% to 80% of people have communicating radial and ulnar bursae. This occurs via multiple variations of connections

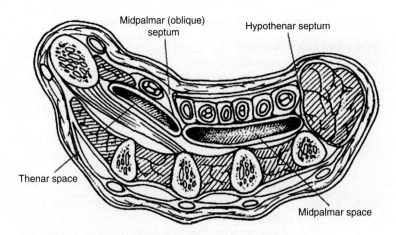

FIGURE 47.1 Anatomy of deep palmar spaces. Cross-section of hand demonstrates thenar, midpalmar, and hypothenar spaces. From Abrams RA, Botte MJ. Hand infections : treatment recommendations for specific types. *J Am Acad Orthop Surg.* 1996;4(4):219-230.

between the index, middle, ring, and small finger tendon sheaths, as well as the FPL tendon sheath with the ulnar and radial bursa.[7,8] Infections involving the thumb flexor tendon or small finger flexor tendon can thus result in a "horseshoe abscess."[7,8]

- Infection of the index finger flexor tendon sheath can spread to the thenar space, as this sheath is the volar boundary of the thenar space.[7]
- Infection involving the thenar space in the interval between the adductor pollicis and first dorsal interossei muscles can cause a "pantaloon" effect.[7]
- Contiguous spread of flexor tenosynovitis can continue proximally to involve Parona's space. The communication that can exist between the radial and ulnar bursa occurs via Parona's space, and thus can extend to the carpal tunnel.[9]
  * Controversy exists whether involvement of the carpal tunnel is from communicating spread or through rupture of the bursa.[9]
- Parona's space can also be involved through spread from an infection within the radiocarpal joint and invasion through the volar joint capsule.[6]

TABLE 47.1 Anatomy of Deep Palmar Spaces

Deep Hand Space	Borders
Thenar space	Dorsal: adductor pollicis
	Volar: index flexor tendon
	Radial: adductor pollicis insertion at proximal phalanx of thumb
	Ulnar boundary: midpalmar (oblique) septum, which separates this from midpalmar space
Midpalmar or deep palmar space	Dorsal: long and ring finger metacarpals, 2nd and 3rd interossei
	Volar: long, ring, and small finger flexor tendons and lumbricals
	Radial: midpalmar/oblique septum
	Ulnar: hypothenar muscles and hypothenar septum
Hypothenar space	Dorsal: periosteum of 5th metacarpal and fascia of deep hypothenar muscles
	Volar: palmar fascia and fascia overlying superficial hypothenar muscles
	Radial: hypothenar septum
Dorsal subaponeurotic space	Dorsal: extensor tendons
	Volar: periosteum of metacarpals and dorsal fascia of interossei
Interdigital subfascial web space	Dorsal: dorsal hand fascia and skin
	Volar: palmar fascia
	Radial and ulnar: digital extensor mechanism, metacarpophalangeal (MCP) joint capsules, ligamentous structures. This is the palmar space between digits and is continuous with the dorsal subcutaneous space between the fingers
Parona's quadrilateral space	Dorsal: digital flexor tendons
	Volar: pronator quadratus
	Radial: flexor pollicis longus
	Ulnar: flexor carpi ulnaris

- Penetrating trauma
  - Hypothenar space infections are very rare and almost always the result of penetrating trauma.[10] Contiguous spread of infection does not occur commonly as the boundaries of the hypothenar space keep this compartment isolated.[6]
- Infected palmar blisters or skin fissures
  - Collar button abscesses occur in the interdigital subfascial space, typically from spread from an infected palmar blister or skin fissure (see Chapter 46).[7] Adherent fascia and palmar skin force the

abscess to extend dorsally into the web space.[7] Additionally, the interdigital web space is contiguous with the dorsal subcutaneous tissue between fingers.[3]

- Microbiology
  - Over 90% of infections are bacterial in origin.[11]
  - *Staphylococcus aureus* and *Streptococcus* species are the most commonly implicated bacteria, with *Staphylococcus* the principal organism in 50% to 80% of infections.[7,12]
    - *S. aureus* tends to cause a suppurative infection that peaks in 3 to 6 days.[12]
    - *Staphylococcus epidermidis* infections tend to be more superficial.[12]
    - Methicillin-resistant *S. aureus* (MRSA) infections are becoming increasingly frequent, with an incidence of 34% to 73% in all hand infections.[5,13]
      - Risk factors for MRSA infections include patients with diabetes or an immunocompromised state, as well as a history of prior antibiotic use. Additionally, risk factors include those patients living in close spaces such as contact sports, military recruits, day cares, prisoners, or homeless patients.
      - Nosocomial MRSA acquisition can occur from prolonged hospital stays, in particular in an intensive care unit.[1]
    - Depending on the mechanism of injury, different bacteria may be present (Table 47.2).
    - Trauma is the most common etiology of hand infections followed by a laceration or puncture wound.[14]
      - Industrial injuries or those within the home typically are a single microbial infection with a Gram-positive organism.[7]
      - Bite wounds, farm injuries, and infections in IV drug users as well as diabetics are often polymicrobial and involve Gram-negative and anaerobic species in addition to Gram-positive organisms.[1]
        - 42 bacterial strains have been isolated in human bite wounds.[7]
        - Although alpha-hemolytic *Streptococci* is the most frequently isolated pathogen, *Eikenella corrodens* is frequent and isolated about one-third of the time.[7,15]
        - *Pasteurella multocida* is found in infections involving dog or cat bites, as this facultative anaerobe is present in two-third of domestic cat and half of domestic dog oral flora.[7,12]

TABLE 47.2 **Antibiotic Recommendations for Specific Clinical Scenario**

Injury/Organism	Antibiotics	Duration of Treatment
Suture line abscess	Cephalexin or sulfamethoxazole/trimethoprim	7-10 d
Abscess	Ampicillin/sulbactam + vancomycin	
	Cefazolin + vancomycin	
	Clindamycin if severe penicillin injury	
Cat or dog bites	Amoxicillin/clavulanic acid (orally) or ampicillin/sulbactam (intravenously)	7-14 d
	If penicillin allergic, ciprofloxacin, ceftriaxone, or doxycycline	
Human bites	Cephalosporins	
	Gentamicin and penicillinase-resistant penicillin	
Osteomyelitis	Vancomycin and piperacillin/tazobactam	6-8 wk
Septic arthritis		3-4 wk
Tenosynovitis		2-3 wk

The antibiotics listed in this chart are first-line antibiotics to be used until cultures dictate treatment.

Reprinted from Osterman M, Draeger R, Stern P. Acute hand infections. *J Hand Surg Am*. 2014;39(8): 1628-1635. Copyright © 2014 American Society for Surgery of the Hand. With permission.

EVALUATION

History

- Inquire about a history of trauma or inoculating injury.
- May have history of other hand infections that have spread to involve the deep spaces including antecedent cellulitis, felon, paronychia, flexor tenosynovitis, septic arthritis, or osteomyelitis
- Inquire about recent surgery or IV drug use.
- May present with fever, pain, malaise
- Risk factors for the development of hand infections include diabetes mellitus and patients who are immunocompromised or on immunosuppressant drugs.[7]

Physical Examination

- The classic signs of flexor tenosynovitis may be present if the deep space infection results from spread from advanced flexor tenosynovitis (see Chapter 44).

- Kanavel signs—fusiform swelling, tenderness over the flexor tendon sheath, finger resting in a flexed position, and pain with passive extension of the finger[16]
- Fever, erythema, and marked pain with palpation as well as range of motion of the fingers, particularly the middle and ring fingers, may be present.[1,17]
- Lymphadenopathy, systemic malaise, and tachycardia may be present in advanced infection.[11]
- Thenar space abscess
  - The most common deep space infection
  - Presents with marked swelling of the thenar eminence and first web space
  - Thumb rests in palmar abduction to minimize pressure within the space.[10,17]
  - Any adduction or opposition of the thumb elicits pain.
  - A "dumbbell" or "pantaloon" infection may be present if infection spreads dorsally over the adductor pollicis and first dorsal interosseous muscles and travels deep to the index finger flexor tendons.[3]
- Midpalmar space infection
  - Presents with marked swelling and loss of normal palmar concavity, causing the palm to be flattened or appear convex.[1,3]
  - There may be pain present with passive extension of the middle and ring fingers.
    - If present, this is typically less than with a pyogenic flexor tenosynovitis involving those digits.[6]
- Hypothenar space infection
  - May have fullness and pain over the hypothenar eminence
  - Due to the strict boundaries of this space, there is usually no swelling of the remainder of the palm or fingers.
- Dorsal subaponeurotic space infection
  - Typically occurs from local penetration and signs of trauma may be present.
  - Due to its superficial location, purulence may be found emanating from the wound.
  - Finger extension may be painful.
  - Infections in this space may appear similar to cellulitis.[3]
- Interdigital web space infection
  - Collar-button abscesses can present with dumbbell-shaped swelling involving both the dorsal and volar web space, and abduction of the fingers.[1,17]

- Abscess tends to be more pronounced dorsally, as the thick attachments of the palmar fascia prevent the abscess from tracking significantly volarly.
■ Parona's space infection
  - Tenderness and swelling in the distal volar forearm
  - May have pain with finger flexion
  - Evaluate for signs of median nerve compression.[18]

Imaging

■ Diagnosis can often be made without the need for advanced imaging in cases of obvious superficial infections.
■ Radiographs are necessary in the initial workup to rule out the presence of a foreign body or fracture.
■ Ultrasound can be helpful to evaluate for fluid collections.
  - Operator-dependent and has limited availability depending on the center
■ Magnetic resonance imaging (MRI) offers improved visualization of soft tissues and deep infections.
  - Time-consuming, expensive, and may not be available at all hospitals
■ Recently, computed tomography (CT) is being used for the evaluation of deep or complicated infections due to its wide availability and quick processing.[9]

Laboratory Studies

■ Complete blood count, C-reactive protein, and erythrocyte sedimentation rate are helpful to establish the presence of an infection and assess severity.
■ Glucose should be obtained in diabetic patients.
■ Cultures should be obtained prior to initiating antibiotic treatment. This can be obtained from a draining wound or abscess, or intraoperatively at the time of debridement.
  - Aerobic and anaerobic cultures are adequate in acute uncomplicated infections.[3]
■ Chronic or complicated infections may require specialized stains or culture medium.

ACUTE MANAGEMENT

Nonoperative Treatment

■ Early infections, if detected within 24 hours, can be treated with an attempt at nonoperative management that includes IV antibiotics, rest, elevation, and observation.[12,17]
■ Tetanus prophylaxis should be initiated if indicated.

Antibiotics

- Empiric antibiotics should be started after obtaining an initial culture (Table 47.3).
  - Recent evidence recommends empiric treatment for MRSA infections if local prevalence exceeds 10% to 15%, due to the delay in proper treatment if incorrect antibiotic is selected.[1,13]
- Depending on the mechanism, different empiric antibiotics may also be advisable (Table 47.2).

TABLE 47.3 Antibiotic Recommendations for Common Organisms

Organism	Antibiotic	Additional information
Methicillin-sensitive *Staphylococcus aureus*	Cephalexin, amoxicillin clavulanate (orally)	
Methicillin-resistant *S. aureus*	Trimethoprim/sulfamethoxazole (orally), linezolid (orally or IV) If sulfa allergy, clindamycin or doxycycline Vancomycin (IV), daptomycin (IV) Quinupristin/dalfopristin (IV) Tigecycline (IV) Ceftaroline (IV)	Linezolid: expensive, avoid in endocarditis or meningitis, weekly complete blood cell monitoring Daptomycin: weekly creatinine phosphokinase monitoring
Vancomycin-resistant Enterococci	Daptomycin, linezolid (orally or IV), tigecycline (IV), quinupristin/dalfopristin (IV)	
Gram-negative	Piperacillin/tazobactam Ceftriaxone Ertapenem Quinolones/ciprofloxacin	
Pseudomonas	Piperacillin/tazobactam Cefepime Meropenem	
Anaerobic infections	Ampicillin/sulbactam, Piperacillin/tazobactam, ertapenem, meropenem Metronidazole Clindamycin Tigecycline	

TABLE 47.3 Antibiotic Recommendations for Common Organisms (*continued*)

Organism	Antibiotic	Additional information
Vibrio vulnificus	Ceftriaxone and doxycycline	
	Imipenem and doxycycline	
Nocardia	Trimethoprim/sulfamethoxazole	6 mo of treatment in immunosuppressed patients
	If sulfa allergy: imipenem, ceftriaxone, amikacin	
Sporothrix schenckii	Itraconazole	
	Fluconazole and voriconazole	
Mycobacterium marinum	Clarithromycin/azithromycin	
	Trimethoprim/sulfamethoxazole, minocycline	
	Ethambutol	
Aeromonas hydrophila	Ciprofloxacin	
	Imipenem	
	Trimethoprim/sulfamethoxazole	
Cutaneous anthrax	Ciprofloxacin	Treatment for 60 d to treat any remaining spores
	Doxycycline	
Tularemia	Gentamicin and doxycycline	

Reprinted from Osterman M, Draeger R, Stern P. Acute hand infections. *J Hand Surg Am*. 2014;39(8): 1628-1635. Copyright © 2014 American Society for Surgery of the Hand. With permission.

DEFINITIVE TREATMENT

Operative Treatment

- If no improvement is seen within 24 hours of nonoperative management, or if presentation occurs 24 hours after injury, operative treatment is recommended.[17]
- Formal incision and drainage in the operating room is the mainstay of operative treatment.

General Principles

- Primary goal is evacuation of pus.
- Straight incisions are preferred to prevent flap necrosis.[17]
- In the palm, incisions should be parallel to the distal palmar crease.[19]

- Avoid incisions over tendons or neurovascular structures.
- Irrigate thoroughly intraoperatively with either bulb syringe or pulsed irrigation.[3]
- Leave contaminated wounds open to granulate in and allow daily wet-dry dressings.[17]
- Loosely approximate wounds over an irrigating catheter or a drain.[17]
- Through-and-through drains should not be used in the palm.[6]
- If performing continuous irrigation, typical irrigation amount is 100 mL/h for 24 to 48 hours.[3]
- Immobilize digits in the "intrinsic-plus" position.
- Maintain space between the web spaces with dressing to avoid contractures.[17]
- Multiple debridements may be necessary before wounds are clean enough for closure.[17]
- If there is no improvement after surgical treatment and antibiotics, additional debridement and reexploration may be necessary.[3]
- Negative-pressure wound therapy may be used.[17]
- Avoid constricting bandages. Moist bulky dressings with immobilization are preferred.[12]
- Whirlpool or soaks may promote drainage.[17]
- Dakin's solution can be used for large open wounds.[12]
- Hand therapy is key to maintain range of motion.

Surgical Approaches

- Thenar space
  - Dorsal, palmar, combined dorsal and palmar, and transcommissural incisions can be used (Figures 47.2 and 47.3).[17]
    - If a dumbbell or pantaloon abscess is present, avoid use of a single dorsal approach as access to volar deep tissue planes can be difficult. A combined volar-dorsal or single volar incision is preferred for these abscesses.[3]
  - Thenar crease (volar) approach (Figure 47.3C)
    - Incision is parallel to the thenar crease. Protect the neurovascular structures and perform blunt dissection through the palmar fascia toward the adductor pollicis.[6] Continue distal to the adductor pollicis to access the dorsal compartment between the adductor pollicis and first dorsal interosseous compartment.[3]
  - Dorsal transverse incision (Figure 47.2B)
    - Incision is in the middle of the dorsal web space at the base of the thumb metacarpophalangeal (MCP).

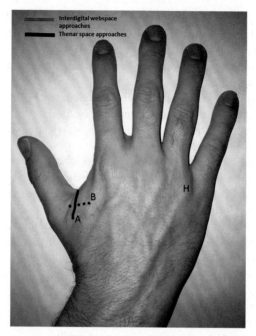

FIGURE 47.2 Dorsal hand incisions. A—Dorsal longitudinal incision to access thenar space; B—Dorsal transverse incision to access thenar space; H—Interdigital web space dorsal incision, to be used in combination with a volar incision.

- Dorsal longitudinal incision (Figure 47.2A)
    - Incision is from the dorsum of the first web space and extended proximal to the web.[6] Blunt dissection is performed between the interval between the first dorsal interosseous and adductor muscle.[3]
- Dangers
    - Palmar cutaneous branch of the median nerve as well as the recurrent motor branch of the median nerve are at risk for injury using both of these incisions.[3]
    - Avoid incisions parallel to the first web space to avoid contracture.[17]
    - Terminal branch of the ulnar motor nerve can be injured when exposing the deep portion of adductor pollicis.[19]

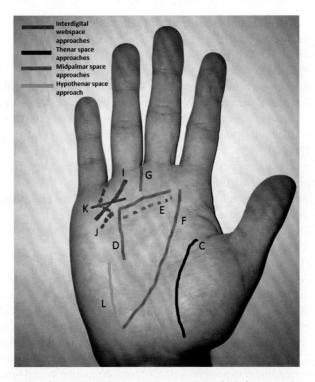

FIGURE 47.3 Volar hand incisions. C—Thenar crease (volar) approach to thenar space; D—Combined volar transverse and longitudinal incision to midpalmar space; E—Transverse volar incision to midpalmar space; F—Curved longitudinal volar incision to midpalmar space; G—Lumbrical approach to midpalmar space; I—Volar curved longitudinal incision to access interdigital web space, to be used in combination with a dorsal incision; J—Volar zigzag incision to access interdigital web space; K—Volar transverse incision to access interdigital web space; L—Volar longitudinal incision to hypothenar space.

- Midpalmar space infection
  - Volar transverse incision (Figure 47.3E)
    - Incision is distal to the distal palmar crease, along the width of the middle and ring finger. Divide the palmar fascia, protect neurovascular bundles, and then dissect on either side of the flexor tendons until the abscess is reached.[3]
  - Can also use a longitudinal curved incision (Figure 47.3F), or a combined longitudinal and transverse incision (Figure 47.3D).[3] Longitudinal

incisions should be made ulnar to the middle finger and parallel to the thenar crease.[19]

- Lumbrical approach (Figure 47.3G)
  - ◆ Used for infections that involve the lumbrical canal
  - ◆ Incision is made proximal to the 3rd web space just distal to the midpalmar crease. Do not cross the web space. A hemostat can be passed retrograde and dorsal to the flexor tendons and down the lumbrical canal to access the space.[3]
- Dangers
  - ◆ Common digital nerve, arteries, superficial palmar arch
- Hypothenar space infection
  - Accessed through a longitudinal incision proximal and ulnar to the midpalmar crease (Figure 47.3L)[3]
  - Divide hypothenar fascia directly underneath incision to access the abscess.
- Dorsal subaponeurotic space infection
  - A longitudinal incision over a localized region can be used. More diffuse infections may require the use of two linear incisions overlying the 2nd metacarpal and between the 4th and 5th metacarpals.[3]
    - ◆ Maintain an adequate skin bridge and do not place incision directly over the extensor tendons. Incise the dorsal hand fascia between the extensor tendons, but maintain the paratenon and juncturae tendinum to preserve extensor tendon vascularity and function.[3]
- Interdigital web space
  - Volar zigzag, curved longitudinal, volar transverse, or dorsal longitudinal incisions can be used (Figures 47.2 and 47.3). Straight longitudinal incisions do not have adequate exposure.[3]
  - Volar incisions alone can be used if excision of the tethering palmar fascia is performed to allow decompression of the dorsal extent of the infection.[17]
    - ◆ If the palmar fascia is not excised, both dorsal and volar incisions are necessary to perform drainage along both sides of the palmar fascia.[3]
  - Volar curved longitudinal approach and dorsal approach (Figures 47.2H and 47.3I)
    - ◆ Incision is made along the radial border of the affected web space and ends distal to the midpalmar crease. Divide subcutaneous tissue and dissect until the abscess is found. The dorsal incision is then made proximal to the involved web space and tissues are dissected until the abscess is encountered.[6]

- Volar zigzag approach (Figure 47.3J)
  - Begin incision proximal to the involved web and end distal to the midpalmar crease. Expose the dorsal and volar longitudinal spaces by incising the palmar fascia and superficial transverse metacarpal ligaments. Ensure protection of neurovascular bundles.
    - An additional dorsal incision at the level of the MCPs can be performed if adequate decompression is not achieved after milking of the dorsal region through the volar approach.[3]
  - Dangers
    - Transverse incisions can cause contracture and loss of finger abduction.[3,17]
- Parona's space
  - Wide exposure is necessary to decompress this region.
  - Volar curvilinear or longitudinal incision
    - Incision is proximal to the wrist crease and radial to the flexor carpi ulnaris. Incise through skin and antebrachial fascia with gentle retraction of the flexor tendons and median nerve.[3]
    - Carpal tunnel release may also be indicated if there is involvement of this region.
    - If there is involvement of the midpalmar region, consider placement of a catheter into the midpalmar region for continuous retrograde irrigation into both regions.[17]
    - Dangers
      - Avoid placement of incisions over tendons and the median nerve.

Complications

- Delayed treatment can result in adverse outcome.[20]
- Prolonged infection can affect tendon vascularity. This can result in tendon ischemia and necrosis, adhesions, continuous spread of the infection, and sepsis.[17]
- Stiffness and contracture may result if range of motion therapy is not initiated or incisions are placed within web spaces.
- Iatrogenic neurovascular injury during surgery is uncommon but can occur.
- Worse outcomes are seen in diabetic patients.
  - Slower resolution of infection (greater than 8 days) is seen.[20]
  - Amputation rates range from 16% to 39%.[21]
  - 50% rate of repeat surgical treatment[20]

Postoperative Care

- Most wounds are left open with moist, soft bulky dressing. A removable splint can be used in between range of motion exercises and soaks.
- IV antibiotics and elevation are indicated. IV antibiotics are recommended until the infection is controlled and then can be transitioned to oral antibiotics as dictated by cultures.[6]
- Tight glycemic control is necessary in diabetic patients.
- First dressing change within 24 hours and soaks begun
- Early range of motion is encouraged with active range of motion exercises initiated during soaks.[19]
- If there is no improvement after 24 to 36 hours, repeat debridement may be needed with an especially low threshold to return to the operating room with immunocompromised or diabetic patients.[6]

MANAGEMENT ALGORITHM

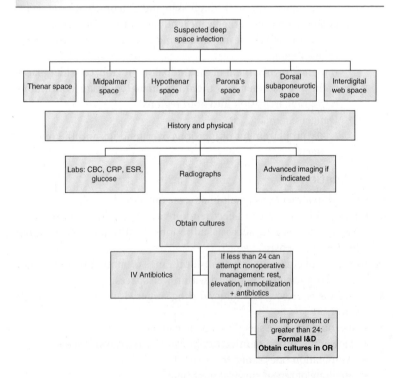

REFERENCES

1. McDonald LS, Bavaro MF, Hofmeister EP, Kroonen LT. Hand infections. *J Hand Surg Am*. 2011;36(8):1403-1412. doi:10.1016/j.jhsa.2011.05.035.
2. Ong YS, Levin SL. Hand infections. *Plast Reconstr Surg*. 2009;124(4):225e-233e. doi:10.1097/PRS.0b013e3181b458c9.
3. Jebson PJ. Deep subfascial space infections. *Hand Clin*. 1998;14(4):557-566, viii.
4. Crosswell S, Vanat Q, Jose R. The anatomy of deep hand space infections: the deep thenar space. *J Hand Surg Am*. 2014;39(12):2550. doi:10.1016/j.jhsa.2014.10.015.
5. Osterman M, Draeger R, Stern P. Acute hand infections. *J Hand Surg Am*. 2014;39(8):1628-1635. doi:10.1016/j.jhsa.2014.03.031.
6. Stevanovic MV, Sharpe F. Acute infections. In: Wolfe SW, Hotchkiss RN, Pederson WC, Kozin SH, eds. *Green's Operative Hand Surgery*. 6th ed. Philadelphia, PA: Elsevier/Churchill Livingstone; 2011:41-84.
7. Abrams RA, Botte MJ. Hand infections: treatment recommendations for specific types. *J Am Acad Orthop Surg*. 1996;4(4):219-230.
8. Draeger, RW, Bynum DK. Flexor tendon sheath infections in the hand. *J Am Acad Orthop Surg*. 2012;20:373-382.
9. Ahlawat S, Corl FM, LaPorte DM, Fishman EK, Fayad LM. MDCT of hand and wrist infections: emphasis on compartmental anatomy. *Clin Radiol*. 2017;72(4):338.e1-338.e9. doi:10.1016/j.crad.2016.11.020.
10. Patel DB, Emmanuel NB, Stevanovic MV, et al. Hand infections: anatomy, types and spread of infection, imaging findings, and treatment options. *Radiographics*. 2014;34(7):1968-1986. doi:10.1148/rg.347130101.
11. Thornton DJA, Lindau T. Hand infections. *Orthop Trauma*. 2010;24(3):186-196. doi:10.1016/j.mporth.2010.03.016.
12. Hausman MR, Lisser SP. Hand infections. *Orthop Clin North Am*. 1992;23:171-185.
13. Tosti R, Ilyas AM. Empiric antibiotics for acute infections of the hand. *J Hand Surg Am*. 2010;35(1):125-128. doi:10.1016/j.jhsa.2009.10.024.
14. Houshian S, Seyedipour S, Wedderkopp N. Epidemiology of bacterial hand infections. *Int J Infect Dis*. 2006;10(4):315-319. doi:10.1016/j.ijid.2005.06.009.
15. Goldstein EJC, Citron DM, Wield B, Finegold SM, Vera L. Bacteriology of human and animal bite wounds. *J Clin Microbiol*. 1978;8(6):667-672.
16. Kanavel AB. The classic. Infections of the hand. Allen Buchner Kanavel. *Clin Orthop Relat Res*. 1974;(104):3-8.
17. Franko OI, Abrams RA. Hand infections. *Orthop Clin North Am*. 2013;44(4):625-634. doi:10.1016/j.ocl.2013.06.014.
18. Sharma KS, Rao K, Hobson MI. Space of Parona infections: experience in management and outcomes in a regional hand centre. *J Plast Reconstr Aesthet Surg*. 2013;66(7):968-972. doi:10.1016/j.bjps.2013.03.020.
19. Linscheid RL, Dobyns JH. Common and uncommon infections of the hand. *Orthop Clin North Am*. 1975;6(4):1063-1104.
20. Glass J. Factors related to the resolution of treated hand infections. *J Hand Surg Am*. 1982;7(4):388-394.
21. Jalil A, Barlaan PI, Kwok B, et al. Hand infection in diabetic patients. *Hand Surg*. 2011;16(3):307-313. doi:10.1142/S021881041100559X.

Julie Johnson and John R. Fowler

INTRODUCTION

- **Pathoanatomy**—It is infection of dermis and subcutaneous tissue without associated abscess.
- **Mechanism**—Infection is through bacterial breach of cutaneous surface, however, a break in the skin is not required for spread of bacteria
- **Epidemiology** in the United States is about 14.5 million cases annually with approximately 12% in the upper extremity, with a slight male predominance
- **Risk factors** include trauma, IV drug use, immunocompromised patients, diabetes mellitus, steroid use, skin disorders (eczema, shingles), obesity

EVALUATION

- **History** reveals pain, fever, abrasion, puncture wound, or insect bite, expanding erythema
- **Physical examination** shows erythematous, swollen, painful hand, which may have associated lymphangitis
- **See** Figure 48.1
- **Laboratory studies** present elevated WBC, ESR, CRP, and lactate (lack specificity), <5% have a positive blood culture, skin biopsy yields a pathogen in 20% to 30% of cases—culture and biopsy are not recommended
- **Imaging**—Radiographs will show soft tissue swelling without bony pathology
  - Should be ordered to rule out osteomyelitis and/or foreign body
- **Classification**—Infection is classified as mild (no systemic signs), moderate (has systemic signs), severe (has systemic signs, purulence, and is rapidly evolving)

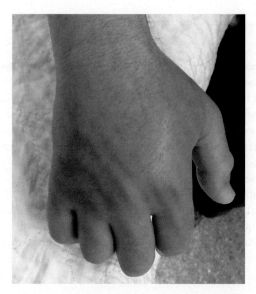

FIGURE 48.1 Cellulitis over dorsum of hand with erythema and swelling.

ACUTE MANAGEMENT

- Rule out more serious disease
  - Necrotizing fasciitis, gas gangrene, abscess, osteomyelitis
- Initiate antibiotics (see Table 48.1 of antibiotics based on severity)
  - Most common organisms: β-hemolytic *Streptococcus*, *Staphylococcus aureus*, mixed flora
- Immobilize hand
- Strict elevation
- Low threshold for admission and IV antibiotics

TABLE 48.1 Suggested Antibiotic Therapy for Cellulitis

Antibiotic Therapy	
Mild	Oral Rx: Pen VK, Cephalosporin, Dicloxacillin, or Clindamycin
Moderate	IV Rx: Penicillin, Ceftriaxone, Cefazolin, or Clindamycin
Severe	IV Rx: Vancomycin PLUS Piperacillin/Tazobactam
Methicillin-resistant *Staphylococcus aureus* suspected	PO Rx: Clindamycin, SMX-TMP/IV Rx: Vancomycin

DEFINITIVE TREATMENT

- **Nonoperative**—Oral or IV antibiotics for 5 to 14 days (see Table 48.1 of antibiotic therapy)
- **Surgical indications**—Surgery is rarely indicated unless purulence or deeper infection develops; however, associated bite or puncture wounds may necessitate incision and drainage.
  - **Relative contraindications** include mild or moderate cellulitis without fluid collection.
- **Operative technique**
  - Irrigation and debridement as needed
- **Potential complications** include abscess formation, gas gangrene, necrotizing fasciitis.
- **Postoperative care** comprises 4 to 6 weeks of IV and/or oral antibiotics, possible repeat incision and drainage if patient is not responding to antibiotic treatment.

SUGGESTED READINGS

Osterman M, Draeger R, Stern P. Acute hand infections. *J Hand Surg Am*. 2014;39(8):1628-1635.

Stevanovic M, Sharpe F. Acute infections. In: Wolfe SW, Hotchkiss DP, Pederson RN, Kozin SH, Cohen MS, eds. *Green's Operative Hand Surgery*. 6th ed. Philadelphia, PA: Elsevier Churchill Livingstone; 2011:41-45.

Stevens DL, Bisno AL, Chambers HF, et al; Infectious Diseases Society of America. Practice guidelines for the diagnosis and management of skin and soft tissue infections: 2014 update by the Infectious Diseases Society of America. *Clin Infect Dis*. 2014;59(2):e10-e52.

49 Bite Wounds

Mark Henry

INTRODUCTION

- Pathoanatomy[1-5]
  - Skin wound—mixed pattern of crush, cut, tear damage to margins (Figure 49.1)
  - Deep structural injury to bone, tendon, nerve with powerful bites (dog, larger birds, human)
  - Introduction of oral bacteria to varying depths
    - Skin only
    - Deep space, nonsynovial
    - Joint (septic arthritis)
    - Tendon sheath (septic tenosynovitis)

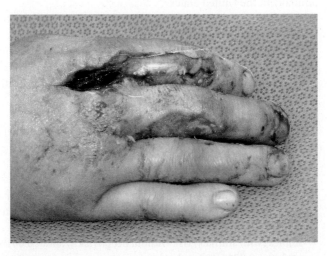

FIGURE 49.1 Dogs are capable of creating large tearing wounds with extensive soft tissue damage.

- Human bites also may transmit HIV, hepatitis B, hepatitis C
- Clinical infection depends on burden of microorganisms and capacity of immune system to overcome it (greatest at the skin level, least in a contained synovial space), up to 50% in cat bites, 41% in dog bites.
- Risk factors: smoking, immunocompromised status, diabetes, depth of penetration, delay in treatment >24 hours, wound closure[6]
- Additional tissue necrosis is proportionate to the duration of infection prior to debridement and spread of infection along anatomic planes (along the course of tendon sheath, from joint cavity into bone)
- Mechanism of injury[7-9]
  - Sharp penetration to deep target with little structural injury (cats and small dogs)
  - Crushing (2000 lb/sq in) and avulsion of soft tissue with fracture seen in up to 30% of large dog bites.
  - Cutting through tendon to bone or joint with impaction fracture (human bites: up to 62% metacarpophalangeal joint penetration and 20% tendon injury).
- Epidemiology[10-12]
  - 4.9 million animal bites annually in the United States
  - Domestic pet bites 2 million/300 000 emergency department visits annually in the United States
  - 80% of animals are known to the victim; 50% are an attempt by the victim to break up animal fight.
  - Middle-aged Caucasian women (cat bites = 10%–15% of all animal bites)
  - Wide demographic distribution (dog bites = 80%–90% of all animal bites)
  - Young males (human bites)
  - Veterinary professionals (often present late having ignored initial bite)
  - Bacterial profile
    - *Pasteurella multocida* 80% (dog, cat)
    - *Eikenella corrodens* (human)
    - *Staphylococcus, Streptococcus, Bartonella, Prevotella, Fusobacterium, Peptococcus, Peptostreptococcus, Bacteroides, Pseudomonas, Proteus, Salmonella, Escherichia coli*, mixed.
    - Rabies (wild animals) risk without prophylaxis, about 0.001% for cat bites, 0.00001% for dog bites

EVALUATION

- History[13]
  - Identify source of bite—human, domestic cat, or dog (species or approximate weight of dog), undomesticated cat or dog, wild animal species
  - Variables increasing likelihood of underlying structural injury—that is, large dog clamped down and held on, punch to mouth of human
  - Compromising medical variables—diabetes, vascular disease, smoking
- Physical examination (Figure 49.2)
  - Locate all bite sites—rate each for depth of penetration and signs of infection
    - Redness
    - Warmth
    - Tenderness
    - Swelling

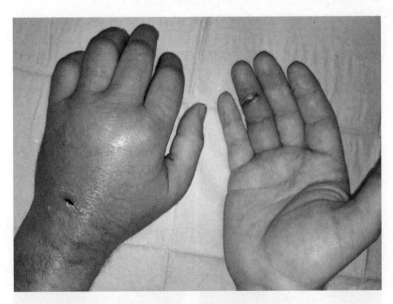

FIGURE 49.2 Regardless of the size of the original penetration, local signs of infection (erythema, swelling, warmth, tenderness, drainage) indicate the need for treatment, especially when overlying synovial structures.

- - Purulence
  - Fluctuance
  - Lymphangitic proximal spread and/or enlarged lymph node
  - Test function of tendons and nerves in zone of bite
- Imaging (Figure 49.3)
  - Examine for complete fracture (large dogs, human punch impact)
  - Seek subtle findings (retained tip of small cat tooth, cortical penetration, early signs of osteomyelitis in delayed presentation cases)
- Classification
  - No formal classification
  - Categorize each bite site as not infected, cellulitis only, deep space infection (with particular emphasis on synovial spaces—joint, tendon sheath).

ACUTE MANAGEMENT

- Rabies prophylaxis immune globulin[14] days 0, 3, 7, 14
- No deep penetration, no infection

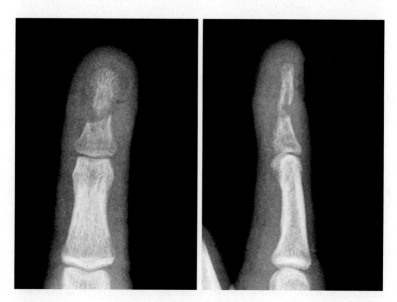

FIGURE 49.3 Open fractures with delay in treatment can lead to osteomyelitis and bone loss.

- Wash wounds externally with warm soapy water and cover openings with a simple external dressing
- No controlled data to indicate that the addition of antibiotics will necessarily prevent progression to infection, but low risk with potential efficacy

DEFINITIVE TREATMENT

- Nonoperative treatment[2]
  - No deep penetration, cellulitis evident, no signs of deep infection
  - Oral antibiotics for 7 to 10 days
  - Augmentin is drug of choice (except if allergic to penicillin); quinolone plus clindamycin or doxycycline
  - Monitor closely for signs of deep infection, failure to resolve on time
- Surgical indications[15]
  - Deep penetration (particularly if joint or tendon sheath breached) within days of original bite as prophylaxis against development of infection—early intervention reduces risk of infection to 2% from 50% (cat) and 41% (dog)
  - Established deep space infection following previous bite
  - Contraindications—patient refuses surgery
- Surgical approach
  - Elliptically excise bite track along axis of wound (longitudinally if no clear axis)
  - Protect all functional structures (tendon, nerve, artery, ligament)
  - Excise all necrotic/purulent tissues
  - Curette/rongeur any bone penetrations
  - Pack wound fully open with gauze (do not close, even partially)
- Potential complications
  - Injury to functional structure while attempting debridement
  - Incomplete debridement results in persistent infection.
- Postoperative care
  - Begin open wound care within 48 to 72 hours
    - Daily damp-to-dry dressing changes two to three times a day for smaller wounds
    - Serial operative debridement every 48 to 72 hours for more extensive wounds

- Secondary closure once wound is clean in 5 to 10 days, depending on the extent of the initial infection
  - ◆ Spontaneous healing by secondary intention (no exposed tendon or joint)
  - ◆ Repeat debridement and definitive suture closure (recut dermis)

MANAGEMENT ALGORITHM

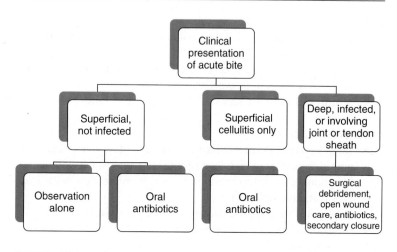

REFERENCES

1. Babovic N, Cayci C, Carlsen BT. Cat bite infections of the hand: assessment of morbidity and predictors of severe infection. *J Hand Surg.* 2014;39:286-290.
2. Henton J, Jain A. Cochrane corner: antibiotic prophylaxis for mammalian bites. *J Hand Surg Eur Vol.* 2012;47:804-806.
3. Kwo S, Agarwal JP, Meletiou S. Current treatment of cat bites to the hand and wrist. *J Hand Surg.* 2009;36:152-153.
4. Nygaard M, Dahlin LB. Dog bite injuries to the hand. *J Plast Surg Hand Surg.* 2011;45:96-191.
5. Meyer CI, Abzug JM. Domestic bird bites. *J Hand Surg Am.* 2012;37:1925-1927.
6. Speirs J, Showery J, Abdou M, Pirela-Cruz MA, Abdelgawad AA. Dog bites to the upper extremity in children. *J Pediatr Child Health.* 2015;51:1172-1174.
7. Benson LS, Edwards SL, Schiff AP, Williams CS, Visotsky JL. Dog and cat bites to the hand: treatment and cost assessment. *J Hand Surg.* 2006;31:468-473.
8. Chadaev AP, Jukhtin VI, Butkevich AT, Emkuzhev VM. Treatment of infected clench-fist human bite wounds in the area of metacarpophalangeal joints. *J Hand Surg.* 1996;21:299-303.

9. Benfield R, Plurad DS, Lam L, et al. The epidemiology of dog attacks in an urban environment and the risk of vascular injury. *Am Surg.* 2010;76:203-205.

10. Gonzalez MH, Papierski P, Hall RF. Osteomyelitis of the hand after a human bite. *J Hand Surg.* 1993;18:520-522.

11. Alluri RK, Pannell W, Heckmann N, Sivasundaram L, Stevanovic M, Ghiassi A. Predictive factors of neurovascular and tendon injuries following dog bites to the upper extremity. *Hand.* 2016;11(4):469-474.

12. Vaidya SA, Manning SE, Dhankhar P, et al. Estimating the risk of rabies transmission to humans in the U.S. *BMC Public Health.* 2010;10:278.

13. Kennedy SA, Stoll LE, Lauder AS. Human and other mammalian bite injuries of the hand: evaluation and management. *J Am Acad Orthop Surg.* 2015;23:47-57.

14. Ellis R, Ellis C. Dog and cat bites. *Am Fam Physician.* 2014;90:239-243.

15. Shewring DJ, Trickett RW, Subramanian KN, Hnyda R. The management of clenched fist 'fight bite' injuries of the hand. *J Hand Surg Eur Vol.* 2015;40: 819-824.

Julie Johnson and John R. Fowler

INTRODUCTION

- **Pathoanatomy**—bony infection caused by microbial invasion characterized by inflammation and destruction of bone
- **Mechanism**—contiguous spread (abscess, septic joint), direct inoculation (trauma, surgery, foreign body), or indirect (hematogenous seeding)
- **Epidemiology**—24 cases per 100 000 person-years, more male patients than female, greater incidence with age, occurs more in lower extremity than in upper extremity, 1% to 6% of all hand infections involve bone, most often in the distal phalanx
- **Risk factors** include recent surgery or trauma, IV drug use, immune deficiency/suppression, diabetes, vascular insufficiency.

EVALUATION

- **History**—pain, fever, chills, fatigue, exposure to risk factors
- **Physical examination**—tenderness, erythema, edema, warmth, fluctuance, exposed bone, sinus tract (Figure 50.1)
- **Laboratory studies**—elevated white blood cell count, erythrocyte sedimentation rate, and C-reactive protein (lack specificity), positive blood cultures in 50% of cases; laboratory findings can be normal in osteomyelitis of the small bones of the hand and wrist
- **Imaging**—Radiograph (Figure 50.2) (lytic lesion, surrounding sclerosis, periosteal thickening) may not show changes for 2 weeks, MRI positive up to 90% sensitivity and specificity (distinguish between soft tissue and bone infection), CT scan is rarely used in diagnosis (may be helpful for guided needle biopsy)

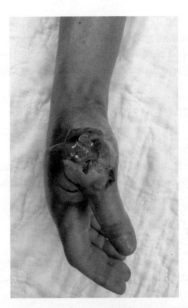

FIGURE 50.1 Abscess over thumb metacarpophalangeal joint tracks to bone with osteomyelitis.

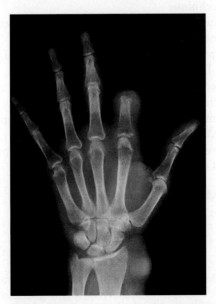

FIGURE 50.2 Index finger amputation secondary to osteomyelitis. Now with soft tissue swelling and early osteomyelitis over the distal radius.

- **Classification**—acute (within 2 weeks), subacute (between 2 weeks and several months), and chronic (after several months); 10% to 30% acute turn chronic; chronic osteomyelitis characterized by sequestrum (necrotic bone) and involucrum (new bone formation)

ACUTE MANAGEMENT

- Identify organism (see Table 50.1)
  - Bone biopsy is the gold standard (sinus tract culture unreliable)
  - Broad-spectrum antibiotics pending cultures and sensitivities

DEFINITIVE TREATMENT

- **Nonoperative**—IV or oral antibiotics for 4 to 6 weeks (see Table 50.2)
- **Surgical indications**—localized or diffuse osteomyelitis, abscess, sinus tract
  - **Relative contraindications**—acute hematogenous or superficial osteomyelitis
- **Operative technique**
  - Debridement—remove all devitalized tissue and sequestrum
  - Remove hardware and any foreign bodies
  - Fill dead space with vascular tissue (grafts, flaps, wound vacuum-assisted closure), if needed
  - Stabilize bone
  - Amputation if necessary
- **Potential complications**—persistent infection, sepsis, malignant transformation (Marjolin's ulcer)
- **Postoperative care**—4 to 6 weeks of IV and/or oral antibiotics, repeat debridement as necessary

TABLE 50.1 **Most Common Organisms**

Neonate (<4 mo)	*Staphylococcus aureus, Enterobacter*, groups A and B *Streptococcus*
Children (4 mo-4 y)	*S. aureus*, group A Streptococci, *Kingella kingae*, *Enterobacter*
Children to adolescents (4 y+)	*S. aureus*, group A Streptococci, *Enterobacter*
Adult	*S. aureus, Enterobacter, Streptococcus*
Sickle cell anemia patient	*S. aureus* most common, *Salmonella* is pathognomonic

TABLE 50.2 Antibiotic Therapy

S. aureus (MSSA)	First-generation cephalosporin, nafcillin
S. aureus (MRSA)	Vancomycin
Enterobacter	Quinolone, Piperacillin/tazobactam
Streptococcus	Pen G
Anaerobes	Clindamycin
Mixed aerobe/anaerobe	Amoxicillin-clavulanic acid

Abbreviations: MRSA, methicillin-resistant *Staphylococcus aureus*; MSSA, methicillin-sensitive *Staphylococcus aureus*.

SUGGESTED READINGS

Kremers H, Nwojo M, Ransom J, Wood-Wentz C, Melton L, Huddleston P. Trends in the epidemiology of osteomyelitis: a population-based study, 1969 to 2009. *J Bone Joint Surg Am*. 2015;97(10):837-845.

Stevanovic M, Sharpe F. Acute infections. In: Wolfe SW, Pederson WC, Hotchkiss RN, Kozin SH, Cohen MS, eds. *Green's Operative Hand Surgery*. 6th ed. Philadelphia, PA: Elsevier Churchill Livingstone; 2011:69-71.

Walter G, Kemmerer M, Kappler C, Hoffmann R. Treatment algorithms for chronic osteomyelitis. *Deutsches Ärzteblatt Int*. 2012;109(14):257-264.

CHAPTER

51 Compartment Syndrome

Roshan Melvani and Christopher M. Jones

INTRODUCTION

- Acute compartment syndrome (ACS) is an increase in tissue pressure within an osseofascial compartment above tissue perfusion pressure, resulting in diminished local circulation and eventual tissue necrosis.
- Operative intervention can decrease the degree of permanent muscle and nerve injury in the initial stages of compartment syndrome.
- Volkmann ischemic contracture is a delayed finding of compartment syndrome and represents a continuum of static muscle contractures secondary to fibrosis and neurologic injury.
- Pathoanatomy
  - ACS results from a nonelastic constrictive element, such as muscle fascia, casts, or tight dressings, which decreases venous outflow and arterial inflow in the setting of bleeding or muscle swelling.
  - Elevated intracompartmental pressure, when left untreated, results in a decrease in arterial perfusion to a level that is not compatible with tissue viability (Figure 51.1).
  - Continued cellular anoxia leads to activation of apoptosis via up-regulated lysosomal pathways.
  - Permanent dysfunction of muscle occurs after 4 to 12 hours of anoxia.
- Mechanism of injury
  - External causes: extracompartmental compression by tight dressings or casts
  - Internal causes: bleeding or swelling from fractures, penetrating injuries, blunt soft tissue trauma or crush injuries, ischemia-reperfusion injuries, deep burns, animal/insect bites, intravenous fluid extravasation, infection, and bleeding secondary to coagulopathy

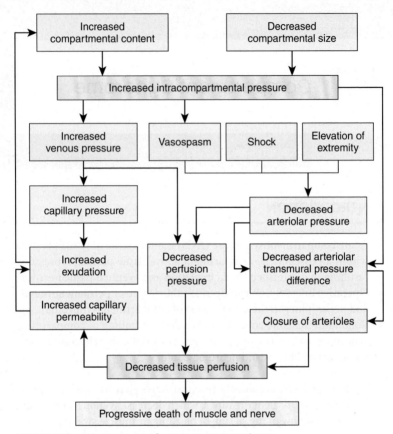

FIGURE 51.1 Pathoanatomy of compartment syndrome.

- Epidemiology
  - The incidence of compartment syndrome in pediatric upper extremity fractures is as low as 1%. Pediatric fractures most associated with forearm compartment syndrome are both bone forearm fractures and floating elbow injuries.
  - In adults, the most frequent upper extremity fractures correlated with compartment syndrome are both bone forearm fractures and distal radius fractures. Compartment syndrome is more commonly reported in males younger than 35 years, penetrating trauma, open fractures, and elbow dislocations.
  - Compartment syndrome of the hand is most strongly associated with intravenous injections.

EVALUATION

- Patient history
  - A high index of suspicion must be present when there is pain out of proportion to injury.
  - Increasing analgesic demands must be closely monitored and may be the most reliable symptom of evolving compartment syndrome in children.
  - Loss of consciousness, altered mental status, diverting polytraumatic injuries, or regional anesthesia pose challenges in accurate diagnosis and may require objective tests such as compartment pressure measurements.
- Physical examination
  - Compartment syndrome is a clinical diagnosis that may in certain circumstances be confirmed based on objective findings.
  - Consider the six P's associated with ACS: pain, paresthesias, pallor, paralysis, pulselessness, and poikilothermia.
  - Unrelenting pain is the earliest and most sensitive finding.
  - Compartments will generally be tense on palpation, and passive stretch of the involved compartment will create intolerable discomfort.
  - Compartment pressure can be measured if physical examination findings are ambiguous. The patient should be supine, with the affected extremity at heart level.
  - An arterial line monitor or a handheld pressure-monitoring device (Stryker) may be used after appropriate calibration to avoid falsely elevated readings.
  - Threshold pressures include 30 to 40 mm Hg or within 30 mm Hg of diastolic blood pressure. In patients with bleeding disorders, diffuse thrombocytopenia, or cellulitis, obtaining pressure measurements may pose additional risk. See Table 51.1.
- Imaging
  - Radiographs of affected portion of upper extremity should be obtained to evaluate for fracture, foreign bodies, subcutaneous air, or other pathologies that may be contributing to the disease process.
- Classification
  - ACS: tissue pressures increase within an osseofascial compartment, resulting in tissue ischemia.
  - Exertional compartment syndrome: transient tissue ischemia secondary to nonelastic fascial compartment unable to acclimate to

TABLE 51.1 Myofascial Compartments of the Upper Extremity and Their Contents

	Compartment	Muscle	Artery	Nerve
Arm	Anterior	Biceps, brachialis, coracobrachialis	Brachial	Musculocutaneous
	Posterior	Triceps	Profunda brachii	Radial
	Deltoid	Deltoid	–	Axillary
Forearm	Volar		Radial and ulnar	Median, ulnar, and anterior interosseous
	Superficial	Pronator teres, flexor carpi radialis, palmaris longus, flexor digitorum superficialis, flexor carpi ulnaris		
	Deep	Flexor pollicis longus, flexor digitorum profundus, pronator quadratus		
	Dorsal		Posterior interosseous	Posterior interosseous
	Superficial	Extensor digitorum communis, extensor digiti minimi, extensor carpi ulnaris		
	Deep	Abductor pollicis longus, extensor pollicis brevis, extensor pollicis longus, extensor indicis proprius, supinator		
	Mobile wad	Brachioradialis, extensor carpi radialis longus, extensor carpi radialis brevis	–	Radial
Hand	Thenar	Abductor pollicis brevis, opponens pollicis, flexor pollicis brevis	Digital	Recurrent motor
	Hypothenar	Abductor digiti minimi, opponens digiti minimi, flexor digiti minimi	–	Ulnar
	Adductor	Adductor pollicis	–	Ulnar
	Interosseous	Four dorsal and three palmar interosseous muscles	–	Ulnar
	Carpal tunnel	Flexor digitorum profundus, flexor digitorum superficialis, flexor pollicis longus	–	Median
	Digit		Digital	Digital

Reprinted from Chung KC. *Operative Techniques: Hand and Wrist Surgery*. 2nd ed. Philadelphia, PA: Elsevier Saunders; 2013:615-616, with permission from Elsevier.

muscle amplification during increased activity. Patients report pain beginning as a slow ache within the first half-hour of beginning a specific activity until cessation and rest.

- Neonatal compartment syndrome: newborns may have upper extremity swelling with distinctive skin lesions known as "sentinel lesions of neonatal compartment syndrome."

ACUTE MANAGEMENT

- Surgical release
  - All external causes of compression must be eliminated including casts and circumferential dressings.
  - It is important to raise the limb only to the heart level to achieve a balance between edema control and appropriate perfusion.
  - Inquire about a history of coagulopathy and correct as necessary.
  - In crush injuries, urine myoglobin and serum electrolytes should be closely monitored and treated to avoid shock, acidosis, renal failure, or arrhythmias.
  - Fasciotomy is the treatment for ACS. Treatment within 8 hours of diagnosis is necessary to reduce the prospect of long-term functional deficits.
  - Indications for fasciotomy include: presence of positive history and physical examination findings, compartment pressures greater than 30 mm Hg, or compartment pressures within 30 mm Hg of the diastolic pressure.
  - Necrotic tissue must be resected intraoperatively to avoid becoming a nidus for infection or becoming fibrosed and leading to contractures.

DEFINITIVE MANAGEMENT

- Surgical technique
  - Release of compartments of the arm
    - Anterior and posterior compartments of the arm may be released through a single incision along the medial aspect of the humerus. This approach permits access to the neurovascular structures, the biceps and brachial fascia of the anterior compartment, and the triceps fascia of the posterior compartment (Figure 51.2).
    - Alternatively, a two-incision approach to anterior and posterior compartments is an option if access to neurovascular structures

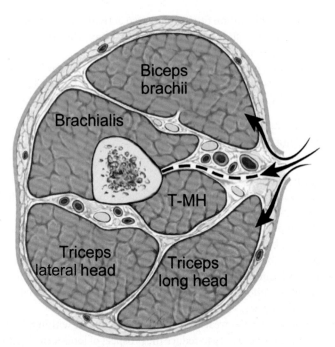

FIGURE 51.2 Cross-sectional anatomy of the arm. The dotted line represents the plane of dissection for decompression of the anterior and posterior compartments through a medial incision. The intermuscular septum can be excised, which further decompresses both compartments. Alternatively, a straight anterior and posterior incision may be used to separately decompress the anterior and posterior compartments. T-MH, triceps medial head. Reprinted from Wolfe SW, Pederson WC, Hotchkiss RN, Kozin SH, Cohen MS. *Green's Operative Hand Surgery*. 7th ed. Philadelphia, PA: Elsevier; 2017:1763-1787, with permission from Elsevier.

is not needed. Whatever approach is taken, it is crucial to release anterior, middle, and posterior subcompartments of the deltoid as necessary.

- Release of compartments of the forearm
  - In the forearm, superficial and deep flexor compartments and the extensor compartments must be decompressed.
  - In a typical approach to the volar forearm, a central incision is made along the lateral humeral epicondyle extending to the radial styloid. Division of the fascia between the palmaris longus and flexor carpi radialis, and the deep fascia overlying the anterior surface of the flexor digitorum superficialis should be completed to access the deep flexor compartment (Figures 51.3 and 51.4).

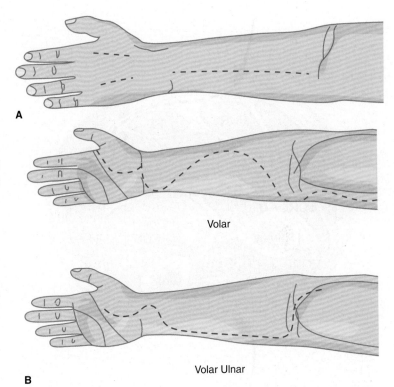

FIGURE 51.3 Incision placement for (A), standard dorsal surgical approach and (B), standard volar surgical approaches for forearm compartment decompression.

- ◆ Alternatively, an ulnar incision can be made along the medial humeral epicondyle to the ulnar styloid process and the fascia divided between the flexor carpi ulnaris and medial side of the flexor digitorum superficialis; the ulnar neurovascular bundle must be retracted with the flexor digitorum superficialis so that the deep fascia of the flexor compartment can be incised.
- ◆ The extensor compartment is decompressed by making an incision from the lateral humeral epicondyle to Lister tubercle. The fascia may be incised in line with the skin incision. To prevent bowstringing of the extensor tendons, the extensor retinaculum at the level of the wrist should be preserved whenever possible.
- • Release of compartments of the hand
  - ◆ The hand has 10 compartments, which may all require release depending on mechanism of injury and location of swelling.

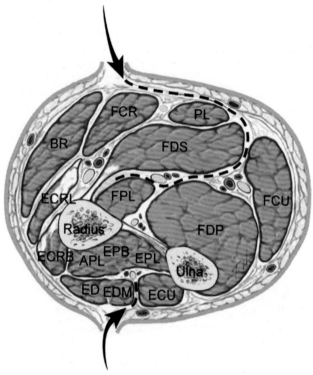

FIGURE 51.4 Cross-sectional anatomy of the forearm. The dotted lines represent the plane of dissection for dorsal and volar compartments. The superficial flexor compartment can be released in the midline or any location, trying to avoid an incision over the radial or ulnar artery or median nerve. The deep flexor compartment is best released by opening the interval between flexor carpi ulnaris and the flexor digitorum superficialis. APL, abductor pollicis longus; BR, brachioradialis; ECRB, extensor carpi radialis brevis; ECRL, extensor carpi radialis longus; ECU, extensor carpi ulnaris; ED, extensor digitorum; EDM, extensor digiti minimi; EPB, extensor pollicis brevis; EPL, extensor pollicis longus; FCR, flexor carpi radialis; FCU, flexor carpi ulnaris; FDP, flexor digitorum profundus; FDS, flexor digitorum superficialis; FPL, flexor pollicis longus; PL, palmaris longus. Reprinted from Wolfe SW, Pederson WC, Hotchkiss RN, Kozin SH, Cohen MS. *Green's Operative Hand Surgery.* 7th ed. Philadelphia, PA: Elsevier; 2017:1763-1787, with permission from Elsevier.

- Release of the volar compartments should begin with carpal tunnel release, which also releases the ulnar neurovascular bundle within Guyon's canal. This incision can be extended to the second volar webspace to release the volar fascia of the adductor pollicis longus. The palmar fascia is opened to release the volar interosseous musculature.

- The thenar and hypothenar musculature can be released via isolated incisions as deemed necessary.
  - Release of the dorsal compartments and their associated interosseous muscles is accomplished via incisions between the second-third metacarpals and fourth-fifth metacarpals (Figures 51.5 and 51.6).
- Release of the fingers
  - Release of tense fingers can be done via a midaxial approach to avoid contractures. This should be done on the side of the finger that will minimize irritation during pinch or grasp (Figure 51.7).
- Postoperative care
  - Incisions are generally not closed acutely, as there will typically be continued swelling.
  - Use of a wound vac, packing with moist gauze, or retention sutures may keep wounds clean and protected until definitive closure can safely be performed.
  - Depending on the amount of necrotic tissue present, revision irrigation and debridement are often necessary.
  - It is important to begin physical and occupational therapy postoperatively to maximize finger range of motion and prevent stiffness.
- Potential complications
  - The result of untreated compartment syndrome is Volkmann ischemic contracture, which has varied presentations based on severity.

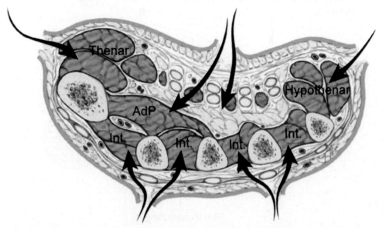

FIGURE 51.5 Cross-sectional anatomy of the hand. The arrows show the planes of dissection for decompression of the compartments of the hand. AdP, adductor pollicis; Int, interosseous muscles. Reprinted from Wolfe SW, Pederson WC, Hotchkiss RN, Kozin SH, Cohen MS. *Green's Operative Hand Surgery*. 7th ed. Philadelphia, PA: Elsevier; 2017:1763-1787, with permission from Elsevier.

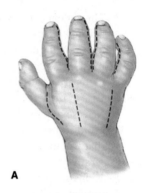

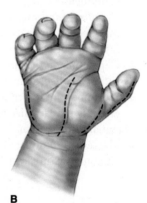

FIGURE 51.6 A, Dorsal incision for fasciotomy of the hand and dermotomies of the fingers. B, Volar incision for release of the thenar and hypothenar compartments, carpal tunnel release, and dermotomy of the thumb. Reprinted from Wolfe SW, Pederson WC, Hotchkiss RN, Kozin SH, Cohen MS. *Green's Operative Hand Surgery*. 7th ed. Philadelphia, PA: Elsevier; 2017:1763-1787, with permission from Elsevier.

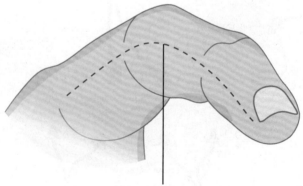

Skin incision, finger

FIGURE 51.7 Incision placement for midaxial surgical approaches for digital compartment decompression. From Hammert WC, Bozentka DJ, Calfee RP, Boyer MI. *ASSH Manual of Hand Surgery*. Philadelphia, PA: Wolters Kluwer Health; 2010.

- A mild contracture generally represents incomplete ischemia of the flexor digitorum profundus or flexor pollicis longus with flexion contractures of a few fingers and minimal sensory dysfunction. Treatment includes dynamic splinting and therapy with possible eventual surgical lengthening.
- A moderate contracture involves not only finger flexors, but also wrist flexors with moderate sensory dysfunction and an intrinsic minus deformity of the hand. This requires tendon transfers, muscle slides, and neurolysis of affected nerves.
- A severe contracture involves forearm extensors in addition to finger and wrist flexors with significantly diminished sensation. This condition may require free muscle transfer for treatment.

SUGGESTED READINGS

Bae DS, Kadiyala RK, Waters PM. Acute compartment syndrome in children: contemporary diagnosis, treatment, and outcome. *J Pediatr Orthop*. 2001;21:680-688.

Blakemore L, Cooperman D, Thompson G, et al. Compartment syndrome in ipsilateral humerus and forearm fractures in children. *Clin Orthop Relat Res*. 2000;376:32-38.

Boody AR, Wongworawat MD. Accuracy in the measurement of compartment pressures: a comparison of three commonly used devices. *J Bone Joint Surg Am*. 2005;87A:2415.

Branco BC, Inaba K, Barmparas G, et al. Incidence and predictors for the need for fasciotomy after extremity trauma: a 10-year review in a mature level I trauma centre. *Injury*. 2011;42(10):1157-1163.

Capo JT, Renard RL, Moulton MJ, et al. How is forearm compliance affected by various circumferential dressings? *Clin Orthop Relat Res*. 2014;472:3228.

Chan PSH, Steinberg DR, Pepe MD, Beredjiklian PK. The significant of the three volar spaces in forearm compartment syndrome: a clinical and cadaveric correlation. *J Hand Surg*. 1998;23A:1077-1081.

Dente CJ, Feliciano DV, Rozycki GS, et al. A review of upper extremity fasciotomies in a level I trauma center. *Am Surg*. 2004;70(12):1088-1093.

Diesselhorst MM, Deck JW, Davey JP. Compartment syndrome of the upper arm after closed reduction and percutaneous pinning of a supracondylar humerus fracture. *J Pediatr Orthop*. 2014;34:e1.

Duckworth AD, Mitchell SE, Molyneux SG, White TO, Court-Brown CM, McQueen MM. Acute compartment syndrome of the forearm. *J Bone Joint Surg Am*. 2012;94(10):e63.

Franz RW, Skytta CK, Shah KJ, et al. A five-year review of management of upper-extremity arterial injuries at an urban level I trauma center. *Ann Vasc Surg*. 2012;26(5):655-664.

Grottkau B, Epps H, Di Scala C. Compartment syndrome in children and adolescents. *J Pediatr Surg*. 2005;40(4):678-682.

Kalyani B, Fisher B, Roberts C, et al. Compartment syndrome of the forearm: a systematic review. *J Hand Surg Am*. 2011;36:535-543.

Lipschitz AH, Lifchez SD. Measurement of compartment pressures in the hand and forearm. *J Hand Surg Am*. 2010;35A:1893.

Matsen FA III. Compartmental syndrome. An unified concept. *Clin Orthop Relat Res*. 1975;113:8-14.

McQueen M, Gaston P, Court-Brown C. Acute compartment syndrome. Who is at risk? *J Bone Joint Surg Br*. 2000;82:200-203.

Ouellette E, Kelly R. Compartment syndromes of the hand. *J Bone Joint Surg Am*. 1996;78(10):1515-1522.

Ragland RI, Moukoko D, Ezaki M, et al. Forearm compartment syndrome in the newborn: report of 24 cases. *J Hand Surg Am*. 2005;30(5):997-1003.

Royle SG. Compartment syndrome following forearm fracture in children. *Injury*. 1990;21(2):73-76.

Yuan PS, Pring ME, Gaynor TP, Mubarak SJ, Newton PO. Compartment syndrome following intramedullary fixation of pediatric forearm fractures. *J Pediatr Orthop*. 2004;24(4):370-375.

52 Nail Bed Injury

Andrew D. Sobel

INTRODUCTION

Fingertip injuries, and injuries to the nail bed specifically, are common problems that vary widely in mechanism and severity. Injuries to the nail can involve any combination of the nail plate, nail bed, germinal matrix, eponychium, or bone of the distal phalanx. Nail bed injuries in the pediatric population may have different management than those in the adult population, depending on a variety of factors including involvement of the growth plate. Proper evaluation and identification of the injury and timely management is critical to preventing a painful, sensitive, or cosmetically unappealing outcome.

- Anatomy (see Figure 52.1)[1,2]
  - Perionychium[3]—the nail and its surrounding structures
    - Nail plate
      - * Made of onchyn, a keratin-like material
      - * Protects the nail bed and distal tissue. Improves sensory feedback of the fingertip
    - Eponychium
      - * Fold of tissue dorsally and proximally over nail
      - * Serves to smooth the nail plate as it grows
    - Sterile matrix
      - * Contains one to two layers of germinal cells that contribute to nail plate thickness as it grows and moves distally
    - Lunula
      - * White arc on the proximal nail
      - * Nail bed distal to the lunula is the sterile matrix; proximal to and including the lunula is the germinal matrix
    - Germinal matrix
      - * Extends from ventral floor to lunula. Immediately superficial to distal phalanx periosteum

- ∗ Ventral floor
  - ▲ Three to four germ cell layers thick. Produces 90% of the nail plate volume through "gradient parakeratosis"
- ◆ Dorsal root/roof
  - ∗ Contributes to the nail plate formation. Source of shiny quality of nail plate
- ◆ Hyponychium
  - ∗ Site at which the sterile matrix stops and epithelial skin starts at the distal tip. A keratin plug at this site acts as a barrier between the nail and sterile matrix to prevent contamination/infection
- ◆ Paronychium
  - ∗ Folds of skin on sides of nail that can tear ("hangnail") and become infected ("paronychia")
- ● Pulp[4]
  - ◆ Distributes force placed on the palmar finger
  - ◆ Contains sensory receptors such as Pacinian and Meissner corpuscles, Merkel cell-neurite complexes
- ● Extensor tendon (terminal slip)
  - ◆ Inserts approximately 2 mm proximal to the germinal matrix on the distal phalanx
- ● Flexor digitorum profundus (FDP) tendon
  - ◆ Inserts on the distal phalanx just proximal to the distal palmar digital arterial anastomosis
- ● Vasculature[5]
  - ◆ Dorsal vein—overlies the distal phalanx and is important for anastomosis in amputations
  - ◆ Digital arteries—send major branches to the pulp, paronychium, and nail fold. Smaller branches go to the nail bed
- ● Nerves
  - ◆ Digital nerves send branches to the paronychium, pulp, and fingertip
  - ◆ Located palmar to the digital arteries
- ● Zones—see Classification
  - ◆ Tamai
  - ◆ Allen
  - ◆ Fassler
- ■ Mechanism of injury[6]
  - ● Crush
    - ◆ Most common mechanism for nail bed injuries
  - ● Sharp laceration

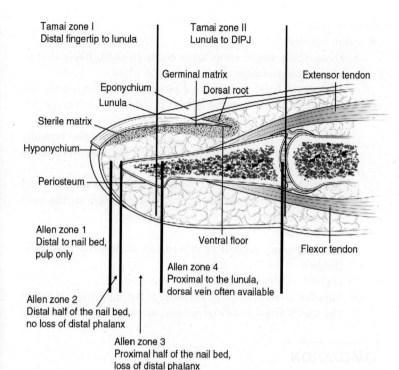

FIGURE 52.1 Anatomy of the finger distal to the distal interphalangeal joint (DIPJ). Pertinent structures and classifications of zone anatomy (Tamai and Allen) are labeled. From Lee DH, Mignemi ME, Crosby SN. Fingertip injuries: an update on management. *J Am Acad Orthop Surg.* 2013;21(12):756-766.

- Avulsion
  - Nail bed avulsions with the loss of matrix tissue result in some of the worst outcomes as they often result in permanent deformity.
  - Fingertip avulsion (including the nail bed) may result in a more proximal injury as tension can be placed on the neurovascular structures.
- Bite
  - May result in inoculation with flora from the mouth of the animal
    * *Eikenella* sp. (human bites)—adjunctively treat with amoxicillin-clavulanic acid[7]
    * *Pasteurella* sp. (dog or cat bites)—adjunctively treat with amoxicillin-clavulanic acid[8]

- Epidemiology
  - Adult injuries[6]
    - ◆ Historically occur more commonly in men, likely due to occupational hazards
      - ∗ Powered hand tools or fixed powered machines are the top contributors to fingertip injuries in industries such as agriculture, manufacturing, and construction.[9]
      - ∗ Injuries at home in patients >15 years old are also typically caused by power tools (power saws, lawn mowers, snow blowers, etc.).[10]
    - ◆ The middle finger is most commonly injured as are the distal and middle portions of the nail bed because these are the most exposed/unprotected by the rest of the hand.
  - Pediatric injuries[11,12]
    - ◆ Nail bed injury present in 15% to 24% of fingertip injuries in children
    - ◆ Highest incidence in children <5 years old
    - ◆ Most commonly caused by jamming or crushing finger in a door
    - ◆ The middle finger and distal nail bed are most commonly injured.

EVALUATION

- History
  - Patient-related factors are important to determine the need and amount of intervention
    - ◆ Functional need
      - ∗ Hand dominance
      - ∗ Occupation
      - ∗ Hobbies
    - ◆ Medical history
      - ∗ Age
      - ∗ Diabetes
      - ∗ Tobacco use
      - ∗ Vasospastic disorders
      - ∗ Tetanus prophylaxis
    - ◆ Cosmetic concerns
  - Injury-related issues
    - ◆ Work-related mechanism
    - ◆ Involvement of chemicals, toxic substances, electricity
    - ◆ Timing of injury

- Physical examination (Figure 52.2)[13]
  - Inspection
    - In the setting of active bleeding inadequately managed by compression alone, visualization may be improved by the placement of a tourniquet proximally on the digit or an inflated blood pressure cuff on the arm or forearm. It is crucial to remove this when control of bleeding is obtained to prevent ischemia.
    - Integrity of nail plate. Eponychial hematomas suggest avulsions of the plate at that site.
    - Nail bed/subungual hematoma
      * If hematoma takes up >50% nail bed surface area, there is a 60% chance of a laceration to the nail bed requiring repair.[14]
    - Pulp/tissue defect
    - Injury pattern to the nail bed (avulsion and/or tissue loss vs other types amenable to direct repair)
    - Open fracture
      * In pediatrics, evaluate for avulsion of the proximal nail bed (Figure 52.3A)
  - Palpation
    - If crush mechanism, palpate all compartments of the hand/forearm, consider compartment syndrome
    - Assess the sensation to the radial and ulnar borders of the finger. Perform this portion of the examination before any local analgesic is administered.
  - Range of motion (ROM)
    - May be limited by pain, and therefore better assessed after a digital block with local anesthetic
      * Epinephrine has been shown to be safe in patients without vascular disease.[15]
    - Check active flexion and extension of the distal interphalangeal (DIP) joint for integrity of the FDP and terminal slip of the extensor tendon, respectively.
    - Assess ROM of proximal interphalangeal and metacarpophalangeal joint as motion of these joints may be important when considering treatment of tissue loss with local flaps in the hand/palm.
  - Pediatric considerations
    - Patients may be unable to comply with examination, depending on age and anxiety. Conscious sedation can aid in the examination.
    - Use the tenodesis effect to gauge the integrity of flexor and extensor tendons.
    - Ensure that all tissue, even if avulsed, is saved in moist gauze.

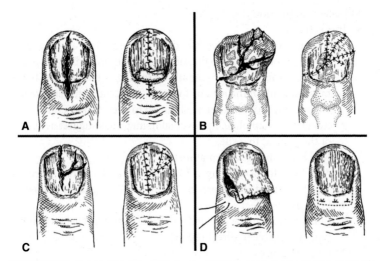

FIGURE 52.2 Types of nail bed injuries and their repairs. A, Laceration. B, Crush injury (with fracture). C, Stellate laceration. D, Avulsion of proximal matrix. Note repair is completed with horizontal mattress suturing. Adapted from Ashbell TS, Kleinert HE, Putcha SM, et al. The deformed finger nail, a frequent result of failure to repair nail bed injuries. *J Trauma*. 1967;7(2):177-190.

- Imaging
  - Anteroposterior and lateral x-rays of the affected digit are necessary element of evaluation.
  - If there is avulsion or amputation of tissue, x-rays of the amputated part may be helpful.
  - Tuft fracture
    - Fracture of the distal phalanx of the affected digit is common in crush mechanisms.
  - Seymour fracture[16,17] (Figure 52.3B)
    - A juxta-epiphyseal fracture pattern in children in which the distal phalanx metaphysis slips off of the epiphysis and the nail bed becomes entrapped in the physis, preventing reduction. These are frequently identified by wide/asymmetric appearance of the physis on lateral x-ray.
- Classification
  - Adult injuries
    - Allen[18]
      - Based on anatomic structures
      - See Figure 52.1 for zones

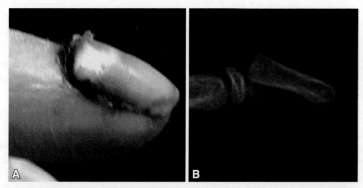

FIGURE 52.3 A, Clinical photo of a Seymour fracture. Note the avulsion of the nail plate and nail bed from beneath the eponychial fold. B, Lateral radiograph of an unreduced Seymour fracture. Adapted from Reyes BA, Ho CA. The high risk of infection with delayed treatment of open Seymour fractures: Salter-Harris I/II or Juxta-epiphyseal fractures of the distal phalanx with associated nailbed laceration. *J Pediatr Orthop.* 2015;37(4):247-253.

- Fassler[19]
  * Zones describe the injury pattern
    ▲ Zone 1—volar oblique (no nail bed involvement)
    ▲ Zone 2—volar oblique (nail bed involved)
    ▲ Zone 3—transverse
    ▲ Zone 4—dorsal oblique
- Tamai[20]
  * Levels are based on vascular anatomy.
    ▲ Zone I—distal to lunula. Central artery repair necessary
    ▲ Zone II—between DIP joint and lunula. Digital artery repair possible
- Pulp-nail-bone[21]
  * Most descriptive in terms of what component of the distal fingertip is involved, but has a low intraobserver reliability.

MANAGEMENT (SEE ALGORITHM)

- Surgical indications
  - Injuries involving the nail bed require replantation, repair, or revision amputation.
    - Repair of the nail bed requires adequate suture repair of the sterile matrix.

- ◆ Care must be taken with revision amputation to either leave enough distal phalanx to support nail growth or ablate the germinal matrix to prevent hook nail deformity.
- Regardless of size and presence of fracture, subungual hematomas with an intact nail plate can be treated with trephination alone. Nail plate removal and direct nail bed repair are unnecessary.[22-26]
- Obvious nail bed injuries or nail bed hematomas with disruption of the nail plate should be repaired.
- Seymour fractures should be treated operatively, with removal of the germinal matrix from the physis and realignment of the physis with or without K-wire fixation.
- Nonoperative treatment
  - Trephination can be performed with a specialized trephination device or with a heated paperclip.
    - ◆ The hole should be adequate in size to decompress the hematoma.
    - ◆ Needles are not recommended because of potential trauma they can induce to the nail bed.
  - Tuft fractures resulting from a crush mechanism often do not need to be surgically stabilized or splinted if not significantly displaced, despite comminution.
- Surgical approach
  - Curved scissors or an elevator should be used to break up adhesions between the nail plate and nail bed as proximally as possible. The nail can be gripped and withdrawn from the eponychial fold when loose.
  - Simple nail bed lacerations may be repaired with small (eg, 6-0 or 7-0) chromic gut or another fast-absorbing suture (Figure 52.2).
  - Eponychial and paronychial folds should be repaired with 5-0 nylon or with chromic sutures. When repairing fingertip injuries in pediatric patients, it is advisable to use absorbable sutures to avoid suture removal in the office.
  - Closure of a laceration to the nail bed with 2-octyl cyanoacrylate is as efficacious at producing good cosmesis as suture repair and can be faster.[27]
  - Nail bed injuries in the setting of amputations must be managed based on the type of amputation.
    - ◆ Nonreplantable injuries through the nail bed may result in a short segment of remaining nail bed.
    - ◆ Coverage of exposed bone may necessitate a flap.

- Nail bed avulsions[28]
  - ◆ Sterile matrix avulsion
    - ∗ If the matrix tissue is still adhered to the nail plate, removal and free tissue grafting with the avulsed tissue is indicated
    - ∗ Split thickness nail matrix grafts from uninjured portions of the same digit or other digits (including the great toe) are the treatment of choice if the avulsed tissue is lost.
  - ◆ Germinal matrix avulsion
    - ∗ Bipedicled flaps of germinal and sterile matrices or distally based flaps may be used for small linear germinal matrix defects.
    - ∗ Wide germinal matrix defects may be grafted from the great toe.
- Replacement of the nail after cleaning is not necessary to "splint open" the eponychial fold.[29]
- Composite grafting can be a reasonable option for pediatric patients with amputations involving the nail bed.[30-32]
  - ◆ The amputated tip is sutured back onto the remaining distal phalanx.
- Seymour fractures require extraction of the incarcerated nail matrix from the physis, reduction of the fracture, and proximal nail matrix repair under the eponychial fold.[33]
  - ◆ The partially avulsed nail plate should not be removed. Removal can cause more instability of the fracture.
  - ◆ K-wire fixation across the physis and DIP joint is indicated for fracture instability after reduction.
- Nonadherent gauze with or without a bolster should be placed on the repaired matrix. Gauze and a finger splint can be used for additional coverage and protection.

POSTOPERATIVE CARE

- ■ Postoperative care
  - Oral antibiotics (typically a cephalosporin) are recommended for open fractures.
  - It is recommended to check the patient's wound within 1 week of the procedure.

- Most patients with injuries that do not involve flap coverage or bony repair can return to work/function about 2 weeks after injury.
- Patients should be counseled that nail growth may be irregular for approximately 100 days.[3]
■ Potential complications
  - Infection
    ◆ Especially common for open fractures and Seymour fractures treated in delayed fashion[17]
  - Nail deformities[1] (Figure 52.4)
    ◆ Hook nail
      ✳ Occurs from the lack of bony support from a shortened distal phalanx
      ✳ Can cause pain. Treatment involves removal of the nail and ablation of the germinal matrix.
    ◆ Nail ridging
      ✳ Occurs from uneven sterile matrix or bony support
    ◆ Split nails
      ✳ Occurs from a scar between the dorsal roof and germinal matrix or a loss of the matrix
  - Painful neuromas
    ◆ Can occur if a transected nerve is not repaired or revised truncation very proximal to the laceration
  - Cold intolerance
    ◆ Incidence can be as high as 85% to 100%.[34,35]
  - Joint stiffness

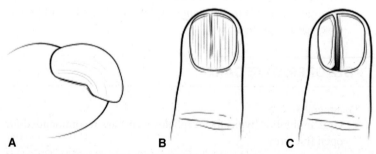

FIGURE 52.4 A, Hook nail. B, Nail ridging. C, Split nail. From Lee DH, Mignemi ME, Crosby SN. Fingertip injuries: an update on management. *J Am Acad Orthop Surg.* 2013;21(12):756-766.

MANAGEMENT ALGORITHM

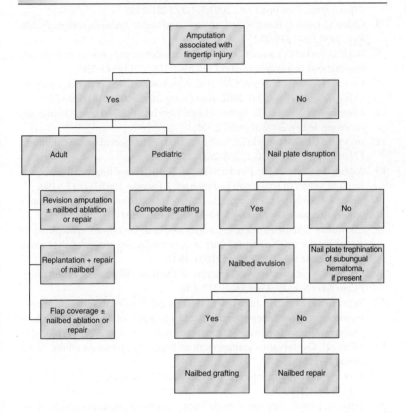

REFERENCES

1. Lee DH, Mignemi ME, Crosby SN. Fingertip injuries: an update on management. *J Am Acad Orthop Surg.* 2013;21(12):756-766.
2. Peterson SL, Peterson EL, Wheatley MJ. Management of fingertip amputations. *J Hand Surg Am.* 2014;39(10):2093-2101.
3. Zook EG. Anatomy and physiology of the perionychium. *Clin Anat.* 2003;16(1):1-8.
4. Murai M, Lau HK, Pereira BP, et al. A cadaver study on volume and surface area of the fingertip. *J Hand Surg Am.* 1997;22(5):935-941.
5. Strauch B, de Moura W. Arterial system of the fingers. *J Hand Surg Am.* 1990;15(1):148-154.
6. Zook EG, Guy RJ, Russell RC. A study of nail bed injuries: causes, treatment, and prognosis. *J Hand Surg Am.* 1984;9(2):247-252.

7. Talan DA, Abrahamian FM, Moran GJ, et al. Clinical presentation and bacteriologic analysis of infected human bites in patients presenting to emergency departments. *Clin Infect Dis*. 2003;37(11):1481-1489.

8. Glaser C, Lewis P, Wong S. Pet-, animal-, and vector-borne infections. *Pediatr Rev*. 2000;21(7):219-232.

9. Boyle D, Parker D, Larson C, et al. Nature, incidence, and cause of work-related amputations in Minnesota. *Am J Ind Med*. 2000;37(5):542-550.

10. Conn JM, Annest JL, Ryan GW, et al. Non-work-related finger amputations in the United States, 2001-2002. *Ann Emerg Med*. 2005;45(6):630-635.

11. Doraiswamy NV, Baig H. Isolated finger injuries in children—incidence and aetiology. *Injury*. 2000;31(8):571-573.

12. Inglefield CJ, D'Arcangelo M, Kolhe PS. Injuries to the nail bed in childhood. *J Hand Surg Br*. 1995;20(2):258-261.

13. Ashbell TS, Kleinert HE, Putcha SM, et al. The deformed finger nail, a frequent result of failure to repair nail bed injuries. *J Trauma*. 1967;7(2):177-190.

14. Simon RR, Wolgin M. Subungual hematoma: association with occult laceration requiring repair. *Am J Emerg Med*. 1987;5(4):302-304.

15. Chowdhry S, Seidenstricker L, Cooney DS, et al. Do not use epinephrine in digital blocks: myth or truth? Part II. A retrospective review of 1111 cases. *Plast Reconstr Surg*. 2010;126(6):2031-2034.

16. Seymour N. Juxta-epiphysial fracture of the terminal phalanx of the finger. *J Bone Joint Surg Br*. 1966;48(2):347-349.

17. Reyes BA, Ho CA. The high risk of infection with delayed treatment of open Seymour fractures: Salter-Harris I/II or Juxta-epiphyseal fractures of the distal phalanx with associated nailbed laceration. *J Pediatr Orthop*. 2015;37(4):247-253.

18. Allen MJ. Conservative management of finger tip injuries in adults. *Hand*. 1980;12(3):257-265.

19. Fassler PR. Fingertip injuries: evaluation and treatment. *J Am Acad Orthop Surg*. 1996;4(1):84-92.

20. Tamai S, Hori Y, Tatsumi Y, et al. Microvascular anastomosis and its application on the replantation of amputated digits and hands. *Clin Orthop Relat Res*. 1978;133:106-121.

21. Evans DM, Bernardis C, Bernadis C. A new classification for fingertip injuries. *J Hand Surg Br*. 2000;25(1):58-60.

22. Dean B, Becker G, Little C. The management of the acute traumatic subungual haematoma: a systematic review. *Hand Surg*. 2012;17(1):151-154.

23. Batrick N, Hashemi K, Freij R. Treatment of uncomplicated subungual haematoma. *Emerg Med J*. 2003;20(1):65.

24. Meek S, White M. Subungual haematomas: is simple trephining enough? *J Accid Emerg Med*. 1998;15(4):269-271.

25. Seaberg DC, Angelos WJ, Paris PM. Treatment of subungual hematomas with nail trephination: a prospective study. *Am J Emerg Med*. 1991;9(3):209-210.

26. Roser SE, Gellman H. Comparison of nail bed repair versus nail trephination for subungual hematomas in children. *J Hand Surg Am*. 1999;24(6):1166-1170.

27. Strauss EJ, Weil WM, Jordan C, et al. A prospective, randomized, controlled trial of 2-octylcyanoacrylate versus suture repair for nail bed injuries. *J Hand Surg Am*. 2008;33(2):250-253.

28. Shepard GH. Management of acute nail bed avulsions. *Hand Clin*. 1990;6(1):39-56; discussion 57-58.

29. O'Shaughnessy M, McCann J, O'Connor TP, et al. Nail re-growth in fingertip injuries. *Ir Med J*. 1990;83(4):136-137.

30. Butler DP, Murugesan L, Ruston J, et al. The outcomes of digital tip amputation replacement as a composite graft in a paediatric population. *J Hand Surg Eur Vol*. 2016;41(2):164-170.

31. Eberlin KR, Busa K, Bae DS, et al. Composite grafting for pediatric fingertip injuries. *Hand*. 2015;10(1):28-33.

32. Moiemen NS, Elliot D. Composite graft replacement of digital tips. 2. A study in children. *J Hand Surg Br*. 1997;22(3):346-352.

33. Krusche-Mandl I, Köttstorfer J, Thalhammer G, et al. Seymour fractures: retrospective analysis and therapeutic considerations. *J Hand Surg Am*. 2013;38(2):258-264.

34. van den Berg WB, Vergeer RA, van der Sluis CK, et al. Comparison of three types of treatment modalities on the outcome of fingertip injuries. *J Trauma Acute Care Surg*. 2012;72(6):1681-1687.

35. Ni F, Appleton SE, Chen B, et al. Aesthetic and functional reconstruction of fingertip and pulp defects with pivot flaps. *J Hand Surg Am*. 2012;37(9):1806-1811.

53 Fingertip Amputations

Robert Ryu and Hisham M. Awan

INTRODUCTION

- Fingertip injuries are the most common hand injuries presenting to emergency departments.
- Fingertip injuries with soft tissue loss may be time-intensive and challenging to treat.
- Goals of management include preserving finger length, restoring a sensate, durable tip, and preserving bony support for nail growth when possible.
- Anatomy
  - Fingertip anatomy (Figure 53.1)
    - Eponychium—also known as the cuticle, soft tissue at distal margin of proximal nail fold
    - Paronychium—lateral margins of nail fold
    - Hyponychium—barrier to microorganisms where nail bed meets skin of fingertip
    - Lunula—crescent-shaped structure seen at junction between sterile and germinal matrices
    - Nail bed
      - * Sterile matrix—lies directly beneath the nail plate where it adheres to the nail bed
      - * Germinal matrix—just proximal to the sterile matrix, responsible for majority of nail growth

EVALUATION

- History and physical examination
  - Determine mechanism of injury, including avulsion, crush, or laceration.
  - Assess zone of injury and characteristics of laceration and presence or absence of exposed bone, which will ultimately guide management (Figure 53.2).

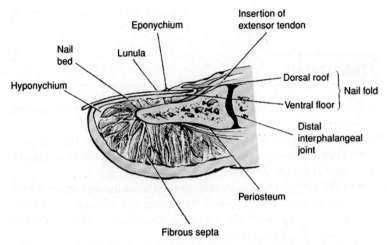

FIGURE 53.1 Sagittal section of fingertip anatomy. Reprinted with permission from Wolfson A, Cloutier R, Hendey G, et al. *Harwood-Nuss' Clinical Practice of Emergency Medicine*. Philadelphia, PA: Lippincott Williams & Wilkins; 2014.

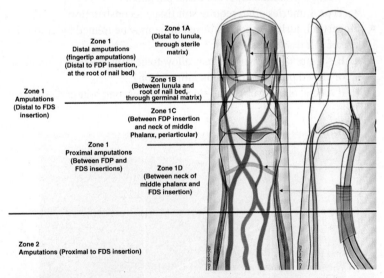

FIGURE 53.2 A new classification system for digital amputations distal to flexor digitorum superficialis tendon. FDP, flexor digitorum profundus; FDS, flexor digitorum superficialis. From Sebastin SJ, Chung KC. A systematic review of the outcomes of replantation of distal digital amputation. *Plast Reconstr Surg.* 2011;128:725, with permission.

- Evaluate range of motion to determine flexor or extensor tendon involvement.

TREATMENT

- Accurate categorization of fingertip injuries is critical for guiding treatment.
- These injuries can be classified into four main patterns (Figure 53.3):
  - **Type 1** transverse tip amputations without exposed bone may be treated with healing by secondary intention.
  - **Type 2** injuries with more extensive soft tissue loss and exposed bone may be treated with skeletal shortening and primary closure, but are often associated with nail plate abnormalities, especially when >50% of nail plate is removed.
  - **Type 3** injuries near distal interphalangeal (DIP) joint may be considered for replantation or revision amputation. Replantation is most successful when amputation is proximal to area of paronychium through proximal aspect of distal phalanx.
  - **Type 4** injuries often require soft tissue reconstruction.
- Fingertip injuries without exposed bone may be treated based on the size of soft tissue deficit:
  - If <1 cm^2 of tip involved, may allow to heal by secondary intention or closed primarily (revision amputation)
  - If >1 cm^2 of tip involved, full-thickness skin or composite grafts required

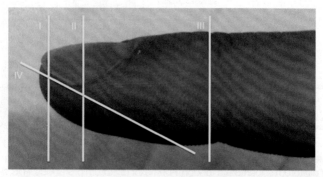

FIGURE 53.3 Classification system for fingertip amputations. With permission from Biswas D, Wysocki RW, Fernandez JJ, Cohen MS. Local and regional flaps for hand coverage. *J Hand Surg Am.* 2014;39(5):992-1004.

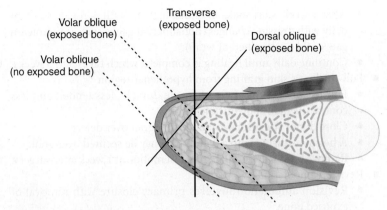

FIGURE 53.4 Orientation of fingertip amputations. Redrawn with permission from Lister GD. The theory of the transposition flap and its practical application in the hand. *Clin Plast Surg.* 1981;8:115-128.

- Fingertip injuries with exposed bone are treated based on orientation of tissue loss (Figure 53.4):
  - Volar oblique injury
    - Cross-finger flap
    - Thenar flap
    - Neurovascular island flaps
    - Distant flaps (chest, abdomen, or groin)
    - Moberg advancement flap for volar oblique thumb injury
  - Transverse injury
    - V-Y advancement flap
    - Kutler paired V-Y lateral advancement flaps
    - Moberg advancement flap for transverse thumb injury
  - Dorsal oblique injury
    - V-Y advancement flap
    - Reverse cross-finger flaps
    - First dorsal metacarpal artery "kite" flap or heterodigital island flap for dorsal thumb injury

TECHNIQUES

- Secondary intention
  - Perform initial irrigation and debridement and soft dressing.

- After 1 week, start soaks in dilute, half-strength peroxide solution daily with dressing changes (nonadherent gauze such as petroleum gauze and a self-adherent wrap).
- Continue daily until healing is complete, which takes 3 to 5 weeks.
- Full-thickness skin grafting from hypothenar region
  - Full-thickness skin grafts are more durable, less tender, and less contractile than split-thickness grafts.
  - Close donor site primarily and suture graft over defect.
  - A bolster dressing with a cotton ball may be secured over graft.
  - Remove bolster and initiate range of motion at 1 week after surgery.
- Revision amputation
  - Revision amputation involves primary closure with removal of exposed bone.
  - Ablate remaining nail matrix to prevent formation of irritating nail fragments.
  - If flexor or extensor tendon insertions are irreparable, then disarticulate DIP joint.
  - Transect remaining tendons and nerves as proximal as possible.
  - Advance volar over bone and suture to dorsal skin.
- V-Y advancement flap
  - V-Y advancement flaps preserve length and provide coverage for transverse or dorsal oblique fingertip injuries.
  - Elevate a wide V-shaped, full-thickness volar flap off distal phalanx with a tapered base at level of DIP joint (Figure 53.5A).
  - Advance flap over fingertip toward dorsal side with a tension and kink-free closure.
  - The repair converts the V-shaped incision into a Y-shaped wound.
  - Kutler popularized the paired lateral V-Y advancements using two separate smaller V-Y advancement flaps from lateral aspects of finger to cover a transverse fingertip amputation (Figure 53.5B).
- Cross-finger flap (Figure 53.6)
  - Preferred for large volar defects in patients >30 years of age.
  - Elevate dorsal skin and subcutaneous tissue superficial to the paratenon from adjacent finger to create a bed for the injured fingertip.
  - Raise a rectangular flap from three sides of dorsal surface of middle phalanx, typically based on radial side.
  - Cutting Cleland's ligament will extend the flap up to 20% longer.
  - Rotate flap outward on its hinge and suture in place.
  - Cover donor site with a split-thickness skin graft.
  - Divide flap within 2 weeks to avoid stiffness.

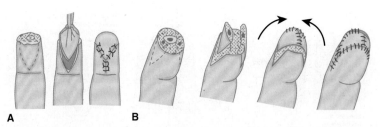

FIGURE 53.5 A, V-Y advancement flap. B, Kutler advancement flap. Redrawn with permission from Singh AP. Fingertip injuries to the hand. http://boneandspine.com/fingertip-injuries-of-the-hand. Accessed August 29, 2018.

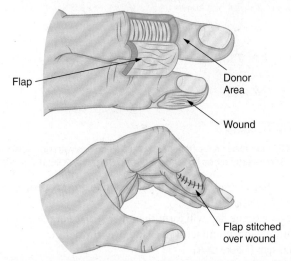

Flap

Donor Area

Wound

Flap stitched over wound

FIGURE 53.6 Cross-finger flap. Redrawn with permission from Singh AP. Fingertip injuries to the hand. http://boneandspine.com/fingertip-injuries-of-the-hand. Accessed August 29, 2018.

- Reverse cross-finger flap (Figure 53.7)
  - Indicated for deep dorsal finger wounds
  - Also indicated for reconstruction of an eponychial skinfold and coverage of an exposed extensor tendon near DIP joint.
  - Elevate a full-thickness, obliquely oriented skin flap with intact subdermal vascular plexus on dorsum over adjacent middle phalanx about 1 cm longer and 4 to 5 mm wider than the defect.

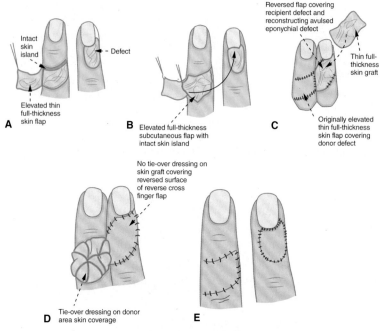

FIGURE 53.7 Reverse cross-finger flap (A-E). Redrawn with permission from Atasoy E. The reverse cross finger flap. *J Hand Surg Am.* 2016;41(1):122-128.

- Raise flap at level of extensor paratenon to preserve dorsal veins and arteries with the flap.
- Reversing the flap will form the inner surface of the eponychium.
- Suture flap with intact skin island over the defect.

■ Thenar flap (Figure 53.8)
- Preferred for volar oblique fingertip injuries to index or long finger in patients <30 years of age.
- Involves flexing affected finger and suturing wound into a flap in the thenar eminence at base of thumb.
- A rectangular flap, slightly wider and longer than defect, is lifted parallel to proximal thumb crease with base on proximal side of flap.
- Finger is flexed, and flap is loosely sutured into the defect, and this is ultimately split after 2 to 3 weeks. Donor site can be covered with skin graft or allowed to heal by secondary intention.
- Advantage of thenar flap is improved cosmesis.
- Complications include possible proximal interphalangeal joint contraction.

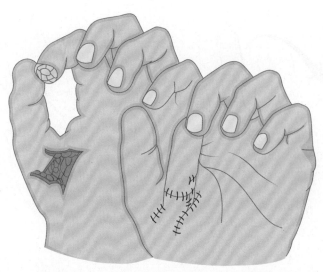

FIGURE 53.8 Thenar flap. Redrawn with permission from Singh AP. Fingertip injuries to the hand. http://boneandspine.com/fingertip-injuries-of-the-hand. Accessed August 29, 2018.

- Neurovascular island flaps
  - Homodigital island flap
    - Best axial pattern flap for volar oblique or transverse fingertip amputations
    - Raised on digital artery of involved digit
    - Maintains sensory innervation to finger.
  - Heterodigital island flap (Figure 53.9)
    - Flap raised on ulnar aspect of long or ring finger and tunneled in the palm to cover defect on thumb
- Distant flaps
  - Includes chest, abdomen, and groin
  - Disadvantages: flaps cumbersome and too bulky for fingertips
- Moberg advancement flap (Figure 53.10)
  - Useful for thumb amputations distal to interphalangeal (IP) joint.
  - The entire volar surface of thumb with its corresponding neurovascular bundle is advanced and is raised from distal to proximal at level of flexor tendon sheath.
  - Slight flexion of thumb IP joint assists in soft tissue defect coverage with advancement flap.
  - Complications include possible flap necrosis and thumb IP joint contracture.

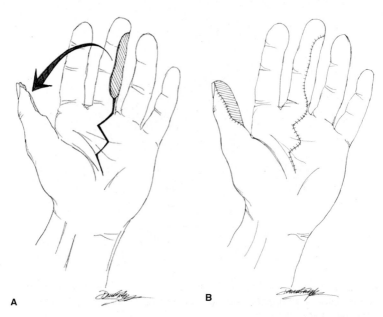

A   B

FIGURE 53.9 Heterodigital neurovascular island flap (A and B). With permission from Thorne CH, Gurtner, GC, Chung K, et al. *Grabb and Smith's Plastic Surgery*. Philadelphia, PA: Lippincott Williams & Wilkins; 2013.

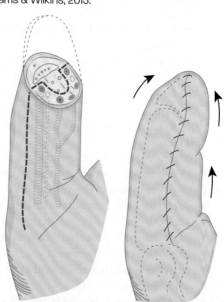

FIGURE 53.10 Moberg advancement flap. Redrawn with permission from Lister GD. The theory of the transposition flap and its practical application in the hand. *Clin Plast Surg.* 1981;8:115-128.

- First dorsal metacarpal artery "kite" flap (Figure 53.11)
  - For dorsal thumb amputations or volar thumb amputations >2 cm
  - Based off first dorsal metacarpal artery ulnar branch to index finger
  - Elevate flap from dorsoradial aspect of hand at level of index finger metacarpal head
  - Full-thickness flap is elevated including underlying fascia of first dorsal interosseous muscle on which lies the corresponding neurovascular structures.
  - Raise aponeurosis with the perivascular fat and take radial nerve branches and accompanying artery.
  - Once pedicled flap is raised, tunnel it subcutaneously to thumb without tension or kinking.
  - Donor site may be repaired primarily or covered with skin graft.
- Postoperative management
  - Patients to be seen 5 to 7 days after surgery.
  - Gently remove dressing, soak finger with normal saline to ease removal of dressing.
  - Any bolster should be removed at that time as well.
  - Check nail for subungual seroma or hematoma. If present, raise nail or place hole to facilitate drainage.
  - Any suture used to hold nail or sheet holding nail fold should be removed 5 to 7 days after surgery to avoid sinus tract formation.
  - Sutures placed in hyponychium or paronychium may remain until 14 days after surgery.

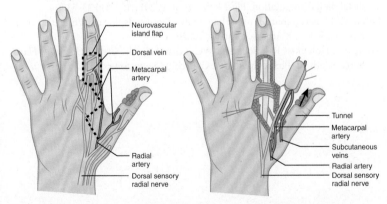

FIGURE 53.11 First dorsal metacarpal artery "kite" flap. Redrawn with permission from Al-Balushi F. Hand flaps & micro surgery. Dr Fawaz Albalushi/ Plastic & Micro Reconstructive Surgery. August 2009. http://drfawazalbalushi. blogspot.com. Accessed August 29, 2018.

- Protect nail bed repairs and any distal phalanx fractures with immobilization with splint dressing for first 3 to 4 weeks.
- Distal phalanx fractures are followed by radiographic evaluation at 4 weeks.
- Complications
  - Flap failure
    - Result of inadequate arterial inflow (vasospasms, thrombosis) or inadequate venous outflow.
    - Also prone to failure from shear stresses and hematoma formation.

SUGGESTED READINGS

Al-Balushi F. Hand flaps & micro surgery. Dr. Fawaz Albalushi/Plastic & Micro Reconstructive Surgery. August 2009. http://drfawazalbalushi.blogspot.com. Accessed August 29, 2018.

Atasoy E. The reverse cross finger flap. *J Hand Surg Am*. 2016;41(1):122-128.

Biswas D, Wysocki RW, Fernandez JJ, Cohen MS. Local and regional flaps for hand coverage. *J Hand Surg Am*. 2014;39(5):992-1004.

Hansen SL, Lang P, Sbitany H. Soft tissue reconstruction of the upper extremity. In: *Plastic Surgery*: chap 73. Also available at http://doctorlib.info/surgery/plastic/73.html.

Lister GD. The theory of the transposition flap and its practical application in the hand. *Clin Plast Surg*. 1981;8:115-128.

Ramirez MA, Means KR Jr. Digital soft tissue trauma: a concise primer of soft tissue reconstruction of traumatic hand injuries. *Iowa Orthop J*. 2011;31:110-120.

Sebastin SJ, Chung KC. A systematic review of the outcomes of replantation of distal digital amputation. *Plast Reconstr Surg*. 2011;128(3):723-737.

Singh AP. Fingertip injuries to the hand. http://boneandspine.com/fingertip-injuries-of-the-hand. Accessed August 29, 2018.

Wolfe SW, Hotchkiss RN, Pederson WC, Kozin SH, eds. *Green's Operative Hand Surgery*. 6th ed. Philadelphia, PA: Churchill Livingstone; 2011.

54 Replantation

Michael S. Gart

INTRODUCTION

- The first upper extremity replantation was performed in Boston, MA by Dr Ronald Malt in 1962.[1]
- Three years later, Komatsu and Tamai reported the first successful digital replantation.[2]
- In order to be truly "successful," a replanted part must function as well as or better than the available prosthetic technology.
- Although surgeons can now technically replant nearly any severed part, recent focus has been on identifying patients who will have excellent functional outcomes following replantation.[3]

Pathoanatomy

- An amputation in the upper extremity severs soft tissue, muscle/tendon, nerve, blood vessels, and bone.
- The status of each of these structures will dictate the functional outcome of the replanted part(s).
  - In particular, severe nerve injury may preclude replantation, particularly with proximal upper extremity amputations, because an insensate extremity without motor function will ultimately be less useful than a prosthetic.
- In digital amputations, the neurovascular bundles run volar to the mid-axis of the digit, between Grayson's (volar) and Cleland's (dorsal) ligaments.
- Digital veins can be reliably located in the dorsal subcutaneous tissue.
- Knowledge of the flexor tendon anatomy is critical because amputations through zone II will often have poor functional outcomes due to a high incidence of postoperative adhesions.
- The thumb is responsible for nearly half of all hand function and, even with poor range of motion, a replanted thumb will provide the best functional outcome.[4]

Mechanism of Injury

- Mechanism of injury is among the most important determinants of replantation success rates and ultimate functional outcomes.
- Tool injuries (saws, agricultural machinery) are a common source of digital or hand/wrist level amputations.
  - New table-saw technology can stop a saw blade immediately upon contact with skin to reduce the potential for amputation.[5]
- Polytrauma patients may present with crush or avulsion amputations.
- Sharply amputated parts have higher rates of replantation success than crush or avulsion injuries.[6-8] Ring avulsion injuries present a particular spectrum of injury and will be discussed elsewhere.

Epidemiology

- In the United States, digits and thumbs account for the vast majority of upper extremity amputations; however, several hundred patients suffer more proximal amputations each year.
- More than 45 000 traumatic digital amputations occur each year in the United States.[9]
- Most patients suffering amputation are males, with a mean age of 40 years.[10]
- Patients treated at large urban hospitals and/or academic medical centers are more likely to undergo replantation.[10]
- African-American patients and uninsured patients are less likely to undergo replantation than Caucasian or privately insured patients.[11]

EVALUATION

History

- If possible, the patient's age, handedness, smoking status, medical comorbidities, and time of injury should be obtained.
- The time since amputation and method of preservation of the amputated part(s) should be noted.
- The patient's occupation and need for timely return to work may be important in determining treatment (ie, replantation vs revision amputation).
  - Age > 45 to 50, heavy smoking, diabetes, avulsion or crush injury, and prolonged ischemia time are associated with failure of replantation.[6,12]
  - Some data suggest that smoking and medical comorbidities may not have the detrimental effects on replantation success that were once thought.[13]

Physical Examination

- Every effort should be made to minimize the time from injury to definitive treatment.
- The amputated parts and distal stump should be photographed and x-rays obtained prior to any attempted replantation (Figure 54.1).

ACUTE MANAGEMENT

Acute Patient Management

- Patients presenting with traumatic amputations must be thoroughly evaluated by a trauma service for other life-threatening injuries, which take treatment priority.
  - Replantation is only considered in medically stable patients after appropriate resuscitation.
- Any ongoing hemorrhage from the proximal stump should be controlled with external compression because vessel ligation or clamping can cause additional vessel damage.
- Patients should be started on prophylactic antibiotics and given tetanus prophylaxis preoperatively.

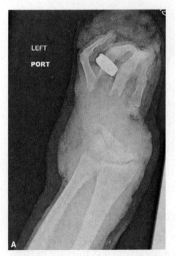 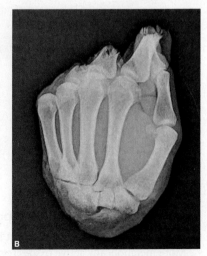

FIGURE 54.1 Preoperative radiographs (A, B) and intraoperative photos (C, D) of multilevel hand and multiple digit amputation. Photos courtesy of Jason H. Ko, MD.

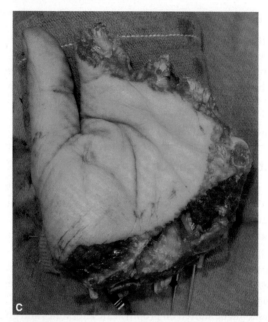

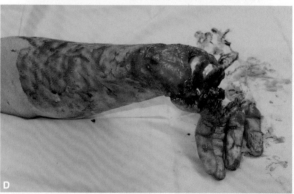

FIGURE 54.1 (*continued*)

Acute Management of the Amputated Part(s)

- Preservation of the amputated part is critical to replantation success. More metabolically active tissues (eg, muscle) are less tolerant of ischemia than tendon, bone, etc.

- Generally accepted ischemia times for reliable replantation are <12 hours of warm or <24 hours of cold ischemia for digital amputations and <6 hours of warm or 12 hours of cold ischemia for major upper extremity amputations.[14]
  - Ideally, amputated parts are wrapped in saline-soaked gauze and immediately placed on ice or in a plastic bag and submerged in an ice water bath at 4°C.
  - Amputated parts should not be placed directly on ice or in water because this may cause freezing or further damage to the tissues.
- While the patient is being evaluated, the amputated part(s) should be taken to the operating room to identify and prepare important structures for replantation[15,16] (Figure 54.2).

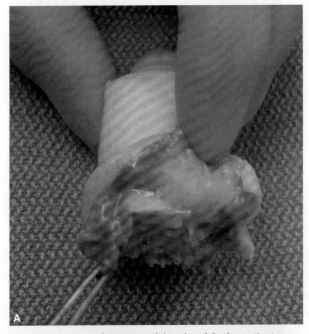

FIGURE 54.2 Preparation of amputated thumb. While the patient was prepared for surgery, a second team identifies the radial digital artery (A), flexor pollicis longus tendon (B), and ulnar digital nerve (C).

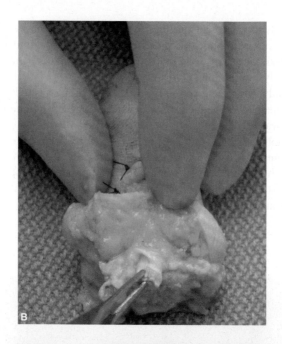

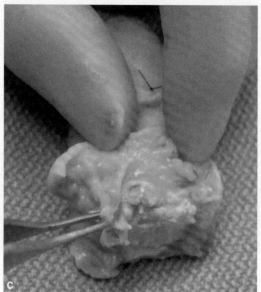

FIGURE 54.2 *(continued)*

DEFINITIVE TREATMENT

- The definitive treatment for amputation, when possible, is replantation.
  - The decision to undergo replantation depends on a number of economic, social, and psychological factors, which must all be considered in the context of the patient's overall health, mechanism of injury, status of the amputated part(s), and expected functional outcome.
  - Patients who are unwilling or unable to comply with an extensive postoperative rehabilitation program or who require the most expeditious treatment to return to work may elect for revision amputation, particularly with amputations of single, nonthumb digits.
    - Return to gainful employment is usually >24 months for manual laborers.[17]
- A final decision to attempt replantation usually depends on the state of the amputated parts under evaluation in the operating room.
- Bones, tendons, nerves, and blood vessels must be suitable for repair, and soft-tissue coverage must be possible with local or free tissue transfer.[18]

Surgical Indications

- Each patient should be considered individually, but the following are general indications to attempt replantation:
  - Pediatric amputations (any)
  - Thumb or multiple digit amputations
  - Single digit amputations distal to the insertion of the flexor digitorum superficialis (FDS tendon; preserved proximal interphalangeal [PIP] joint)
  - Any amputation at or proximal to the palm

Contraindications

- Contraindications to replantation are generally related to poor functional outcomes or patients who are unsuitable for replantation surgery.
- Absolute contraindications[3]
  - Multilevel amputations
  - Severe crush injury
  - Tendon avulsion from muscle belly (extreme avulsive force)
  - Prolonged warm ischemia time
  - Massive contamination

- Nonviable proximal stump
- Concomitant life-threatening injuries that require immediate treatment
■ Relative contraindications[3]
  - Amputations unlikely to pose a significant functional deficit (ie, border digit amputations, single digit amputations of non-dominant hand)
  - Replantations likely to result in poor functional outcome (ie, single digit amputations through zone II, ring avulsion injuries, severe destruction of PIP joint)

Surgical Approach

■ Replantation surgery can be performed with regional blockade and/or general anesthesia, with the former providing long-lasting analgesia and sympathetic blockade, which may reduce vasospasm and microvascular complications.
■ While the patient is being evaluated for surgery, another surgical team can prepare the amputated part(s) in the operating room.
  - Placement of core tendinous sutures and K-wires can be positioned before the patient arrives to the operating room to reduce ischemia time.[15]
  - Once the amputated part has been prepared, it should be maintained in a saline ice bath to minimize warm ischemia time.
  - Digits or other parts deemed nonreplantable should not be discarded; these can be valuable sources of graft material (nerve, tendon, artery/vein, bone, skin).[19]
■ A multiteam approach is preferred to allow one team to begin working on the amputated part(s) while the other works on the proximal stump.
  - The amputated part and proximal stump must be thoroughly irrigated and debrided of any nonviable tissue.
■ Exposure must be obtained proximal and distal to the level of amputation to identify any severed structures that have retracted and/or to facilitate nerve or vein grafts.
■ One or both feet should be prepped into the surgical field as a source for vein graft material as needed. Alternatively, veins can be marked out on the forearm for potential sources of graft.
■ If ischemia time has exceeded 6 hours preoperatively or will exceed 6 hours intraoperatively, a temporary vascular shunt should be utilized

to reestablish flow to the amputated parts and allow accumulated metabolites to drain through unrepaired veins.[17]

- Fasciotomies should be considered in every case, depending on the amount of warm ischemia time and tissue damage; they are almost always required in proximal amputations to reduce the risk of reperfusion-related compartment syndrome.

Operative Technique

- The exact approach and sequence of repair will differ for every surgeon and patient, but general themes are common to all replants:
  - Minimize warm ischemia time with early arterial repair or shunting.
  - Achieve bony stability before microsurgical anastomosis or nerve repair is attempted.
  - When possible, perform arterial anastomoses and nerve repair before venous anastomosis.
    - Deflation of the tourniquet may facilitate identification of veins after the severed part is revascularized.
  - When possible, two veins should be repaired for each arterial repair to allow adequate venous drainage of the replanted part.
  - Aggressive debridement is essential to avoid postoperative necrosis and subsequent infection.
  - Nerves and blood vessels should be resected to healthy edges. This may require resecting structures beyond the zone of injury, and require the use of vein grafts or nerve grafts.
- Our preferred sequence for digital replantation is: osteosynthesis, flexor tendon repair, arterial anastomosis, nerve repair, extensor tendon repair, and venous anastomosis.
  - This sequence typically enables arterial and nerve repair under a single tourniquet run, saving tourniquet time.
- Artery and vein
  - Arteries must be carefully evaluated for signs of intimal damage, including the "red line" and "ribbon signs," which are predictive of replantation failure.[20]
  - Any segment of artery that appears damaged should be resected back to healthy vessel architecture with liberal use of vein grafts from the volar forearm or dorsal foot.
  - If there are no veins suitable for repair, medicinal leeches can be used, or, in the case of a digital replantation, the nail plate or volar

pulp can be removed and scrubbed with heparin-soaked gauze postoperatively to establish venous outflow.

- For thumb replantation, vein graft can be sewn to the ulnar digital artery on the back table to greatly reduce the technical difficulty of this specific vessel anastomosis.[15]

■ Osteosynthesis

- In nearly every case, the bone should be shortened to enable tension-free vascular anastomoses, nerve coaptation, and primary soft-tissue closure.
- Osteosynthesis should proceed as rapidly as possible, but must be secure enough to initiate early postoperative motion.
- When amputation is through an interphalangeal joint, primary arthrodesis should be considered.

■ Tendon repair

- Avulsion of tendons from their musculotendinous junction is suggestive of an extreme avulsive force, and the vessels should be closely examined for evidence of intimal injury.
- In amputated digits, repair of both the flexor digitorum profundus and FDS has demonstrated improved outcome.[21]
- For segmental tendon losses, immediate grafting can be performed using traditional tendon grafts (palmaris longus, plantaris, etc.).
- If there is concern for the viability of soft-tissue coverage, delayed tendon repair or placement of a silicone rod is also an acceptable alternative.
- Digital flexor tendons should be repaired with 4 to 6 core sutures; we prefer three Tsuge sutures with a 3-0 looped Supramid, which is a rapid, 6-strand technique.

■ Nerve repair

- Nerves should be evaluated for their viability prior to proceeding with replantation.
- Particularly with proximal upper extremity amputations, if the nerves are severely damaged, even a successful replantation will have no sensory or motor function, and the patient will ultimately be best served by a prosthetic.
- Debridement of the nerve back to healthy-appearing, bleeding fascicular architecture **is more important** than achieving primary repair.
  - This should be done with an operating microscope to ensure adequate debridement.

- When possible, nerves should be repaired primarily with epineurial sutures, provided they are not placed under excessive tension.
  - As a general rule, if the nerve cannot be held in coaptation with a single 9-0 epineurial suture, there is too much tension for primary repair.
- If a nerve gap exists, processed nerve allografts or autograft from a nonreplantable digit, or from an expendable donor nerve (medial antebrachial cutaneous nerve, lateral antebrachial cutaneous nerve, posterior interosseous nerve, sural nerve) can be used.
  - If there is questionable soft-tissue coverage or concern for infection, processed nerve allografts may be preferred to avoid potential loss of autograft.
- Soft tissues
  - Skin should be loosely approximated with judicious use of skin grafts to avoid closure under excessive tension.
  - The microanastomoses and nerve coaptation should be covered, but other areas may be left open or covered with skin grafts.
  - Large soft-tissue defects or situations without adequate coverage of critical structures may require immediate free flap coverage.[18,19]
  - If the proximal stump is nonviable or massively contaminated, temporary ectopic implantation is an option to allow the proximal stump to be reconstructed before orthotopic replantation.[22-24]

Potential Complications

- Replantation failure
  - Usually due to microvascular thrombosis.
  - All thumb or nondigit amputations should be emergently reexplored for potential microvascular salvage.
  - Amputated parts showing evidence of venous congestion may be salvaged with medicinal leeches.
    - In digital replantation, nail plate or volar pulp can be removed and scrubbed with heparin-soaked gauze to achieve venous outflow.
- Postoperative stiffness
  - Often due to tendinous adhesions, particularly with digital amputations through zone II
  - May require secondary tenolysis

- Nonunion/Malunion/Posttraumatic arthritis
  - May require corrective osteotomies, bone grafting, or arthroplasty/arthrodesis
- Neuroma formation or poor sensory recovery
- Cold intolerance
- Poor functional outcome
  - May hinder overall function and patient may elect for secondary amputation and prosthesis

Postoperative Care

- Prevention of peripheral vasospasm
  - Adequate analgesia and IV hydration
  - Avoidance of nicotine, including patches
  - Consider indwelling catheter for regional blockade
- Maintaining perfusion to replanted part
  - Elevation and loose dressings
  - IV toradol and prophylactic low molecular weight heparin while inpatient
  - Postoperative anticoagulation remains controversial—some surgeons may consider prescribing 81 mg aspirin daily for 1 month following discharge.
    - No standard regimen exists for postoperative anticoagulation.[25]
- Monitoring for microvascular thrombosis
  - Pulse oximeter on replanted part to objectively monitor oxygenation
  - Clinical monitoring of temperature, color, turgor, and bleeding with pinprick
    - Signs of arterial thrombosis: reduced temperature, pale color, diminished tissue turgor, minimal bleeding with pinprick
    - Signs of venous thrombosis: purple color, swollen, increased tissue turgor, rapid release of deoxygenated blood with pinprick
- Rehabilitation
  - Immobilization and initiation of movement typically dictated by bone and/or tendon repairs
    - Microvascular anastomoses and nerve coaptations should not be under tension throughout a full range of motion
  - Early active motion rehabilitation protocols for replanted digits unless otherwise contraindicated[21]

MANAGEMENT ALGORITHM

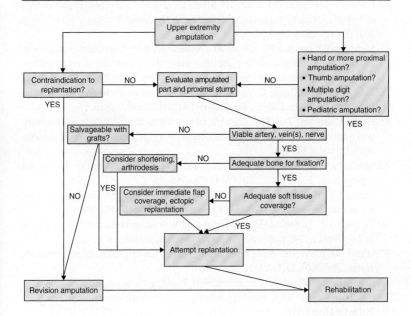

REFERENCES

1. Malt RA, McKhann C. Replantation of severed arms. *JAMA.* 1964;189:716-722.
2. Komatsu S, Tamai S. Successful replantation of a completely cut-off thumb. *Plast Reconstr Surg.* 1968;42(4):374-377.
3. Prucz RB, Friedrich JB. Upper extremity replantation: current concepts. *Plast Reconstr Surg.* 2014;133(2):333-342.
4. Janezic TF, Arnez ZM, Solinc M, Zaletel-Kragelj L. Functional results of 46 thumb replantations and revascularisations. *Microsurgery.* 1996;17(5):264-267.
5. Chung KC, Shauver MJ. Table saw injuries: epidemiology and a proposal for preventive measures. *Plast Reconstr Surg.* 2013;132(5):777e-783e.
6. Dec W. A meta-analysis of success rates for digit replantation. *Tech Hand Up Extrem Surg.* 2006;10(3):124-129.
7. Li J, Guo Z, Zhu Q, et al. Fingertip replantation: determinants of survival. *Plast Reconstr Surg.* 2008;122(3):833-839.
8. Sebastin SJ, Chung KC. A systematic review of the outcomes of replantation of distal digital amputation. *Plast Reconstr Surg.* 2011;128(3):723-737.

9. Maroukis BL, Chung KC, MacEachern M, Mahmoudi E. Hand trauma care in the United States: a literature review. *Plast Reconstr Surg.* 2016;137(1):100e-111e.

10. Friedrich JB, Poppler LH, Mack CD, Rivara FP, Levin LS, Klein MB. Epidemiology of upper extremity replantation surgery in the United States. *J Hand Surg.* 2011;36(11):1835-1840.

11. Mahmoudi E, Swiatek PR, Chung KC, Ayanian JZ. Racial variation in treatment of traumatic finger/thumb amputation: a national comparative study of replantation and revision amputation. *Plast Reconstr Surg.* 2016;137(3):576e-585e.

12. Zhu X, Zhu H, Zhang C, Zheng X. Pre-operative predictive factors for the survival of replanted digits. *Int Orthop.* 2017;41(8):1623-1626.

13. He JY, Chen SH, Tsai TM. The risk factors for failure of an upper extremity replantation: is the use of cigarettes/tobacco a significant factor? *PLoS One.* 2015;10(10):e0141451.

14. Maricevich M, Carlsen B, Mardini S, Moran S. Upper extremity and digital replantation. *Hand (N Y).* 2011;6(4):356-363.

15. Chang J, Jones N. Twelve simple maneuvers to optimize digital replantation and revascularization. *Tech Hand Up Extrem Surg.* 2004;8(3):161-166.

16. Kleinert HE, Jablon M, Tsai TM. An overview of replantation and results of 347 replants in 245 patients. *J Trauma.* 1980;20(5):390-398.

17. Hanel DP, Chin SH. Wrist level and proximal-upper extremity replantation. *Hand Clin.* 2007;23(1):13-21.

18. Sabapathy SR, Elliot D, Venkatramani H. Pushing the boundaries of salvage in mutilating upper limb injuries: techniques in difficult situations. *Hand Clin.* 2016;32(4):585-597.

19. Morrison WA, McCombe D. Digital replantation. *Hand Clin.* 2007;23(1):1-12.

20. Van Beek AL, Kutz JE, Zook EG. Importance of the ribbon sign, indicating unsuitability of the vessel, in replanting a finger. *Plast Reconstr Surg.* 1978;61(1):32-35.

21. Ross DC, Manktelow RT, Wells MT, Boyd JB. Tendon function after replantation: prognostic factors and strategies to enhance total active motion. *Ann Plast Surg.* 2003;51(2):141-146.

22. Cavadas PC, Landin L, Thione A. Secondary ectopic transfer for replantation salvage after severe wound infection. *Microsurgery.* 2011;31(4):288-292.

23. Godina M, Bajec J, Baraga A. Salvage of the mutilated upper extremity with temporary ectopic implantation of the undamaged part. *Plast Reconstr Surg.* 1986;78(3):295-299.

24. Higgins JP. Ectopic banking of amputated parts: a clinical review. *J Hand Surg.* 2011;36(11):1868-1876.

25. Buckley T, Hammert WC. Anticoagulation following digital replantation. *J Hand Surg.* 2011;36(8):1374-1376.

55 The Mangled Hand

Jason S. Lipof and John C. Elfar

INTRODUCTION

- The mangled extremity, by definition, exhibits injury to three or more of the four limb systems: (1) soft tissue, (2) nerves, (3) vessels, and (4) bone (Figure 55.1).
- It is marked by significant tissue damage and loss, these injuries are physically and psychologically devastating.
- Del Piñal's "acceptable hand" concept is defined as a hand with three fingers of near-normal length, near-normal proximal interphalangeal (PIP) joint motion, good sensibility, and a functional thumb. This may be helpful in determining a surgical plan for reconstruction.
- Due to modern advances in surgical reconstruction, limb salvage, nerve repair and transfer, internal fixation capabilities, soft-tissue handling and transfer, and microvascular reconstruction, injuries previously treated with amputation are now salvaged.
- The decision to attempt salvage of a mangled extremity is complex and involves the surgeon, patient, their support system, and resources available.
- Surgical salvage of a mangled limb is often time and resource consuming for the surgeon and patient, plagued by reoperations, complications, infection, pain, and morbidity.
- The ability to manage a mangled limb is often based on the state of the remaining tissues.
- Mechanism and severity of injury, the initial operative assessment and debridement, reconstruction, patient compliance, and their involvement in rehabilitation have a direct impact on outcome.

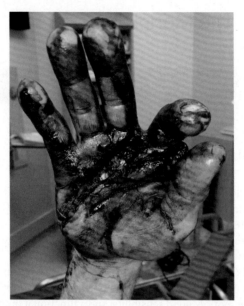

FIGURE 55.1 A 35-year-old male status-post table saw injury to his right palm. Despite soft-tissue attachments, all flexors, digital nerves, and digital arteries to the lesser four digits were severed. Emergent revascularization, nerve, and tendon repair were undertaken.

Mechanism

- Often caused by industrial or agricultural equipment, explosion, power tool injury, motor vehicle accidents, and high-velocity firearms.
- Higher energy → increased four-system tissue-type damage → decreased viability and vascularity of tissues → increased risk of infection and poor outcome.
- Typically, these injuries involve a significant crush component and may also exhibit degloving, avulsion, friction burn, abrasion, and partial amputation.
- Mangling injuries are often severely contaminated, especially those caused by farming and industrial equipment.
- For severely contaminated limbs, serial and extensive irrigation and debridement are necessary, as well as appropriate antibiotic selection.

Pathoanatomy and Pathophysiology

- Crush, explosion, and destruction of soft tissues cause endothelial injury, devascularization, and direct cell disruption. Resultant ischemia, depletion of oxygen, ATP, and glucose in turn cause increased CO_2 and lactic acid to accumulate. These increase superoxide free radicals and begin a cascade of chemotaxis causing local inflammation, increased endothelial injury, worsening microvascular flow, and eventually necrosis.

- Direct crush injury affects tissues differently. From most to least severe, tissues affected include skin > muscle > fat > vessels > nerve.
- Tendon, ligament, and bone are relatively crush resistant, depending on mechanism and force of crush.
- Reperfusion injury is caused by two mechanisms: (1) superoxide radicals interact with endothelial membranes, causing lipid peroxidation, increased permeability of endothelium, and edema. (2) Chemotaxis causes polymorphonuclear infiltration of tissues which causes microvascular occlusion, local tissue destruction, and necrosis. The latter mechanism is typically responsible for the characteristic "zone of injury" associated with these injuries.

EVALUATION

History

- Key questions include:
  - Is this an agricultural injury? Does it involve caustic substances? Is there significant contamination? Is the injury work-related?
  - This information may direct antibiotic choices, decision for acute versus delayed closure, and nature and extent of debridement.
- Timing of injury:
  - Important to discern warm or cold ischemia time for dysvascular tissue.
  - Increased time from injury to operation is associated with increased infection rate and poor outcome.
- Mechanism:
  - May help elucidate extent of energy imparted to soft tissues
  - Can define zone of injury
- Past medical history:
  - Important information includes: age, hand dominance, cardiac and vascular comorbidities, and diabetes.
  - Prior surgeries and injuries to affected extremity
  - Medication list and allergies

- Social history:
  - History of smoking, alcohol, substance use
  - Patient occupation
  - Support system/living situation
  - Ability to comply with postoperative rehabilitation

Physical Examination

- Due to the extensive and usually very painful nature of these injuries, it is often impossible to fully evaluate a mangled extremity in the emergency room, and injuries are most thoroughly assessed under anesthesia in the operating room.
- Emergency room evaluation:
  - It is important to obtain a brief examination to assess the four systems—soft tissue, nerves, vessels, and bone (Figure 55.1)
  - Gross assessment of vascular status
    - Capillary refill and dorsal paronychial refill are useful in determining gross vascularity.
    - If the patient is anesthetized, and vascularity is not obvious, 18-gauge needle stick may be useful to check for immediate return of bright red blood.
    - Doppler ultrasound of large vessels and of palmar arch may be useful.
  - Assessment of sensation
    - Assess two-point discrimination along the radial and ulnar aspects of each digit if nerve injury is suspected.
    - Assess sensation within the distribution of median (volar long finger), radial (1st dorsal web space), and ulnar (volar small finger) nerves.
    - Assess light touch versus pinprick
  - Assessment of gross motor and tendon function, if possible
    - Assess active flexion and extension of digits and at each joint.
    - Thumb extension can be tested to check for function of the posterior interosseous nerve, thumb flexion at the IP joint can be used to check for the anterior interosseous nerve, and finger abduction and adduction can check for the ulnar nerve. Depending on the nature of the injury, initial examination may be limited due to patient discomfort or distress.
    - In situations of possible tendon injury, checking tenodesis (passive tendon function through joint motion) may be helpful.

- Consideration should be given to concomitant compartment syndrome.
- Dress all wounds with saline-soaked gauze, grossly align the limb and digits and apply an appropriate splint for immobilization.

Imaging

- Radiographic studies
  - Plain radiographs are useful in the acute setting—anteroposterior, lateral, and oblique x-rays, as well as stress, traction, or special views are often needed. Some x-rays may be deferred until the patient is under anesthesia in the operating room, to minimize patient discomfort.
  - CT and MRI are rarely used in the acute setting.
  - If there is an avulsed or amputated part, obtain radiographs to discern foreign bodies and fractures.

Classification

- Attempts at classifying and predicting outcomes of mangled extremities have been largely unfruitful.
  - The Mangled Extremity Severity Score[1] utilized objective data to predict probability of amputation of lower extremity.
    - This score has not universally been adopted in upper extremity trauma.

ACUTE MANAGEMENT

- Initial presentation
  - Following typical advanced trauma life support (ATLS) protocol, control of hemorrhage may be obtained by using several techniques:
    - Direct pressure
    - Compressive dressing
    - Tie off hemorrhaging vessels under direct visualization
    - Tourniquet use, will worsen existing ischemia to distal tissues
  - Assess and manage life-threatening injuries.
  - Ensure adequate resuscitation per ATLS protocol.
  - ATLS secondary survey to rule out other injuries

- Administer antibiotics as soon as possible, with consideration of gentamicin or penicillin depending on extent of contamination.
- Administer tetanus vaccination/booster if not up-to-date or unknown.
- Emergent formal operative assessment, vascular repair, irrigation, and debridement.
  - Adequate initial debridement is of paramount importance to ultimate outcome.
  - Assess digital, radial, ulnar, brachial, and axillary artery flow.
  - Restoration of vascular supply, if necessary, with primary repair or temporary shunt should be attempted before time-consuming debridement and fixation.
  - Debridement is the vital step
    - Debridement of nonviable tissue decreases the risk of early and late infection. Attempts should be made to preserve viable tendon and nerve.
    - Debridement initially performed under tourniquet control, later released to assess for viable margins.
    - Remove of all foreign material (Figure 55.2).
    - Use tag sutures or vessel loops to identify key nerves and vessels.
    - Utilize nonpulsatile lavage and mechanical debridement using curettes, rongeurs as indicated.

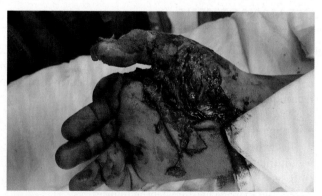

FIGURE 55.2 A 29-year-old female status-post all-terrain vehicle rollover with right hand crush and degloving injury, sustaining multiple comminuted metacarpal and phalanx fractures and neurologic injury with severe contamination.

- Assess need for antibiotic cement beads or vacuum-assisted closure device.
- Preserve bridging skin if viable.
- Assess need for early amputation
  - Unreconstructable osseous, soft-tissue, or skin defects and damage may be an indication for primary amputation.
  - Irreparable and severe vascular injury may indicate need for amputation.
  - Amputations should be performed at the most distal level possible.
  - Surgeons may save "spare parts" for reconstruction.
- Skeletal management
  - Stabilize sharp fracture fragments and restore bone length.
  - Restore articular congruency when joints are involved.
  - Minimize further periosteal stripping.
  - Utilize minimally invasive internal fixation and external fixation when appropriate.
  - Assess need for shortening osteotomy to obtain soft-tissue coverage.
- Soft-tissue management
  - Utilize soft-tissue friendly dissection techniques.
  - Assess flexor digitorum superficialis and profundus and repair if possible.
  - Assess need for delayed secondary procedures.
  - Reassess vascularity without tourniquets.
  - Perform formal repair or reconstruction of radial and ulnar arteries when possible.
  - Determine need for fasciotomy.
  - Identify injured nerves encountered during debridement.
  - Sharply remove crushed or frayed nerve ends and primarily repair severed nerves with appropriate sutures for repair (eg, epineurial, fascicular, etc.)
  - Shortening osteotomies and nerve graft or conduit may be used to assure the repair is not at risk of tension failure. Nerves should not be repaired with joints in flexed positions, and should be repaired without tension throughout a range of motion.
- Soft-tissue coverage
  - May be delayed until after serial debridements, once clean wound bed is attained (Figure 55.3)
  - Soft-tissue coverage is vital to protecting underlying repairs and reconstructions and decreases infection risk.

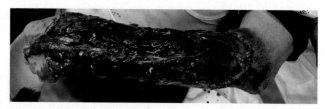

FIGURE 55.3 A 66-year-old female with severe left forearm crush and degloving injury after rollover motor vehicle collision with arm outside the vehicle. She underwent staged soft-tissue reconstruction after multiple debridements and skeletal stabilization.

- Maintain a moist environment with sterile saline-soaked sponges, vessel-loupe assisted closure, or negative pressure therapy (vacuum-assisted closure) until definitive soft-tissue closure.
- Provide vascularized tissue coverage over poorly vascularized structures including joints, tendons, and stripped bone.
- Utilize split-thickness skin grafts when appropriate.

POSTOPERATIVE CARE

- Most injuries benefit from well-molded and padded splints. Care should be taken to fashion splints to allow for any continued monitoring deemed necessary, including vascular checks.
- Position wrist in a neutral position with digits in intrinsic-plus (if grafts, repairs, and reconstructions allow).
- Begin an individualized, early passive motion therapy program to prevent contractures, scarring, loss of tendon excursion, and stiffness.
- Assess and document a physical examination regularly.
- Provide resources for psychological support and assess for psychiatric comorbidities after traumatic event.

SECONDARY RECONSTRUCTIVE PROCEDURES

- Reconstructive procedures may be considered after the limb has been appropriately managed in the acute setting.
- These procedures include:
  - Toe-to-hand transfer or pollicization of digit
  - Z-lengthening of contracted scars

- Vascularized bone grafts
- Nerve grafting
- Tendon grafting and tendon transfers
- Corrective osteotomies, restoration of articular congruency

MANAGEMENT ALGORITHM

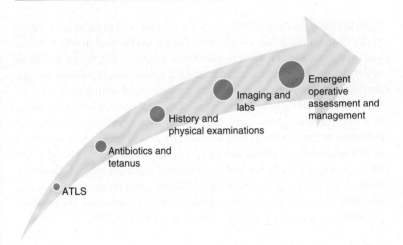

Emergent operative assessment and management

Imaging and labs

History and physical examinations

Antibiotics and tetanus

ATLS

REFERENCE

1. Helfet DL, Howey T, Sanders R, Johansen K. Limb salvage versus amputation: preliminary results of the mangled extremity severity score. *Clin Orthop Relat Res*. 1990;256:80-86.

SUGGESTED READINGS

Alphonsus CK. Principles in the management of a mangled hand. *Indian J Plast Surg*. 2011;44(2):219.

Bumbasirevic M, Stevanovic M, Lesic A, et al. Current management of the mangled upper extremity. *Int Orthop*. 2012;36(11):2189-2195.

del Piñal F. Severe mutilating injuries to the hand: guidelines for organizing the chaos. *J Plas Reconstr Aesthet Surg*. 2007;60(7):816-827.

Gupta A, Wolff TW. Management of the mangled hand and forearm. *J Am Acad Orthop Surg*. 1995;3(4):226-236.

Prasarn ML, Helfet DL, Kloen P. Management of the mangled extremity. *Strategies Trauma Limb Reconstr*. 2012;7(2):57-66.

Wolfe SW, Hotchkiss RN, Green DP. *Green's Operative Hand Surgery*. 6th ed. Philadelphia, PA: Elsevier Churchill Livingstone; 2011:chap 43.

56 High-Pressure Injection Injuries

Erez Avisar

High-pressure injection (HPI) injury has the potential to cause devastating injury to the limb. It has a high risk of being overlooked due to its often benign presentation. Failure to accurately diagnose this injury results in undertreatment and potentially devastating consequences. Patients usually present to the emergency room or to an outpatient setting soon after an injury occurs. Often, patients report an accidental or unexpected discharge of a high-pressure paint gun, after which they experienced a stinging sensation in the finger or hand followed by a disproportionate sensation of pain and swelling. Physicians can be misled by early objective physical findings, which may be limited to a minimal puncture wound. However, when recognized appropriately, early diagnosis and proper treatment can minimize the sequelae of injury including soft-tissue ischemia. The reported amputation rate of these injuries is between 30% and 48%.[1]

EPIDEMIOLOGY

It is estimated that annually 1 of 600 traumatic hand injuries involves an HPI injury.[1,2] Commonly, young manual workers sustain injury to the upper limb, usually to the tip of the index finger. The most common scenario occurs while the worker is using his nondominant hand for testing or cleaning the tip of a paint gun.

PATHOPHYSIOLOGY

The type of material injected (gas, liquid, plastic paint, grease, paraffin, fuel, paint thinner) and the pressure of the instrument used have a substantial influence on the soft-tissue damage and the injury zone. A pressure of 100 psi is the minimum needed to penetrate the skin. Oil-based paint and turpentine are associated with the worst outcomes, whereas latex paint is associated with more favorable outcomes.[3] The primary insult to the digit is related to the volume and pressure of the material injected. Subsequent to the mechanical damage, the material's inherent toxicity creates an inflammatory response that leads to edema and tissue ischemia. High-pressure air and water injections present with similar mechanisms of injury to material injections, but do not have the same inflammatory effect. Pain after these injuries is usually mild and disproportionate to the subcutaneous emphysema that rapidly spreads proximally. The prognosis is usually benign compared with material HPI injury from paint or oil.[4]

The initial management of an HPI injury includes urgent hand surgery consultation. The patient should be sent for a toxoid vaccine in the case of radiopaque material or gas HPI injury. Radiographs can help in the estimation of the zone of injury (Figure 56.1).

Nonsurgical treatment may be considered in cases of air and water HPI injury, but patients should be admitted for close observation, and water injection in particular should be closely monitored for compartment syndrome.

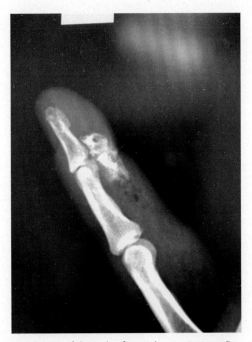

FIGURE 56.1 Lateral X ray of the index finger demonstrate radio-opaque injected material to soft tissue.

HPI injuries to the upper extremity are a true surgical emergency. Early surgical intervention includes open debridement through an extensive surgical exposure. Bruner incisions are typically used to access the entire flexor tendon sheath. Debridement should be done to minimize foreign material left in the tendon sheath or around the neurovascular bundles. It may be performed under regional or general anaesthesia. Delayed surgical intervention more than 6 hours after the HPI injury is associated with a high level of complications and amputation.[2,5-7] Surgeons should make every effort to irrigate and remove the injected material that usually adheres to the soft tissue, but it is often impossible to entirely remove all of the foreign substance (Figures 56.2 and 56.3).

Steroid administration is controversial. Hogan and Ruland reported that 8 of 15 patients who received steroid therapy eventually required amputation.[8] The surgical wound may be loosely closed over a drain when appropriate or may be packed and left open if repeat surgical debridement is deemed necessary.[7] Retained necrotic tissue can be a substrate for

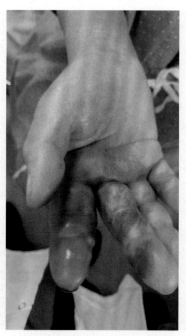

FIGURE 56.2 Delayed presentation of high-pressure injection injury—presented as infectious flexor tenosynovitis.

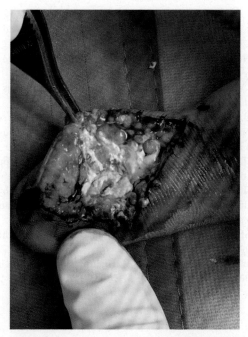

FIGURE 56.3 Finger incision demonstrates oil-based white paint in the soft tissue.

secondary infection, and therefore broad-spectrum antibiotic administration is indicated. The secondary infection rate in HPI injury varies between 1.6% and 60%[4,9-11] and when infection occurs it is usually found to be polymicrobial.

Once the initial injury has stabilized, early evaluation and treatment by a hand therapist is mandatory to maximize outcome. Therapy is designed to enhance tendon gliding and avoid adhesions and joint stiffness. Patients should be aware of the modest functional outcome following an HPI injury.

REFERENCES

1. Verhoeven N, Hierner R. High-pressure injection injury of the hand: an often underestimated trauma. Case report with study of the literature. *Strategies Trauma Limb Reconstr.* 2008;3(1):27-33.
2. Neal NC, Burke FD. High-pressure injection injuries. *Injury.* 1991;22(6):467-470.
3. Schoo MJ, Scott FA, Boswick JA Jr. High-pressure injection injuries of the hand. *J Trauma.* 1980;20(3):229-238.

4. Bekler H, Gokce A, Beyzadeoglu T, Parmaksizoglu F. The surgical treatment and outcomes of high-pressure injection injuries of the hand. *J Hand Surg Eur Vol*. 2007;32:394-399.

5. Stark HH, Ashworth CR, Boyes JH. Paint-gun injuries of the hand. *J Bone Joint Surg Am*. 1967;49(4):637-647.

6. Pai CH, Wei DC, Hou SP. High-pressure injection injuries of the hand. *J Trauma*. 1991;31(1):110-112.

7. Chaput B, Nouaille de Gorce H, et al. The role of a systematic second look at 48-72 hours in high pressure injection injuries to the hand: a retrospective study [in French]. *Chir Main*. 2012;31(5):250-255.

8. Hogan CJ, Ruland RT. High-pressure injection injuries to the upper extremity: a review of the literature. *J Orthop Trauma*. 2006;20:503-511.

9. Pinto MR, Turkula-Pinto LD, Cooney WP, Wood MB, Dobyns JH. High pressure injection injuries of the hand: review of 25 patients managed by open wound technique. *J Hand Surg Am*. 1993;18(1):125-130.

10. Schnall SB, Mirzayan R. High-pressure injection injuries to the hand. *Hand Clin*. 1999;15(2):245-248, viii.

11. Gelberman RH, Posch JL, Jurist JM. High-pressure injection injuries of the hand. *J Bone Joint Surg Am*. 1975;57(7):935-937.

57 Ring Avulsion Injuries

Evan H. Horowitz, Michael Guju, and
Francisco A. Schwartz-Fernandes

INTRODUCTION

- Definition
  - Acute trauma to a finger caused by a sudden force on a ring, leading to skin and soft tissue damage.[1]
  - Ring avulsion injuries vary in severity, ranging from bruising to traumatic amputation of the finger.[1]
  - Such injuries often occur to people who work with machinery while wearing a ring.[1]
- Incidence and risk factors
  - Incidence
    - Wearing a ring or wedding band accounts for 90% of finger avulsion cases that are treated in hospital departments and 13% to 15% of digit amputations per year.[2]
    - Average ratio of 300 cases per year for a population of 60 million in industrialized countries.[2]
  - Risk factors/epidemiology
    - Young men, average age 31 years at highest risk[2]
      - * Majority of patients of age 21 to 40 years, commonly working men[3]
    - Occupational hazards involving the use of hands to operate machinery and/or lift heavy objects

CLASSIFICATION OF AVULSION INJURIES

See Table 57.1
- Mechanism
  - Ring gets caught and anchored on a heavy, moving object such as a door, fence, or piece of heavy machinery. As the object continues to move, the ring may avulse the underlying tissues.

543

TABLE 57.1 The Urbaniak Classification of Avulsion Injuries and the Kay Classification With Adani Modifications[1,5,7,14]

Urbaniak Classification	
I	Avulsion injury with adequate circulation
II	Incomplete avulsion injury with inadequate circulation
III	Avulsion injury with complete degloving or amputation
Kay Classification as Modified by Adani	
I	Avulsion injury with adequate circulation
II	Incomplete avulsion injury with inadequate arterial or venous circulation, no skeletal injury
	IIa Arterial circulation inadequate only
	IIv Venous circulation inadequate only
III	Incomplete avulsion injury with inadequate arterial or venous circulation, fracture or joint injury present
	IIIa Arterial circulation inadequate only
	IIIv Venous circulation inadequate only
IV	Avulsion injury with complete degloving or amputation
	IVp Complete avulsion injury with amputation proximal to FDS insertion
	IVd Complete avulsion injury with amputation distal to FDS insertion

FDS, flexor digitorum superficialis.

- Biomechanics (Table 57.2)
  - The average maximum force resulting in class I injuries is 80 N.[4]
  - The average maximum force producing amputation in class III injuries was 154 N. Force measurements for class II injuries were nearly identical to those of class III.[4]

TABLE 57.2 Tensile Strengths of Rings Based on Their Type and Material, and the Common Classes of Injuries Associated With Different Rings[2]

Type of Ring	Material	Average Tensile Strength (N)	Type of Injuries
Open ring	Nickel-free alloy or silver	21-52.5	Class I injuries
Bejeweled, squared closed, or signet ring	Steel, resin Plexiglas, or Sumac wood	147-203	Class I-III Injuries (at up to 351 N, risk of severe impairment, or class III and IV, is limited to 14% of cases)
Closed, three-strand braided, or signet ring	Jade, aluminum, silver, gold-plate, or steel	624-999	Very high risk of class IV injuries

- Prognosis
  - The extent of artery, vein, and nerve involvement varies and can be used to classify these injuries and determine prognosis.[1,18]
  - Recent advancements in microsurgery,[5] such as revascularization and replantation, have improved prognosis and outcomes.[6]
  - Kay et al concluded that extent of skeletal injury is a significant prognostic factor and proposed a revision of the Urbaniak et al classification.[7]

IMAGING

- Radiographs should be taken of the injured digit and the amputated part[8] (Figure 57.1).

TREATMENT[9]

- Early[8]
  - Appropriate first aid
  - Analgesia
  - The amputated part is preserved appropriately and the wound is assessed. Amputated specimen should be retained and stored at cold temperature.
  - Admission for elevation, analgesia, intravenous antibiotics, and tetanus prophylaxis should be initiated.

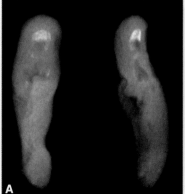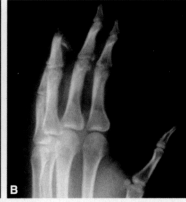

FIGURE 57.1 (A) AP (anterior-posterior) and lateral views, (B) oblique view.

- Surgical
  - Replantation
    - Indications[10]
      - * Amputation distal to the insertion of the flexor digitorum superficialis (FDS)
      - * Ring injuries type II and IIIa
      - * Amputations at the level of or distal to the proximal interphalangeal (PIP) joint (Proximal to the PIP joint in patients who are willing to accept a poor functional result)[19] (Figure 57.2)
    - Contraindication
      - * PIP joint avulsion and fracture of proximal phalanx[3,7,11-13]
      - * Amputation proximal to PIP joint and proximal to FDS insertion[11,14]

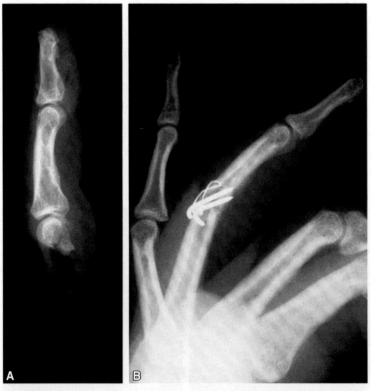

FIGURE 57.2 Avulsion injury just proximal to the proximal interphalangeal (PIP) joint (A) with successful arthrodesis of the PIP joint (B).

- Outcomes
  - Digit survival
    - Overall digit survival ~81%[3]
    - No significant statistical difference among class II, III, and IV injuries regarding digit survival and total arc of motion (TAM).[3]
    - Smoking has not been shown to affect survival rates.[3]
  - Sensibility
    - Primary neuronal repair leads to poor sensory recovery[15]
    - 66% of repaired nerves present with a two-point discrimination greater than 8 mm.[3]
    - 86% of digits examined at last follow-up evaluation may be free of pain.[3]
    - 60% of the patients who finally have their fingers amputated are free of pain at the last follow-up appointment, as opposed to 87% of those who have successful revascularization.[3]
  - Range of motion
    - Mean TAM of complete finger avulsions after successful replantation is 174°.[5]
    - The final TAM (including metacarpophalangeal [MCP] joint motion) of fingers that had MCP, proximal phalanx, and PIP joint injury was even superior to fingers that had more distal skeletal injuries. However, a high proportion of patients have arthrodesis of the distal interphalangeal joint (DIPJ) when the middle phalanx and DIPJ are affected. Therefore, level of bone injury is not always an accurate predictor of TAM outcomes.
- Amputation
  - Indications
    - PIP joint avulsion and fracture of the proximal phalanx[3]
    - Amputation proximal to PIP joint and proximal to FDS insertion[11,14]

SURGICAL TECHNIQUE

Replantation/Revascularization

- Approach
  - Ideal situation—two teams working simultaneously. One preparing the stump, one the amputated part. The goal is to be able to debride and tag all the structures to facilitate the surgery.
  - Both teams working under operating microscope midlateral approach to digit.

- May need extensive approach. It's an avulsion injury so the damage is likely to be proximal.
■ Technique
  - Bone
    ◆ If amputation occurs at DIPJ, perform primary arthrodesis of DIPJ (Figure 57.3).
    ◆ Fixation with K-wires, cerclage, or combined. Microplates can also be used.
  - Arteries
    ◆ Thorough debridement of nonviable tissue
    ◆ Thorough arterial debridement (inadequate debridement leads to failure)
    ◆ Repair using vein grafts because of significant vascular damage
    ◆ May need another step-down vein graft because of difficulty in arterial size matching (small artery, large vein graft)
    ◆ May reroute arterial pedicle from adjacent digit
      ✳ Disadvantage is this sacrifices major artery from adjacent digit.
  - Veins
    ◆ Repair at least two veins
    ◆ Can use flow-through grafts
    ◆ Important factor in revascularization failure

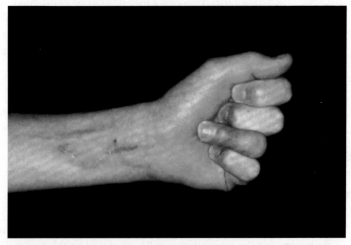

FIGURE 57.3 Arthrodesis of the distal interphalangeal joint (DIPJ)—a common surgical treatment when avulsion is at the DIPJ or distal middle phalanx.

- Nerves
  - ◆ Thorough debridement of nonviable tissue
  - ◆ Repair using nerve grafts or nerve tube (vein, collagen, etc.). Gaps up to 2.0 cm can be repaired with vein tubes. Any defect bigger than that requires nerve grafting.
  - ◆ Repair without tension.
  - ◆ Sources—posterior interosseous nerve, medial antibrachial cutaneous nerve, cadaver (Axogen).
- Skin
  - ◆ Split-thickness skin graft, free venous flaps, and reversed vascularized cross-finger flaps.
  - ◆ The arterialized venous flow-through flap is a reliable solution for the complex ring avulsion injury that requires simultaneous soft tissue and digital vessel reconstruction[16] (Figure 57.4).
  - ◆ Full-thickness skin grafts to prevent tight closure or may utilize commercially available synthetic acellular dermal matrix.

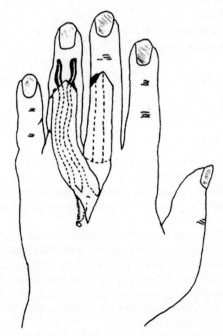

FIGURE 57.4 Arterialized venous flow-through flap.

- Surgical complications
  - In unsuccessful cases thrombosis usually occurs in the *first 3 days* (71%).[3] The mechanism of injury does not influence the timing of thrombosis.[17]
  - Artery and vein thromboses are implicated equally as the cause of failure.[3]

COMPLICATIONS

- Complications after successful revascularization include
  - Pain
  - Hypersensitivity
  - Flexion contracture
  - Cold intolerance
  - Malunion
  - Boutonniere deformity
  - Fungal infection
  - Nonunion
  - Osteomyelitis
  - PIP joint arthritis
- Complications after amputation
  - Pain
  - Hypersensitivity
  - Neuroma
  - Quadriga syndrome

REFERENCES

1. Kay S, Werntz J, Wolff TW. Ring avulsion injuries: classification and prognosis. *J Hand Surg.* 1989;14A:204-213.
2. Institut National de la Consommation. Consumer safety commission. Paris. December 2005. http://www.securiteconso.org/rings-and-wedding-bands/. Accessed February 13, 2017.
3. Sanmartin M, Fernandes F, Lajoie AS, Gupta A. Analysis of prognostic factors in ring avulsion injuries. *J Hand Surg Am.* 2004;29(6):1028-1037.
4. Kupfer DM, Eaton C, Swanson S, McCarter MK, Lee GW. Ring avulsion injuries: a biomechanical study. *J Hand Surg Am.* 1999;24(6):1249-1253.
5. Sears ED, Chung KC. Replantation of finger avulsion injuries: a systematic review of survival and functional outcomes. *J Hand Surg Am.* 2011;36(4):686-694. doi:10.1016/j.jhsa.2010.12.023.
6. Brooks D, Buntic RF, Kind GM, Schott K, Buncke GM, Buncke HJ. Ring avulsion: injury pattern, treatment, and outcome. *Clin Plast Surg.* 2007;34:187-195.

7. Urbaniak JR, Evans JP, Bright DS. Microvascular management of ring avulsion injuries. *J Hand Surg.* 1981;6:25-30.

8. Jones M, Gujral S. Ring avulsion injuries. *Eplasty.* 2016;16:ic5. Also available at www.ePlasty.com.

9. Rawles RB, Deal DN. Treatment of the complete ring avulsion injury. *J Hand Surg.* 2013;38(9):1800-1802. doi:10.1016/j.jhsa.2013.06.002.

10. Soucacos PN, Beris AE, Touliatos AS, Vekris M, Pakos S, Varitimidis S. Current indications for single digit replantation. *Acta Orthop Scand Suppl.* 1995;264:12-15. doi:10.3109/17453679509157157.

11. Beris AE, Soucacos PN, Malizos KN, Xenakis TA. Microsurgical treatment of ring avulsion injuries. *Microsurgery.* 1994;15:459-463.

12. Foucher G. Technique of ring injuries replantation. *Plast Reconstr Surg.* 1988;81:996-997.

13. Tsai T-M, Manstein C, DuBou R, Wolff TW, Kutz JE, Kleinert HE. Primary microsurgical repair of ring avulsion amputation injuries. *J Hand Surg.* 1984;9A:68-72.

14. Adani R, Castagnetti C, Busa R, Caroli A. Ring avulsion injuries: microsurgical management. *J Reconstr Microsurg.* 1996;12:189-194.

15. Mafi P, Hindocha S, Dhital M, Saleh M. Advances of peripheral nerve repair techniques to improve hand function: a systematic review of literature. *Open Orthop J.* 2012;6:60-68. doi:10.2174/1874325001206010060.

16. Brooks D, Buntic RF, Taylor C. Use of the venous flap for salvage of difficult ring avulsion injuries. *Microsurgery.* 2008;28(6):397-402. doi:10.1002/micr.20527.

17. Betancourt FM, Mah ET, McCabe SJ. Timing of critical thrombosis after replantation surgery of the digits. *J Reconstr Microsurg.* 1998;14:313-316.

18. Waikakul S, Sakkarnkosol S, Vanadurongwan V, Unnanuntana A. Results of 1018 digital replantations in 552 patients. *Injury.* 2000;31:33-40.

19. Fujioka M, Hayashida K. Proximal interphalangeal replantation with arthrodesis facilitates favorable esthetics and functional outcome. *J Trauma Manag Outcomes.* 2015;9:7. doi:10.1186/s13032-015-0028-z.

58 Upper Extremity Gunshot Wounds

Alex C. Lesiak and John R. Fowler

INTRODUCTION

- Mechanism of injury
  - Penetration of the upper extremity by a bullet or other missile projected by a firearm
- Pathoanatomy
  - Small entrance wound and larger exit wound
  - Tissue damage occurs due to the passage of the bullet/missile through the tissue, a secondary shock wave, and the cavitation created by the missile.
  - The injury can cause blood vessel, bone, muscle, and other soft-tissue damage.
  - Extent of injury is determined by the type of firearm, projectile velocity, and projectile mass.
- Epidemiology
  - 33 599 deaths from firearms in 2014 (63.5% from suicide and 32.6% from homicide)
  - 11 101 firearm-related homicides in 2011
  - 70% to 80% of firearm homicides and 90% of nonfatal firearm victimizations were committed with a handgun from 1993 to 2011.

EVALUATION

- History
  - Type of firearm when known
  - Timing of injury
  - Injuries to other extremities or organ systems
  - Associated symptoms
    - Pain
    - Numbness and/or tingling

- Physical examination
  - Inspection—identify entrance and exit wounds
  - Assess for wound contamination (clothing, or other debris that may have entered the wound)
  - Detailed neurovascular examination
    - If concern for vascular injury: perform an Allen test and consider use of a doppler machine to evaluate vasculature
  - Evaluate bony stability to assess for fracture/dislocation
- Diagnostic data
  - Radiographs of the involved area as well as the joint above and below zone of injury
  - CT scan or saline injection challenge can assist in determining intra-articular involvement if suspected
  - Vascular injury suspected
    - Doppler ultrasonography
    - Arteriography—CTA versus intraoperative angiogram depending on situation and injury
  - EMG/nerve conduction velocity cannot distinguish between neuropraxia and transection in the early postinjury period
- Classification
  - Low velocity (<2 000 ft/s)
  - High velocity (>2 000 ft/s)
  - Shotgun (Type 0 to Type III)
    - 0: >20 yards away and causes very minimal damage
    - I: >7 yards and often does not produce major soft-tissue injury due to pellet scatter
    - II: <3 to 7 yards
    - III: <3 yards
      * Types II and III associated with high rates of associated injury
        ▲ 32% to 48% comminuted fractures
        ▲ 43% to 59% major soft-tissue disruption
        ▲ 23% to 45% vascular injury
        ▲ 21% to 58% peripheral nerve damage

ACUTE MANAGEMENT

- Initial trauma evaluation: check airway, breathing, and ciculation (ABCs)
- Thorough history and physical examination
- Tetanus prophylaxis (Table 58.1)

TABLE 58.1 Tetanus Prophylaxis Recommendations for Gunshot Wound Patients

Number of Previous Tetanus Vaccinations	Give Td	Give TIG
Uncertain	Yes	Yes
Less than 3	Yes	Yes
3 or more	No	No
Adults and children 7 years of age or older: Td preferred to tetanus toxoid alone.		
Children less than 7 years of age: diphtheria, tetanus, pertussis (DTP; DT, if pertussis vaccine is contraindicated) is preferred to tetanus toxoid alone.		
If only three doses of fluid toxoid have been received: give a fourth dose of toxoid, preferably an adsorbed toxoid.		
If greater than 5 years since last dose: give a booster.		
Abbreviations: Td, adult-type tetanus and diphtheria toxoid; TIG, tetanus immune globulin.		

Adapted from Centers for Disease Control and Prevention. Diptheria, tetanus, and pertussis: recommendations for vaccine use and other preventive measures: recommendations of the Immunization Practices Advisory Committee (ACIP). *MMWR Morb Mortal Wkly Rep.* 1991;40(RR-10):1-28.

- May consider initial dose of antibiotics (1 g cefazolin)
- Initial debridement
  - Cleanse wounds with povidone/normal saline and debride in emergency department (E.D).
  - Apply sterile dressing
  - Splint/cast

DEFINITIVE TREATMENT (DICTATED BY ENERGY/ WOUND CONTAMINATION/JOINT INVOLVEMENT/ FRACTURE STYLE)

- Nonoperative treatment
  - Low energy, uncontaminated, and no evidence of neurovascular injury
    - ◆ Acute management as earlier
    - ◆ ± antibiotics: Cephalexin 500 mg QID × 5–7 days
    - ◆ Closure by secondary intention
    - ◆ If bony injury sustained that does not require surgical stabilization, it should be treated like a closed injury and reduced/splinted/ casted when appropriate
    - ◆ Neuropraxic injury is common, and nerve dysfunction may be monitored without early intervention unless there is a strong suspicion of transection.

- Surgical indications
  - High energy
  - Severe soft-tissue damage
  - Vascular injury
  - Gross contamination
  - Compartment syndrome
  - Unstable fracture
  - Tendon injuries
- Contraindications
  - Hemodynamic instability
- Surgical approach
  - Operative technique
    - Wound
      - Aggressive irrigation and debridement
        - Excise margin of entrance and exit wound
        - Enlarge incision
        - Excise any and all devitalized/necrotic tissue
          - Skin
          - Subcutaneous tissue/fat
          - Muscle
          - Bone
      - Fasciotomy if required
      - Avoid primary closure if contamination is a concern
      - Hand wounds may be primarily closed
    - Vascular injury
      - Transect and debride vessel ends
        - Extremity perfused: tie off vessel
        - Extremity not perfused
          - Primary repair
          - Reversed autogenous saphenous vein graft
    - Joint involvement
      - Arthrotomy and fragment removal if bullet fragment in joint
      - No need for routine arthrotomy if no fragments are retained
    - Fracture care
      - Fracture pattern dictates fracture care
        - Consider temporary stabilization/external fixator in con-taminated, high-energy wounds.
        - Definitive fracture care can be performed at initial debride-ment if contamination is not an issue.
    - Peripheral nerve injury
      - Complete

▲ If wound exploration performed:
  ◈ Consider primary repair and/or grafting.
▲ If facilities not capable of neural repair/grafting:
  ◈ Clean, tag, and cover neural injury with soft tissue.
  ◈ Do not debride neural structures.
* Incomplete/lesion-in-continuity
  ▲ Consider delayed exploration to allow for resolution of any neurapraxia.
    ◈ Radial nerve injury associated with a gunshot wound (GSW) and a humeral shaft fracture can be treated nonoperatively
      O Electrodiagnostic studies at 6 weeks and again at 3 months and if no return function identified:
        ◇ Can wait ~6 months postinjury for neuropraxia resolution
■ Potential complications
  ● Infection
  ● Loss of function
  ● Stiffness
  ● Amputation
■ Postoperative care
  ● Wound care
  ● Early mobilization
  ● Hand therapy

SUGGESTED READINGS

Bartlett CS, Helfet DL, Hausman MR, Strauss E. Ballistics and gunshot wounds: effects on musculoskeletal tissues. *J Am Acad Orthop Surg.* 2000;8(1):21-36.

Planty M, Truman JL, Bureau of Justice Statistics. *Firearm Violence, 1993-2011.* Special tabulation from the Bureau of Justice Statistics, National Crime Victimization Survey; 2013. NCJ 241730.

Kline DG. Timing for exploration of nerve lesions and evaluation of the neuroma-in-continuity. *Clin Orthop.* 1982;163:42-49.

Kline DG, Hackett ER, Happel LH. Surgery for lesions of the brachial plexus. *Arch Neurol.* 1986;43:170-181.

Deitch EA, Grimes WR. Experience with 112 shotgun wounds of the extremities. *J Trauma.* 1984;24:600-603.

Omer GE Jr. Injuries to nerves of the upper extremity. *J Bone Joint Surg Am.* 1974;56:1615-1624.

Magalon G, Bordeaux J, Legre R, Aubert JP. Emergency versus delayed repair of severe brachial plexus injuries. *Clin Orthop.* 1988;237:32-35.

Nichols JS, Lillehei KO. Nerve injury associated with acute vascular trauma. *Surg Clin North Am.* 1988;68:837-852.

59 Burns

Ryan M. Garcia and Michael S. Gart

INTRODUCTION

- Demographics
  - 1 200 000 burn cases in the United States per year
  - Increased survival secondary to critical care measures has led to an increased need for reconstruction.
- Criteria for patient transfer to a burn center based on guidelines from the American Burn Association
  - Any burn to the hands, feet, genitalia, perineum
  - Chemical or electric burns
  - Third-degree burns or second-degree burns of >10% total body surface area (TBSA)
  - Burns associated with additional trauma or associated medical comorbidities
  - Burns in children
- Burn histology (moving from central area to the periphery)
  - Zone of coagulation—tissue necrosis, nonviable, requires excision and grafting
  - Zone of stasis—surrounds the zone of coagulation, viable, requires aggressive resuscitation to avoid transitioning to tissue necrosis
  - Zone of hyperemia—peripheral most zone, viable, preserved with resuscitation

EVALUATION

- History
  - Timing of injury
  - Type of burn (chemical, electrical, flame, contact, etc.)

- Physical examination
  - Airway assessment
  - TBSA burned
  - Depth of burn
  - Evaluate for compartment syndrome and for circumferential eschars that diminish limb perfusion
    - Consideration of deep compartment syndrome in electrical burn patients given the pathway of injury
- Imaging
  - None indicated unless concomitant injuries are present
- Classification of burns
  - Based on depth of penetration (superficial to deep penetration)
    - First degree
      - Epidermis only—behaves like a sunburn
      - Erythema, digital pressure leads to blanching, no blisters
    - Second degree (subclassified into superficial and deep)
      - Superficial
        - ▲ Papillary dermis involved
        - ▲ Skin appendages (ie, hair follicles) spared, blistering, sensate
      - Deep
        - ▲ Reticular dermis involved
        - ▲ White in color without capillary refill, blistering, diminished sensation
    - Third degree
      - Entire dermis involved
        - ▲ Insensate, black to brown in color, no blistering

ACUTE MANAGEMENT

- Initial evaluation and management
  - Advanced trauma life support protocol
  - Airway management
    - Inhalation injury requires intubation and intensive care management
      - Carbonaceous material in the oral or nasal airway
      - Arterial blood gas/elevated carboxyhemoglobin
      - Diagnosis confirmed with bronchoscopy
  - Compartment syndrome
    - Tense/firm compartments
    - 5 "P"s evaluation (**P**ain with stretch and palpation, **P**allor, **P**aresthesia, **P**ulselessness, **P**oikilothermic)

- Clinical examination versus pressure monitoring
  - Difference of 30 mm Hg or less between compartment and diastolic blood pressure suggestive of compartment syndrome
- Chemical burn antidotes
  - Hydrofluoric acid—treat with topical or injection of calcium gluconate
  - Phenol—irrigate with polyethylene glycol
  - Phosphorus—treat with copper
- Electrical injuries
  - Cardiac monitoring/EKG
  - Check creatinine kinase and renal function
  - IV fluid hydration

- Resuscitation
  - Parkland formula
    - TBSA calculated by the "rule of 9's"
      - Head/neck—9%, arm—9% each, anterior and posterior torso—18% each, leg—18% each
    - 4 mL/kg × %TBSA burned × kg = total fluid administered in first 24 hours after injury
      - 50% given within first 8 hours from time of burn injury (not time of presentation)
      - 50% given over next 16 hours
  - Urine output goal—0.5 to 1.0 mL/kg/h
- Antibiotics
  - No role for empiric IV or oral antibiotics
  - Topical antibiotics
    - Silver sulfadiazine—gram (+) and (−) coverage
      - Caution—leukopenia
    - Sulfamylon—gram (+) coverage
      - Caution—metabolic acidosis (carbonic anhydrase inhibition)
    - Silver nitrate—*Staphylococcus* and *Pseudomonas* coverage
      - Caution—hyponatremia

DEFINITIVE MANAGEMENT

- Treatments based on classification
  - First-degree burn—soothing lotions (ie, aloe), typically heals without other intervention
  - Second-degree burn (superficial)—apply silver sulfadiazine, Vaseline-impregnated gauze, typically heals without surgery

- Second-degree burn (deep)—apply silver sulfadiazine, portions may require surgical excision and grafting
- Third-degree burn—apply silver sulfadiazine during period of resuscitation, early excision, and grafting
- Surgical treatments
  - Escharotomies/fasciotomies
    - Performed in the emergent setting
    - Relief of advancing soft tissue compression and pressures
  - Surgical excision and grafting
    - Only performed in a stable, resuscitated patient
    - For questionable areas in the zone of stasis or second-degree (deep) burns—allow the burn to completely demarcate prior to excision and grafting
      - Goal is to get wounds closed with skin graft by 3 weeks
        - Reduces incidence of hypertrophic scarring
    - Tangential excision
      - Use of a Watson or Weck/Goulian knife or the Versajet hydro dissector
      - Layered excisions continue until bleeding tissue is visualized
      - Expect high blood losses and the need for transfusion therapy
    - Grafting
      - Typically autografting for the hand and upper extremity
      - Full thickness
        - Increased primary contracture, decreased late contracture
      - Split-thickness
        - Decreased primary contracture, increased late contracture
        - Sheet grafts (without meshing) are typically used on the hand and upper extremity
          - Superior function and cosmetic results
        - Meshing (from ratios of 1:1 to 1:4)
          - Decreases hematoma, seroma formation, and graft loss
          - Increases the surface area coverage
          - Greater ratios create increased scars and contractures
      - Dermal regeneration
        - Integra (Integra Life Sciences Co, Plainsboro, New Jersey)—off-the-shelf dermal regeneration product

▲ Bilayer construct
  ◆ Dermal layer allows for fibroblast and endothelial ingrowth along with angiogenesis
    ○ Requires a noninfected, viable, and vascularized wound bed
  ◆ Silicone/silastic layer acts as a protective barrier against infection and evaporation
- Complications
  ◆ Graft loss (hematoma, seroma, shear, infection)
  ◆ Wound breakdown
  ◆ Wound contracture
- Postoperative care
  ◆ Application of hydrant/moisturizer to the graft for 3 to 4 weeks
  ◆ Occupational therapy for stretching
  ◆ Upper extremity splinting—avoidance of contracture development
    ∗ Elbow—Extension, wrist—extension, hand—intrinsic plus position
  ◆ Scar treatments
    ∗ Silicone sheeting, massage, laser therapy, contracture releases

SUGGESTED READINGS

Cope O, Langohr JL, Moore FD, et al. Expeditious care of full-thickness burn wounds by surgical excision and grafting. *Ann Surg.* 1947;125:1-22.

Dantzer E, Queruel P, Salinier L, et al. Dermal regeneration template for deep hand burns: clinical utility for both early grafting and reconstructive surgery. *Br J Plast Surg.* 2003;56:764-774.

Herndon DN, Barrow RE, Rutan RL, et al. A comparison of conservative versus early excision: therapies in severely burned patients. *Ann Surg.* 1989;209:547-552.

Herndon D. ed. *Total Burn Care.* 2nd ed. London, England: WB Saunders; 2002.

Ryan CM, Shoenfeld DA, Thorpe WP, et al. Objective measurements of the probability of death from burn injuries. *N Engl J Med.* 1998;338:362-366.

CHAPTER

60   Frostbite

Michael S. Gart

INTRODUCTION

- Frostbite is an injury that occurs in tissues exposed to extreme cold temperatures, often as a result of inadequate protection from the environment.
  - The severity of the injury is related to several host and environmental factors, including but not limited to: ambient temperature, wind speeds (commonly referred to as "wind chill"), altitude, duration of exposure, amount of moisture on tissues, patient's underlying vascular status, and the conditions of tissue rewarming.
- Historically, frostbite injuries were associated with military campaigns; however, increasing participation in winter sports and socioeconomic factors have caused a dramatic increase in the incidence of civilian frostbite injuries over the last 30 years.

Mechanism of Injury

- Frostbite occurs when tissues are subjected to temperatures low enough to form intracellular ice crystals, typically $-2°C$ and below.
- Tissues with "terminal" blood supply that contain little fat and are difficult to shield from the cold (fingers, toes, ears, nose) are the most susceptible to frostbite injury.
- More recently, it was recognized that tissue injury occurs not only during freezing, but also during (and often as a result of) rewarming.
- Tissue damage from frostbite can be described as direct cellular injury and progressive tissue ischemia.
- Direct cellular injury—formation of both intracellular and extracellular ice crystals, leading to osmotic imbalances and resulting cellular de-hydration, electrolyte imbalances, enzyme denaturation, and ultimate cell death.
  - Ice crystal formation in the intracellular space can directly damage cell membranes leading to cell lysis.

- Progressive tissue ischemia occurs secondary to vasoconstriction, shunting of blood away from the extremities, blood flow stasis, and thrombosis.
  - Initial exposure to cold temperatures results in vasospasm, which is followed shortly (in many, but not all individuals) by the "hunting response," cycles of vasodilation and vasoconstriction aimed at restoring extremity blood flow.
    - However, this response also returns cooled blood from the extremities and results in decreased core body temperature.
  - As exposure continues, the core temperature will drop sufficiently that the body will begin shunting blood away from the extremities to preserve life over limb.
  - Progressive decreases in temperature cause ice crystal formation in the plasma, leading to increased blood viscosity and diminished blood flow, ultimately resulting in thrombosis and microcirculatory failure.
- Tissue damage also occurs during rewarming because the freezing process is reversed.
  - Endothelial cells become highly permeable, leading to edema and blistering.
  - Reperfusion injury leads to oxygen free radial formation and initiation of the arachidonic acid cascade.
    - Proinflammatory mediators have been found in similar levels in blister fluid from burns and frostbite.

Epidemiology

- Increased participation in winter sports such as skiing and mountain climbing, as well as a vulnerable homeless population has caused a dramatic rise in the incidence of frostbite injuries in civilian populations over the last few decades.
  - Homelessness in urban environments that have harsh winters (ie, Chicago) is a leading cause of frostbite injuries in these areas.
- Laborers whose work requires prolonged periods in freezing temperatures are also at risk for frostbite.
- In part because such manual laborers are more commonly working-age males, frostbite occurs more commonly in men (10:1 M:F), with a peak incidence between ages 30 and 50 years.
- Both patient and environmental factors can affect the severity of frostbite injury.
- Patient factors—alcohol abuse/intoxication, psychiatric illness, smoking, peripheral vascular disease, history of frostbite injury, and overall health and functional status.

- Alcohol abuse and/or psychiatric illness can predispose to prolonged exposures and/or inadequate protection.
  - The incidence of alcoholism in patients admitted for frostbite is more than twice that of those admitted for other diagnoses.
- Peripheral vascular disease limits blood flow to the extremities and compounds the risk of smoking when present in combination.
  - Vasospastic disorders (Raynaud disease, scleroderma) may also potentiate the effects of cold exposure.
- A history of even one cold-related injury leaves that area at increased risk for reinjury with additional exposures.
- Chronically ill or malnourished patients have impaired thermoregulation at baseline and are more susceptible to frostbite injuries.
- Ethnicity and acclimation to cold climates may also play a role.
  - Individuals of African descent appear to be more susceptible to cold-induced injury than Caucasians, possibly due to differences in cold-induced vasodilation.
  - Whether or not populations indigenous to arctic climates are able to accommodate to extreme cold temperatures is controversial.
- Environmental factors—ambient temperature, wind speeds (commonly referred to as "wind chill"), altitude >17 000 ft, and duration of exposure.
  - Tissue freezing occurs more rapidly when tissues are in contact with a conducting surface (ie, water or metal) due to more rapid heat loss from the body.

EVALUATION

History

- When possible, the presence or absence of patient/environmental factors outlined earlier should be determined.
  - Ideally, the patient's medical history and the conditions of the exposure (time exposed, protective gear, temperatures) should be obtained.
  - Intoxication, psychiatric illness, or associated hypothermia/altered mental status will limit the amount of history provided.

Physical Examination (Figure 60.1)

- In addition to the affected part(s), the physical examination of the patient will focus on identifying any associated hypothermia and electrolyte or acid–base derangements that can be life threatening.

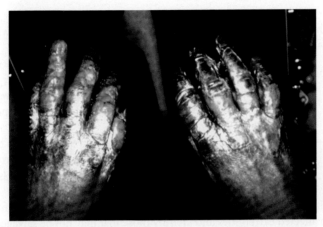

FIGURE 60.1 Acute presentation of frostbite injury to right hand. Note the hemorrhagic blisters distally and mottled appearance of the digits, consistent with deep frostbite injury. (Photo courtesy of Gregory A. Dumanian.)

- Vital signs and laboratory tests (complete blood count, chemistry panel) should be obtained in all patients, with more focused testing on a case-by-case basis.
- Focused physical examination should identify any areas affected by superficial or deep frostbite injury and a neurovascular evaluation of each area.
  - Patient may complain that an affected part feels cold, numb, or "clumsy."
  - Appearance can range from yellowish discoloration to blue and mottled, with obvious freezing of tissues.
  - Blisters are often, but not always, present.
  - Clear or cloudy fluid-filled blisters with deformable soft tissue likely represent a more superficial injury with better prognosis; hemorrhagic blisters and stiff tissues are more likely to represent a deeper injury with poorer prognosis.
- Initial clinical examination is often unreliable in determining the ultimate level of tissue loss.

Imaging

- Photographs of the initial presentation may be useful in following the progression of tissue damage over time.
- Recently, advanced imaging modalities have been employed to determine the eventual level of tissue loss in an effort to expedite treatment of frostbite injuries.

- Triple-phase bone scans have been shown to reliably predict the likelihood and level of eventual amputation in a frostbite injury within 2 to 3 days of rewarming.
  - The time from rewarming appears to affect the positive predictive value (PPV) of bone scans, with more time elapsed leading to a higher PPV.
  - Many centers are now routinely using bone scans soon after rewarming to determine if patients are candidates for additional therapeutic measures for limb salvage.
  - Single-photon emission computed tomography scans utilize a combination of bone scan and computed tomography scan to provide better anatomic detail to a conventional bone scan and may also be useful in determining which tissues are nonviable.
- Magnetic resonance angiography (MRA) is also able to evaluate perfusion to affected extremities and identify those that may not be salvageable.
  - MRA has the advantage of directly visualizing vessels to clearly determine areas lacking blood flow and may more clearly delineate viable from nonviable tissue.

Classification

- Historically, cold injuries have been classified in a "degree" system, similar to burn injuries:
  - First degree (partial thickness skin)—edema, erythema, hyperemia, no blistering, or tissue loss
  - Second degree (full thickness skin)—erythema, clear or cloudy blister formation, and superficial skin slough
  - Third degree (full thickness skin, superficial subcutaneous tissues)—edema with gray-blue discoloration, full thickness skin loss with exposed subcutaneous tissues
  - Fourth degree (full thickness skin and subcutaneous tissues)—deep blue discoloration, no edema or blistering, necrosis of skin and subcutaneous tissues to the level of muscle, tendon, or bone
- A simplified and more useful system has largely replaced the "degree" system, classifying frostbite injuries as superficial or deep, which appears to be more useful for predicting outcomes.
  - Superficial frostbite presents with erythema, numbness, blisters filled with clear or cloudy fluid.
    - The tissue bed is characteristically supple and painful once rewarming has occurred.
    - This roughly corresponds to first- and second-degree frostbite.

- ◆ Superficial frostbite results in minimal or no tissue loss.
- Deep frostbite presents as a blue extremity with hemorrhagic blisters, indicating extension through the full thickness of the dermis, with cold, insensate, stiff "woody" tissues.
  - ◆ After thawing, seep injuries tend to remain insensate from nerve damage.
  - ◆ This roughly corresponds to third- and fourth-degree frostbite.
  - ◆ Deep frostbite results in severe tissue loss.

ACUTE MANAGEMENT

- ■ Life-threatening conditions that may accompany frostbite (ie, hypothermia and severe acid–base or electrolyte disturbances) require immediate treatment.
  - Hypothermia must be treated before addressing the frostbitten extremity.
    - ◆ If a frozen extremity is rewarmed before core body temperature reaches 95°F, core temperature may drop rapidly as cooled blood from the extremity is returned to the circulation.
      - ✳ This is known as "afterdrop."
  - Acid–base status and electrolyte levels must be corrected before rewarming and monitored during rewarming.
    - ◆ If the blood returning from an affected extremity is acidotic and hyperkalemic, arrhythmias and hypotension can occur.
      - ✳ This is known as "rewarming shock."
- ■ Cardiac monitoring should be used during rewarming.
- ■ Restoring core body temperature is achieved with a combination of warm intravenous fluids, warm gastric lavage, warm rectal irrigation, or total body immersion in warm water.
  - In very extreme cases, extracorporeal membrane oxygenation may be necessary.
- ■ Acute management of the frostbite injury should focus on limiting progression of tissue injury by avoiding additional cold exposure and rewarming tissues.
  - Rewarming of the affected extremity should not begin until the patient can be maintained in a warm environment.
    - ◆ Repeated freeze–thaw cycles lead to significantly greater tissue damage.

- Rewarming is performed rapidly, with immersion in a water bath between 104°F and 107.6°F (40°C and 42°C).
  - Lower temperatures will reduce tissue survival, where higher temperatures may cause thermal injury.
- Rewarming is successful if the tissue becomes pliable and assumes a reddish-purple coloration within 15 to 30 minutes.
  - Tissue that remains "woody," dark, and anesthetic is unlikely to recover.
- Following rewarming, patients must be observed for development of compartment syndrome and treated with immediate fasciotomy or escharotomy should one develop.
- Clear or cloudy blisters should be debrided to remove the blister fluid, which is high in proinflammatory and procoagulant factors.
- Aside from debridement of blisters or infected necrotic tissues, acute surgical intervention is rarely required in the treatment of frostbite injuries.

DEFINITIVE TREATMENT

Nonoperative Treatment

- The effect of proinflammatory mediators should be minimized following rewarming.
- Topical aloe vera has been shown to be efficacious in inhibiting thromboxane.
  - Oral or intravenous nonsteroidal anti-inflammatory drugs are administered for several days.
- Tetanus prophylaxis and antibiotic coverage are typically administered.
- Adequate analgesia is important in recovery to allow patients to tolerate any dressing changes and/or therapy that may be required.
- Tissue plasminogen activator (tPA) has been shown to reduce the need for digital amputations if given within the first 24 hours after cold exposure.
  - However, many patients presenting with frostbite injuries have contraindications to tPA treatment.
    - Notably alcoholics, because of the risk for concomitant head injury and variceal bleeding
    - May not be effective in patients with repeated freeze–thaw cycles or warm ischemia times >6 hours
- Hyperbaric oxygen therapy has been anecdotally reported to be effective, but there is no evidence supporting its use.

Surgical Indications

- Surgery is generally reserved for late treatment of frostbite.
- The adage "frostbite in January, amputation in July" was often used to describe the treatment of these injuries, highlighting the time required for full demarcation of devitalized tissues (Figure 60-2).
  - Several months are often necessary for the areas of tissue loss to fully demarcate.
  - Debridement typically performed at 1 to 3 months unless evidence of ongoing healing.
- As frostbite injuries tend to affect the digits in a circumferential manner, revision amputation is a mainstay of treatment with emphasis on preserving length when possible (Figure 60.3).
- If the amount of tissue resection would be devastating to hand function, limb salvage techniques should be considered.
  - With multiple digit or subtotal hand loss, grafts and flaps can be used in an attempt to maintain limb length.
  - For complete thumb loss, standard techniques for thumb reconstruction can be employed.

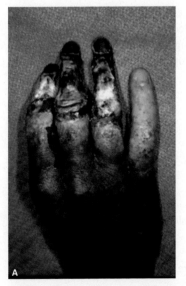 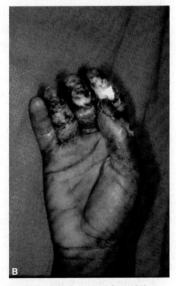

FIGURE 60.2 (A) Dorsal and (B) volar view of right hand of patient from (A) after 2 months of observation. Note the clear demarcation between healthy tissue and dry gangrene. (Photos courtesy of Dr. Gregory A. Dumanian.)

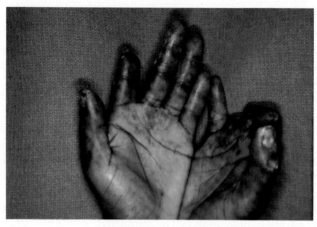

FIGURE 60.3 Final postoperative appearance following revision amputations. (Photo courtesy of Dr. Gregory A. Dumanian.)

- Patients suffering from chronic digital vasospasm may benefit from surgical sympathectomy.
- Patients with peripheral neuropathies and abnormal electrodiagnostic studies may benefit from surgical decompression.
- With severe bone or joint pathology as a result of frostbite injury, standard techniques such as arthroplasty, arthrodesis, or corrective osteotomy may be required.

Potential Complications

- Chronic pain
- Vasomotor dysfunction
  - Cold insensitivity
  - Discoloration
  - Hyperhidrosis
- Neuropathy
- Increased susceptibility to future cold-related injury
- Musculoskeletal problems
  - Osteopenia
  - Subchondral bone loss ("frostbite arthropathy")
  - Joint contractures
- Growth disturbances (children)
  - Typically manifest years later

Postoperative Care

- In the case of amputation, surgical incisions are cared for in the standard fashion, with scar management techniques once adequate healing has occurred.
- Patients should be sent to physical and/or occupational therapy to maintain and maximize joint range of motion.

MANAGEMENT ALGORITHM

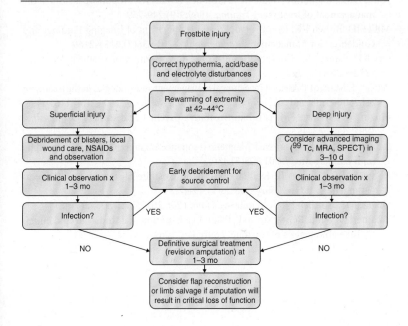

SUGGESTED READINGS

Barker JR, Haws MJ, Brown RE, Kucan JO, Moore WD. Magnetic resonance imaging of severe frostbite injuries. *Ann Plast Surg.* 1997;38(3):275-279.

Britt LD, Dascombe WH, Rodriguez A. New horizons in management of hypothermia and frostbite injury. *Surg Clin North Am.* 1991;71(2):345-370.

Cauchy E, Marsigny B, Allamel G, Verhellen R, Chetaille E. The value of technetium 99 scintigraphy in the prognosis of amputation in severe frostbite injuries of the extremities: a retrospective study of 92 severe frostbite injuries. *J Hand Surg.* 2000;25(5):969-978.

Cauchy E, Chetaille E, Marchand V, Marsigny B. Retrospective study of 70 cases of severe frostbite lesions: a proposed new classification scheme. *Wilderness Environ Med.* 2001;12(4):248-255.

Golant A, Nord RM, Paksima N, Posner MA. Cold exposure injuries to the extremities. *J Am Acad Orthop Surg.* 2008;16(12):704-715.

Handford C, Thomas O, Imray CHE. Frostbite. *Emerg Med Clin North Am.* 2017;35(2):281-299.

Hutchison RL. Frostbite of the hand. *J Hand Surg.* 2014;39(9):1863-1868.

Jones LM, Coffey RA, Natwa MP, Bailey JK. The use of intravenous tPA for the treatment of severe frostbite. *Burns.* 2017;43(5):1088-1096.

Knize DM, Weatherley-White RC, Paton BC, Owens JC. Prognostic factors in the management of frostbite. *J Trauma.* 1969;9(9):749-759.

Millet JD, Brown RK, Levi B, et al. Frostbite: Spectrum of Imaging Findings and Guidelines for Management. *Radiographics.* 2016;36(7):2154-2169.

Orr KD, Fainer DC. Cold injuries in Korea during winter of 1950-51. *Medicine.* 1952;31(2):177-220.

Petrone P, Kuncir EJ, Asensio JA. Surgical management and strategies in the treatment of hypothermia and cold injury. *Emerg Med Clin North Am.* 2003;21(4):1165-1178.

Pinzur MS, Weaver FM. Is urban frostbite a psychiatric disorder? *Orthopedics.* 1997;20(1):43-45.

Raman SR, Jamil Z, Cosgrove J. Magnetic resonance angiography unmasks frostbite injury. *Emerg Med J.* 2011;28(5):450.

Robson MC, Heggers JP. Evaluation of hand frostbite blister fluid as a clue to pathogenesis. *J Hand Surg.* 1981;6(1):43-47.

Shenaq DS, Gottlieb LJ. Cold injuries. *Hand Clin.* 2017;33(2):257-267.

Weatherley-White RC, Sjostrom B, Paton BC. Experimental studies in cold injury. II. The pathogenesis of frostbite. *J Surg Res.* 1964;4:17-22.

CHAPTER

61 Hand and Wrist Anatomy

Mark K. Solarz and Robert C. Matthias, Jr.

INTRODUCTION

- Comprehensive knowledge of upper extremity anatomy is the foundation for the diagnosis and treatment of hand and wrist pathology.

SURFACE ANATOMY (Figure 61.1)

- **Kaplan's cardinal line (KCL)**—originally described in 1953 as the line from the "apex of the interdigital fold between the thumb and index finger . . . parallel with the middle crease of the hand"
  - However, several differing lines have been described using the same name with no consensus among hand surgeons as to which is correct.[1]
  - **Using the original description as a surgical landmark**
    - The motor branch of the median nerve lies 15 mm ulnar and proximal to the intersection of KCL and a longitudinal line drawn from the 2nd webspace.[1]
    - The superficial palmar arch (SPA) lies 14 mm distal to the intersection between KCL and a longitudinal line drawn from the 3rd webspace.[1]
      - The SPA was no closer than 11 mm from any of the four lines considered as KCL in a cadaveric study by Vella et al.[1]
    - The distal extent of the transverse carpal ligament lies 5 mm proximal to the intersection of KCL and a longitudinal line drawn from the 3rd webspace.[1]
- **Distal and proximal palmar creases**—palmar creases are used by some to estimate the level of the A1 pulley.
  - Ring and small at the crease[2]

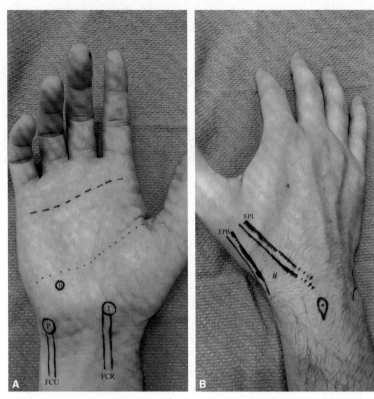

FIGURE 61.1 A and B, Surface anatomy of the hand and wrist. The dotted line represents the original description of Kaplan's cardinal line. The dashed line denotes the distal palmar crease. On the palmar view, the superficial flexor carpi radialis (FCR) and flexor carpi ulnaris (FCU) tendons are easily palpable on their respective sides of the wrist. The FCU continues to the pisiform (P), and the hook of the hamate (H) is palpable in the palm distal and radial to the pisiform. The FCR tendon continues to its groove in the trapezium (T). On the dorsal wrist view, Lister tubercle (asterisk) is palpable on the distal radius. The anatomic snuffbox (hash) is noted between the extensor pollicis longus (EPL) and extensor pollicis brevis (EPB) tendons.

- Long between the distal and proximal creases
- Index at the proximal crease
- The distance from the proximal edge of the A1 pulley to the palmodigital crease can be estimated by the distance from the palmodigital crease to the proximal interphalangeal (PIP) crease.[3]

- **Pisiform**—sesamoid bone within the flexor carpi ulnaris (FCU) tendon, forms the ulnar border of Guyon canal, serves as an attachment point for the transverse carpal ligament
- **FCU tendon**—ulnar artery is palpable deep and radial to the tendon as the artery enters Guyon canal.
- **Hook of hamate**—forms the radial border of Guyon canal and the ulnar border of the carpal tunnel, provides a fulcrum for small and ring finger flexors
- **Flexor carpi radialis (FCR)**—runs through the groove of trapezium, which is palpable along with distal pole of scaphoid, radial artery located immediately radial to the tendon
- **Lister's tubercle**—Bony prominence on the dorsum of the distal radius, which serves as a fulcrum for the extensor pollicis longus (EPL) tendon, which is located on its ulnar side and curves radially as it passes distal to the tubercle
  - The scapholunate (SL) ligament is located about 1 cm distal to Lister's tubercle.
- **Anatomic snuffbox**—bordered by the EPL and extensor pollicis brevis (EPB), location of the scaphoid

BONES (Figure 61.2)

Distal Radius (Figure 61.3)
- Average radiographic parameters[4]
  - Inclination: 23.6°
    - Angle formed by the line between the tip of the radial styloid and the central reference point (CRP: midpoint between the volar ulnar corner and dorsal ulnar corner) and a line perpendicular to the radial shaft
  - Height: 11.6 mm
    - Axial length from the tip of the radial styloid and CRP
  - Volar tilt: 11°
    - Angle formed on the lateral view between the line connecting the volar and ulnar dorsal corners and the line perpendicular to the radial shaft
  - Ulnar variance: 0.6 mm
    - Axial length from the ulnar head and CRP

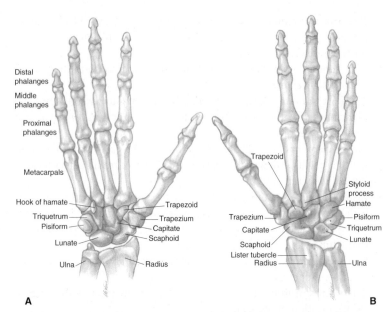

FIGURE 61.2 A,B, Bones of the wrist and hand. Reprinted with permission from Doyle JR, Tornetta P, Einhorn TA. *Hand and Wrist*. Philadelphia, PA: Lippincott Williams & Wilkins; 2006.

- Teardrop angle: 70°
  - Angle formed from a line parallel to the subchondral bone of the volar rim of the lunate facet and the radial shaft
- Scaphoid facet
- Lunate facet—radius of curvature[5] 10.9 mm
- Sigmoid notch—articulates with ulnar head at distal radial ulnar joint (DRUJ), radius of curvature 50% to 100% larger than ulnar head
  - Articular contact provides about 20% DRUJ stability[6]

Distal Ulna

- Ulnar styloid—base serves as the attachment point for the triangular fibrocartilage complex (TFCC)
- Extensor carpi ulnaris (ECU) groove—located at the dorsal-ulnar aspect of the ulnar head
  - Average depth of 1.4 mm and width[7] of 9.0 mm
- Ulnocarpal ligament complex—composed of the ulnotriquetral, ulnocapitate, and ulnolunate ligaments
  - Originates adjacent to the ulnar styloid at the volar foveal region and the individual ligaments fan out to their respective insertions

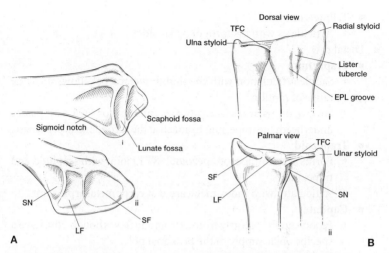

FIGURE 61.3 A and B, Osseous anatomy of the distal radius. EPL, extensor pollicis longus; LF, lunate facet; SF, scaphoid facet; SN, sigmoid notch; TFCC, triangular fibrocartilage complex. From Cooney WP. *The Wrist: Diagnosis and Operative Treatment.* 2nd ed. Philadelphia, PA: Lippincott Williams & Wilkins, a Wolters Kluwer Business; 2010. Used with permission of Mayo Foundation for Medical Education and Research. All rights reserved.

Carpus

- Proximal row
  - **Scaphoid**
    - Serves as crutch to stabilize the proximal and distal rows
    - Blood supply—dorsal carpal branch of the radial artery makes up the primary vascular supply
      - Retrograde pattern predisposes scaphoid to avacsular necrosis (AVN) particularly with proximal pole fractures
      - Superficial palmar branch of the radial artery supplies distal pole
    - SL angle—formed by the longitudinal axis of the scaphoid and the line intersecting the body of the lunate on a lateral radiograph
      - Normal—30° to 60°, DISI deformity: >60°, VISI deformity: <30°
  - **Lunate**
    - Blood supply variants[8]: Y-pattern (59%), X-pattern (10%), I-pattern (31%)
    - Radius of curvature[5] 10.4 mm
    - Variable distal medial facet for hamate articulation (type 1: absent, type 2: present)

- **Triquetrum**
  - Articulates with pisiform on volar side
- Distal row
  - **Trapezium**
    - Saddle articulation with the thumb metacarpal allows for wide range of motion.
    - Groove on volar surface provides fulcrum for FCR as it passes underneath the trapezium to attach at the second metacarpal base.
  - **Trapezoid**
    - Forms scaphotrapezotrapezoidal (STT) joint with scaphoid and trapezium
    - Articulates with index metacarpal at carpometacarpal joint
  - **Capitate**
    - Blood supply—largely from retrograde flow, though 70% have a specific volar supply to the proximal pole[9]
    - Radius of curvature[5] 6.1 mm
    - Articulates with long metacarpal at carpometacarpal joint
  - **Hamate**
    - Hook projects volarly—serves as attachment point for transverse carpal ligament, pisohamate ligament, hypothenar muscles
    - Articulates with type 2 lunates
    - Articulates with ring and small metacarpals at carpometacarpal joint

Metacarpals

- Medial and lateral sides are concave to serve as attachment points for adjacent interosseous muscles (four dorsal and three palmar).
- Metacarpal bases serve as the site of attachment for the abductor pollicis longus (APL; thumb), extensor carpi radialis longus (ECRL; index), extensor carpi radialis brevis (ECRB; middle), extensor carpi ulnaris (small), flexor carpi radialis (index and middle), flexor carpi ulnaris (small).

Phalanges

- Each digit has three phalanges (proximal, middle, and distal), other than thumb (proximal and distal).
  - Proximal phalanx serves as attachment site for interosseous muscles.
  - Middle phalanx serves as attachment site for flexor digitorum superficialis (FDS) and central slip.
  - Distal phalanx serves as attachment site for flexor digitorum profundus (FDP) and terminal tendon of the extensor mechanism.

LIGAMENTS

Metacarpophalangeal (MCP) Joint of the Thumb

- **Ulnar collateral ligament**
  - Stabilizes the thumb during pinch and grasp
  - Origin is 4.2 mm from the dorsal cortex and 5.3 mm from the articular surface on the thumb metacarpal head.
  - Insertion is 2.8 mm from the volar surface and 3.4 mm from the articular surface of the proximal phalanx.[15]
  - Proper collateral ligament is the main stabilizer in midflexion while the accessory collateral ligament and volar plate stabilize the joint in extension.
- **Radial collateral ligament**
  - Origin is 3.5 mm from the dorsal cortex and 3.3 mm from the articular surface on the thumb metacarpal head.
  - Insertion is 2.8 mm from the volar cortex and 2.6 mm from the articular surface.

MCP Joints of the Fingers (Figure 61.4)

- **Proper collateral ligaments**
  - Origin is dorsal to the axis of rotation on the metacarpal head.
    - Along with an increasing diameter of the metacarpal head in the sagittal plane from dorsal to volar, the resulting cam effect tightens the proper collateral ligament in 70° to 90° flexion.
    - Proper collateral ligament is lengthened by 15% when flexing[10] from 0° to 90°.

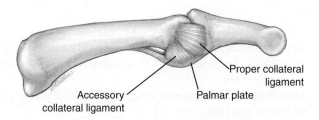

FIGURE 61.4 Collateral ligaments of the digits. Proper collateral ligament, which inserts onto bone, is dorsal to the accessory collateral ligament, which inserts onto the volar plate. Reprinted with permission from Doyle JR, Tornetta P, Einhorn TA. *Hand and Wrist*. Philadelphia, PA: Lippincott Williams & Wilkins; 2006.

- **Accessory collateral ligament**
  - Inserts onto and suspends the volar plate
  - Along with the volar plate, provides stability in extension
- **Deep transverse metacarpal ligaments**
  - Attach adjacent volar plates of the index through small MCP joints to prevent ray separation

PIP Joints

- **Proper collateral ligaments**
  - Crescent-shaped origin is dorsal and proximal within the concavity on the head of the proximal phalanx.
  - Insertion includes the majority of the base of the middle phalanx.
  - Dorsal fibers of the ligament extend parallel to the axis of the middle phalanx and the volar fibers run in an oblique manner, giving the ligament its fan shape.[11]
  - Proper collateral ligament is tensioned throughout the interphalangeal (IP) range of motion.
- **Accessory collateral ligament**
  - Volar to the proper collateral ligament, inserts onto the volar plate
  - Tensioned with IP joint extension and relaxes in flexion
  - Results in contracture with prolonged immobilization in flexion
- **Intrinsic-plus splinting**
  - "Position of Safety"
  - MCP joints placed in 70° to 90° of flexion to tension proper collateral ligament, and IP joints placed in full extension to tension accessory collateral ligament and volar plate
  - Failure to maintain this position during prolonged splinting results in joint contracture and limitations in motion.

Wrist

- Extrinsic ligaments (Figure 61.5)
  - **Dorsal radiocarpal ligament**—distal radius to lunate and triquetrum
    - Stabilizes lunotriquetral (LT) articulation and acts as sling for proximal row
  - **Dorsal intercarpal ligament**—triquetrum to distal pole of scaphoid, trapezoid, and trapezium
    - Stabilizes midcarpal joint
  - **Radioscaphocapitate (RSC) ligament**—volar distal radius, across scaphoid waist, to proximal pole of capitates

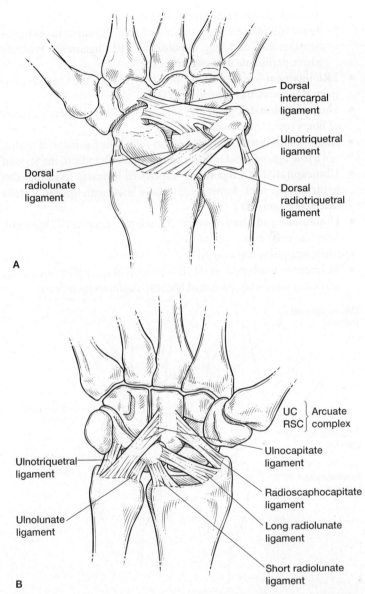

FIGURE 61.5 A and B, Extrinsic ligaments of the wrist. From Cooney WP. *The Wrist: Diagnosis and Operative Treatment*. 2nd ed. Philadelphia, PA: Lippincott Williams & Wilkins, a Wolters Kluwer Business; 2010. Used with permission of Mayo Foundation for Medical Education and Research. All rights reserved.

- ◆ Acts as fulcrum for scaphoid flexion
- ◆ **Space of Poirier**—weak portion of volar ligamentous complex between RSC and long radiolunate (LRL) ligaments, typically where perilunate dislocations occur
- **LRL ligament**—ulnar to RSC, fibers blend with the volar lunotriquetral interosseous ligament (LTIL)
- **Short radiolunate ligament**—adjacent to LRL, vertical orientation of fibers resist hyperextension
- **Radioscapholunate ligament**—also called the ligament of Testut, not a true ligament but rather a neurovascular bundle to the SL joint
- **Ulnocapitate (UC) ligament**—superficial ligament from the ulna to the capitate neck, forms confluence of fibers with the RSC distally (**arcuate ligament**)
- **Ulnolunate and ulnotriquetral ligaments**—deep to UC ligament, form the volar aspect of the TFCC
- ■ Intrinsic ligaments (Figure 61.6)
  - **SL interosseous ligament** (SLIL)—consists of three portions (dorsal and volar ligaments, proximal fibrocartilaginous membrane)

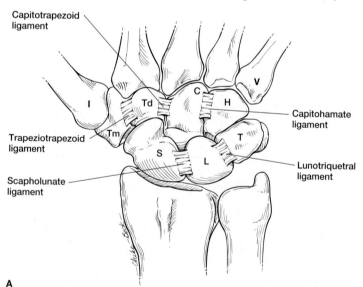

A

FIGURE 61.6 A and B, Intrinsic ligaments of the wrist. From Cooney WP. *The Wrist: Diagnosis and Operative Treatment*. 2nd ed. Philadelphia, PA: Lippincott Williams & Wilkins, a Wolters Kluwer Business; 2010. Used with permission of Mayo Foundation for Medical Education and Research. All rights reserved.

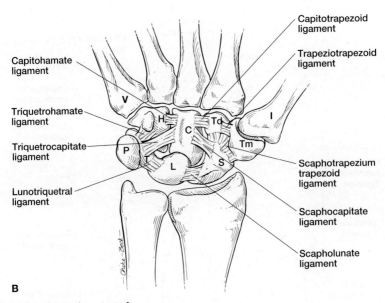

Capitotrapezoid ligament

Trapeziotrapezoid ligament

Capitohamate ligament

Triquetrohamate ligament

Triquetrocapitate ligament

Lunotriquetral ligament

Scaphotrapezium trapezoid ligament

Scaphocapitate ligament

Scapholunate ligament

B

FIGURE 61.6 (*continued*)

- ◆ Dorsal SL ligament is the strongest.
- **LTIL**—consists of three portions (dorsal and volar ligaments, proximal fibrocartilaginous membrane)
  - ◆ Volar LT ligament is the strongest.
- ■ **TFCC** (Figure 61.7)
  - Interposed between the ulnar head and the proximal carpal row
  - Stabilizes the DRUJ while allowing the sigmoid notch to rotate around the ulnar head
  - Blood supply—anterior interosseous and ulnar arteries, supply only outer 15% of articular disk
  - Components
    - ◆ **Radioulnar ligaments**[6,12]—primary stabilizers of the DRUJ, each have superficial and deep limbs
    - ◆ **Palmar**—tight in supination, main constraint to dorsal ulnar translation
    - ◆ **Dorsal**—tight in pronation, main constraint to volar ulnar translation
    - ◆ **Articular disk**—extends from the sigmoid notch and blends ulnarly with the converging radioulnar ligaments
      - ✳ Composed of fibrocartilage to transmit compressive loads

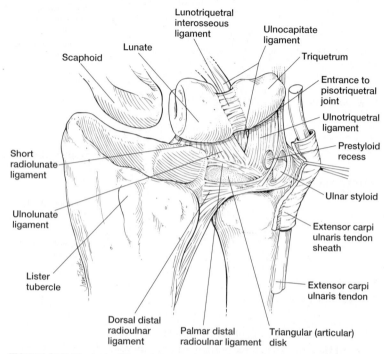

FIGURE 61.7 Triangular fibrocartilage complex. From Cooney WP. *The Wrist: Diagnosis and Operative Treatment.* 2nd ed. Philadelphia, PA: Lippincott Williams & Wilkins, a Wolters Kluwer Business; 2010. Used with permission of Mayo Foundation for Medical Education and Research. All rights reserved.

- ◆ **ECU sheath**
- ◆ **Ulnotriquetral** and **ulnolunate** ligaments
- ◆ **Meniscus homologue**—vascular synovial fold from the dorsal radius to the volar triquetrum

MUSCLES

Wrist and Finger Flexors (Table 61.1; Figures 61.8 and 61.9)

Pulley System (Figure 61.10)

- ■ **Annular pulleys**
  - • Prevent bowstringing, **especially A2 and A4**

TABLE 61.1 Flexors of the Wrist and Digits

Muscle	Innervation	Origin	Insertion
PT	Median	Medial supracondylar ridge, proximal ulna	Proximal radial shaft
FCR	Median	Medial epicondyle	Volar base of II/III metacarpal
PL	Median	Medial epicondyle	Transverse carpal ligament
FCU	Ulnar	Medial epicondyle, proximal ulna	Pisiform, volar base V metacarpal
FDS	Median	Medial epicondyle, proximal radius	Volar base of middle phalanx
FDP	AIN (II and III), ulnar (IV and V)	Proximal ulna, IOM	Volar base of distal phalanx
FPL	AIN	Volar radius, IOM	Volar base thumb distal phalanx
PQ	AIN	Distal ulna	Volar surface distal radius

Abbreviations: AIN, anterior interosseous nerve; FCR, flexor carpi radialis; FCU, flexor carpi ulnaris; FDP, flexor digitorum profundus; FDS, flexor digitorum superficialis; FPL, flexor pollicis longus; IOM, interosseous membrane; PL, palmaris longus; PQ, pronator quadratus; PT, pronator teres.

- A1, A3, and A5 originate from the volar plates of the MCP, PIP, and distal interphalangeal (DIP) joints, respectively.
- A2 and A4 pulleys originate from the proximal and middle phalanges, respectively.
- **Oblique pulley** is most important in thumb to prevent bowstringing.
- **Cruciate pulleys**
  - Allow the sheath to shorten and lengthen with flexion and extension of the digit

Extensor Muscles of the Wrist and Digits (Table 61.2; Figures 61.11 and 61.12)

Extensor Mechanism (Figure 61.13)

- Extensor indicis proprius (EIP) and extensor digiti minimi (EDM) tendons both ulnar to extensor digitorum communis (EDC) tendons of index and small finger, respectively
- **Juncturae tendinae**
  - Tendinous interconnections proximal to the MCP joints between EDC tendons

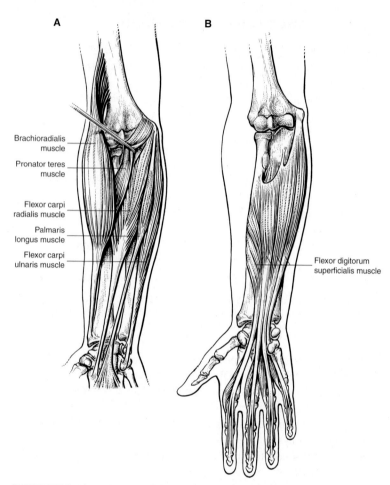

FIGURE 61.8 A to D, Extrinsic finger flexors. Reprinted with permission from Clemente CD. *Clemente's Anatomy Dissector*. 3rd ed. Baltimore, MD: Lippincott Williams & Wilkins; 2011.

- Maintain some active extension if tendon is lacerated proximal to the juncturae
- **Sagittal bands**
  - Extend MCP joints via sling effect
  - Serve as check reins to centralize extensor tendon
  - Insert onto volar plate

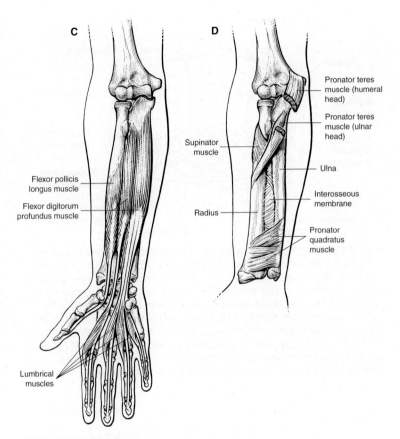

FIGURE 61.8 (*continued*)

- ■ **Central slip**
  - ● Inserts onto base of middle phalanx to extend PIP joint
- ■ **Lateral bands**
  - ● Formed by the tendons of the lumbricals and interossei, are joined by the lateral portions of the EDC after trifurcation
  - ● **Triangular ligament** prevents volar subluxation of the bands before forming the terminal tendon.
  - ● **Transverse retinacular ligament** prevents dorsal subluxation of the bands at the level of the PIP joint.
- ■ **Terminal tendon**
  - ● Formed by convergence of the two lateral bands
  - ● Extends the DIP joint

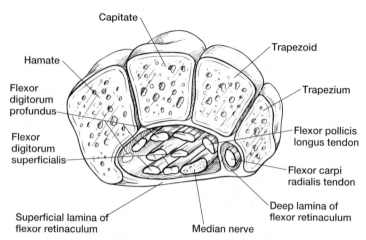

FIGURE 61.9 Contents of the carpal tunnel. Carpal bones form an osseous arch at the floor of the carpal tunnel and the transverse carpal tunnel forms the roof. The flexor pollicis longus (FPL) is most radial. The flexor digitorum superficialis (FDS) tendons are oriented middle and ring over index and small. The flexor digitorum profundus (FDP) tendons are adjacent to one another at the floor. The median nerve is superficial and radial to the FDS tendons. The flexor carpi radialis (FCR) tendon is adjacent to but outside the carpal tunnel. From Cooney WP. *The Wrist: Diagnosis and Operative Treatment*. 2nd ed. Philadelphia, PA: Lippincott Williams & Wilkins, a Wolters Kluwer Business; 2010. Used with permission of Mayo Foundation for Medical Education and Research. All rights reserved.

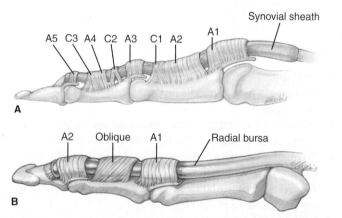

FIGURE 61.10 A and B, Pulley system of the digits and thumb. Reprinted with permission from Doyle JR, Tornetta P, Einhorn TA. *Hand and Wrist*. Philadelphia, PA: Lippincott Williams & Wilkins; 2006.

TABLE 61.2 Extensors of the Wrist and Digits

Muscle	Innervation	Origin	Insertion
BR	Radial	Lateral epicondyle	Radial styloid
ECRL	Radial	Lateral epicondyle	Dorsal base II metacarpal
ECRB	Radial/PIN	Lateral epicondyle	Dorsal base III metacarpal
APL	PIN	Dorsal proximal radius/ulna, IOM	Base thumb metacarpal
EPB	PIN	Dorsal radius	Base thumb proximal phalanx
EPL	PIN	Dorsal ulna, IOM	Base of thumb distal phalanx
EDC	PIN	Lateral epicondyle	Extensor hood
EIP	PIN	Dorsal ulna, IOM	Extensor hood index finger, ulnar to EDC
EDM	PIN	Lateral epicondyle	Extensor hood small finger, ulnar to EDC
ECU	PIN	Lateral epicondyle	Dorsal base V metacarpal

Abbreviations: APL, abductor pollicis longus; BR, brachioradialis; ECRB, extensor carpi radialis brevis; ECRL, extensor carpi radialis longus; ECU, extensor carpi ulnaris; EDC, extensor digitorum communis; EDM, extensor digiti minimi; EIP, extensor indicis proprius; EPB, extensor pollicis brevis; EPL, extensor pollicis longus; IOM, interosseous membrane; PIN, posterior interosseous nerve.

- **Oblique retinacular ligament** (Landsmeer ligament)
  - From the flexor sheath at the PIP joint to the terminal tendon
  - Allows for DIP extension with PIP extension

Intrinsics

- Thenar and hypothenar muscles (Table 61.3; Figure 61.14)
- **Lumbricals**
  - Originate from the FDP tendons in the palm
  - Pass volar to the intermetacarpal ligaments and insert onto the radial-sided lateral bands
  - Act to flex the MCP joints while extending the IP joints

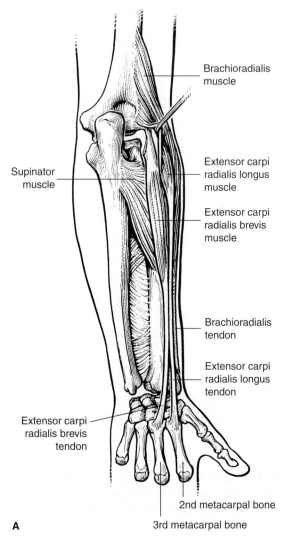

A

FIGURE 61.11 A–C, Extrinsic hand and wrist extensors. Reprinted with permission from Clemente CD. *Clemente's Anatomy Dissector*. 3rd ed. Baltimore, MD: Lippincott Williams & Wilkins; 2011.

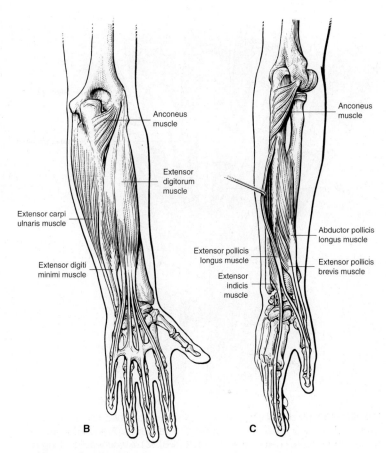

FIGURE 61.11 (*Continued*)

- Index and middle finger lumbricals
    - **Unipennate**, innervated by the **median** nerve
- Ring and small finger lumbricals
    - **Bipennate**, innervated by the **ulnar** nerve
- Dorsal and palmar **interossei**
    - All innervated by the motor branch of the **ulnar** nerve
    - Tendons pass dorsal to the intermetacarpal ligament.
    - Act to flex MCP joints and extend IP joints and to abduct and adduct the fingers
    - Four bipennate dorsal interossei abduct away from the long finger.
    - Three unipennate palmar interossei adduct the digits toward the long finger.

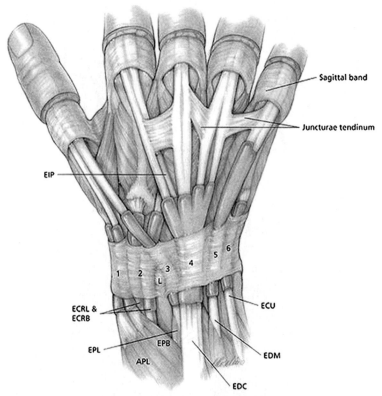

FIGURE 61.12 Six dorsal compartments of the wrist: (1) abductor pollicis longus (APL) and extensor pollicis brevis (EPB), (2) extensor carpi radialis longus (ECRL) and extensor carpi radialis brevis (ECRB), (3) extensor pollicis longus (EPL), (4) extensor digitorum communis (EDC) and extensor indicis proprius (EIP), (5) extensor digiti minimi (EDM), (6) extensor carpi ulnaris (ECU). Extensor retinaculum prevents bowstringing of tendons. EIP is most distal muscle belly in the 4th compartment. Reprinted with permission from Hammert WC, Boyer MI, Bozentka DJ, Calfee RP. *ASSH Manual of Hand Surgery*. Philadelphia, PA: Lippincott Williams & Wilkins; 2010.

VASCULAR

- **Radial artery**
  - Runs radial and deep to the FCR tendon before dividing at the radial styloid

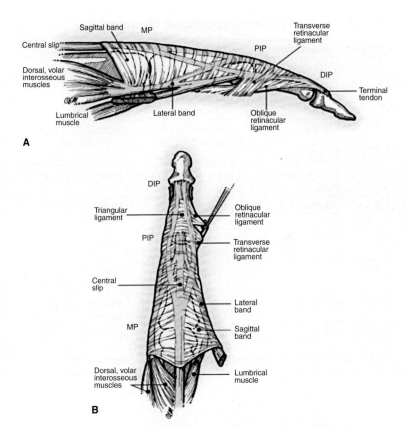

FIGURE 61.13 A and B, Extensor mechanism of the digits. DIP, distal interphalangeal; MP, metacarpophalangeal; PIP, proximal interphalangeal. Reprinted with permission from Maschke S, Graham TJ, Evans P. *Master Techniques in Orthopaedic Surgery: The Hand*. 3rd ed. Philadelphia, PA: Wolters Kluwer; 2016.

- Deep branch courses dorsally under the first dorsal compartment tendons before passing between the bellies of the first dorsal interosseous muscle.
- Forms **princeps pollicis** artery and **radialis indicis** artery before forming the **deep palmar arch**
  * Deep palmar arch is complete 98.5%.[13]
- Superficial branch passes through thenar compartment to complete SPA.

TABLE 61.3 Thenar and Hypothenar Muscles

Muscle	Innervation	Origin	Insertion
AP	Ulnar	Oblique head: II and III metacarpal Transverse head: III metacarpal	Ulnar base of thumb proximal phalanx, ulnar sesamoid
APB	Median	Distal pole scaphoid, trapezium	Radial base of thumb proximal phalanx
FPB	Superficial head: median, deep head: ulnar	Transverse carpal ligament, trapezium	Base of thumb proximal phalanx, radial sesamoid
OP	Median	Trapezium	Radial aspect of thumb metacarpal
PB	Ulnar (zone III)	Transverse carpal ligament	Palm
ADM	Ulnar	Pisiform	Ulnar base of small prox phalanx, extensor hood
FDMB	Ulnar	Hook of hamate	Volar base small prox phalanx
ODM	Ulnar	Hook of hamate	Ulnar small metacarpal

Abbreviations: ADM, abductor digiti minimi; AP, adductor pollicis; APB, abductor pollicis brevis; FDMB, flexor digiti minimi brevis; FPB, flexor pollicis brevis; ODM, opponens digiti minimi; OP, opponens pollicis; PB, palmaris brevis.

- **Ulnar artery**
  - Runs deep to FCU tendon on the radial side of the ulnar nerve
  - Divides at Guyon canal to form the deep and superficial branches
  - Deep branch anastomoses with the radial artery to complete the deep palmar arch.
  - Superficial branch gives off the proper ulnar digital artery to the small finger before continuing on as the **SPA.**
    - Arch sends off **common digital arteries** to supply the 2nd, 3rd, and 4th webspaces.
    - SPA is complete 78.5%.[13]
- **Proper digital arteries**
  - Run dorsal to digital nerves in the finger
  - Proper digital arteries to the thumb form from the princeps pollicis.
  - Radial proper digital artery to the index finger forms from the radialis indicis.

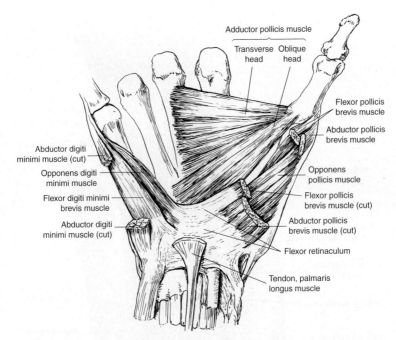

FIGURE 61.14 Thenar and hypothenar muscles. Reprinted with permission from Clemente CD. *Clemente's Anatomy Dissector*. 3rd ed. Baltimore, MD: Lippincott Williams & Wilkins; 2011.

- Ulnar proper digital artery to the small finger arises directly from the superficial arch.
- Common digital arteries to the 2nd to 4th webspaces bifurcate to form the remainder of the proper digital arteries.

NERVES

Cutaneous Sensation of the Forearm (Figure 61.15)

- **Lateral antebrachial cutaneous nerve**—continuation of the musculocutaneous nerve, supplies the radial aspect of the forearm
- **Medial antebrachial cutaneous nerve**—originates from the medial cord of the brachial plexus, supplies the ulnar aspect of the forearm
- **Posterior antebrachial cutaneous nerve**—originates from the radial nerve, supplies the dorsum of the forearm

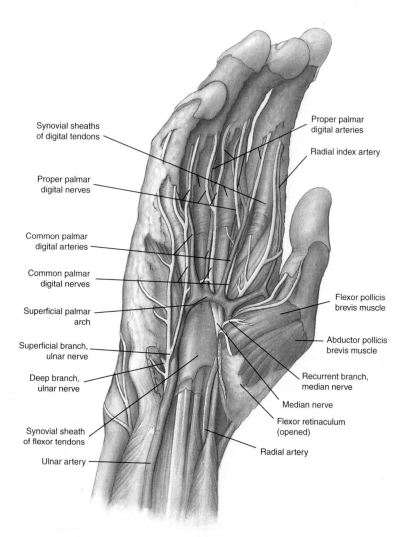

Synovial sheaths
of digital tendons

Proper palmar
digital nerves

Common palmar
digital arteries

Common palmar
digital nerves

Superficial palmar
arch

Superficial branch,
ulnar nerve

Deep branch,
ulnar nerve

Synovial sheath
of flexor tendons

Ulnar artery

Proper palmar
digital arteries

Radial index artery

Flexor pollicis
brevis muscle

Abductor pollicis
brevis muscle

Recurrent branch,
median nerve

Median nerve

Flexor retinaculum
(opened)

Radial artery

FIGURE 61.15 Arterial supply of the hand. Note that the superficial palmar arch and common digital arteries are superficial to the nerves in the palm, but this relationship switches at the level of the metacarpophalangeal joints so that proper digital nerves are superficial in the digits. Reprinted with permission from Clemente CD. *Clemente's Anatomy Dissector*. 3rd ed. Baltimore, MD: Lippincott Williams & Wilkins; 2011.

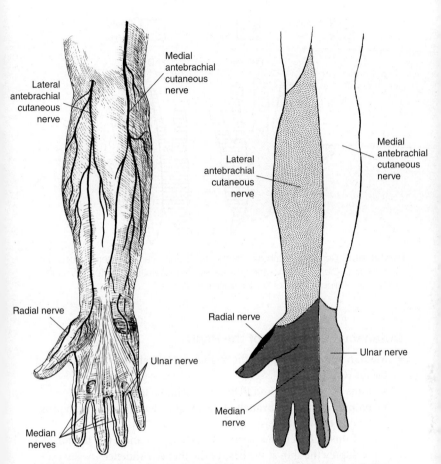

FIGURE 61.16 Sensory distribution of the forearm. Reprinted with permission from Clemente CD. *Clemente's Anatomy Dissector*. 3rd ed. Baltimore, MD: Lippincott Williams & Wilkins; 2011.

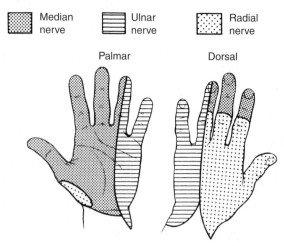

FIGURE 61.17 Sensory distribution of the hand. Reprinted with permission from Clemente CD. *Clemente's Anatomy Dissector*. 3rd ed. Baltimore, MD: Lippincott Williams & Wilkins, a Wolters Kluwer business; 2011.

Cutaneous Sensation of the Hand

- **Median nerve**—formed by the medial and lateral cords of the brachial plexus (C5-T1)
  - Runs between FDS and FDP muscles in the forearm
  - **Palmar cutaneous branch** of the median nerve divides 5 cm proximal to the wrist crease.
    - Runs between the palmaris longus (PL) and FCR tendons to supply the skin at the base of the thenar eminence
  - Divides into common digital nerves in the palm to supply the thumb, index, middle, and radial side of the ring finger
- **Radial nerve**—formed by the posterior cord of the brachial plexus (C5-T1)
  - **Dorsal radial sensory nerve** runs beneath the brachioradialis (BR) and emerges between the BR and ECRL 8 to 9 cm proximal to the radial styloid.
  - Supplies the dorsum of the hand to the thumb IP joint and PIP joint of the index, middle, and radial aspect of ring fingers (distal supplied by the median nerve)

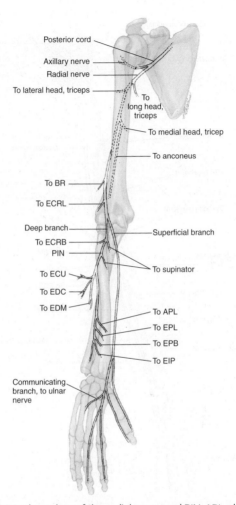

FIGURE 61.18 Motor branches of the radial nerve and PIN. APL, abductor pollicis longus; BR, brachioradialis; ECRB, extensor carpi radialis brevis; ECRL, extensor carpi radialis longus; ECU, extensor carpi ulnaris; EDC, extensor digitorum communis; EDM, extensor digiti minimi; EIP, extensor indicis proprius; EPB, extensor pollicis brevis; EPL, extensor pollicis longus; PIN, posterior interosseous nerve. Reprinted with permission from Doyle JR, Tornetta P, Einhorn TA. *Hand and Wrist*. Philadelphia, PA: Lippincott Williams & Wilkins; 2006.

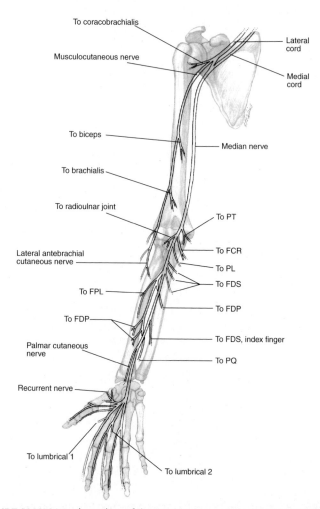

FIGURE 61.19 Motor branches of the median nerve and anterior interosseous nerve. FCR, flexor carpi radialis; FDP, flexor digitorum profundus; FDS, flexor digitorum superficialis; FPL, flexor pollicis longus; PL, palmaris longus; PQ, pronator quadratus; PT, pronator teres. Reprinted with permission from Doyle JR, Tornetta P, Einhorn TA. *Hand and Wrist*. Philadelphia, PA: Lippincott Williams & Wilkins; 2006.

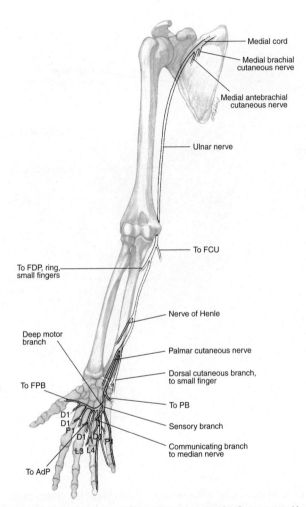

FIGURE 61.20 Motor branches of the ulnar nerve to the forearm and hand. AdP, adductor pollicis; FCU, flexor carpi ulnaris; FDP, flexor digitorum profundus; FPB, flexor pollicis brevis; PB, palmaris brevis. Reprinted with permission from Doyle JR, Tornetta P, Einhorn TA. *Hand and Wrist*. Philadelphia, PA: Lippincott Williams & Wilkins; 2006.

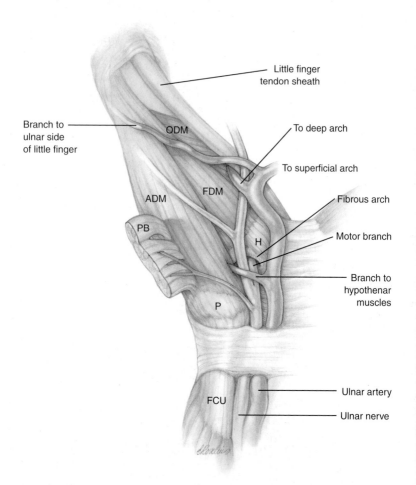

FIGURE 61.21 Guyon canal. ADM, abductor digiti minimi; FCU, flexor carpi ulnaris; FDM, flexor digiti minimi; H, hamate; ODM, opponens digiti minimi; P, pisiform; PB, palmaris brevis. Reprinted with permission from Doyle JR, Tornetta P, Einhorn TA. *Hand and Wrist*. Philadelphia, PA: Lippincott Williams & Wilkins; 2006.

- **Ulnar nerve**—formed by the medial cord of the brachial plexus (C7-T1)
  - Runs under the FCU in the forearm before entering Guyon canal at the wrist
  - **Dorsal ulnar sensory nerve** divides 5 cm proximal to the wrist and courses from volar to dorsal at the ulnar styloid (Figure 61.16)
  - Supplies the small and ulnar side of the ring finger

Motor Supply of the Forearm and Hand

- **Radial nerve** (Figure 61.17)
  - Innervates BR, ECRL, +/− ECRB before branching of posterior interosseous nerve (PIN) at the elbow
  - PIN (proximal to distal innervation)—+/− ECRB, supinator, ECU, EDC, EDM, APL, EPL, EPB, EIP
- **Median nerve** (Figures 61.18 and 61.19)
  - Pronator teres, FCR, PL, FDS before branching of **anterior interosseous nerve** (AIN), then innervates the index and middle lumbrical muscles in the palm
  - AIN—FDP to index and middle fingers, flexor pollicis longus, and pronator quadratus
  - **Motor (thenar) branch**—opponens pollicis, abductor pollicis brevis, flexor pollicis brevis (superficial head)
    - Variability of location—extraligamentous 46%, subligamentous 31%, and transligamentous 23%[14]
- **Ulnar nerve** (Figure 61.20)
  - FCU, FDP to ring and small fingers before entering Guyon canal
  - **Guyon canal** (Figure 61.21)
    - Zone 1—mixed motor and sensory
    - Zone 2—**deep motor branch** (abductor digiti minimi, flexor digiti minimi brevis, opponens digiti minimi, palmar and dorsal interossei, lumbricals to the ring and small fingers, adductor pollicis, and flexor pollicis brevis (deep head)
    - Zone 3—Motor to **palmaris brevis** and digital nerves to small finger and ulnar side of ring fingers

REFERENCES

1. Vella JC, Hartigan BJ, Stern PJ. Kaplan's cardinal line. *J Hand Surg Am*. 2006;31(6):912-918.
2. Lyu SR. Closed division of the flexor tendon sheath for trigger finger. *J Bone Joint Surg Br*. 1992;74(3):418-420.

3. Fiorini HJ, Santos JB, Hirakawa CK, Sato ES, Faloppa F, Albertoni WM. Anatomical study of the A1 pulley: length and location by means of cutaneous landmarks on the palmar surface. *J Hand Surg Am.* 2011;36(3):464-468.

4. Medoff RJ. Essential radiographic evaluation for distal radius fractures. *Hand Clin.* 2005;21(3):279-288.

5. Hawkins-Rivers S, Budoff JE, Ismaily SK, Noble PC, Haddad J. MRI study of the capitate, lunate, and lunate fossa with relevance to proximal row carpectomy. *J Hand Surg Am.* 2008;33(6):841-849.

6. Stuart PR, Berger RA, Linscheid RL, An KN. The dorsopalmar stability of the distal radioulnar joint. *J Hand Surg Am.* 2000;25(4):689-699.

7. Iorio ML, Bayomy AF, Huang JI. Morphology of the extensor carpi ulnaris groove and tendon. *J Hand Surg Am.* 2014;39(12):2412-2416.

8. Gelberman RH, Bauman TD, Menon J, Akeson WH. The vascularity of the lunate bone and kienbock's disease. *J Hand Surg Am.* 1980;5(3):272-278.

9. Kadar A, Morsy M, Sur YJ, Laungani AT, Akdag O, Moran SL. The vascular anatomy of the capitate: new discoveries using micro-computed tomography imaging. *J Hand Surg Am.* 2017;42(2):78-86.

10. Dy CJ, Tucker SM, Kok PL, Hearns KA, Carlson MG. Anatomy of the radial collateral ligament of the index metacarpal joint. *J Hand Surg Am.* 2013;38(1):124-128.

11. Allison, DM. Anatomy of the collateral ligaments of the proximal interphalangeal joint. *J Hand Surg Am.* 2005;30:1026-1031.

12. Ward LD, Ambrose CG, Masson MV, Levaro F. The role of the distal radioulnar ligaments, interosseous membrane, and joint capsule in distal radioulnar joint stability. *J Hand Surg Am.* 2000;25(2):341-351.

13. Coleman SS, Anson BJ. Arterial patterns in the hand based upon a study of 650 specimens. *Surg Gynecol Obstet.* 1961;113:409-424.

14. Lanz U. Anatomical variations of the median nerve in the carpal tunnel. *J Hand Surg Am.* 1977;2(1):44-53.

15. Carlson MG, Warner KK, Meyers KN, Hearns KA, Kok PL. Anatomy of the thumb metacarpophalangeal ulnar and radial collateral ligaments. *J Hand Surg Am.* 2012;37(10):2021-2026.

James D. Bedford and Sarah Turner

INTRODUCTION

- All decisions regarding rehabilitation should be customized to the injury and to the patient.
- It is important for the hand surgeon to have clear and effective communication with a team of hand therapists and to communicate with each patient the importance of compliance with rehabilitation.

PRINCIPLES OF REHABILITATION

- Early goals: reduce edema, manage pain, promote healing, prevent deformity, and maximize functional motion while protecting injured structures
- Late goals: allow return to activities of daily living, allow return to work, manage mechanical dysfunction, and manage pain, scar tissue and hypersensitivity

PRINCIPLES OF SPLINTING

- Immobilization for protection and pain relief
  - Following nerve injury: decrease tension on repair
  - After fracture: reduce risk of displacement or reinjury
- Immobilization to allow healing
  - Maintain alignment of well-reduced fractures
  - Soft tissue injuries: protect and prevent overuse
  - Following repair/reconstruction: Immobilization protocols should be tailored to the specific procedure
    - Tendon repairs should be protected, and early therapy initiated for appropriate patients
  - Provide passive stretch

605

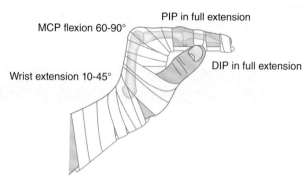

FIGURE 62.1 The position of safe immobilization. DIP, distal interphalangeal; MCP, metacarpophalangeal; PIP, proximal interphalangeal.

- Prevent joint contracture
- Overcome established contracture
- The position of safe immobilization (POSI)
  - The POSI is designed to place the joints of the hand in positions that reduce the risk of contractures. It is typically referred to as the intrinsic plus position (Figure 62.1).
■ Functional splinting
- Improve function by correcting deformity, such as in nerve palsy or tendon dysfunction (e.g. swan neck deformity)

EDEMA CONTROL AND MANAGEMENT

■ Edema is the pathologic accumulation of extracellular fluid. In the hand, soft tissues may develop edema following injury or surgery, with a variety of effects:
- Subcutaneous edema leads to obvious swelling, with greater capacity for swelling on the dorsum of the hand in nonglabrous skin
- Edema within tendon sheaths produces increased gliding resistance, which is especially important in the context of tendon repairs.
- Edema may cause nerve compression symptoms, including altered sensation in affected digits.
- Generalized edema in the hand produces a typical posture of metacarpophalangeal joint (MCPJ) hyperextension, interphalangeal joint (IPJ) flexion, and thumb adduction; this is known as the intrinsic minus position.
- The consequences of edema are contrary to the goals of surgery and therapy:
  - Impaired wound healing and increased susceptibility to infection

- ◆ Resistance to passive and active joint motion
- ◆ Risk of fibrosis and permanent joint contracture
- The specific consequence of the intrinsic minus position is proximal interphalangeal joint (PIPJ) flexion contracture because of fibrosis of the volar plate in its shortened position and MCPJ extension contracture as a result of fibrosis of the collateral ligaments in their shortened positions.

- Management
  - Elevation
  - Active and passive range of motion (ROM) exercises
  - Retrograde massage and/or compression via bandaging or garments/gloves
  - Contrast bathing: alternating between warm and iced water baths

REHABILITATION PROTOCOLS

- Hand surgery centers have their own protocols for the rehabilitation of common injuries. These protocols have coevolved in recent decades with the surgical techniques of repair and reconstruction for hand injuries.
- This phenomenon is perhaps most notable in the treatment of flexor tendon injuries. Tendon repairs have evolved to improve strength of repair by increasing number of core strands from two to four or six. This has allowed for the development and use of early active motion protocols. The importance of reducing bulk and gapping at the repair site with low-profile epitendinous sutures has also become more commonly used, allowing better tendon gliding.
- Given the improved treatment protocols, rehabilitation regimes that place higher demands on surgeons' repairs have developed. As combined passive and early active mobilization has overtaken purely passive regimens as the preferred way to rehabilitate flexor tendons, functional outcomes of tendon repairs have continued to improve.
- Rehabilitation over a period of weeks to months can be helped by consistency of therapy staff and by clearly written patient instructions. Some centers may also consider telephone or video call "clinics," especially if their patient catchment area is wide.
- The rehabilitation protocols described below summarize typical protocols that may be used, but may vary depending on the center, patient factors, and therapist experience.
- The ideal splint material would have the following properties:
  - A balance between durability (to resist breakage) and malleability/formability (to permit construction)

- Affordability
- Breathability
- Resistance to infection
- Nontoxic and hypoallergenic
- Commonly used splint materials:
  - Plaster of Paris (calcium sulfate hemihydrate, $CaSO_4 \cdot 0.5H_2O$), commonly used by surgeons fabricating postoperative splints, and occasionally used by hand therapists when removable splints are contraindicated
  - Resin cast, a formable roll of material commonly used to fabricate cylindrical casts, and which is less brittle and less prone to softening with further exposure to water than plaster of Paris
  - Thermoplastics, which are formable and conformable when heated in a water bath and rapidly set as they cool to room temperature. Commonly used for fabrication of custom splints, fastened by Velcro, and may integrate springs or elastic to provide dynamic effects
  - Neoprene and stretchable woven fabrics may be used for positioning where absolute immobilization is not required.
  - Aluminum with foam backing (AlumaFoam/Zimmer splint) is commonly used to fashion single-digit splints, which are affixed to the affected finger with coban tape, or Elastoplast.
  - Tape or Velcro buddy straps can be used alone for buddy-strapping of an injured digit to its uninjured neighbor.
- Rules common to all protocols:
  - The surgeon must clearly communicate the instructions for rehabilitation to their therapy team, particularly if there is any deviation from a standard protocol.
  - Good outcomes are dependent on a mutual understanding between the therapist and the patient of the level of commitment required and on the goals of therapy.
- Initiation of therapy
  - Most therapy protocols will commence 5 to 7 days postoperatively.
    - Flexor tendon repairs should typically be seen earlier, ideally within 3 days following repair.
  - Early therapy may allow a reduction in postoperative pain and swelling.
  - The first visit typically includes a change from postoperative splint to well-fitted therapeutic splint

Extensor Tendon Injuries

- Zone I (mallet injuries) and zone II
  - Manage in distal interphalangeal joint (DIPJ) hyperextension splint ($-10°$) but avoid skin blanching which can lead to skin necrosis

- Can be commercial (eg, Stack splint) or custom (eg, AlumaFoam/Zimmer or thermoplastic)
- Fit must be snug; check and adjust as initial swelling subsides.
- Splint initially for 6 weeks (surgical repair or bony mallet) or 8 weeks (closed soft tissue); strictly no DIPJ flexion.
- Wean (night wear) for further 2 weeks; this protocol may vary depending on center and therapist experience.
- Commence gentle active motion at 6-8 weeks.
- Graded return to normal activities from 10 to 12 weeks but avoid passive DIPJ flexion until 12-14 weeks
- Maintain PIPJ and MCPJ active range throughout.
- Zone III (central slip injuries)
  - Manage initially in digital volar gutter splint.
  - Surgical repairs for 2 weeks closed tendon injuries for 3 weeks
  - Allow free DIPJ from week 1 to 2 for isolated DIPJ active range exercises.
  - Switch to dynamic PIPJ extension splint (eg, Capener) at 2 to 4 weeks; provide static splint for night wear.
  - Commence active flexion exercises in Capener
    * 5 to 10 repetitions every 1 to 2 hours
    * Aim for 30° at week 2
    * Increase by 10° each week
  - If no PIPJ extensor lag, start to wean splint from week 5
  - Discard splint at week 6 and gradual return to normal activities by week 12
  - Extensor lag of greater than 30° may indicate failure of repair
- Zone IV, V and VI (including sagittal band injuries)
  - Splint options:
    * Merritt yoke splint with 15° hyperextension of affected digit (appropriate for 1-3 digits)
    * Volar splint from mid forearm to PIPJs, with wrist in 30° to 40° extension and MCPJs in neutral
  - Commence active IPJ flexion and extension exercises immediately.
  - Wean splint from 4 to 6 weeks, discard at 6 weeks, build toward normal activities at week 12.
- Zone VII and VIII
  - Manage in a volar splint from forearm to fingertips
    * Wrist in 20° (zone VI) to 45° (zone VIII) extension
    * MCPJs in 0° (neutral) extension
    * IPJs in neutral
  - Commence active IPJ flexion and extension exercises at week 2.

- From weeks 3 to 4, remove splint for gentle wrist flexion/extension exercises.
- Discard splint at week 6 and gradually build to normal activities by week 12.
- Extensor pollicis longus
  - For zone I and distal zone II
    - Manage in an IPJ extension splint (eg, thermoplastic or Zimmer), keeping MCPJ free.
    - Commence isolated thumb flexion to 30° at week 3.
    - Commence active composite thumb flexion from week 6.
    - Avoid isolated passive IPJ flexion before week 8.
    - Discard splint at week 6 (unless there is a lag) and gradually increase exercise.
    - Return to normal activities at week 12.
  - For zone III to zone VIII
    - Manage in a volar splint with wrist in 20°, thumb comfortably abducted and extended, IPJ in neutral.
    - Commence active IPJ thumb flexion from week 4.
    - Avoid composite IPJ and MCPJ flexion (passive or active) before week 6.
    - Discard splint at week 6 and gradually increase exercise.
    - Return to normal activities at week 12.

Flexor Tendon Injuries

- Goals of therapy and types of regimes
  - The ultimate goals of therapy following flexor tendon repair are to allow differential gliding of the flexor digitorum profundus and flexor digitorum superficialis tendons through a competent pulley system, in a finger which has a normal active and passive ROM and is free of pain and swelling.
  - The ideal repair is therefore strong enough to withstand motion at an early stage so that mobilization can occur prior to the onset of fibrosis and stiffness, and it is sufficiently smooth and low profile to eliminate drag as it passes through the tendon sheath.
  - Some tendon repairs will fail to meet at least one of these criteria, and so compromises must be made in rehabilitation. For the best quality repairs in motivated, compliant patients, the early active motion protocol may give the best outcomes. For more tenuous repairs, or repairs done in patients where communication, compliance, or motivation is an issue, there exist less demanding regimes which will also be described.

- Early active movement/controlled active motion (EAM/CAM; Gratton/Sheffield/Belfast)
  - This is appropriate for repairs using four or more core strands plus an epitendinous suture, where the surgeon has indicated that there is no gapping and minimal bunching, and there is a good glide through the pulley system on-table.
  - Forearm-based dorsal splint to fingertips with wrist in 20° extension, MCPJs 30° flexion, IPJs in extension
  - Commence hourly exercises on days 3 to 5
    - 10× passive flexion of IPJs and MCPJ
    - When good passive range, 10× active extension into splint, 10× gentle active flexion
    - Aim for one-quarter range in week 1, one-half range in week 2, full range in week 3
  - From week 3, concentrate on differential glide if passive range good using graduated hook grip and wrist tenodesis movements
  - At week 6, begin to discard splint, but consider night extension splinting in the presence of any flexion deformity.
  - Commence light activities from week 6.
  - Return to normal activities at week 12.
  - Flexion contractures are common and can be managed safely with finger gutter splints at night without significant increase in rupture rate
- Alternative regimes
  - Delayed mobilization
    - May be appropriate in children or unreliable adults
    - Immobilize the hand with wrist in 20° flexion, MCPJs 40° flexion, and IPJs in neutral or slightly flexed.
    - At 3 weeks, convert to dorsal splint with wrist in neutral, MCPJs 40° flexion, and IPJs extended; initiate gentle active flexion exercises out of splint with wrist in slight extension.
    - At 6 to 8 weeks, discard splint and concentrate on extensor lag and tendon gliding.
  - Early passive motion (based on Duran protocol)
    - May be indicated where repairs are delicate or insubstantial (eg, two strand repairs, poor quality tendon)
    - Forearm-based dorsal splint with wrist in 20° flexion, MCPJs in 50° to 70° flexion, and IPJs in neutral
    - From day 3, commence passive flexion and active extension of injured digit.
    - Add gentle "place and hold" with MCPJ, PIPJ, and DIPJ each at 45° flexion from week 2 or when edema has subsided and passive range is full.

* Note: place and hold in modern flexor tendon rehabilitation is contentious, with many authors arguing that it increases rupture rate
  - Add active digital flexion exercises at week 4, out of splint
  - Add wrist and composite (fist) flexion at week 5
  - Aim to discard splint at weeks 6 to 8.
  - Graduated return to normal activities from week 6 to week 10.
- Zone IV and zone V
  - Immobilize in slight wrist flexion for 4 weeks.
  - Begin active wrist flexion/extension, pronosupination and radial and ulnar deviation at week 3, provide splint for support
  - Gradually return to normal activities and discard splint from week 6.
- Wrist flexors
  - Follow protocol for zone IV / V flexors, but splint in wrist-based splint excluding fingers.
- Flexor pollicis longus
  - Splint with thumb in radial abduction and palmar abduction with slight MCPJ flexion, leaving uninjured fingers free
  - Commence exercises as per finger flexor EAM/CAM regime.

FRACTURES AND JOINT INJURIES

- Splinting of fractures may be indicated as a primary treatment for cases in which the fracture deformity has been corrected satisfactorily and any dislocation has been reduced. The surgeon must monitor their patients carefully for signs of malposition, such as rotational deformities or scissoring of neighboring digits, and for the duration of conservative therapy.
- In some cases, hand fractures treated with open reduction and internal fixation can be considered stable enough to permit early active exercises. Splints in these cases may be provided for comfort.
- Closed reduction and Kirschner wire fixation are less likely to produce a rigid construct, and so splints may be used to provide additional immobilization to protect the repair and permit fracture healing, but wherever possible (i.e. where there is adequate stability) early active mobilisation should be a priority.
- The choice of whether to splint for immobilization or comfort will, in all cases, remain with the operating surgeon.
- Detailed guidance on the closed manipulation of hand fractures and the application of plaster of Paris splints is beyond the scope of this text.

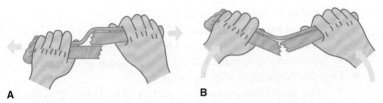

A **B**

FIGURE 62.2 Fracture reduction maneuvers. A, Longitudinal traction and (B) reversing the mechanism of injury can help to realign fragments.

The AO Foundation provides excellent online resources and courses that cover the details of these techniques. The basic principles include:

- Perform manual reduction, involving a combination of traction to disimpact and pressure to correct displacement (Figure 62.2).
- Screen the fracture (using an image intensifier) to check position prior to casting.
- Apply stockinette and cast padding, concentrated over bony prominences.
- Using plaster of Paris immersed in cold water (to prevent burns because of exothermic reaction), fashion the splint, aiming for 10 to 12 thicknesses.
- Apply three-point pressure to maintain the reduction (Figure 62.3).

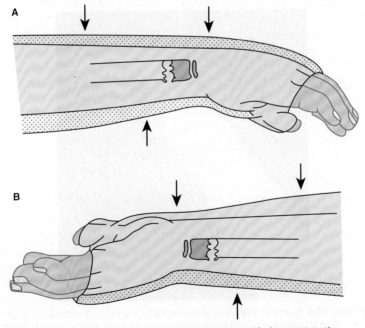

FIGURE 62.3 A and B, An example of a three-point molded cast. Note the dorsal periosteal bridge. The three compression points act to maintain reduction.

- Phalangeal and metacarpal fractures
  - Metacarpal base fractures (see also Chapter 11)
    - Volar splint from forearm to MCPJs with wrist in 20° extension
    - Start to mobilize from 4 weeks, discard splint at 6 weeks
  - Unstable Metacarpal shaft fractures
    - Volar splint from forearm to finger tips with wrist in 20° extension and MCPJs in 50° to 90° flexion, IPJs in neutral
    - Stable metacarpal shaft fractures
      * May be treated with minimal splinting, for example a removable Futuro splint
    - Maintaining the position can be difficult; use of a dorsal hood is possible to assist in three-point molding (dorsal pressure over the fracture, volar pressure proximal and distal to the fracture).
    - Ring or little metacarpals can be treated in an ulnar gutter splint covering only those two fingers, freeing the index and middle (Figure 62.4). A similar radial gutter can be used for index or middle metacarpal fractures.
      * Start to mobilize from 5 weeks, discard splint at 6 weeks.
  - Unstable Metacarpal neck fractures

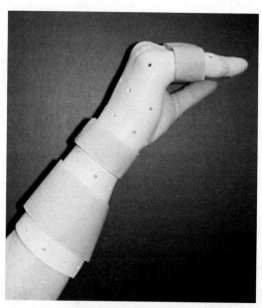

FIGURE 62.4 Example of an ulnar gutter splint for managing a metacarpal shaft fracture. With permission from Hammert W, Boyer M, Bozentka D, Calfee R. *ASSH Manual of Hand Surgery.* Philadelphia, PA: Lippincott Williams & Wilkins; 2010.

- ◆ Volar splint from forearm to MCPJs with wrist in 20° extension. Dorsal splint component over hand and fingers, with MCPJs in 90° flexion, IPJs in neutral (Burkhalter splint).
- ◆ Mobilize MCPJ and IPJs early, goal to discard splint at 4 weeks
- ◆ Many metacarpal neck fractures are stable, impacted fractures. These may be managed with minimal splinting, e.g. Futuro splint for comfort
- Phalanx fractures (see also Chapter 5)
  - ◆ The range of possible fracture patterns is as broad as the range of methods of reduction and fixation.
  - ◆ For nonarticular phalangeal fractures that are minimally displaced, with no rotation or angulation:
    - ✳ Dorsal or volar hand-based splint with MCPJs in 70-90° flexion and IPJs in neutral.
    - ✳ Begin gentle active flexion and extension exercises early, aiming to discard the splint by 4 to 6 weeks.
    - ✳ Note that some undisplaced, stable phalangeal fractures may be managed appropriately with simple neighbor-strapping, with splints only for comfort or protection at night or in busy surroundings.
- Thumb fractures and ulnar collateral ligament injuries (see also Chapters 10 and 11)
  - ◆ Stable, extra-articular thumb metacarpal and proximal phalangeal fractures and partial skier's thumb/ulnar collateral ligament injuries may be managed in a spica splint (Figure 62.5).
    - ✳ Leave IPJ free.
    - ✳ Immobilize thumb in slight radial abduction and slight palmar abduction to prevent first web contracture.
    - ✳ Mobilize IPJ and fingers early.
    - ✳ Aim to discard splint at 3 to 4 weeks.
- ■ Scaphoid fractures (see also Chapter 14)
  - Apply a scaphoid cast, with wrist in 20° extension and thumb in slight radial abduction and slight palmar abduction (Figure 62.6).
  - While some biomechanical studies suggest that thumb immobilization may reduce motion at a scaphoid fracture, clinical data suggest that inclusion of the thumb may not affect union rates.
  - Mobilize the thumb and fingers, leaving IPJ free.
  - At 6 weeks, consider repeat imaging and examination out of cast.
- ■ Forearm fractures: casting may be appropriate in stable, nondisplaced (or reduced), extra-articular fractures.
  - Distal radius and ulnar fractures (see also Chapters 26 and 28)
    - ◆ Cast using the principles of three-point molding, with the wrist in 20° to 30° extension, and the MCP and IPJs free (Figure 62.7).

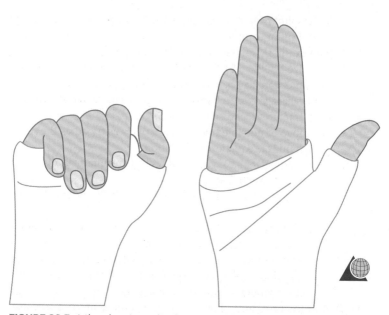

FIGURE 62.5 A thumb spica splint, keeping the finger metacarpophalangeal (MCP) and interphalangeal joints (IPJs) free, and the thumb IPJ free. This splint immobilizes the basal thumb joint and the thumb MCP joint and provides some stability to the proximal phalanx.

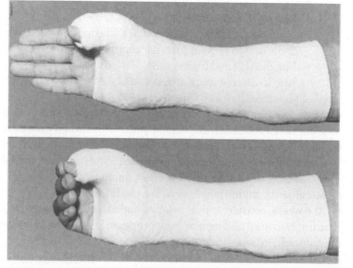

FIGURE 62.6 Example of a scaphoid plaster. With permission from Salter R. *Textbook of Disorders and Injuries of the Musculoskeletal System*. Philadelphia, PA: Lippincott Williams & Wilkins; 1998.

  ✳ Be careful not to apply casts too tightly, as tight casts may be associated with the development of chronic regional pain syndrome (CRPS)
- ◆ Mobilize the digits immediately.
- ◆ At 4 to 6 weeks, consider repeat imaging and examination out of cast (see Chapter 26).
  - ✳ If concern for possible displacement, consider repeat imaging in cast before this point.
  - ✳ Initial displacement is best predictor of late displacement and can be used to determine whether earlier imaging is required.
- ◆ If both forearm bones are involved and casting is appropriate, consider a sugar-tong splint or Muenster cast to prevent prono-supination (Figure 62.8).

SPLINTING AFTER PERIPHERAL NERVE INJURY

- Ulnar nerve palsy
  - Static anti-claw splint
    - ◆ Counteracts MCPJ hyperextension, correcting intrinsic minus position of ring and little fingers (all four fingers can be included in cases of combined median and ulnar nerve injuries). Results in improved cylinder grip performance
    - ◆ Suitable as a functional (daytime) splint for patients who can't actively overcome MCPJ hyperextension
- Median nerve palsy
  - Night thumb abduction splint to prevent first web space adduction contracture

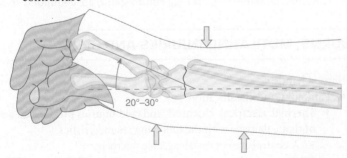

FIGURE 62.7 Example of a below-elbow distal radius cast demonstrating the principle of three-point molding.

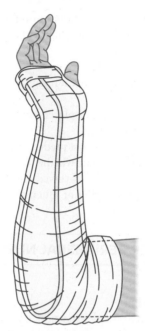

FIGURE 62.8 Example of a sugar-tong splint to limit pronosupination.

- Functional abduction splint (eg, neoprene opponens strap) for day-time wear to allow opposition against a weak thumb
- High lesions
■ Radial nerve or posterior interosseous nerve palsy
- Static, volar splint at night to immobilize wrist in 15° to 30° extension to prevent shortening of long flexors
- Commercial splints (eg, the long Futuro splint) are commonly used.

BURNS, MUTILATING INJURIES AND CRPS

■ Burned hands
- Pathology and classification
  ◆ Thermal, electrical, chemical, and cold injuries produce an area of tissue damage with the following characteristics:
    ∗ A central area of unsalvageable necrosis
    ∗ A surrounding area of stasis that may survive if treated well or become necrotic if it suffers further insult
    ∗ A peripheral area of hyperemia that will return to normal
  ◆ The severity and duration of the insult will influence the breadth and depth of tissue injury.

* Superficial/first-degree injuries produce erythema only, with no necrosis.
* Partial thickness/second-degree injuries cause necrosis of varying depth within the epidermis and dermis, with no deep structural injury and the capacity for full skin healing.
* Full thickness/third-degree injuries cause necrosis of subcutaneous tissues, which may include longitudinal structures and minimal or no capacity for healing without surgery.
- Natural history of burn contractures
  - An intrinsic minus position (hyperextended MCPJs, flexed IPJs, flexed wrist, adducted thumb, extended thumb IPJ) develops rapidly because of edema.
  - High concentrations of inflammatory mediators provoke scarring and fibrosis.
  - Scar contractures, particularly of the dorsal hand, exacerbate MCPJ hyperextension, leading to a characteristic burn claw.
  - Contributors to reduced ROM include:
    * Edema
    * Undebrided eschar
    * Neocollagen formation (scar contracture)
  - Depending on the depth of injury, many deformities can result, including boutonnière, swan-neck, adduction contractures, and pseudosyndactyly.
- Early therapy
  - The surgeon should be aware of the risk of compartment syndrome and the indications for escharotomies.
  - Elevate burned upper limbs in slings or on foam wedges.
  - Splint the hand in POSI
    * Mobilize joints early in superficial burns.
    * In deeper burns over PIPJs, some advocate prolonged immobilization to reduce risk of boutonnière.
    * Finger IPJs maybe immobilized in gutter splints, permitting MCPJ mobilization.
  - Splint the elbow in extension to prevent flexion contracture; mobilize regularly to prevent fixed extension deformity.
  - Splint the shoulder in abduction to prevent axillary contracture.
  - ROM exercises (active or passive) should be performed opportunistically at dressing changes whether the patient is awake or anesthetized. Active ROM exercises are less painful than passive ROM exercises.
  - Goals of early therapy:
    * Full fist closure
    * Full digital extension
    * Thumb opposition, abduction, and extension

- Late therapy
  - The scar remodeling and maturation phase in burns is prolonged.
  - Splinting must continue until scar activity reduces.
    - Active scars are erythematous, itchy, raised, and firm.
    - Scar activity may reduce over time, or following scar release surgery.
    - Splinting may be required long term (months to years).
  - Established contractures tend to be refractory to splinting.
  - Surgery is the mainstay.
  - Serial casting at maximal stretch may increase ROM.
    - Check neurovascular status after casting.
    - Change casts frequently (from daily to weekly depending on the patient).
  - Conforming thermoplastic splints may be used to prevent web space contracture, especially the first web space.
  - When tolerated, the patient should begin resistive exercises and activities that encourage finger dexterity.
  - Scar massage can help soften contracture bands or sheets of scar.
  - Other components of scar management:
    - Pressure therapy, including the incorporation of acrylic plates within splints
    - Topical silicone therapy
- Therapy after surgery
  - Grafts require immobilization for the first 5 to 7 days to prevent shear and graft loss.
  - Mobilization should begin as soon as graft take is identified.
  - Minor graft loss should be tolerated in favor of early motion.
- Mutilating hand injuries
  - Mutilating injuries present specific challenges to rehabilitation because they may affect multiple structures, including long flexors and extensors, bone and joints, nerve supply, vascularity, and the skin.
  - Early phase
    - Clear communication between the surgeon and therapist
    - Control of edema and pain
      - Analgesia and resting splints for pain
      - Elevation for edema
    - Balance the requirement for mobilization against the need to immobilize certain structures.
    - Mobilize uninvolved joints.
    - Protect repaired structures.
    - Facilitate wound healing (allow for dressings).
  - Intermediate phase

- Document ROM and sensibility.
- Modify splinting and mobilization regime regularly.
- Permit tendon gliding and joint ROM when permitted by tendon or fracture healing.
- Identify and treat hypersensitivity and joint contractures.
- Late phase (3 weeks to scar maturation)
  - Document ROM and sensibility.
  - Aggressive scar management; moisturize, massage, and pressure; surgery if indicated
  - Compressive but unrestrictive wraps for control of edema if persistent
  - Identify limitations of ROM by adhesions and contracture because of prior immobilization or rupture of repaired structures
    - Consider increasing intensity of active ROM exercise, versus further surgical intervention
    - After 6 weeks or depending on structures repaired may require night splinting or serial casting if significant joint contractures exist
    - Create targeted goals for regaining activities of daily living and function required for employment (strength, endurance, and dexterity)
    - Consider social support and alternative employment
- Complex regional pain syndrome (CRPS)
  - Definition and diagnosis
    - The Budapest criteria define CRPS as persistent pain that is disproportionate to the severity of injury.
    - To make the diagnosis, the patient must have symptoms in three of four, and clinical signs in two of four of the following categories, and no other plausible diagnosis:
      - Motor or trophic change (decreased ROM or power, tremor, altered hair or nail growth, skin changes)
      - Sensory (hypersensitivity, allodynia, or hyperpathia)
      - Sudomotor (edema, sweating asymmetry)
      - Vasomotor (temperature or color asymmetry)
    - CRPS is a clinical diagnosis.
    - Investigations may be useful in exploring differential diagnoses.
    - There is no investigation to confirm the diagnosis of CRPS.
  - Management
    - The mainstay of treatment for CRPS is hand therapy, comprising many of the elements previously discussed.
    - Early and regular therapy is most likely to be effective.
    - Functional goal setting and psychological support, including relaxation techniques

- Reduce edema through elevation, active exercises, massage, taping techniques (eg, Kinesio taping), and pressure garments.
- Desensitization techniques
- Active and passive range of movement exercises within the patient's tolerance
- Graded motor imagery
  * A proprietary technique involving multiple stages
  * Laterality training (reeducating the discrimination between left and right)
  * Explicit motor imagery (imagining joint and limb positions, progression to imagining active movements)
  * Sensory discrimination (retraining of the associations between sensory perception and different textures)
  * Mirror therapy (cortical retraining by watching the mirror image of the unaffected limb perform movements and interact with objects)
- Management of neuropathic pain with gabapentin or pregabalin
- There is weak evidence in favor of topical local anesthetics (eg, patches), transcutaneous electrical neurostimulation, and invasive techniques such as sympathetic blocks, epidurals, and spinal cord or peripheral nerve stimulators.

SUGGESTED READINGS

Star HM, Snoddy M, Hammond KE, Seiler JG. Flexor Tendon Repair Rehabilitation Protocols: A Systematic Review. *J Hand Surg*. 2013;38(9):1712-1717.

Tang JB. Recent evolutions in flexor tendon repairs and rehabilitation. *J Hand Surg Eur*. 2018;43(5):469-473.

Glasgow C, Tooth L, Fleming J. Which Splint? Dynamic versus Static Progressive Splinting to Mobilise Stiff Joints in the Hand. *Hand Therapy*. 2008;13(4):104-110.

Higgins A, Lalonde DH. Flexor Tendon Repair Postoperative Rehabilitation: The Saint John Protocol. *Plast Reconstr Surg Glob Open*. 2016;4(11):e1134.

Miller LK, Jerosch-Herold C, Shepstone L. Effectiveness of edema management techniques for subacute hand edema: A systematic review. *J Hand Ther*. 2017;30(4):432-446.

Gülke J, Leopold B, Grözinger D, Drews B, Paschke S, Wachter NJ. Postoperative treatment of metacarpal fractures - Classical physical therapy compared with a home exercise program. *J Hand Ther*. 2018;31(1):20-28.

Peck FH, Roe AE, Ng CY, Duff C, McGrouther DA, Lees VC. The Manchester short splint: A change to splinting practice in the rehabilitation of zone II flexor tendon repairs. *Hand Therapy*. 2014;19(2):47-53.

Cooper C. *Fundamentals of Hand Therapy*. 2nd ed. Philadelphia, PA: Elsevier; 2014

Wolfe S, Pederson W, Kozin SH, Cohen M. *Green's Operative Hand Surgery*. 7th ed. Philadelphia, PA: Elsevier; 2016.

63 How to Remove a Tight Ring

John C. Elfar and David J. Ciufo

INTRODUCTION

- Constrictive rings are a common problem encountered in acute care settings.
- A tight ring may occur either in isolation or in the setting of trauma.
- Constricting items may include metal hardware (nuts and washers) in addition to jewelry.
- Patients often try home-based methods of removal before presentation.
- The hand is often the dependent portion of the upper extremity, predisposing it to swelling in the setting of trauma or edema due to medical diagnoses.
- Edema coupled with outflow obstruction leads to a cycle of increasing venous congestion.
- Arterial obstruction can lead to digital ischemia in severe cases.
- Rings should prophylactically be removed in the setting of upper extremity trauma.

EVALUATION

- Identification of potentially constricting jewelry is a critical first step in the setting of trauma.
- Previous attempts at removal and duration of constriction are important elements of a thorough history.
- Neurologic and vascular examination of the entire extremity is critical, along with documentation of the examination findings, before and after removal of constricting devices.
- A focused neurologic and vascular examination of the affected digit should be performed.

- The type of material causing constriction may affect the management (soft vs. hard metal vs. ceramic or stone).

PATIENT MANAGEMENT

- Attempts to remove a ring are sometimes destructive of the ring itself, and patients should be warned of this possibility.
- If vascular status is compromised (absent capillary refill, mottling of the digit), the ring should be removed emergently.
- Provide a field block if indicated for the patient to better tolerate removal.
  - This should be avoided if removal methods would benefit from protective sensation for feedback from the patient.
  - Injection of local anesthetic should be performed with caution because this could add fluid and increase swelling of the affected digit.
- Efforts should be made to repeat imaging studies after removal to avoid missed injuries to the affected digit.
- Rings should never be left in place under splints or other forms of immobilization.
- Avoid intravenous access in an injured extremity when possible.

METHODS OF RING REMOVAL

Edema Management

- Compression of the entire digit by wrapping it with an elastic tourniquet (such as those used for intravenous access) may be used to reduce edema.
- Ice and elevation may be sufficient to reduce minor edema and allow the ring to slide off.
- These are some of the simplest methods and often have been attempted before presentation in isolated tight-ring situations.

Lubricants

- Apply lubricant such as soap or surgical lubricating jelly in the area of obstruction, as well as around and distal to the ring, then rotate the ring to coat the undersurface.

- Once the ring and finger are sufficiently lubricated, an attempt to slide the ring past the obstructing region can be made.
- Rotating the ring while sliding it distally is the most successful strategy.
- The goal is reduction of friction to allow the ring to slide past an obstruction.

String Wrap

- **This is the authors' preferred method.**
- This can be completed with string, heavy suture, or ribbon gauze (ie, packing gauze).
- One end of the string is passed under the ring to provide a several-inch tail proximally.
  - This may require a hemostat/forceps depending on tightness at the position of the ring.
- The string is wrapped in a spiral fashion starting at the proximal end of the constricted digit and proceeding toward the distal aspect.
  - It is important to overlap the wrap to obtain sufficient tissue compression.
  - The wrap should bypass the obstruction as seen in Figure 63.1.
- The string is then unwound from the proximal end, pulling it toward the distal end as it is unwrapped.
- The unwrapping process should spiral around the finger, with a distally directed force.

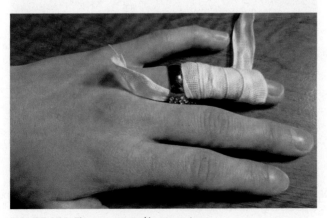

FIGURE 63.1 Finger wrapped in gauze tape.

- The ring will be carried distally with the string as it unwinds, bypassing the obstruction, as seen in Figure 63.2.
- This occasionally requires the string to be rewrapped and the process repeated because the ring may not completely pass the obstruction in the first attempt.

Glove Slide

- A surgical glove is used, with stronger gloves being more effective, for this technique.
- A finger from the glove is cut at both ends to produce a cylindrical sleeve.
- The sleeve is pulled over the affected digit, with the proximal end slipped under the ring using forceps or a hemostat.
- The proximal portion of the glove is grasped at two points and pulled distally, carrying the ring with it.

Ring Cutting or Breakage

- Commercial manual ring cutters

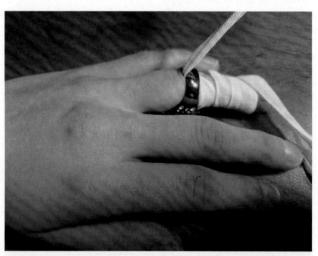

FIGURE 63.2 Removal of ring over proximal interphalangeal (PIP) joint by pulling gauze tape distally in spiral fashion.

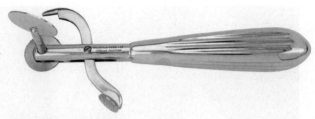

FIGURE 63.3 Commercial ring cutter.

- These work best on thinner rings and can be used on most metal rings. A basic example can be seen in Figure 63.3.
- The device has a smooth edge for protection of the underlying skin.
- The protective edge is placed between the ring and digit, and the thumb piece is pressed to squeeze the cutting blade against the ring.
- The handle is manually rotated to cut through the ring.
- This technique is unable to cut tungsten carbide or other hardened rings.
- Ring cutting via electric rotary tool
  - These are less often available in most health care settings.
  - Requires use of a grinding or cutting attachment
  - There is a risk of abrasive or heat damage to the affected digit, which can be avoided by the use of saline or water irrigation
  - The process will produce debris, which could contaminate wounds.
  - Eye protection should be used by the health care practitioner and patient.
  - Nerve blocks should be avoided for this procedure to allow for patient feedback to minimize the risk of thermal injury.
- Ring breakage for removal
  - Tungsten carbide or other hard rings (ie, ceramic, stone) that cannot be cut can be broken off.
  - A vice grip can be used to compress the ring at multiple points along its circumference to fracture or weaken the ring, as demonstrated in Figure 63.4.
  - After several sequential compressions, the ring should break off the digit.
  - Adjustable locking pliers or vice grips are most effective because they allow finer adjustment of the force applied to the ring.
  - Care should be taken not to crush the underlying digit.

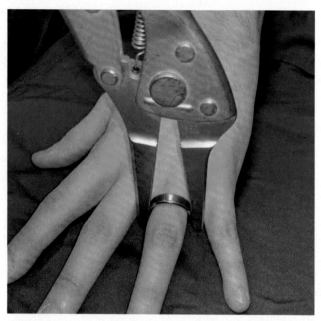

FIGURE 63.4 Use of vice grip to compress ring for breakage.

SUGGESTED READINGS

Allen KA, Rizzo M, Sadosty AT. A method for the removal of tungsten carbide rings. *J Emerg Med*. 2012;43:93.

Baker A, Rylance K, Giles S. The occasional ring removal. *Can J Rural Med*. 2010;15:26.

Belliappa PP. A technique for removal of a tight ring. *J Hand Surg Br*. 1989;14:127.

Cresap CR. Removal of a hardened steel ring from an extremely swollen finger. *Am J Emerg Med*. 1995;13:318.

Greenspan L. Tourniquet syndrome caused by metallic bands: a new tool for removal. *Ann Emerg Med*. 1982;11:375.

64 Vascular Evaluation of the Hand

Christopher M. Jones and Beatrice L. Grasu

INTRODUCTION

- A diagnosis of vascular insufficiency of the upper extremity begins with taking a thorough history and performing a physical exam.
- Hand held doppler ultrasounds are useful to audibly and visually evaluate normal or obstructed vessels throughout the upper extremity (UE).
- The vascular laboratory includes several crucial tests to evaluate vascular insufficiency including Doppler fluxometry, plethysmography, cold stress testing, and nail fold capillaroscopy.
- Angiography is the **gold standard for evaluation of vasculature,** but the evolution of CT and magnetic resonance imaging (MRI) has improved visualization of upper limb vessels in a noninvasive manner.

VASCULAR PATHOLOGY IN THE UPPER EXTREMITY

- Vascular disorders are much more common in the lower limb than in the upper limb; however, UE vascular disorders may be just as debilitating.
- May present as part of a systemic disorder affecting both extremities or as a specific injury to one UE
  - Upper extremity bloodflow is both thermoregulatory and nutritional with symptoms of
    - cold sensitivity
    - signs of ulceration
    - skin changes such as hair loss
    - numbness, pain, and/or gangrene[1]
- *Vaso-occlusive disease*
  - Physical obstruction
  - Structural abnormalities
  - Vasospastic disease
  - Combination

- Primary goal of treatment—restore pulsatile blood flow to nutritional capillary beds

VASCULAR ANATOMY OF THE UPPER EXTREMITY

- **Arterial supply** is derived from the *subclavian artery*
  - Originates from the brachiocephalic (innominate) artery on the right
  - Directly from the aortic arch on the left
  - The subclavian artery branches to the head and neck before it becomes the *axillary artery* at the level of the first rib
    - First supplies branches to both the shoulder and scapula
  - The axillary artery then becomes the *brachial artery* just below the axilla.
  - The brachial artery travels medially down the arm and elbow to give off a deep branch and collateral vessels that provide an arterial anastomosis to the elbow.
    - Terminates just distal to the elbow in its bifurcation to the *radial and ulnar arteries*, which course along their respective sides of the forearm
  - The ulnar and radial arteries give off recurrent arteries to also provide collateral circulation around the elbow.
    - The ulnar artery also gives off an *interosseous branch* that trifurcates into posterior, recurrent, and anterior branches
    - Further distally, the ulnar artery becomes the *superficial palmar arch*.
    - The radial artery becomes the *deep palmer arch*.
    - Both arches of the hand give off arterial branches to supply the thumb and fingers.[2]
- **Venous system** of the UE includes a superficial and deep network.
  - Superficially, the *cephalic vein* is located more lateral in the upper arm; the *basilic vein* is located more medially.
    - These two veins typically join just distal to the elbow at the *median antecubital vein*.
  - The deep system includes the *radial and ulnar veins* in the forearm, which unite caudal to the elbow to form the *brachial veins*.
  - The brachial veins join the basilic vein typically at the level of the teres major muscle and continue as the *axillary vein*.
  - The axillary vein passes through the axilla and crosses the first rib before becoming the lateral portion of the *subclavian vein*.
    - The medial portion of the subclavian vein includes the *external and internal jugular vein*, which all flow into the *brachiocephalic vein*.

HISTORY AND PHYSICAL EXAMINATION

- Crucial portion of the evaluation and must include:
  - Past medical history, cardiac history, smoking use
  - Any similar symptoms in the contralateral extremity or lower extremities
  - Patients may not report any symptoms from mild vascular disease; however, they may describe pain from repetitive use of their UEs causing intermittent claudication.
- As the disease progresses, skin, nail, and hair changes and pain may occur.
- Evaluate patient's general appearance and perform a cardiovascular examination followed by examination of the affected extremity.
  - Compare the affected upper limb to the contralateral limb.
  - Palpate the radial, ulnar, and brachial pulses for intact arterial flow.
  - Inspect skin for color or pallor, ulcerations, hair loss, or fingernail changes that may display hallmark signs of embolic or other signs of chronic ischemia (Figure 64.1).
- Specific physical examination tests for vascular pathology
  - Allen test (Figure 64.2)
    - Physical exam maneuver that can identify specific arterial patency.[1]
    - Unlike ulnar artery aneurysms, radial artery aneurysms do not generally cause arterial occlusion.
      - Test might demonstrate normal flow through the radial artery despite pathology.
    - Performing the test
      - Elevate the hand and ask the patient to make a fist for 30 seconds to 1 minute.
      - Apply pressure to both the radial and ulnar arteries to occlude them.
      - With hand still elevated, ask the patient to open the fist. Observe hand pallor.
      - Release pressure off one of the arteries, but maintain pressure on the other.
      - Determine how long it takes for the color to return to the hand.
      - Repeat the examination but reverse which artery remains occluded.
      - A normal exam is observed when color returns within six seconds

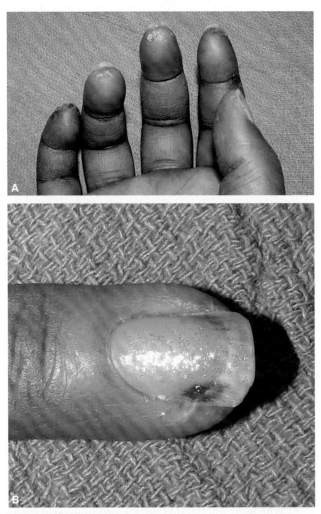

FIGURE 64.1 Ischemic ulcerations at the tips of second through fifth digits prior to revascularization (A). Nail changes also known as *splinter hemorrhages* indicating digital vessel emboli and capillary ischemia (B). Originally printed in Grasu BL, Jones CM, Murphy MS. Use of diagnostic modalities for assessing upper extremity vascular pathology. *Hand Clin*. 2015;31(1):1-12. Courtesy of R.D. Katz, MD, Baltimore, Maryland.

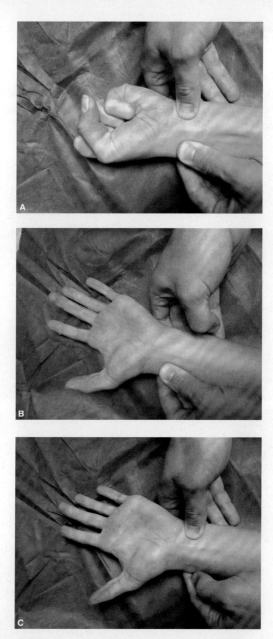

FIGURE 64.2 Perform the Allen test to assess for ulnar versus radial dominance by compressing both the ulnar and radial arteries until the hand becomes pale (A). Then release pressure on the ulnar artery while maintaining compression on the radial artery (B). Evaluate for capillary perfusion and then repeat the test by reversing the compressed vessel (C). Originally printed in Grasu BL, Jones CM, Murphy MS. Use of diagnostic modalities for assessing upper extremity vascular pathology. *Hand Clin.* 2015;31(1):1-12.

- Digital Allen test (Figure 64.3)
  - Elevate hand/perform digital artery occlusion at base of digit.
  - Flex the finger several times to cause blanching and then the hand is lowered.

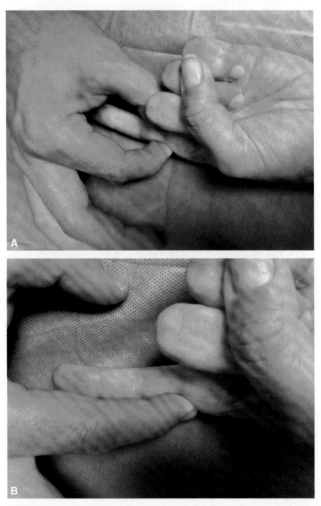

FIGURE 64.3 A,B, The Allen test can also be performed in the hand to assess radial and ulnar digital artery circulation. Originally printed in Grasu BL, Jones CM, Murphy MS. Use of diagnostic modalities for assessing upper extremity vascular pathology. *Hand Clin.* 2015;31(1):1-12.

- ◆ If the finger remains blanched after lowering the hand and releasing compression of one digital artery, then the released digital artery is considered compromised.[1]
- Handheld Doppler evaluates blood flow or velocity through the radial and ulnar arteries at the wrist and the digital arteries.
  - ◆ Allows "mapping" of the arterial network
  - ◆ Several types of Doppler transducers to match specific requirements for physiologic application
    - ∗ Suction-on Doppler flow probes or suture-down transducers
    - ∗ Extravascular Doppler flow transducer is most commonly seen for evaluation of the UE in particular
      - ▲ Stainless steel tube with a 1 mm diameter piezoelectric crystal mounted at a 45° angle inside
      - ▲ Angle the probe at 45° to the vascular bed while using conductive gel and avoiding excessive compression (Figure 64.4)
      - ▲ The reflected sound waves result from the movement of blood cells and vary with blood flow velocity. This velocity is visualized in a triphasic flow pattern if it is normal, whereas

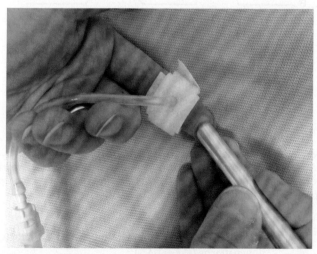

FIGURE 64.4 Using a conductive gel, angle the Doppler probe about 45° to the vessel being studied. Originally printed in Grasu BL, Jones CM, Murphy MS. Use of diagnostic modalities for assessing upper extremity vascular pathology. *Hand Clin.* 2015;31(1):1-12.

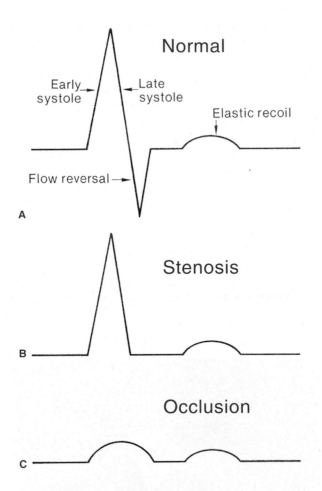

FIGURE 64.5 Normal arterial waveform patterns of the Doppler signal have a triphasic pattern (A) while obstructed (B) and stenotic (C) vessels have these characteristic patterns. Reprinted with permission from Koman LA. Diagnostic study of vascular lesions. *Hand Clin.* 1985;1(2):221. Copyright © Elsevier.

areas of occlusion or compression also have characteristic flow patterns (Figure 64.5).

▲ There is no correlation between the arterial Doppler signal and systolic blood pressure or actual blood volume.[1]

▲ The Allen test may be performed while using the handheld Doppler to assess the arterial flow in the digits (Figure 64.6).

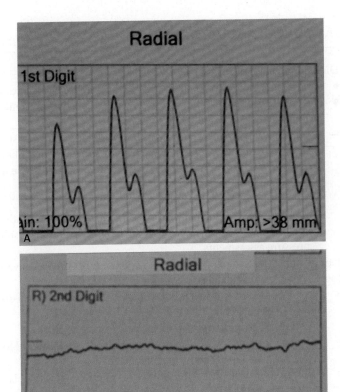

FIGURE 64.6 Normal triphasic Doppler signal of the first digit while performing the Allen test and obstructing the radial artery (A). Evaluation of the second digit during Allen testing revealed an obstruction in the ulnar digital artery with this Doppler signal (B). Originally printed in Grasu BL, Jones CM, Murphy MS. Use of diagnostic modalities for assessing upper extremity vascular pathology. *Hand Clin.* 2015;31(1):1-12, copyright Elsevier.

- Adson maneuver
  - Arm abduction and extension while rotating the patient's head to the ipsilateral elevated arm and extending the neck after deep inspiration
  - Palpate the radial pulse before and during the maneuver. If pulse decreases or is completely absent, the maneuver is positive for diagnosis of thoracic outlet obstruction
  - Patients frequently complain of vague, diffuse arm pain or fatigue with activity, especially overhead exercises

VASCULAR LABORATORY

- Digital brachial index (DBI)
  - Ratio of the systolic pressure of the digit to the systolic brachial pressure
  - Place a miniature blood pressure cuff on the respective digit and the systolic value is obtained (Figure 64.7).
  - Abnormally large pressure gradients between the two suggest structural, obstructive disease such as stenosis, thrombosis, or embolus.
    - A ratio <0.7 is indicative of significant vascular disease and treatment is encouraged.[1]
    - A DBI of 0.5 suggests imminent digital gangrene.
    - Be cautious of a normal or elevated index in diabetic patients because their vessels may be calcified, falsely elevating absolute pressure assessments.
- Laser Doppler fluxometry and perfusion imaging are other noninvasive tools available to evaluate vascular flow of the UE.
  - Laser Doppler uses laser lights to measure the flux or real-time cutaneous perfusion.
    - Quantitative measurement of surface skin blood flow
  - Flow measurements reflect movement of capillary cells and blood flow in the peripheral thermoregulatory bed.[1]
  - A color-coded image of the tissue perfusion distribution is reproduced on a computer screen, which provides mean perfusion values.[1]
- Color Duplex ultrasound provides real-time structural and functional vascular anomalies.
- Ultrasound is the initial imaging modality to evaluate the UE venous system.
  - Differentiate between deep and superficial veins
    - Deep veins have arteries running with them in the upper limb.
    - Deep venous system is clinically important in cases of obstruction or thrombosis.
  - Indications
    - Assessment of dialysis access and intravenous access
    - Venous mapping before harvest for arterial bypass
    - Determine or follow-up of venous thrombosis, aneurysm, or hematoma[3,4]
  - The overlying clavicle and first rib make UE ultrasound more technically challenging than the lower extremity.

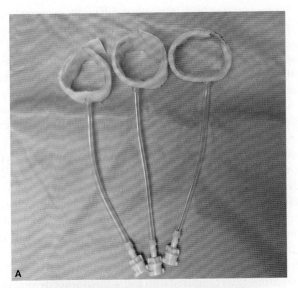

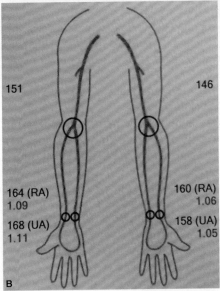

FIGURE 64.7 A, Blood pressure cuffs to obtain systolic digital blood pressure. B, Useful in calculating digital brachial index. Originally printed in Grasu BL, Jones CM, Murphy MS. Use of diagnostic modalities for assessing upper extremity vascular pathology. *Hand Clin.* 2015;31(1):1-12.

- Valsalva maneuver or brisk inspiratory sniff results in normal venous collapse or narrowing and may assist in determining significant stenosis or obstruction of the deep, central venous system.[3]
- Color images may be acquired to appreciate real-time venous or arterial blood flow and a corresponding Doppler signal can be obtained (Figure 64.8).
- If sonographic findings are equivocal or nondiagnostic, especially in studies of the central deep veins, further imaging such as magnetic resonance venography may be useful.[4]

- Plethysmography is the study of changes in volume of an organ from the fluctuations in blood or air it contains.
  - Study of changes in digital blood volume
  - Air-filled cuffs connected to pressure transducers and photoplethysmographs
  - Pulse volume recording (PVR) is a *functional* test, meaning that it evaluates all the blood flow to the examined extremity, not just a specific blood vessel.
    - The surface area under the PVR waveform is entered into a spreadsheet and compared with and without arterial compression to calculate the pulse–volume ratio.
    - A pulse–volume ratio close to 0 indicates that this compressed artery is required for pulsatile flow to the digit, whereas a ratio of 1 or greater suggests that this artery is not required for digital blood flow.[5]
  - Transmitter–receiver unit usually <1 cm^2 is placed on the pulp of the tested digit to obtain PVRs
    - Using a light-emitting diode, infrared light signals are transmitted and received from moving erythrocytes (Figure 64.9).[6]
    - Varies with changes in digital artery blood content and lumen dimension[1,6]
    - Similar to Doppler readings, the tracing of a normal artery should produce a triphasic wave pattern.
      * Stenotic and occluded vessels will produce classic, pathognomonic waveform patterns (Figure 64.10).
    - Pre- and postoperative plethysmographs may be obtained to evaluate effectiveness of interventions, such as digital periarterial sympathectomy for scleroderma or severe Raynaud disease.
- Digital temperature evaluation is a crude method to assess vascular flow.
  - Cutaneous surface temperature of the digit is directly proportional to blood flow and normally ranges between 20°C and 30°C.[1]

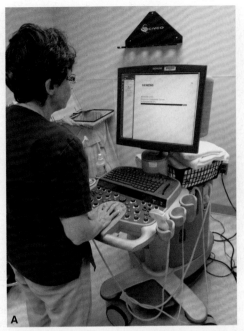

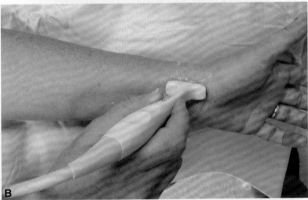

FIGURE 64.8 Ultrasound is often the first noninvasive vascular study to evaluate pathology and is typically performed in the vascular suite by a trained technician (A). To obtain an image, use conductive gel and place the probe at about a 45° angle (B).

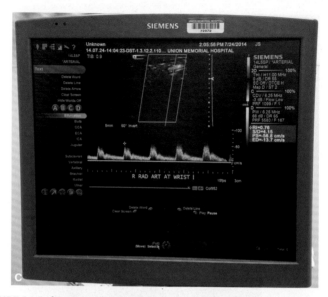

FIGURE 64.8 *(continued)* Color ultrasound images may be acquired to appreciate real-time venous or arterial blood flow and a corresponding Doppler signal can be obtained (C). Originally printed in Grasu BL, Jones CM, Murphy MS. Use of diagnostic modalities for assessing upper extremity vascular pathology. *Hand Clin.* 2015;31(1):1-12.

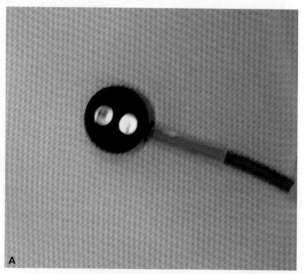

FIGURE 64.9 Photoplethysmography is performed using a light-emitting diode sensor (A) that is placed on the examined digit (B).

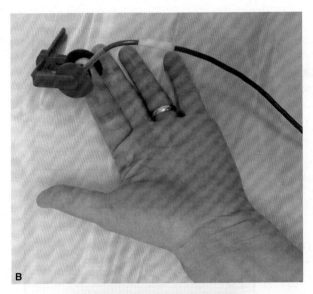

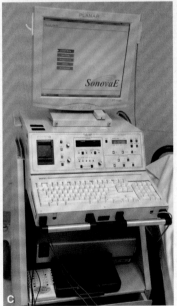

FIGURE 64.9 (*continued*) The signal is transmitted–received into a computer software (C). Originally printed in Grasu BL, Jones CM, Murphy MS. Use of diagnostic modalities for assessing upper extremity vascular pathology. *Hand Clin.* 2015;31(1):1-12.

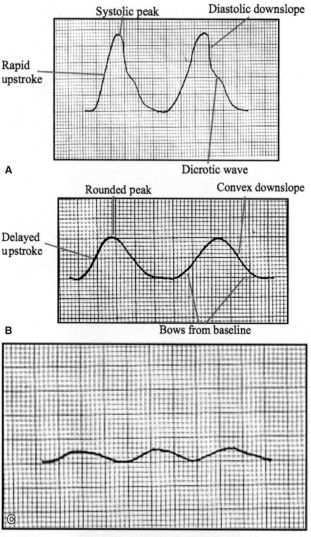

FIGURE 64.10 Plethysmography pulse volume recordings: normal (A), stenotic (B), occlusion (C). Originally printed in Grasu BL, Jones CM, Murphy MS. Use of diagnostic modalities for assessing upper extremity vascular pathology. *Hand Clin.* 2015;31(1):1-12.

- By measuring digital temperature, the thermoregulatory ability of the vascular bed is evaluated.
- Isolated cold stress testing studies the ability of a vascular bed to respond and recover to physiologic stress.
- Three phases to the test
  - Baseline phase with the hand at room temperature
  - Cooling phase by submerging the hand in water and exposed to 5°C to 8°C for approximately 3 to 5 minutes (Figure 64.11)[1]
  - Rewarming phase with the hand back at room temperature for 20 minutes
- Normal responses display temperature readings that parallel the curve for laser Doppler fluxometry.
- Abnormalities present as cold or warm responses
  - A cold response, often seen in women, is a decrease in digital temperature and microvascular perfusion when the hand is stressed to cold temperatures.
  - A warm response, seen twice as often in men as women, is a sympathetic dysfunction where few modulations in vascular tone occur.[7]

RADIOGRAPHIC STUDIES

- Three-phase bone scan (scintigraphy)
  - Useful for soft tissue damage and bone devitalization in cases of frostbite
  - Technetium-99m (Tc-99m) is a nuclear isomer that is taken up by osteoblasts.
    - Active bone growth including bone tumors, metastasis, and fractures is detected.
  - Three phases: flow phase, blood pool image, and delayed phase
    - The first phase detects perfusion of a lesion as scans are obtained within seconds of Tc-99m injection.
    - Blood pool images are obtained about 5 minutes after injection, evaluating the vascularity of the region.
    - Delayed phase: 3 hours after injection when most of the radioisotope has metabolized and bone turnover associated with lesion/region is assessed
    - In 19 patients with frostbite, Zera et al found that Tc-99m bone scanning was an accurate predictor of potential digital loss and level of digit amputation such that more invasive testing is unnecessary.[8]

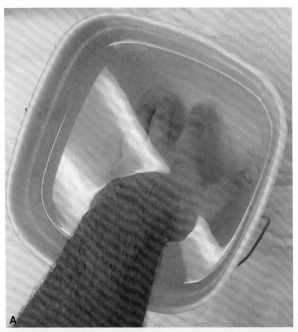

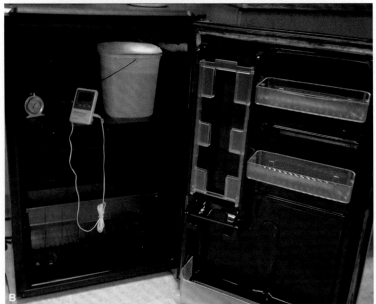

FIGURE 64.11 Stress testing is performed by submerging the hand (A) in water cooled to 5° to 8°C (40°F–50°F) (B).

- Angiography (arteriography)
  - Gold standard to evaluate vascular pathology
  - Invasive but can be both diagnostic and therapeutic
  - Arterial system is accessed and radiopaque contrast agent injected, the blood vessels are then visualized using fluoroscopy
  - Digital subtraction angiography, however, uses computer processing to manipulate the acquired data and subtract osseous structures or enhance vascular ones in real time (Figure 64.12).[9]
    - Can diagnose the cutoff level (Figure 64.13) or segmental defect (Figure 64.14)
  - The interventional radiologist or vascular surgeon may dilate a lumen with balloon angioplasty, maintain vessel patency with a stent, or perform thrombolysis or thrombectomy for revascularization.[10]
- CT angiogram
  - High-resolution vascular images and cross-sectional slices of soft tissue structures adjacent to vascular ones such as bones and ligaments
  - Iodine contrast dye must first be injected into the patient's venous system to achieve arterial enhancement.
  - Surrounding tissues are subtracted to isolate vascular structures, and the rapid speed of image acquisition is vital in polytrauma patients.[11]

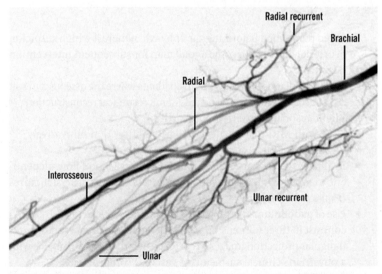

FIGURE 64.12 Arterial anatomy of the forearm appreciated on digital subtraction angiography. Originally printed in Grasu BL, Jones CM, Murphy MS. Use of diagnostic modalities for assessing upper extremity vascular pathology. *Hand Clin.* 2015;31(1):1-12.

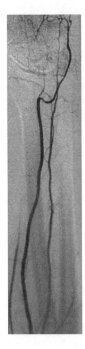

FIGURE 64.13 Digital subtraction angiography visualizing radial artery cutoff. Originally printed in Grasu BL, Jones CM, Murphy MS. Use of diagnostic modalities for assessing upper extremity vascular pathology. *Hand Clin.* 2015;31(1):1-12.

- Often performed before angiography when there is a high suspicion of arterial injury to become a road map for subsequent intervention (Figure 64.15)
- Facilitates diagnosis in polytrauma patients where the osseous and soft tissue detail is exceptional and aids in microsurgical reconstruction[11,12]
■ Magnetic resonance arteriography (MRA)
  - Used with MRI to evaluate vascularity of the UE noninvasively
  - Eliminate the risks of radiation
  - Evaluates the UE's arterial/venous systems in a blood flow–dependent manner while also evaluating adjacent soft tissue structures (Figure 64.16)
  - Use of gadolinium-diethylenetriaminepentaacetic acid (Gd-DTPA) contrast in three-dimensional pulse sequences enhances these multiangular projection images to correlate obstruction or embolus with a physician's clinical suspicion of vascular compromise.[1,13]
  - Gd-DTPA contrast elicits no allergic response and is typically injected in the contralateral antecubital vein.

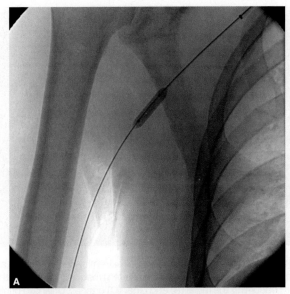

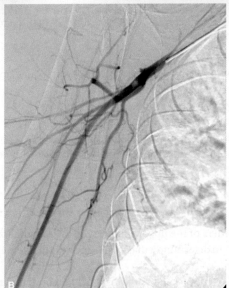

FIGURE 64.14 A, Guide wire threading for dye injection. B, Once the dye is injected and fluoroscopy is performed, an axillary thrombus and intimal tear are visualized. Originally printed in Grasu BL, Jones CM, Murphy MS. Use of diagnostic modalities for assessing upper extremity vascular pathology. *Hand Clin.* 2015;31(1):1-12.

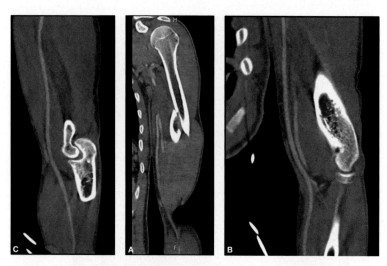

FIGURE 64.15 A, CT angiogram of the left upper extremity demonstrating a midshaft humerus fracture and intact brachial artery medially. Imaging of the brachial artery becoming the radial (B) and ulnar (C) arteries. Originally printed in Grasu BL, Jones CM, Murphy MS. Use of diagnostic modalities for assessing upper extremity vascular pathology. *Hand Clin*. 2015;31(1):1-12. Courtesy of C.C. Sexton, MD, Baltimore, Maryland.

- The portion of UE being imaged must be positioned appropriately in the gantry to ensure adequate coverage.
- MRA has physical limitations.
  - Maximum coverage: 40 to 50 cm
  - Contrast has variable circulation times
  - Overlap of the arteries and veins in the hand makes diagnosis difficult.

SUMMARY

- Vascular disorders of the upper limb can be devastating for a patient.
- It is important to determine a diagnosis quickly and intervene urgently when needed
- The diagnosis of UE vascular pathology includes both noninvasive and invasive examinations.
- Begin with thorough patient interview and continue with pertinent physical examination findings.
- Suspected diagnoses can be confirmed using instruments available at the bedside, vascular lab, or radiology suite.

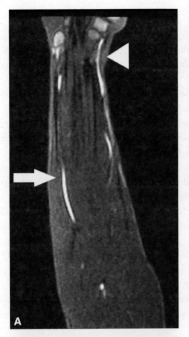

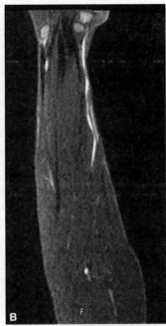

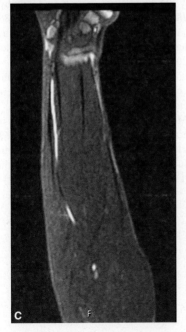

FIGURE 64.16 (A), Multiple slices from a MR angiography of the left forearm demonstrating intact ulnar (arrow) and radial (arrowhead) arteries. (B), continuation of radial artery, and (C), continuation of ulnar artery. Originally printed in Grasu BL, Jones CM, Murphy MS. Use of diagnostic modalities for assessing upper extremity vascular pathology. *Hand Clin.* 2015;31(1):1-12.

REFERENCES

1. Chloros GD, Smerlis NN, Li Z, Smith TL, Smith BP, Koman LA. Noninvasive evaluation of upper-extremity vascular perfusion. *J Hand Surg Am.* 2008;33(4):591-600.

2. Thompson JC. *Netter's Concise Orthopaedic Anatomy.* 2nd ed. Philadelphia, PA: WB Saunders; 2010.

3. Weber TM, Lockhart ME, Robbin ML. Upper extremity venous Doppler ultrasound. *Radiol Clin North Am.* 2007;45(3):513-524, viii-ix.

4. Millet JD, Gunabushanam G, Ojili V, Rubens DJ, Scoutt LM. Complications following vascular procedures in the upper extremities: a sonographic pictorial review. *Ultrasound Q.* 2013;29(1):33-45.

5. Dumanian GA, Segalman K, Buehner JW, Koontz CL, Hendrickson MF, Wilgis EF. Analysis of digital pulse-volume recordings with radial and ulnar artery compression. *Plast Reconst Surg.* 1998;102(6):1993-1998.

6. Whiteley MS, Fox AD, Horrocks M. Photoplethysmography can replace hand-held Doppler in the measurement of ankle/brachial indices. *Ann R Coll Surg Engl.* 1998;80(2):96-98.

7. Pollock FE Jr, Koman LA, Smith BP, Holden M, Russell GB, Poehling GG. Measurement of hand microvascular blood flow with isolated cold stress testing and laser Doppler fluxmetry. *J Hand Surg Am.* 1993;18(1):143-150.

8. Twomey JA, Peltier GL, Zera RT. An open-lable study to evaluate the safety and efficacy of tissue plasminogen activator in treatment of severe frostbite. *J Trauma.* 2005;59(6):1350-1354.

9. Harrington DP, Boxt LM, Murray PD. Digital subtraction angiography: overview of technical principles. *AJR Am J Roentgenol.* 1982;139(4):781-786.

10. Islam A, Edgerton C, Stafford JM, et al. Anatomic findings and outcomes associated with upper extremity arteriography and selective thrombolysis for acute finger ischemia. *J Vasc Surg.* 2014;60(2):410-417.

11. Bozlar U, Ogur T, Norton PT, Khaja MS, All J, Hagspiel KD. CT angiography of the upper extremity arterial system: part 1-anatomy, technique, and use in trauma patients. *AJR Am J Roentgenol.* 2013;201(4):745-752.

12. Bogdan MA, Klein MB, Rubin GD, McAdams TR, Chang J. CT angiography in complex upper extremity reconstruction. *J Hand Surg.* 2004;29B(5):465-469.

13. Disa JJ, CHung KC, Gellad FE, Bickel KD, Wilgis EF. Efficacy of magnetic resonance angiography in the evaluation of vascular malformations of the hand. *Plast Reconstr Surg.* 1997;99(1):136-144.

Index

NOTE: Page numbers those followed by "*f*" denote figures and those followed by "*t*" denote tables.

A

Abductor digiti minimi (ADM), 10, 594*t*, 595*f*
Abductor pollicis brevis (APB), 10, 594*t*, 595*f*
Abductor pollicis longus (APL), 7, 90, 589*t*, 591–592*f*
Abscess, 452*t*
    collar button. *See* Web space infections
    horseshoe, 449
    incision and drainage, 40
    paronychial infections. *See* Paronychial infections
Accessory collateral ligament, 579*f*, 580
Acute Boutonniere injury. *See* Proximal interphalangeal (PIP) joint, volar simple dislocations
Acute compartment syndrome (ACS). *See* Compartment syndrome
Acute open mallet finger, 328
Adductor pollicis (AP), 9–10, 594*t*, 595*f*
Adductor pollicis longus (AdPL), 90
ADM (abductor digiti minimi), 10, 594*t*, 595*f*
AdPL (adductor pollicis longus), 90
Adson maneuver, 391, 637
Advanced trauma life support (ATLS), 533
Afterdrop, 567
AIN (Anterior interosseous nerve), 600*f*, 603
Airway management, burns, 558
Allen classification of nail bed injury, 496
Allen test, 11
    for upper extremity, 631, 633*f*
    digital, 634–635, 634*f*
Allergies, local anesthetics, 25–26
Allograft
    for digital nerve injury, 374
    for lunotriquetral ligament reconstruction, 198
    for peripheral nerve injury and repair principles, 362
Aloe vera, for frostbite, 568
AlumaFoam/Zimmer splint, 608
Alumifoam extension splint, 326*f*
Amikacin, 456*t*
Aminoglycoside, 410

Amitriptyline, 395
Amoxicillin, 452*t*
Amoxicillin-clavulanate (Augmentin), 418, 456*t*
Ampicillin, 452*t*, 456*t*
Anaerobic infections, 455*t*
Analgesia, for frostbite, 568
Anatomic snuffbox, 575
Anconeus muscle muscle, 591*f*
Anesthesia
    digital block techniques, 27–29, 28–29*f*
    general anesthesia, 33
    general considerations, 24
    intravenous regional anesthesia, 30–31
    keys to success, 24
    local anesthesia, 26–27
    local anesthetics, 25–26
    local plus intravenous sedation, 29–30
    regional nerve block, 31–33, 32*f*
    types, 24
Angiography. *See also* Digital subtraction angiography; Magnetic resonance angiography (MRA)
    for upper extremity, 647, 647–649*f*
Angular deformity, 128, 129–130
Animal bites, 44
Annular pulleys, 584–585
Anterior interosseous nerve (AIN), 600*f*, 603
Anterior oblique ligament (AOL), 92
Anteroposterior drawer test, 13*t*
Anthrax, cutaneous, 456*t*
Antibiotics
    for bite wounds, 471
    for burns, 559
    for cellulitis, 465, 465*t*, 466
    for open fractures, 408
    for osteomyelitis, 477*t*
    for palmar space infections, 452*t*, 455
    for paronychial infections, 420
    for pulp space infections, 416
    for pyogenic flexor tenosynovitis, 430–431
    for septic arthritis, 440
AOL (Anterior oblique ligament), 92

AP (Adductor pollicis), 9–10, 594*t*, 595*f*
APB (abductor pollicis brevis), 10, 594*t*, 595*f*
Ape hand, 379, 380*f*
APL (abductor pollicis longus), 7, 90, 589*t*, 591–592*f*
Arterial supply, upper extremity, 630
Arterialization, 181
Arteriography. *See* Angiography
Arthroplasty, for proximal phalanx fractures, 53
Arthroscopic multidirectional stress testing, 187, 187*t*
Arthroscopic repair, 236
    acute tears, 235
Articular fractures, 50
ATLS (advanced trauma life support), 533
Atrophy, hand and wrist, 3
Augmentin (amoxicillin-clavulanate), 418, 456*t*
Autogenic cancellous graft, 247
Autograft
    for digital nerve injury, 374
    for lunotriquetral ligament reconstruction, 198
    for peripheral nerve injuries, 361–362
    of ulnar nerve injuries, 394–395
Avascular necrosis (AVN), 20, 53
    capitate, 212–213
    groups, 205
    hamate, 212–213
    lunate, 208–212
        anatomy, 209
        blood supply pattern, 209*f*
        clinical presentation, 210
        core decompression, 210
        imaging, 210*t*, 211*f*
        Kienbock's disease, 208
        morphologic classification, 209
        pathophysiology, 209
        phenotype, 210
        physical examination, 210
        proximal row carpectomy, 211
        radial shortening osteotomy, 211
        treatment, 212*t*
        wrist fusion, 211–212
    pisiform, 212–213
    scaphoid, 205–208
        anatomy, 205–206
        causes, 205
        classification/imaging, 207, 207*t*
        clinical history, 206
        pathophysiology, 206
        physical examination, 206
        Preiser's disease, 207, 207*t*

        scaphoid stress test, 206
        treatment, 208
        Watson (scaphoid shift) test, 206
    trapezium, 212–213
    trapezoid, 212–213
    triquetrum, 212–213
AVN. *See* Avascular necrosis (AVN)
Axial carpal instability, 162
Axonotmesis. *See also* Median nerve, injuries, Ulnar nerve, injuries
    with damage to endoneurium, 358
    with damage to endoneurium and perineurium, 358
    electromyography findings, 354*t*, 355
    with intact endoneurium, 358
Axons, 353
Azithromycin, 456*t*

B

Baclofen, 395
Bacteroides, 468
Bactrim (trimethoprim-sulfamethoxazole), 418
Ballottement test, 10, 11*f*
Barely discernible subluxation, 332
Barton fracture, 256, 258
Bartonella, 468
Benedict hand, 380, 381*f*
Bennett fractures, 89, 89*f*
    classification, 94
    closed reduction percutaneous pinning, 95, 95*f*
    nonoperative treatment, 94–95
    open reduction internal fixation for, 95–96
    pathoanatomy, 92
    Wagner approach, 96
Bicolumnar intercarpal arthrodesis, 247
Bicondylar fractures, 50, 53
Bier block. *See* Intravenous regional anesthesia
Bite wounds, 43–44. *See also* Animal bites; Human bites
    acute management, 470–471
    classification, 470
    definitive treatment, 471–472
    epidemiology, 468
    history, 469
    imaging, 470, 470*f*
    management algorithm, 472
    mechanism of injury, 468
    pathoanatomy, 467–468
    physical examination, 469–470, 469*f*
    soft tissue damage, 467*f*
Bones, 576*f. See also specific bones*

carpus, 577–578
distal radius, 575–576, 577*f*
distal ulna, 576
grafting, 411
metacarpals, 576*f*, 578
phalanges, 576*f*, 578
scans, 196
for frostbite, 566
for upper extremity, 645
Bony mallets. *See* Mallet fractures
Boxer's knuckle, 329
Brachial plexus/elbow blocks, 32–33
Brachioradialis muscle, 586*f*, 590*f*
Bridge plating, of distal radius fractures, 263–264
Brunner incision, of digital nerve injury, 375, 375*f*
Bunnell–Littler test, 13*t*
Bupivacaine (Marcaine), 25
Burns
acute management, 558–559
airway management, 558
antibiotics, 559
chemical burn antidotes, 559
compartment syndrome, 558–559
electrical injuries, 559
initial evaluation and management, 558
Parkland formula, 559
resuscitation, 559
classification, 558, 618–619
criteria, American Burn Association, 557
definitive management, 559–561
complications, 561
escharotomies/fasciotomies, 560
grafting, 560
postoperative care, 561
surgical excision and grafting, 560
surgical treatments, 560
tangential excision, 560
treatments based on classification, 559–560
demographics, 557
histology, 557
zone of coagulation, 557
zone of hyperemia, 557
zone of stasis, 557
history, 557
imaging, 558
natural history, 619
pathology, 618–619
physical examination, 558
therapy for, 619–620

C

Cain-CMC fracture dislocation, 164, 165*f*
Camper Chiasm, 337
Capitate, 212–213, 576*f*, 578, 588*f*
fracture, 162
Capitohamate ligament, 582–583*f*
Capitotrapezoid ligament, 582–583*f*
Capsaicin, 395
Carbamazepine, 395
Card test, 13*t*
Carpal bone malunion and nonunion. *See also*
Scaphoid fracture
contraindications, 179
diagnostic data, 177–178, 178*f*
epidemiology, 176
history, 177
management, 179
algorithm, 182
mechanism of injury, 176
nonoperative treatment, 179
pathoanatomy, 176
physical examination, 177
postoperative care, 182
potential complications, 181–182
radiographic classifications
Mack-Lichtman classification, 178
scaphoid nonunion advanced collapse, 178–179
surgical approach, 179–182
arterialization, 181
nonvascularized bone grafting, 179–180
plate fixation, 181
vascularized bone grafting, 180–181
Carpal bones, 4
Carpal tunnel syndrome (CTS), 249, 251
acute, 38–39
distal radius fractures and, 265
Carpometacarpal joints, 4
Carpus bones, 577–578. *See also specific carpus*
bones
Cat bites, 44, 452*t*
CCI (continuous catheter irrigation), 433–434
Cefepime, 456*t*
Ceftaroline, 456*t*
Ceftazidime, 410
Ceftriaxone, 452*t*, 455*t*, 456*t*, 465*t*
Cellulitis
acute management, 465, 465*t*
classification, 464
definitive treatment, 466
over dorsum of hand with erythema and
swelling, 465*f*
epidemiology, 464

Cellulitis (*continued*)
  history, 464
  imaging, 464
  laboratory studies, 464
  mechanism, 464
  pathoanatomy, 464
  physical examination, 464
  risk factors, 464
Central slip, 587
  avulsion. *See also* Extensor tendon injuries
    evaluation, 315*f*
    loss of continuity, 317*f*
    repair, 319*f*
Cephalexin, 418, 452*t*, 456*t*
Cephalosporin (Cefazolin), 373, 408, 410, 430,
    452*t*, 465*t*
Chauffeur fracture, 258
Cheiralgia paresthetica. *See* Wartenberg
    syndrome
Ciprofloxacin, 452*t*, 456*t*
Clarithromycin, 456*t*
Clavulanic acid, 452*t*
Clindamycin, 418, 452*t*, 456*t*, 465*t*
Closed reduction (CR)
  and casting
    for acute ulnar dislocation of DRUJ, 302
    for Bennett fractures, 94–95
    of distal radius fractures, 262
    for thumb metacarpal base extra-articular
        fractures, 121
    for unstable, traumatic TFCC injuries, 299
  for distal ulna fractures, 287
  for dorsal metacarpophalangeal dislocations,
      123–124
  for extra-articular fractures, 94
  for Galeazzi fractures, 309
  for metacarpophalangeal dislocations, 123
  for perilunate dislocations, 148
  for PIP joint dorsal fracture-dislocations, 61
  for PIP joint lateral dislocations, 60
  for Rolando fractures, 96–97, 97*f*
  and splinting
    for base of the thumb fractures, 94
    for DIP joint dislocations, 62
    for distal radius fractures, 261, 262
    for unstable, traumatic TFCC injuries, 299
  for wrist dislocation, 220
Closed reduction and internal fixation (CRIF)
  for scaphoid fractures
    dorsal approach, 141, 142*f*
    volar approach, 140, 140*f*
Closed reduction percutaneous pinning (CRPP)
  for base of thumb fractures, 94

  for Bennett fractures, 95, 95*f*
  for distal radius fractures, 263
  for mallet finger, 327, 327*f*
  for metacarpal neck fractures, 119
  for metacarpal shaft fractures, 120
  for middle phalanx fractures, 53
  for perilunate dislocations, 148
  for thumb metacarpal base extra-articular
      fractures, 121
  for wrist dislocation, 221
Closing wedge osteotomy, 129, 129*f*
  for distal radius malunion, 274, 276, 278*f*
Cold injuries. *See* Frostbite
Cold stress testing, 645, 646*f*
Collar button abscess. *See* Web space infections
Colles fracture, 256, 260*f*
  Frykman classification, 259
Color Duplex ultrasound, 638
Compartment syndrome, 162, 311, 414
  acute management, 483
    surgical release, 483
  burns and, 558–559
  classification, 481
  definitive management, 483–489
    postoperative care, 487
    potential complications, 487, 489
    surgical technique, 483–487, 483–488*f*
  description, 479
  emergent indications for surgery, 36–37
  epidemiology, 480
  history, patient, 481
  imaging, 481
  mechanism of injury, 479
  neonatal, 483
  pathoanatomy, 479
  physical examination, 481, 482*t*
Complex regional pain syndrome (CRPS)
  definition and diagnosis, 621
  management, 621–622
Compression neuropathies, 399
Compression test, 232
Compression wire fixation, 250
Compressive neuropathy, acute, 38–39
Computed tomography (CT), 243
  of avascular necrosis of hand and wrist, 207
  of carpal bone malunions and nonunions,
      177
  for distal radioulnar joint instability, 296–297
  for distal radius fractures, 256
  for distal radius malunion, 271
  for distal ulna fractures, 285
  of hamate body fracture, 163
  of hand and wrist, 21, 22*f*

of hook of hamate fractures, 156, 156*f*
for palmar space infections, 454
for perilunate dislocations, 148
for scaphoid fractures, 136
of scapholunate ligament injury and dorsal
    intercalated segment stability, 185
of ulnar nerve injuries, 392
for web space infections, 445
of wrist dislocation, 218
Computed tomography angiogram
    of median nerve injury, 382
    for upper extremity, 647–648, 650*f*
Computed tomography myelography
    of median nerve injury, 382
    of ulnar nerve injuries, 393
Condylar advancement osteotomy, 130, 131*f*
Congruent arc method, 296–297, 298*f*
Continuous catheter irrigation (CCI), 433–434
Core suture strength, 342
Corticosteroids
    for pyogenic flexor tenosynovitis, 431
    for radial tunnel syndrome, 400
CR. *See* Closed reduction (CR)
CRIF. *See* Closed reduction and internal fixation
    (CRIF)
Cross-finger flap, fingertip and, 508, 509*f*
CRPP. *See* Closed reduction percutaneous
    pinning (CRPP)
CRPS. *See* Complex regional pain syndrome
    (CRPS)
Cruciate pulleys, 585
CT. *See* Computed tomography (CT)
CTS. *See* Carpal tunnel syndrome (CTS)
Custom-molded thermoplastic splint, 107

D

Dalfopristin, 456*t*
Daptomycin, 456*t*
DBI (digital brachial index), 638, 639*f*
Deep transverse metacarpal ligaments, 579
Deformity, hand and wrist, 2
Diabetics, pyogenic flexor tenosynovitis and, 429
Dicloxacillin, 465*t*
Digital Allen test, 634–635, 634*f*
Digital block techniques, 27–29, 28–29*f*
Digital brachial index (DBI), 638, 639*f*
Digital collateral ligament injury. *See* Finger
    proximal interphalangeal joint collateral
    ligaments; Thumb metacarpophalangeal
    ulnar collateral ligament
Digital nerve injuries. *See also* Median nerve,
    injuries; Ulnar nerve, injuries
    acute management, 373

definitive treatment, 373–376, 375*f*
history, 372
imaging, 373
management algorithm, 376
mechanism of injury, 369–370
pathoanatomy, 368–369
physical examination, 372–373
Digital subtraction angiography, 647, 647–648*f*
Digital temperature evaluation, 640, 645, 646*f*
Dinner fork deformity, 270, 271*f*
DIP joint. *See* Distal interphalangeal (DIP) joint
Diprivan (propofol), 29
Direct (end-to-end) repair, 360–361
Direct cellular injury, 562
DISI (dorsal intercalary segment instability), 183
Dislocation, wrist
    acute management, 220
    classification
        Dumontier, 218, 220*f*, 221
        Moneim, 219
    definition, 216
    definitive treatment, 221–223
        contraindications, 222
        goals of treatment, 221
        nonoperative treatment, 221
        operative technique, 222, 223*f*
        outcomes, 223
        postoperative care, 223
        potential complications, 222–223
        radiocarpal dislocations, 221
        surgical indications, 221–222
    epidemiology, 217
    history, 217
    imaging, 218–219*f*
    immediate closed reduction, 220
    management algorithm, 224
    mechanism of injury, 217
    pathoanatomy, 216–217
    physical examination, 217
Displaced distal phalanx shaft fractures, 54
Distal interphalangeal (DIP) joint
    arthrodesis, 350
    deformity, 2
    phalanx dislocations, 62–63
    septic arthritis, 441, 442*f*
    stability, 10
Distal phalanx fractures
    nonoperative treatment for, 54
    surgical indications for, 54, 55–56*f*
Distal radioulnar joint (DRUJ) injuries, 292*t*
    acute ulnar dislocation, 302
    anatomy, 291–292, 293*f*, 294*f*
    classification, 297–298, 298*f*

Distal radioulnar joint (DRUJ) injuries
(*continued*)
  complications, 304
  compression test, 13*t*
  differential diagnosis, 297
  imaging, 295–297, 296*f*, 297*f*, 298*f*
  incidence of instability, 305
  instability, 10, 11*f*, 302–303, 303*f*
  mechanism of injury, 291
  physical examination, 293–295, 295*f*
  postoperative protocol, 303
  presentation, 293
  reduction, operative technique for, 309
  shuck test, 283–284, 283–284*f*
  subluxation, 311
  triangular fibrocartilage complex
    degenerative injuries, 299, 302
    stable, traumatic injuries, 299, 300–301*f*
    unstable, traumatic injuries, 299
Distal radius, 4, 575–576, 577*f*
  fractures
    anatomy, 254
    associated injuries, 255
    classification, 256, 258–261
    closed reduction and splinting, 261
    definition, 254
    epidemiology, 254
    goals of treatment, 262
    history, 255
    imaging, 256, 257–260*f*
    mechanism of injury, 254–255
    nonoperative treatment, 262
    operative techniques, 263–265
    outcomes, 266
    physical examination, 255–256
    postoperative care, 265
    potential complications, 265
    surgical indication, 262–263
  malunion, 268, 269*f*
    classification, 271
    closing wedge osteotomy for, 274, 276, 278*f*
    distraction osteogenesis for, 276
    history, 268, 270
    imaging, 271, 272*f*, 273*f*
    initial treatment, 272
    nonoperative treatment, 272, 274
    opening wedge osteotomy for, 274, 275–276*f*, 277*f*
    physical examination, 270, 271*f*
    postoperative care, 280
    potential complications, 276, 278
    radiographic assessment, 270*t*

sliding osteotomy for, 276, 279*f*
surgical indications and contraindications, 273*t*, 274
trapezoidal osteotomy, for, 276, 279*f*
ulnar-sided procedures, 276
Distal ulna, 4, 576
  fractures
    acute management, 286–287
    anatomy, 281–283, 282*f*
    classification, 285–286, 286*f*
    complications, 289
    differential diagnosis, 285
    epidemiology, 281
    imaging, 284–285, 285*f*
    late management, 288
    management algorithm, 286*f*
    mechanism of injury, 281
    physical examination, 283–284, 283–284*f*
    postoperative protocol, 288–289
    presentation, 283
    stable extra-articular ulnar styloid frac-
      tures, 287
    unstable extra-articular ulnar styloid frac-
      tures, 287, 288*f*
    unstable intra-articular ulnar styloid
      fractures, 287
Distant flaps, fingertip and, 511, 512*f*
Distraction osteogenesis, for distal radius
  malunion, 276
Dog bites, 44, 452*t*
Doppler ultrasound, of ulnar nerve injuries, 392
Dorsal blocking splint
  for dorsal metacarpophalangeal dislocations,
    124
  for jersey finger, 350
Dorsal button technique, 348, 349*f*
Dorsal distal radioulnar ligament, 584*f*
Dorsal intercalary segment instability (DISI),
  183
Dorsal intercarpal ligament, 580, 581*f*
Dorsal interossei muscles, 591
Dorsal laceration, 321
Dorsal ligament complex, 92
Dorsal metacarpophalangeal dislocations,
  123–125
Dorsal oblique injury, fingertip and, 507
Dorsal plating
  of distal radius fractures, 264
  fixation, 250
Dorsal radial sensory nerve, 598
Dorsal radiocarpal ligament, 580, 581*f*
Dorsal radiolunate ligament, 581*f*, 582
Dorsal radiotriquetral ligament, 581*f*

Dorsal subaponeurotic space infection, 453
   surgical approaches for, 460
Dorsal ulnar sensory nerve, 603
Dorsal wrist, physical examination, 4
Doxycycline, 410, 418, 452*t*, 456*t*
Doyle classification of mallet finger, 67, 68*f*,
   323, 326*t*
DRUJ injuries. *See* Distal radioulnar joint
   (DRUJ) injuries
Dumontier classification, wrist dislocation, 218,
   220*f*, 221
Duragesic (fentanyl), 29

E

EAM/CAM (early active movement/controlled
   active motion), 611
Early active movement/controlled active motion
   (EAM/CAM), 611
Ebraheim-coronal body of hamate fracture,
   163, 164*f*
ECRB (extensor carpi radialis brevis), 7, 589*t*,
   590*f*, 592*f*
ECRL (extensor carpi radialis longus), 7, 589*t*,
   590*f*, 592*f*
ECU (extensor carpi ulnaris), 9, 584*f*, 589*t*,
   591*f*, 592*f*
EDC. *See* Extensor digitorum communis (EDC)
Edema management
   control and, 606–607
   for ring removal, 624
EDM (extensor digiti minimi), 7, 585, 589*t*,
   591*f*, 592*f*
Ehlers–Danlos syndrome, 26
Eikenella sp., 493
Eikenella corrodens, 438, 451, 468
EIP (extensor indicis proprius), 7, 585, 589*t*, 592*f*
Electric rotary tool, ring cutting by, 627
Electrical injuries, burns, 559
Electromyelography (EMG), 354–355, 354*t*, 392
Elson test, 13*t*
EMG (electromyelography), 354–355, 354*t*, 392
Endoneurium, 351, 368
Endotracheal tube (ETT), 33
EPB (extensor pollicis brevis), 7, 91, 589*t*, 591*f*,
   592*f*
Epinephrine, 27
Epineural repair, 394
Epineurium, 351, 368
EPL (extensor pollicis longus), 7, 91, 589*t*, 591*f*,
   592*f*, 610
Eponychium, 491, 504
Ertapenem, 456*t*
Escherichia coli, 468

Ethambutol, 456*t*
ETT (endotracheal tube), 33
Extension-block pinning of mallet fracture,
   72–73, 72*f*
Extensor carpi radialis brevis (ECRB), 7, 589*t*,
   590*f*, 592*f*
Extensor carpi radialis longus (ECRL), 7, 589*t*,
   590*f*, 592*f*
Extensor carpi ulnaris (ECU), 9, 584*f*, 589*t*,
   591*f*, 592*f*
Extensor digiti minimi (EDM), 7, 585, 589*t*,
   591*f*, 592*f*
Extensor digitorum communis (EDC), 589*t*,
   592*f*
   dislocation, 329–330
Extensor digitorum muscle, 591*f*
Extensor indicis muscle, 591*f*
Extensor indicis proprius (EIP), 7, 585, 589*t*,
   592*f*
Extensor pollicis brevis (EPB), 7, 91, 589*t*, 591*f*,
   592*f*
Extensor pollicis longus (EPL), 7, 91, 589*t*, 591*f*,
   592*f*, 610
Extensor tendon injuries, 313–319
   acute management, 315
   classification, 318*t*
   definitive treatment of
      complications after, 317
      nonoperative treatment, 315
      postoperative care, 318, 319*t*
      surgical approach, 316–317, 319*f*
      surgical indications, 315–316
   epidemiology, 313
   history, 313–314
   imaging, 19, 20, 314, 316–317*f*
   management algorithm, 318
   mechanism of injury, 313
   pathoanatomy, 313
   physical examination, 314, 314–315*f*
   rehabilitation and splinting, 608–610
External fixation
   of distal radius fractures, 263
   of open fractures, 411
   of proximal phalanx fractures, 52
External neurolysis, 360
Extra-articular fractures of thumb, 89
   nonoperative treatment, 94
   operative treatment, 94
   pathoanatomy, 92

F

Fascicles, 351
Fascicular repair, 394

Fasciotomy, 488*f*
  for acute compartment syndrome, 483
  burns, 560
  replantation and, 523
Fassler classification of nail bed injury, 497
FCR (Flexor carpi radialis), 7, 575, 586*f*, 588*f*
FCU (flexor carpi ulnaris), 7, 173, 575, 586*f*
FDMB (flexor digiti minimi brevis), 594*t*, 595*f*
FDP. *See* Flexor digitorum profundus (FDP)
FDS. *See* Flexor digitorum superficialis (FDS)
Felon, 41. *See also* Pulp space infections
Fentanyl (Duragesic, Sublimaze), 29
Fernandez classification of distal radius
  fractures, 261
Fibrin clot glue, for median nerve injury, 383
Fight bite injuries, 119
Finger proximal interphalangeal joint collateral
  ligaments
  acute management, 84–85
  anatomy, 81
  classification, 84
  definitive treatment of
    complications, 86
    nonoperative treatment, 85
    outcomes, 86
    postoperative care, 86
    surgical approach, 85–86
    surgical indications, 85
  epidemiology, 82
  history, 82
  imaging, 83–84, 83*f*, 84*f*
  management algorithm, 87
  mechanism of injury, 81
  pathoanatomy, 81–82
  physical examination, 82–83
Fingers
  abduction, 13*t*
  magnetic resonance imaging, 19
  radiographs, 16
Fingers and hand malunion and nonunion
  definitive treatment of
    complications, 132
    nonoperative treatment, 128
    postoperative care, 132
    surgical approach, 129–131, 129–132*f*
    surgical indications, 129
  history, 128
  imaging, 128
  mechanism of injury, 127
  pathoanatomy, 127
  physical examination, 128
Fingertip amputations
  anatomy, 504, 505*f*
  complications, 514
  dorsal oblique injury, 507
  history and physical examinations,
    504, 505*f*, 506
  postoperative management, 513–514
  techniques, 507–513
    cross-finger flap, 508, 509*f*
    distant flaps, 511, 512*f*
    first dorsal metacarpal artery "kite" flap,
      513, 513*f*
    heterodigital island flap, 511, 512*f*
    Moberg advancement flap, 511, 512*f*
    neurovascular island flaps, 511
    reverse cross-finger flap, 509–510,
      510*f*
    thenar flap, 510, 511*f*
    V-Y advancement flap, 508, 509*f*
  transverse injury, 507
  treatment, 506–507, 506–507*f*
  volar oblique injury, 507
Finkelstein test, 14*t*
First dorsal metacarpal artery "kite" flap,
  fingertip and, 513, 513*f*
Flexor carpi radialis (FCR), 7, 575, 586*f*,
  588*f*
Flexor carpi ulnaris (FCU), 7, 173, 575,
  586*f*
Flexor digiti minimi brevis (FDMB), 594*t*, 595*f*
Flexor digitorum profundus (FDP), 587*f*, 588*f*
  avulsion injury. *See* Jersey finger
  examination, 7, 9*f*
  test, 339, 339*f*
Flexor digitorum profundus tendon, 492
Flexor digitorum superficialis (FDS), 586*f*, 588*f*
  muscular examination, 7, 9*f*
  test, 339, 339*f*
Flexor pollicis brevis (FPB), 10, 594*t*,
  595*f*
Flexor pollicis longus (FPL), 90, 587*f*
  muscular examination, 7
  rehabilitation and splinting, 612
Flexor retinaculum (pulleys), 19
Flexor tendon injuries, 337–343
  acute management of
    vascular compromise, 340
    well-perfused digit, 341
  anatomy, 337, 338*f*
  classification, 340, 340*f*, 341*t*
  definitive treatment of
    complications after, 342–343
    nonoperative treatment, 341
    surgical indications, 342
    surgical repair, 342

history, 338
imaging, 340
magnetic resonance imaging, 19, 20
mechanism of injury, 338
physical examination of
    inspection, 339
    neurovascular examination, 339–340
    strength/range of motion, 339,
        339*f*
postoperative care, 343
rehabilitation and splinting, 610–612
Flexor tendon sheath
anatomy, 425–426, 426*f*
infections. *See* Pyogenic flexor tenosynovitis
    (PFT)
Flexor tenosynovitis, 448–449, 452
Fluconazole, 456*t*
Fluoroquinolone, 408, 410
Fluoroscopy, 647, 649*f*
Fovea sign, 232
FPB (flexor pollicis brevis), 10, 594*t*, 595*f*
FPL. *See* Flexor pollicis longus (FPL)
Fracture fixation method, 411
Fractures and joint injuries
guidance on closed manipulation,
    612–613, 613*f*
phalangeal and metacarpal fractures
    distal radius or ulnar fractures,
        615, 617, 617*f*, 618*f*
    forearm fractures, 615, 617
    metacarpal base fractures, 614
    metacarpal neck fractures, 614–615
    metacarpal shaft fractures, 614,
        614*f*
    phalanx fractures, 615
    scaphoid fractures, 615, 616*f*
    thumb fractures and ulnar collateral liga-
        ment injuries, 615, 616*f*
Fragment-specific fixation, 264–265
Froment sign, 13*t*, 389, 390*f*
Frostbite
acute management, 567–568
classification, 566–567
defined, 562
definitive treatment
    complications, 570
    nonoperative treatment, 568
    postoperative care, 571
    surgical indications, 569–570, 569–570*f*
epidemiology, 563–564
history, 564
imaging, 565–566
management algorithm, 571

mechanism of injury, 562–563
physical examination, 564–565, 565*f*
Functional abduction splint, 618
Fusobacterium, 468

G
Gabapentin, 395, 622
Galeazzi fractures
acute management, 308
classification, 308, 308*t*
defined, 305
definitive treatment of
    management algorithm,
        309, 310*f*
    nonoperative treatment, 309
    operative management, 309
    postoperative care, 311
    potential complications, 311
    surgical approach, 309, 311
    surgical indications, 309
epidemiology, 306
history, 306
imaging, 306, 307*f*, 308
mechanism of injury, 305, 306*f*
pathoanatomy, 305
physical examination, 306, 307*f*
Gamekeeper's thumb, 103
Geissler grade IV lesions, 197–198
General anesthesia, 33
Gentamicin, 452*t*, 456*t*
Germinal matrix, 491
Glove slide, for ring removal, 626
Grafting, 361–362. *See also specific techniques*
    burns, 560
Gram-negative organisms, 455*t*
Greater arc injury, 162
Gunshot wounds, upper extremity
acute management, 553–554, 554*t*
classification, 553
definitive treatment, 554–556
    contraindications, 555
    nonoperative treatment, 554
    operative technique, 555
    postoperative care, 556
    potential complications, 556
    surgical approach, 555–556
    surgical indications, 555
diagnostic data, 553
epidemiology, 552
history, 552
mechanism of injury, 552
pathoanatomy, 552
physical examination, 553

Gustilo classification for open fracture. *See* Open fractures
Guyon canal, 602*f*, 603

H
Hamate bone, 212–213, 578, 588*f*
hamate body fracture
acute management, 165
blood supply, 161
Cain—CMC fracture dislocation, 164, 165*f*
complications, 168
Ebraheim-coronal body of hamate fracture, 163, 164*f*
epidemiology, 162
evaluation, 162–164
Hirano-hamate fracture, 163, 164*f*
history, 162
imaging, 162–163
ligaments, 161
management, 169*f*
mechanisms of injury, 161–162
Milch-hamate fracture, 163
nonoperative treatment, 165–166
pathoanatomy, 161
physical examination, 162, 163*f*
postoperative care, 169
reduction maneuver for hematometacarpal fracture dislocation., 166*f*
surgical approach, 167–168, 167–168*f*
surgical indications, 167
Hand and wrist
computerized tomography, 21, 22*f*
history, 1–2
magnetic resonance imaging, 18–20, 20–21*f*
physical examination of
inspection, 2–3, 2*f*
muscular examination, 7–10, 8*t*, 9*f*
palpation, 3–5, 3–5*f*
range of motion, 5–7, 6*t*, 6*f*
sensory, 10, 12*f*, 13*t*
specialty tests, 10, 13–14*f*
stability, 10, 11*f*
vascular, 11
radiographs
specialized views, 17–18, 18*f*
standard views, 16–17, 17*f*
ultrasound, 21–22
Hand therapy
for acute triangular fibrocartilage complex tears, 235
for complex regional pain syndrome, 621
for malunion and nonunion of fingers and hand, 128
for scaphoid fractures, 143

Handheld Doppler, for upper extremity, 635–636, 635–636*f*
Hemi-hamate arthroplasty, 61
Hemiarthroplasty, 53
Herbert's classification system of scaphoid fractures, 137
Herpetic whitlow, and paronychia, 423
Heterodigital island flap, fingertip and, 511, 512*f*
High-pressure injection injuries (HPI), 538–542
emergent indications for surgery, 45–46
epidemiology, 538
infectious flexor tenosynovitis and, 540*f*
initial management, 539
pathophysiology, 538–541, 539–541*f*
steroid administration and, 540
High-speed bur, 247
Hirano-hamate fracture, 163, 164*f*
Hook nail, 500, 500*f*
Hook of hamate, 18, 18*f*, 575, 576*f*
fractures. *See also* Hamate bone
anatomy, 151–152, 152–154*f*
biomechanics, 152
blood supply, 152
controversies, 157
imaging, 154–156, 155–156*f*
incidence and epidemiology, 151
management, 156–157
mechanism, 151
signs and symptoms, 154
technique guide, hook of hamate excision, 158, 158*f*
pull test, 154
Horseshoe abscess, 449
HPI. *See* High-pressure injection injuries (HPI)
Human bites, 43–44, 452*t*
Humeral shaft fracture, traction injuries with, 401, 402*f*
"Humpback" deformity, 144
Hunter rod, 342–343
Hyperbaric oxygen therapy, for frostbite, 568
Hypersupination, 232
Hyponychium, 492, 504
Hypothenar space infection, 453
surgical approaches for, 459*f*, 460
Hypothenar wrist pain, 174
Hypothermia, 567

I
Iliac bone graft (IBG), 181
Imipenem, 456*t*
Infections. *See also specific infections*
general principles, 40
incision and drainage, 40

Interdigital web space infection, 453–454
  surgical approaches for, 458f, 459f, 460–461
Intermetacarpal ligaments, anterior and
  posterior, 92
Interossei muscles, 10
Intra-articular deformity, 130–131
Intra-articular fractures of thumb, 89
  Bennett fractures. *See* Bennett fractures
  comminuted, 97
  Rolando fractures. *See* Rolando fractures
Intraosseous wiring, for proximal phalanx
  fractures, 52
Intravenous regional anesthesia, 30–31
Intrinsic-plus splinting, 580
Intrinsics, 589, 591, 594t, 595f
Ischemic ulcerations, 631, 632f
Itraconazole, 456t

J

Jamming finger, 50, 82
Jeanne sign, 389, 390f
Jersey finger, 338, 344–350
  acute management, 347
  anatomic location of injury in, 344, 344f
  complications after flexor repair, 350
  definitive treatment, 347–348
    dorsal button technique, 348, 349f
    late management, 350
    postoperative protocol, 350
    suture anchor technique, 348–349
    type I/II, 348
    type III/IV/V, 349–350
  differential diagnosis, 346
  epidemiology, 344–345
  imaging, 346, 346f
  Leddy and Packer classification system,
    346–347, 347t
  mechanism of injury, 344, 345f
  physical examination, 345–346, 345f
  presentation for evaluation, 345
Juncturae tendinae, 585–586

K

K-wire fixation
  and hamate body fracture, 168–169
  for injuries and instability, 197
  and lunotriquetral ligament injuries,
    197–199
  for proximal phalanx fractures, 52
Kanavel signs, 428, 428t, 429f
Kaplan's cardinal line (KCL), 573
Kienbock's disease, 208, 248f
  procedures for, 210
Kleinman shear test, 14t

L

Laceration, 401, 403–404
Lag screw fixation
  for proximal phalanx fractures, 52
  step-cut osteotomy with, 130, 131f
Lamotrigine, 395
Laryngeal mask airway (LMA), 33
Laser Doppler fluxometry, 638
Lateral antebrachial cutaneous nerve, 595
Leddy and Packer classification system of Jersey
  finger, 346–347, 347t
Lichtman classification and treatment algorithm
  LT ligament injuries, 197t
  lunate, 210t, 211f
Lidocaine (Xylocaine), 25, 395
Ligamentous foveal insertion, 230, 230f
Ligaments. *See also specific ligaments*
  magnetic resonance imaging, 19
  MCP joint of fingers, 579–580, 579f
  MCP joint of thumb, 579
  PIP joints, 580
  wrist, 580–584, 581–584f
Linezolid, 456t
Lister's tubercle, 575, 584f
LMA (laryngeal mask airway), 33
Local anesthesia, 26–27
Local anesthetics
  allergies, 25–26
  duration of action/maximum safe
    dose, 25
  mechanism of action, 25
  resistance, 26
  toxicity, 26
  types, 25
Local plus intravenous sedation, 29–30
Long radiolunate ligament, 581f, 582
LT ligament. *See* Lunotriquetral (LT) ligament
LTIL (lunotriquetral interosseous ligament),
  583, 584f
Lubricants, for ring removal, 624–625
Lumbricals, 10, 589, 591, 593f
Lunate bone, 576, 576–577f, 577
  anatomy, 209
  blood supply pattern, 209f
  clinical presentation, 210
  core decompression, 210
  imaging, 210t, 211f
  Kienbock's disease, 208
  Lichtman classification, 210t, 211f
  morphologic classification, 209
  pathophysiology, 209
  phenotype, 210
  physical examination, 210
  proximal row carpectomy, 211

Lunate bone (*continued*)
    radial shortening osteotomy, 211
    treatment, 212*t*
    wrist fusion, 211–212
Lunotriquetral (LT) ligament, 582–583*f*
    injuries
        arthrodesis, 199
        classification, 195, 195*t*
        clinical presentation, 195
        etiology, 193–194, 194*f*
        functional anatomy, 192
        kinematics, 192
        Lichtman classification and treatment
            algorithm, 197*t*
        LT ballotement test, 195
        pathology and pathomechanics, 193
        radiographic presentation, 195–197, 196*f*
        shear test, 195
        treatment, 197–199
        Viegas classification, 195*t*
Lunotriquetral ballotement test (Reagan test),
    14*t*, 195
Lunotriquetral interosseous ligament (LTIL),
    583, 584*f*
Lunula, 491, 504

M

Mack-Lichtman classification, carpal bone
    malunions and nonunions, 178
Magnetic resonance angiography (MRA)
    for frostbite, 566
    for upper extremity, 648, 650, 651*f*
Magnetic resonance imaging (MRI), 196, 243
    of carpal bone malunions and nonunions,
        177
    of distal radius malunion, 271
    of finger proximal interphalangeal joint
        collateral ligaments, 84, 84*f*
    of hand and wrist, 18–20, 20–21*f*
    of median nerve injury, 382
    of palmar space infections, 454
    of peripheral nerve injury, 356
    of sagittal band rupture, 331
    of scaphoid fractures, 136
    of scapholunate ligament injury and dorsal
        intercalated segment stability, 185
    of thumb metacarpophalangeal ulnar
        collateral ligament, 79
    of triangular fibrocartilage complex tears, 297
    of ulnar nerve injuries, 393
    of web space infections, 445
Magnetic resonance imaging arthrogram,
    232–233, 232–233*f*

Mallet finger/fractures, 321–328
    acute management, 323–324
    classification, 67–69, 68–70*f*, 323, 326*t*
    definitive treatment of
        acute open mallet finger, 328
        closed reduction percutaneous pinning
            vs. open reduction internal fixation,
            327, 327*f*
        nonoperative, 324–326, 326*f*
        operative, 326
    epidemiology, 64–66
    evaluation, 321–322, 323–325*f*
    history, 66
    imaging, 67, 67*f*
    management
        algorithm for, 328
        nonoperative treatment, 70–71, 71*f*
        postoperative care, 73
        potential complications, 73
        surgical approach, 72–73, 72*f*
        surgical indications, 71–72
    mechanisms of injury, 64, 321, 322*f*
    pathoanatomy, 64, 65*f*
    physical examination, 65*f*, 66
    swan-neck deformity, 321, 322*f*
    Wehbe and Schneider classification, 323, 325*t*
Malunion and non-union
    of carpal bone. *See* Carpal bone malunions
        and nonunions
    of fingers and hand. *See* Fingers and hand
        malunion and nonunion
Mangled hand
    acute management, 533–536
        debridement, 534–535
        emergent formal operative assessment,
            534–536, 534–536*f*
        initial presentation, 533–534
        skeletal management, 535
        soft-tissue coverage, 535–536, 536*f*
        soft-tissue management, 535
    classification, 533
    description, 529, 530*f*
    history, 531–532
    imaging, 533
    management algorithm, 537
    mechanism, 530
    pathoanatomy and pathophysiology, 530–531
    physical examination, 532–533
    postoperative care, 536
    secondary reconstructive procedures,
        536–537
Marcaine (bupivacaine), 25
MBG (metacarpal bone graft), 180

Medial antebrachial cutaneous nerve, 595
Medial femoral condyle bone graft (MFCBG),
    180–181
Median nerve, 368, 598
    anatomic course, 369f
    injuries
        acute management, 381–382
        classification, 381, 381t, 382t
        definitive treatment, 382–384
        epidemiology, 379
        history, 379
        mechanism of injury, 379
        physical examination, 379–381, 380f, 381f
    motor branches, 600f, 603
    pathoanatomy, 378–379
Melone classification of intra-articular fractures,
    260
Meniscus homologue, 229
Meropenem, 456t
Metacarpal bone graft (MBG), 180
Metacarpal bones, 576f, 578
    fractures
        acute management, 118
        anatomic classification, 116
        epidemiology, 115
        history, 115
        imaging and classification, 116
        mechanism of injury, 115
        metacarpal base fractures, 120–121
        metacarpal head fractures, 118
        metacarpal neck fractures, 118–119
        metacarpal shaft fractures, 120
        pathoanatomy, 115
        physical examination, 115, 115–116f
        thumb metacarpal base extra-articular
            fractures, 121
Metacarpophalangeal (MCP) joint
    deformity, 2
    dislocations
        acute management, 123
        classification, 123
        dorsal dislocations, 123–125
        epidemiology/background, 122
        history, 122
        imaging/assessment, 123
        mechanism of injury, 122
        pathoanatomy, 122
        physical examination, 122–123
        thumb MCP dislocations, 125–126
        volar dislocations, 125
    of fingers, 579–580, 579f
    septic arthritis, 440, 441f
    stability, 10

    of thumb, 579
Methicillin-resistant *S. aureus* (MRSA),
    414, 451, 455t
Methicillin-sensitive *Staphylococcus aureus*, 455t
Metronidazole, 456t
MFCBG (medial femoral condyle bone graft),
    180–181
Michon classification system of flexor
    tenosynovitis, 430, 430t
Midazolam (Versed), 29
Midcarpal shift test, 14t
Middle phalanx fractures
    nonoperative treatment for, 53
    surgical techniques for, 54
Midpalmar space infection, 453
    surgical approaches for, 459–460, 459f
Milch-hamate fracture, 163
Minimally invasive irrigation and debridement
    of pyogenic flexor tenosynovitis, 432–433,
    433f
Minocycline, 456t
Moberg advancement flap, fingertip and, 511,
    512f
Molded plastic Stack splint, 326f
Moneim classification, wrist dislocation, 219
Monitored anesthesia care (MAC). *See* Local
    plus intravenous sedation
Motion-sparing surgical operations, salvage
    procedure and, 243–244, 244t
MRA. *See* Magnetic resonance angiography
    (MRA)
MRI. *See* Magnetic resonance imaging (MRI)
MRSA (Methicillin-resistant *S. aureus*), 414,
    451, 455t
Muscles. *See also specific muscles*
    extensors, 585, 588f, 589, 589t
        examination, 7–9, 8t
    flexors, 584–585, 585t, 586–587f, 588f
        examination, 7, 8t, 9f
    intrinsics, 589, 591, 594t, 595f
        examination, 9–10
Muscular neurotisation, 365
Mutilating hand injuries, 620–621
Mycobacterium marinum, 456t

N
Nail bed
    anatomy, 3, 4f, 491–492
    avulsions, 499
        germinal matrix avulsion, 499
        sterile matrix avulsion, 499
    injury, 54
        classification, 496–497

Nail bed (*continued*)
dorsal root/roof, 492
epidemiology, 494
eponychium, 491
extensor tendon, 492
flexor digitorum profundus tendon, 492
germinal matrix, 491
history, 494
hyponychium, 492
imaging, 496
injury-related issues, 494
lunula, 491
management algorithm, 501
mechanism of injury, 492–493
nail plate, 491
nerves, 492
nonoperative treatment, 498
paronychium, 492
perionychium, 491
physical examination, 495, 496*f*
postoperative care, 499–500
potential complications, 500
pulp, 492
seymour fracture, 496, 497*f*
sterile matrix, 491
surgical approach, 498–499
surgical indications, 497–498
tuft fracture, 496
vasculature, 492
ventral floor, 492
zones, 492
Nail, physical examination, 3, 4*f*
Nail ridging, 500, 500*f*
NAPs. *See* Nerve action potentials (NAPs)
NCV (nerve conduction velocity), 355
Neonatal compartment syndrome, 483
Neoprene, 608
Nerve action potentials (NAPs)
of median nerve injury, 382
of ulnar nerve injuries, 393
Nerve conduction velocity (NCV), 355
Nerves. *See also specific nerves*
conduits, 362
digital nerve injury, 374
ulnar nerve injuries, 395
cutaneous sensation of forearm, 595–596,
596*f*
cutaneous sensation of hand, 597*f*,
598, 603
motor supply of forearm and hand,
598–602*f*, 603
transfer, 362–365, 363–364*t*
radial nerve reconstruction, 404

Neurapraxia, 356, 357*t*, 358. *See also* Median
nerve, injuries, Ulnar nerve, injuries
electromyography findings, 354*t*, 355
Neurorrhaphy, for digital nerve injury, 373
Neurotmesis, 356, 357*t*, 358. *See also* Median
nerve, injuries, Ulnar nerve, injuries
electromyography findings, 354*t*, 355
Neurovascular injury, 311
Neurovascular island flaps, fingertip and, 511
Neviaser technique, 432, 433*f*
Night thumb abduction splint, 617
Nocardia, 456*t*
Nonsteroidal anti-inflammatory drugs
(NSAIDs)
for degenerative TFCC injuries, 302
for DRUJ instability, 302
for Palmar MCI, 201
Nonvascularized bone grafting (NVBG),
179–180
Novocain (procaine), 25
NSAIDs. *See* Nonsteroidal anti-inflammatory
drugs (NSAIDs)
NVBG (nonvascularized bone grafting),
179–180

O

Oblique pulley, 585
Oblique retinacular ligament, 589, 593*f*
ODM (opponens digiti minimi), 10, 594*t*, 595*f*
"OK" sign, 13*t*
OP (opponens pollicis), 10, 594*t*, 595*f*
Open fractures
acute management, 408, 410
classification, 408, 409*t*
definitive treatment of
fracture fixation, 411
irrigation and debridement of wound, 410
postoperative care, 411
surgical debridement, 410
wound closure, 410–411
emergent indications for surgery, 37–38
history, 407
imaging, 407
physical examination, 407, 408*f*
Open reduction internal fixation (ORIF)
for Bennett fractures, 95–96
for carpal bone malunions and nonunions,
179
for distal ulna fractures, 287
for Galeazzi fractures, 309
for hamate body fracture, 168, 168*f*
for mallet finger, 327
for metacarpal neck fractures, 119

for metacarpal shaft fractures, 120
for middle phalanx fractures, 53
for phalanx dislocations, 61
for Rolando fractures, 97
for scaphoid fractures
dorsal approach, 141–143
volar approach, 140–141
for thumb metacarpal base extra-articular
fractures, 121
for wrist dislocation, 221
Opening wedge osteotomy, 130, 130*f*
for distal radius malunion, 274, 275–276*f*,
277*f*
Opponens digiti minimi (ODM), 10, 594*t*, 595*f*
Opponens pollicis (OP), 10, 594*t*, 595*f*
ORIF. *See* Open reduction internal fixation
(ORIF)
Osseous structures, 19
Osteomyelitis, 44–45, 422, 422*f*, 452*t*
acute management, 476
classification, 476
definitive treatment, 476
nonoperative, 476, 477*t*
operative technique, 476
postoperative care, 476
potential complications, 476
surgical indications, 476
of distal phalanx shaft, 415, 415*f*
epidemiology, 474
history, 474
imaging, 474
laboratory studies, 474
mechanism, 474
organisms, identification, 476, 476*t*
pathoanatomy, 474
physical examination, 474, 475*f*
risk factors, 474
Oval-8 finger splint, 326*f*

P

Palmar beak ligament. *See* Anterior oblique
ligament (AOL)
Palmar creases, distal and proximal, 573–574
Palmar distal radioulnar ligament, 584*f*
Palmar interossei muscles, 591
Palmar midcarpal instability (PMCI)
classification, 200
dorsal, 200
extrinsic, 200
palmar, 200
clinical presentation, 200
etiology, 200
functional anatomy, 199

pathology and pathokinematics, 199–200
perilunate instability, 194*f*
treatment
dorsal, 201
extrinsic, 201
palmar, 201
Palmar plate, 579*f*
Palmar space infections, 43
acute management of
antibiotics, 455, 455–456*t*
nonoperative treatment, 454
definitive treatment of
complications, 461
general principles, 456–457
operative treatment, 456
postoperative care, 462
surgical approaches, 457–461, 458–459*f*
epidemiology, 448
history, 452
imaging, 454
laboratory studies, 454
management algorithm, 462
mechanism of injury, 448–451
microbiology, 451, 452*t*
pathoanatomy, 448, 449*f*, 450*t*
physical examination, 452–454
Palmaris brevis (PB), 594*t*, 595*f*, 603
Palmaris longus, 586*f*
Palmer classification, TFCC injuries and,
233–234, 234*t*
Palpation, hand and wrist, 3–5, 3–5*f*
Pantaloons effect, 449
Parkland formula, burns and, 559
Parona's space, 449
infection, 454
surgical approaches for, 461
Paronychial infections, 41
acute management, 420, 421*f*
classification, 420
definitive treatment of
complications, 422–423, 422*f*
postoperative care, 423
surgical approach, 421–422
epidemiology, 419–420
history, 420
imaging, 420
management algorithm, 423
mechanism, 419
pathoanatomy, 419
physical examination, 420
Paronychium, 492, 504
Passive tenodesis, 5, 6*f*
Pasteurella sp., 493

Pasteurella multocida, 451, 468
PB (palmaris brevis), 594*t*, 595*f*, 603
Pediatric physeal injury, 54
Pediatrics
    digital nerve injury in, 372–373
    pyogenic flexor tenosynovitis in, 429
Pen VK, 465*t*
Penetrating trauma, 450
    pulp space infection from, 413, 413*f*
Penicillin, 373, 410, 430, 465*t*
Penicillinase-resistant penicillin, 452*t*
Peptococcus, 468
Peptostreptococcus, 468
Perfusion imaging, 638
Perilunate dislocations
    acute management, 148
    anatomy, 146
    definitive treatment of
        goals, 148
        nonoperative treatment, 148
        operative technique of acute injuries,
            148–149
        outcomes, 149–150
        postoperative care, 149
        potential complications, 149
        surgical treatment, 148
    epidemiology, 147
    greater arc injuries, 147
    history, 147
    imaging, 147–148
    mechanism of injury, 147
    physical examination, 147
Perineurium, 351, 368
Perionychium, 491
Peripheral nerve injury
    closed injuries, 359
    epidemiology, 352
    factors affecting outcome, 358
    gunshot wounds, 555
    history, 353
    imaging, 354–356, 354*t*
    mechanism of injury, 352
    nerve injury physiology, 352
    nerve regeneration physiology, 353
    nonoperative treatment, 359–360
    open injury with neurologic deficit, 359
    pain control, 359
    pathoanatomy of
        blood supply, 351
        endoneurium, 351
        epineurium, 351
        fascicles, 351

        perineurium, 351
    physical examination, 354
    Seddon classification, 356, 357*t*
    splinting after
        median nerve palsy, 617–618
        radial nerve/posterior
            interosseous nerve palsy, 618
        ulnar nerve palsy, 617
    Sunderland classification, 357*t*, 358
    surgical approaches
        direct (end-to-end) repair, 360–361
        external neurolysis, 360
        nerve grafting, 361–362
        nerve transfer, 362–365, 363–364*t*
        postoperative expectations and care, 365
        surgical complications, 365
    surgical indications, 360
PFT. *See* Pyogenic flexor tenosynovitis (PFT)
Phalangeal neck, 50
    fractures, 53
Phalangeal shaft, 50
Phalanges, 576*f*, 578. *See also specific phalanges*
Phalanx dislocations
    acute management, 58
    classification, 58
    distal interphalangeal joint dislocations,
        62–63
    epidemiology/background, 57
    history, 57
    imaging/assessment, 58
    mechanism of injury, 57
    pathoanatomy, 57
    physical examination, 57–58
    proximal interphalangeal joint
        dorsal fracture-dislocations, 61–62
        dorsal simple dislocations, 59
        lateral dislocations, 60–61
        volar fracture-dislocations, 62
        volar simple dislocations, 59–60
Phalanx fractures
    classification, 50
    distal
        nonoperative treatment for, 54
        surgical indications for, 54, 55–56*f*
    emergency room management, 50–51
    epidemiology, 49
    history, 49–50
    imaging for, 50
    mechanism of injury, 49
    middle
        nonoperative treatment for, 53
        surgical techniques for, 54

pathoanatomy, 49
physical examination, 50
principles of definitive treatment for, 51
proximal
  nonoperative treatment for, 51
  potential complications, 53
  specific fracture patterns, 53
  surgical approach for, 52–53
  surgical indications for, 51–52
Phalen test, 14*t*
Phenytoin, 395
Photoplethysmography, 640, 642–643*f*
Pilon fractures, 50
PIN. *See* Posterior interosseous nerve
  (PIN)
PIP joints. *See* Proximal interphalangeal (PIP)
  joints
Piperacillin, 452*t*, 455*t*, 456*t*
Pisiform, 212–213, 575, 576*f*
  fractures, 173–175
    anatomy, 173
    epidemiology, 173
    history, 173–174
    imaging, 174
    management, 174–175
    mechanism of injury, 173
    nonoperative management, 174
    physical examination, 174
    potential complications, 175
    surgery, 174
    surgical indications, 174
    ulnar nerve, 175
Pisotriquetral grind test, 14*t*
Pivot shift test, 14*t*
Plaster of Paris, 608
Plate fixation, 181
  for proximal phalanx fractures, 52
Plethysmography, 640, 644*f*
PMCI. *See* Palmar midcarpal instability (PMCI)
POSI (position of safe immobilization),
  606, 606*f*
Position of safe immobilization (POSI),
  606, 606*f*
Posterior antebrachial cutaneous nerve, 595
Posterior interosseous nerve (PIN), 397–399
  motor branches, 599*f*, 603
  syndrome, 400
PRC. *See* Proximal row carpectomy (PRC)
Pregabalin, 622
Preiser's disease, 207, 207*t*
Prestyloid recess, 584*f*
Prevotella, 468

Princeps pollicis artery, 593
Procaine (Novocain), 25
Progressive tissue ischemia, 563
Proinflammatory mediators, 568
Pronator quadratus muscle, 587*f*
Pronator teres muscle, 586*f*, 587*f*
Propofol (Diprivan), 29
Proteus, 468
Provocative tests, TFCC tears and, 232
Proximal interphalangeal (PIP) joints, 580
  deformity, 2
  dorsal fracture-dislocations, 61–62
  dorsal simple dislocations, 59
  lateral dislocations, 60–61
  septic arthritis, 440–441, 441*f*
  stability, 10
  volar fracture-dislocations, 62
  volar simple dislocations, 59–60
Proximal phalanx fractures
  nonoperative treatment for, 51
  potential complications, 53
  specific fracture patterns, 53
  surgical approach for, 52–53
  surgical indications for, 51–52
Proximal row carpectomy (PRC), 211, 243
  vs. four-corner fusion with scaphoid excision,
    248–249
  indications, 247
  modifications, 248
  outcomes, 248
  preoperative considerations, 247
  technique pearls, 248
Pseudoclawing, 128
Pseudomonas, 455*t*, 468
Pulley system, 584–585, 588*f*
Pulp-nail-bone, nail bed injury, 497
Pulp space infections
  complications, 418
  definition, 413
  epidemiology, 413
  history, 415
  imaging, 416
  management of
    antibiotic options and duration, 418
    nonoperative treatment, 416
    surgical aftercare, 417–418
    surgical drainage, 416–417, 417*f*
  mechanism of injury, 413, 413*f*
  microbiology, 414
  pathoanatomy, 414–415, 414*f*, 415*f*
  physical examination, 415–416
Pulse volume recording (PVR), 640

PVR (pulse volume recording), 640
Pyogenic flexor tenosynovitis (PFT), 41–42
    antibiotics for, 430–431
    complications, 434–435
    continuous catheter irrigation, 433–434
    in diabetic and immune-compromised
        individuals, 429
    epidemiology, 427
    history, 428
    labs/imaging, 429
    local treatment, 431
    management algorithm for, 435
    Michon classification system, 430, 430t
    minimally invasive irrigation and
        debridement, 432–433, 433f
    open irrigation and debridement, 431, 432f
    operative treatment, 431
    pathogenesis, 426–427
    in pediatrics, 429
    physical examination, 428, 428t, 429f

Q

Quinolones, 456t
Quinupristin, 456t

R

Rabies, 468
Radial artery, 592–593
Radial collateral ligament, 579
Radial nerve, 598
    injuries
        laceration, 401, 403–404
        late reconstruction, 403f, 404–405, 404t
        mechanisms of injury, 399–400
        traction injuries, 401, 402f
    and its branches, anatomy, 397–399, 398f
    motor branches, 599f, 603
Radial shortening osteotomy, 211
Radial styloid fracture. See Chauffeur fracture
Radial tunnel syndrome, 399–400
Radialis indicis artery, 593
Radiocarpal fusion, 222
Radiographic arthrography, 196
Radiolunate arthrosis, 245
Radioscaphocapitate (RSC) ligament, 580, 581f,
    582
Radioscapholunate ligament, 582
Radioulnar ligament reconstruction,
    303, 303f
Radioulnar synostosis, 311
Radius fractures, classification, 308, 308t
Range of motion, 5–7, 6t, 6f
Regional nerve block, 31–33, 32f

Rehabilitation
    principles, 605
    protocols, 607–612
    after surgical repair of extensor tendon
        injuries, 318, 319t
Replantation, upper extremity
    acute management of the amputated part(s),
        518–519, 519–520f
    acute pain management, 517
    contraindications, 521–522
    definitive treatment, 521
    epidemiology, 516
    history, 516
    management algorithm, 527
    mechanism of injury, 516
    operative technique, 523–525
        nerve repair, 524–525
        osteosynthesis, 524
        soft tissues, 525
        tendon repair, 524
    pathoanatomy, 515
    physical examination, 517, 517–518f
    postoperative care, 526
        maintaining perfusion to replanted part,
            526
        monitoring for microvascular thrombosis,
            526
        prevention of peripheral vasospasm, 526
        rehabilitation, 526
    potential complications, 525–526
        cold intolerance, 526
        neuroma formation, 526
        nonunion/malunion/posttraumatic ar-
            thritis, 526
        postoperative stiffness, 525
        replantation failure, 525
    surgical approach, 522–523
    surgical indications, 521
Resuscitation, burns, 559
Revascularization, ring avulsion injuries,
    547–550
Reverse cross-finger flap, fingertip and, 509–510,
    510f
Rewarming shock, 567
Ring avulsion injuries
    biomechanics, 544t
    classification, 544t
    complications, 550
    definition, 543
    imaging, 545, 545f
    incidence and risk factors, 543–544
    mechanism, 543
    prognosis, 545

surgical technique, 547–550, 548–549*f*
    replantation/revascularization, 547–550
  treatment, 545–547
    amputation, 547
    early, 545
    surgical, 546, 546*f*
Ring cutter, 627*f*
Ring removal, 623–628
  evaluation, 623–624
  methods of
    cutting or breakage, 626–627, 627*f*, 628*f*
    edema management, 624
    glove slide, 626
    lubricants, 624–625
    string wrap, 625–626, 625*f*, 626*f*
  patient management, 624
Rolando fractures, 89–90, 89*f*
  closed reduction for, 96–97, 97*f*, 98*f*
  open reduction internal fixation for, 97
  pathoanatomy, 92
Rotational deformity, 130

S

Sagittal band, 586
  bridge, 332, 332*f*
  rupture
    classification, 331, 331*t*
    differential diagnosis, 330, 331*t*
    history and physical examination, 330
    imaging, 331
    mechanism of injury, 330
    nonoperative management, 331–333, 332*f*
    pathoanatomy, 329–330
    reconstruction options, 333–334, 335*f*
    surgical management, 333, 334*f*
Salmonella, 468
Salvage procedures, 181
  goals of treatment, 242
  history and physical examination, 242
  imaging, 242–243, 243*f*
  motion-sparing surgical operations, 243–244, 244*t*
  proximal row carpectomy, 247–248
    vs. four-corner fusion with scaphoid excision, 248–249
    indications, 247
    modifications, 248
    outcomes, 248
    preoperative considerations, 247
    technique pearls, 248
  scaphoid excision with capitate-lunate-hamatetriquetrum fusion (four-corner fusion), 245–247

    fixation techniques, 246, 246*f*
    indications, 245
    modifications, 247
    outcomes, 247
    preoperative considerations, 245
    vs. proximal row carpectomy, 248–249
    technique pearls, 246–247
  total wrist arthrodesis, 249–251
    dorsal plating, technique pearls for, 250–251
    fixation techniques, 250, 250*f*
    indications, 249
    modifications, 251
    outcomes/complications, 251
    preoperative considerations, 249
    rationale, 249
  wrist arthrodesis, 242
Scaphocapitate ligament, 583*f*
Scaphoid bone, 576, 576–577*f*, 577
  anatomy, 205–206
  causes, 205
  classification/imaging, 207, 207*t*
  clinical history, 206
  fracture, 162. *See also* Carpal bone malunions and nonunions
    acute management, 138, 139*f*
    anatomy, 134, 134*f*
    blood supply, 135
    classification, 137
    complications, 144
    differential diagnosis, 136–137
    epidemiology, 135
    imaging, 135–136, 137*f*
    late management, 143
    management algorithm, 143, 143–144*f*
    mechanism of injury, 135
    physical examination, 135, 136*f*
    postoperative protocol, 143
    presentation, 135
    stable distal pole fractures, 138
    stable proximal pole fractures, 138
    stable waist fractures, 138
    unstable (displaced) distal pole or waist fractures, 140–141, 140*f*
    unstable (displaced) proximal pole fractures, 141–143, 142*f*
  pathophysiology, 206
  physical examination, 206
  plaster, 615, 616*f*
  Preiser's disease, 207, 207*t*
  scaphoid excision with capitate-lunate-hamatetriquetrum fusion (four-corner fusion)

Scaphoid bone (*continued*)
  fixation techniques, 246, 246*f*
  indications, 245
  modifications, 247
  outcomes, 247
  preoperative considerations, 245
  vs. proximal row carpectomy, 248–249
  technique pearls, 246–247
 scaphoid stress test, 206
 treatment, 208
 Watson (scaphoid shift) test, 14*t*, 206
Scaphoid nonunion advanced collapse (SNAC), 144, 176, 245, 245*f*
 carpal bone malunions and nonunions and, 178–179
Scapholunate advanced collapse (SLAC), 245
Scapholunate interosseous ligament (SLIL), 183, 582–583
Scapholunate ligament, 582–583*f*
 injury
  acute management, 187
  classification, 187, 187*t*
  epidemiology, 183
  history, 184
  imaging, 185–186*f*
  management algorithm, 190
  mechanism of injury, 183
  nonoperative treatment, 188
  pathoanatomy, 183
  physical examination, 184–185
  postoperative care, 189
  potential complications, 189
  surgical approach, 188, 189*f*
  surgical indications, 188
Scaphotrapezium trapezoid ligament, 583*f*
Schwann cells, 353
Scissoring, 128
Seddon classification, 356, 357*t*
 of digital nerve injury, 369
 of median nerve injury, 381*t*
Septic arthritis, 42, 452*t*
 epidemiology, 438
 history, 438
 imaging, 439
 laboratory evaluation, 439
 management, 439–440
 mechanism of injury, 438
 pathoanatomy, 438
 physical examination, 439
 postoperative complications, 442
 postoperative management, 441–442
 surgical approach
  to distal interphalangeal joints, 441, 442*f*

   to metacarpophalangeal joints, 440, 441*f*
   to proximal interphalangeal joints, 440–441, 441*f*
   to wrist, 440
Seymour fracture, 54, 55–56*f*, 496, 497*f*
Shear test, 195
Shearing impaction fractures, 314, 316*f*
Short radiolunate ligament, 581*f*, 582, 584*f*
Shuck test, 283–284, 283–284*f*, 295, 295*f*
Sigmoid notch, 576, 577*f*
Silver nitrate, 559
Silver sulfadiazine, 559
"SIMPLE" technique, 28–29, 29*f*
Skeletal management, mangled hand, 535
Skin wrinkle test, 373
SLAC (scapholunate advanced collapse), 245
Sliding osteotomy, 276, 279*f*
SLIL (scapholunate interosseous ligament), 183, 582–583
Smith fracture, 256
SNAC. *See* Scaphoid nonunion advanced collapse (SNAC)
Sodium bicarbonate, 27
Soft-tissue
 coverage, mangled hand, 535–536, 536*f*
 management, mangled hand, 535
SPC lateral, 284, 295
Spica splint, 615, 616*f*
Splinting. *See specific injuries*
Split nails, 500, 500*f*
Sporothrix schenckii, 456*t*
Sprained finger, Jersey finger and, 346
Spurling test, 391
Staphylococcus, 468
Staphylococcus aureus, 438, 444, 451
Staphylococcus epidermidis, 451
Static anti-claw splint, 617
Step-cut osteotomy, 130, 131*f*
Steroids, for degenerative TFCC injuries, 302
Streptococcus, 438, 444, 451, 468
Stress testing
 of finger proximal interphalangeal joint collateral ligaments, 82
 scaphoid, 206
String wrap method, for ring removal, 625–626, 625*f*, 626*f*
Subcutaneous digital block technique, 28, 29*f*
Sublimaze (fentanyl), 29
Sugar-tong splint, 617, 618*f*
 for distal radius fractures, 261, 262
Sulbactam, 452*t*, 456*t*
Sulfamethoxazole, 452*t*, 456*t*
Sulfamylon, 559

Sunderland type classification for median nerve
    injury, 382*t*
Superficial branch of radial nerve (SBRN),
    397–398
Superficial palmar arch (SPA), 594
Supinator muscle, 587*f*, 590*f*
Surgery
    emergent indications for
        acute compressive neuropathy, 38–39
        compartment syndrome, 36–37
        high-pressure injection injury, 45–46
        infection. *See specific infections*
        open fracture or dislocation, 37–38
        surgical emergency, 36
        traumatic amputation, 39–40
        vascular injury, 46–47
    principles, 35
    risks, 36
Surgical emergency, 36
Suture anchor fixation technique, 287, 288*f*,
    348–349
Suture line abscess, 452*t*
Swan-neck deformity, 66, 321, 322*f*
    etiologies and pathophysiologies, 66*t*

T
Tamai classification of nail bed injury, 497
Tangential excision, burns, 560
Tazobactam, 452*t*, 455*t*, 456*t*
Tendon necrosis, 434
Tendon transfers, for radial nerve
    reconstruction, 403*f*, 404–405, 404*t*
Tenodesis effect, 339
Tenosynovitis, 452*t*
Tension band fixation technique, 287, 288*f*
Terminal tendon avulsion, 314*f*
Tetracaine (Tetravisc), 25
Thenar and hypothenar muscles, 589, 594*t*, 595*f*
Thenar flap, fingertip and, 510, 511*f*
Thenar space abscess, 453
    surgical approaches for, 457–458, 458*f*, 459*f*
Thermoplastics, 608
Three-point molding, 614, 615, 617, 617*f*
Thumb CMC grind test, 13*t*
Thumb collateral ligament injury
    acute management, 107
    definitive treatment of
        nonoperative treatment, 107
        operative treatment, 107–108
        postoperative care, 112
        potential complications, 112
        surgical approach, 108–112, 109–111*f*
    epidemiology, 103

    history, 103
    imaging, 104–107, 105–106*f*
    management algorithm, 113
    mechanism of injury, 103
    pathoanatomy, 102
    physical examination, 103–104
Thumb fractures
    anatomy, 90–92, 90*f*, 91*f*
    classification, 94
    epidemiology, 90
    extra-articular fractures, 89
        nonoperative treatment, 94
        operative treatment, 94
    history and physical examination, 93
    imaging, 93, 93*f*
    intra-articular fractures, 89
        Bennett fractures. *See* Bennett fractures
        comminuted, 97
        Rolando fractures. *See* Rolando fractures
    management algorithm, 99
    mechanism of injury, 90
    pathoanatomy, 92
    postoperative care for, 98
Thumb metacarpal base extra-articular
    fractures, 121
Thumb metacarpophalangeal dislocations,
    125–126
Thumb metacarpophalangeal ulnar collateral
    ligament
    acute management, 79
    anatomy, 77–78
    classification, 79
    definitive treatment of
        complications, 81
        nonoperative treatment, 79–80
        outcomes, 80
        postoperative care, 81
        surgical approach, 80–81
        surgical indications, 80
    epidemiology, 78
    history, 78
    imaging, 79
    mechanism of injury, 77
    pathoanatomy, 78
    physical examination, 78–79
Thumb spanning external fixator, 97, 98*f*
Thumb spica cast (TSC)
    for perilunate dislocations, 148
    for scaphoid fractures, 138
    for thumb collateral ligament injury, 107
    for thumb collateral ligament injury, 107
    for thumb metacarpal base extra-articular
        fractures, 121

Thumb spica splint (TSS), 615, 616f
 for extra-articular fractures, 94
 for perilunate dislocations, 148
 for scaphoid fractures, 138
Thumb stability, 10
Tigecycline, 456t
Tissue plasminogen activator (tPA), 568
Total wrist arthrodesis
 dorsal plating, technique pearls for, 250–251
 fixation techniques, 250, 250f
 indications, 249
 modifications, 251
 outcomes/complications, 251
 preoperative considerations, 249
 rationale, 249
Toxicity, local anesthetics, 26
Traction injuries, 401, 402f
Transarticular pinning, of mallet fractures, 72
Transmetacarpal digital block technique, 28, 28f
Transmetacarpal pinning, for proximal phalanx
 fractures, 52
Transmitter–receiver unit, 640, 642–644f
Transthecal digital block technique, 28, 28f
Transverse retinacular ligament, 587, 593f
Trapeziometacarpal joint, bony anatomy, 91, 91f
Trapeziotrapezoid ligament, 582–583f
Trapezium, 212–213, 576f, 578, 588f
Trapezoid, 162, 212–213, 576f, 578, 588f
Trapezoidal osteotomy, 276, 279f
Traumatic amputation, 39–40
Traumatic extensor tendon dislocation. *See*
 Sagittal band rupture
Traumatic impaction blow, 321, 322f
Trephination, nail bed injury and, 498
Triangular (articular) disk, 584f
Triangular fibrocartilage complex (TFCC) tears.
 See also Distal radioulnar joint (DRUJ)
 injuries
 articular disk, 227, 229
 blood supply/nerve supply, 227
 classification, 233
 components, 227
 definitive management, 235
  arthroscopic repair acute tears, 235
  contraindications for surgical repair, 235
  indications for operative repair, 235
  nonsurgical treatment, 235
  treatment considerations with stable
   DRUJ, 235
  treatment considerations with unstable
   DRUJ, 235
 ECU subsheath and UCL, 230–231
 exposure, 240

 postoperative care, 240
 surgical technique, 240
general considerations, 227
history, 231
imaging, 19–20, 21f, 232–233, 232–233f
initial management, 234–235
ligamentous foveal insertion, 230, 230f
operative techniques, specific, 236–239
 arthroscopic repair, 236
 contraindications for arthroscopic repair,
  236
 outside in technique, 238–239f
 open repair, 239
 portal placement, 236, 237f
 positioning/setup, 236
 potential complications of arthroscopic
  repair, 239
 surgical technique, 236, 237f, 238
Palmer classification, 233–234, 234t, 297,
 298f
physical examination, 231
provocative tests, 232
 Fovea sign, 232
 hypersupination, 232
 TFCC compression test, 232
structures, 228t
superficial dorsal and volar distal radioulnar
 ligaments, 229–230,
 229f
Trimethoprim, 452t, 456t
Trimethoprim-sulfamethoxazole (Bactrim), 418
Triquetral fracture, 162
Triquetrocapitate ligament, 583f
Triquetrohamate ligament, 583f
Triquetrum, 212–213, 576f, 578, 584f
TSC. *See* Thumb spica cast (TSC)
TSS. *See* Thumb spica splint (TSS)
Tubiana classification of mallet fractures,
 67, 69f
Tuft fracture, 496
Tularemia, 456t
Twin "cutback" incisions, 54
Two-point discrimination, 10, 13t

U

UE. *See* Upper extremity (UE)
Ulna fractures, classification, 308, 308t
Ulnar artery, 594
Ulnar bone graft, 181
Ulnar claw posture of fingers, 388, 389f
Ulnar collateral ligament, 579
Ulnar gutter splint, 614, 614f
Ulnar nerve, 368–369, 603